Advanced Nutrition and Dietetics in Nutrition Support

Edited by

Mary Hickson PhD RD

Sara Smith PhD RD

Series Editor

Kevin Whelan PhD RD FBDA

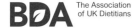

BDA The Association of UK Dietitians

WILEY Blackwell

Registered Office(s)
John Wiley & Sons, Inc., 111 River Street, Hoboken, NJ 07030, USA
John Wiley & Sons Ltd, The Atrium, Southern Gate, Chichester, West Sussex, PO19 8SQ, UK

Editorial Office
9600 Garsington Road, Oxford, OX4 2DQ, UK

For details of our global editorial offices, customer services, and more information about Wiley products visit us at www.wiley.com.

Wiley also publishes its books in a variety of electronic formats and by print-on-demand. Some content that appears in standard print versions of this book may not be available in other formats.

Library of Congress Cataloging-in-Publication data applied for

9781118993859

Cover design: Wiley

Set in 9.5/12pt Times by SPi Global, Pondicherry, India

Printed in Singapore by C.O.S. Printers Pte Ltd

10 9 8 7 6 5 4 3 2 1

Advanced Nutrition and Dietetics in Nutrition Support

ADVANCED NUTRITION AND DIETETICS BOOK SERIES

Nutritional interventions need to be based on solid evidence, but where can you find this information? The British Dietetic Association and the publishers of the *Manual of Dietetic Practice* present an essential and authoritative reference series on the evidence base relating to advanced aspects of nutrition and dietetics in selected clinical areas. Each book provides a comprehensive and critical review of key literature in the area. Each covers established areas of understanding, current controversies and areas of future development and investigation, and aims to address key themes, including:

- mechanisms of disease and its impact on nutritional status, including metabolism, physiology and genetics
- consequences of disease and undernutrition, including morbidity, mortality and patient perspectives
- clinical investigation and management
- nutritional assessment, drawing on anthropometric, biochemical, clinical and dietary approaches
- nutritional and dietary management of disease and its impact on nutritional status.

Trustworthy, international in scope and accessible, *Advanced Nutrition and Dietetics* is a vital resource for a range of practitioners, researchers and educators in nutrition and dietetics, including dietitians, nutritionists, doctors and specialist nurses.

Contents

Preface

Undernutrition is a serious condition that occurs when a person's diet does not contain sufficient energy or nutrients for a healthy and active life. In the past it has been termed malnutrition, but with the rise of obesity and conditions related to overnutrition, it is important to make a clear distinction between the two extremes. This book focuses particularly on undernutrition in economically developed regions of the world, and as such does not cover in any detail undernutrition relating to famine, conflict and long-term food insecurity prevalent in developing countries.

Undernutrition can result from inadequate consumption of nutrients, failure to absorb nutrients, impaired metabolism, excessive loss of nutrients or increased requirements. It generally develops gradually but rapid deterioration in nutritional status can occur in acute disease or starvation. The first changes are to nutrient concentrations in blood and tissues, followed by intracellular changes in biochemical functions and structure. Later, overt symptoms and signs appear, enabling diagnosis by history, physical examination, body composition and dietary analysis, and laboratory tests. The causes of undernutrition can be complex and may involve several interacting factors including physiological, psychological, socioeconomic and institutional. The consequences can be far reaching and affect the optimal functioning of individuals, as well as exacerbating and precipitating disease. Undernutrition commonly occurs concurrently with disease and particular life stages make people more vulnerable to it: childhood, during pregnancy and lactation, and during older age.

Advanced Nutrition and Dietetics in Nutrition Support aims to provide an essential and authoritative reference and review of the evidence base relating to undernutrition. It draws on the experience and expertise of recognised authorities from around the world to bring together the information needed by practitioners, researchers and educators in the area of nutrition and diet. Specialist dietitians and nutritionists will find this to be an essential text, but it will also be valuable for doctors, nurses and other health professionals with a specialist interest in nutrition.

The chapters provide a comprehensive and critical review of the key literature and are split into five sections.

- The background to undernutrition, which examines in detail the causes and consequences of undernutrition. Chapters cover how and why physiological, psychological, socioeconomic and institutional factors can all play a role in the development of undernutrition, and the consequences of these.
- Identification of undernutrition, which covers the range of methods available for screening and assessing levels of undernutrition, including anthropometric, biochemical, clinical and dietary assessment. This section ends with a look at the cutting-edge advanced imaging techniques now available to assess undernutrition.
- Nutritional requirements in nutrition support, which includes fluid, energy, protein, vitamins and minerals in the context of deficiency or when increased requirements exist.
- Nutritional interventions to prevent and treat undernutrition, exploring population-level, community-wide and institutional interventions, as well as looking in detail at oral, enteral and parenteral approaches to managing individuals.

- Undernutrition and nutrition support in a range of clinical specialties. This section incorporates both life stages and clinical conditions where the risk of undernutrition is increased.

The authors have focused on established areas of understanding, current controversies and areas of future development and investigation, and drawn extensively upon the research literature, particularly systematic reviews and meta-analyses. Efforts have been made to highlight the gaps in the literature and specific issues relating to the quality of the evidence in a given specialty. Importantly, the authors have sought to discuss the implications of research findings for practice and the issues to consider when translating research into practice.

Mary Hickson PhD RD
Professor of Dietetics
Plymouth University

Sara Smith PhD RD
Senior Lecturer in Dietetics
Queen Margaret University

Editors
Advanced Nutrition and Dietetics in
Nutrition Support

This book is the fourth title in a series commissioned as part of a major initiative between the British Dietetic Association and the publishers Wiley. Each book in the series provides a comprehensive and critical review of the key literature in a clinical area. Each book is edited by one or more experts who have themselves undertaken extensive research and published widely in the relevant topic area. Chapters are written by experts drawn from an international audience and from a variety of disciplines as required of the relevant chapter (e.g. dietetics, medicine, biomedical sciences).

The editors and I are proud to present this title: *Advanced Nutrition and Dietetics in Nutrition Support*. Undernutrition can have profound impacts on a range of outcomes, including clinical (e.g. mortality, morbidity, complications), patient-centred (e.g. quality of life, patient experience) and economic outcomes (e.g. length of stay, readmission rates, costs). Approaches are needed to both screen and assess undernutrition and to appropriately prevent and manage it, using interventions ranging from public health approaches to parenteral nutrition. We hope that this book will improve health professionals' understanding and application of nutrition and dietetics in these areas and improve outcomes for the patients affected.

Kevin Whelan PhD RD FBDA
Professor of Dietetics
King's College London
Series Editor
Advanced Nutrition and Dietetics Book Series

Foreword

I am delighted to present the foreword for *Advanced Nutrition and Dietetics in Nutrition Support*, edited by two eminent British dietitians and clinical nutritionists, Professor Mary Hickson and Dr Sara Smith. Both of the authors have the advantage of considerable clinical and research experience in actually providing nutrition support as well as a gift for communicating their knowledge of the science and art to others. Together with the experts writing each chapter, they nicely define and set out the problem of undernutrition, the tools for deciding what needs to be done and then what to do, all in a single volume.

This is a book that I, and many other practitioners throughout the world, will welcome as an addition to their core reference libraries that they will turn to repeatedly in their daily work because it manages to convey the essentials succinctly and authoritatively. The information it provides is useful not only in Europe but globally since the comprehensive and critical review of the key literature in nutrition support covers not only basic concepts but current controversies and likely directions for future developments in the field.

The book is well suited to both beginners and master practitioners. Early sections provide a succinct background on undernutrition and how to identify it, followed by a section describing nutritional requirements. In addition to artificial nutrition support (e.g. parenteral, enteral), a welcome addition is a chapter on population and community interventions to prevent and treat undernutrition. The various routes that can be used to provide nutritional support have an entire section of their own. A particularly valuable section of the book is its coverage of over a dozen of the most common diseases and conditions requiring nutrition support. They are tackled in sufficient detail to provide the practitioner with the specific considerations to adequately deal with the patient's problem. Paediatric as well as older adults are considered. In addition to the diseases involving various organ systems and metabolic disease, special and rarely covered problems such as anorexia nervosa, HIV, burns, orthopaedics and spinal cord injury are discussed. The special issues arising in delivering nutrition support in critical care and palliative care are also covered.

I look forward to reading and using this book, and congratulate the authors on a job well done.

Johanna T. Dwyer DSc RD

Professor of Medicine and Community Health, School of Medicine and Friedman School of Nutrition Science and Policy

Senior Nutrition Scientist, Jean Mayer USDA Human Nutrition Research Center, Tufts University

Director, Frances Stern Nutrition Center, Tufts Medical Center, Boston, USA

Editor biographies

Mary Hickson

Mary Hickson is Professor of Dietetics at the University of Plymouth, UK, and leads the Dietetics, Human Nutrition and Health Research group in the Institute of Health and Community. Her research interests include sarcopenia and frailty, hospital nutritional care, and nutrition in older people. Professor Hickson is on the editorial board of the *Journal of Human Nutrition and Dietetics*.

Sara Smith

Sara Smith is a Senior Lecturer in Dietetics and Nutrition at Queen Margaret University in Edinburgh, Scotland, UK. She is particularly interested in nutritional assessment, undernutrition and the effects of treatment interventions on nutritional status. Her own PhD explored the effects of an intradialytic exercise programme on quality of life, functional and nutritional status of individuals receiving haemodialysis therapy. Dr Smith works with the National Health Service in a number of capacities and is actively engaged in the work of the British Dietetic Association. She won the BDA IBEX award in 2016 in recognition of her significant contribution to the dietetic profession.

Kevin Whelan

Kevin Whelan is the Professor of Dietetics and Head of Department of Nutritional Sciences at King's College London. He is a Principal Investigator leading a research programme exploring the interaction between the gut microbiota, diet in health, disease and in patients receiving artificial nutrition support. In 2012 he was awarded the Nutrition Society Cuthbertson Medal for research in clinical nutrition and in 2017 was appointed a Fellow of the British Dietetic Association. Professor Whelan is on the editorial boards of *Alimentary Pharmacology and Therapeutics* and the *Journal of Human Nutrition and Dietetics*.

Contributors

Christine Baldwin PhD RD
Lecturer in Nutrition and Dietetics
King's College London
London, UK

Stephanie Baron PharmD PhD
European Hospital Georges-Pompidou
Paris, France

Danielle Bear MRes RD
HEE/NIHR Clinical Doctoral Research Fellow
Guy's and St Thomas' NHS Foundation Trust
London, UK

Jack J. Bell PhD AdvAPD
Senior Dietitian and Research Fellow
Prince Charles Hospital
Brisbane, Australia

Timothy Bowling MD FRCP
Consultant in Gastroenterology and Clinical Nutrition
Nottingham University Hospitals NHS Trust
Nottingham, UK

Katrina Campbell PhD AdvAPD
Associate Professor of Nutrition and Dietetics
Bond University
Robina, Australia

Stefan G.J.A. Camps PhD
Research Fellow
National University of Singapore
Singapore

Peter F. Collins PhD APD
Senior Lecturer in Nutrition and Dietetics
Queensland University of Technology
Brisbane, Australia

Avril Collinson PhD RD
Associate Professor in Dietetics
Plymouth University
Plymouth, UK

Kevin Conlon MD FRCSI
Professor of Surgery
Trinity College Dublin
Dublin, Ireland

Clare Corish PhD RD FINDI
Associate Professor
University College Dublin
Dubin, Ireland

Marie Courbebaisse MD PhD
Associate Professor
European Hospital Georges-Pompidou
Paris, France

Alison Culkin PhD RD
Research Dietitian
St Mark's Hospital
Harrow, UK

Ronit Das MBBS MRCP
Gastroenterology Registrar
Royal Derby Hospital
Derby, UK

Sinead N. Duggan PhD
Postdoctoral Research Dietitian
Trinity College Dublin
Dublin, Ireland

Alastair Duncan PhD RD
Principal Dietitian and Lecturer in Nutrition
Guy's and St Thomas' NHS Foundation Trust
and King's College London
London, UK

Sarah A. Elliott PhD
Postdoctoral Research Fellow
University of Alberta
Edmonton, Canada

Peter W. Emery PhD
Professor of Nutrition and Metabolism
King's College London
London, UK

Lisa Chiara Fellin PhD
Senior Lecturer in Psychology
University of East London
London, UK

Alastair Forbes MD
Professor of Medicine
University of East Anglia
Norwich, UK

Laura Frank PhD RDN
Clinical Dietitian
Multicare Health System
Tacoma, USA

Gérard Friedlander MD PhD
Professor of Physiology
European Hospital Georges-Pompidou
Paris, France

Maria Gabriella Gentile PhD
Former Director
Eating Disorders Unit
Arese, Italy

Filomena Gomes PhD RD
Nutrition Postdoctoral Researcher
Cereneo AG and Kantonsspital Aarau
Vitznau, Switzerland

Sue M. Green PhD RN
Associate Professor of Nursing
University of Southampton
Southampton, UK

George Grimble PhD
Principal Teaching Fellow
University College London
London, UK

Rosemary Hayhoe RD
Clinical Dietitian
Sunnybrook Health Sciences Centre
Toronto, Canada

C. Jeyakumar Henry PhD
Director of the Clinical Nutrition Research Centre
National University of Singapore
Singapore

Mary Hickson PhD RD
Professor of Dietetics
Plymouth University
Plymouth, UK

Marc Jeschke MD PhD FACS
Professor
University of Toronto
Sunnybrook Health Sciences Centre
Toronto, Canada

Matthieu Joerger MD
Medical Resident, Nutritional Support Unit
Archet University Hospital
Nice, France

Anna Julian MNutr RD
Research Dietitian
Imperial College London
London, UK

Katie Keetarut MSc RD
Specialist Dietitian for IBD
University College London Hospital
London, UK

Lynne Kennedy PhD RNutr (Public Health)
Professor of Public Health and Nutrition
University of Chester
Chester, UK

Ronald L. Koretz MD
Emeritus Professor of Clinical Medicine
UCLA School of Medicine
Los Angeles, USA

Eve M. Lepicard PhD
Scientific Director
Institute for European Expertise in Physiology
Paris, France

Callum Livingstone PhD FRCPath
Consultant Chemical Pathologist
Royal Surrey County Hospital NHS Trust
Guildford, UK

Miranda Lomer MBE PhD RD
Senior Consultant Dietitian and Reader in Dietetics
Guy's and St Thomas' NHS Foundation Trust and
King's College London
London, UK

Angela Madden PhD RD FBDA
Principal Lecturer in Nutrition and Dietetics
University of Hertfordshire
Hatfield, UK

Katelynn Maniatis MHSc RD CNSC
Clinical Dietitian
Sunnybrook Health Sciences Centre
Toronto, Canada

Luise Marino PhD RD
Lead Paediatric Dietitian
University Hospital Southampton Foundation Trust
Southampton, UK

Hilary McCoubrey MSc RD
Specialist Diabetes Dietitian
Birmingham Women's and Children's Hospital
Birmingham, UK

Rosan Meyer PhD RD
Honorary Senior Lecturer
Imperial College London
London, UK

Joao F. Mota PhD
Adjunct Professor
Federal University of Goiás
Goiânia, Brazil

Paula Murphy PhD RD
Nutrition Support Dietitian
Derriford Hospital
Plymouth, UK

Pinal S. Patel PhD RD
Specialist Dietitian for Intestinal Failure
University College London Hospital
London, UK

Emily Player MBBS
Gastroenterologist
Norfolk and Norwich University Hospital
Norwich, UK

Carla M. Prado PhD FTOS
CAIP Chair in Nutrition, Food and Health
University of Alberta
Edmonton, Canada

Claire E. Robertson PhD RNutr
Senior Lecturer in Nutrition and Public Health
University of Westminster
London, UK

Kathryn Rochette MEd RD
Clinical Dietitian
Sunnybrook Health Sciences Centre
Toronto, Canada

Mary Krystofiak Russell MS RDN FAND
Senior Manager for US Nutrition
Baxter Healthcare Corporation
Deerfield, USA

Stéphane M. Schneider MD PhD FEBGH
Professor of Nutrition
Archet University Hospital
Nice, France

Denise Baird Schwartz MS RD FAND
Nutrition Support Co-ordinator
Providence Saint Joseph Medical Center
Burbank, USA

Shahriar Shahrokhi MD FRCSC FACS
Assistant Professor
University of Toronto
Sunnybrook Health Sciences Centre
Toronto, Canada

Clare Shaw PhD RD
Consultant Dietitian
Royal Marsden NHS Foundation Trust
London, UK

Sara Smith PhD RD
Senior Lecturer in Dietetics
Queen Margaret University
Edinburgh, UK

Alan Torrance MSc
Formerly, Head of Newcastle Nutrition
Royal Victoria Infirmary
Newcastle upon Tyne, UK

Liesl Wandrag PhD RD
Principal Critical Care Dietitian
Guy's and St Thomas' NHS Foundation Trust
London, UK

Kevin Whelan PhD RD FBDA
Professor of Dietetics
King's College London
London, UK

Lisa Wilson PhD RPHNutr
Public Health Nutrition Consultant
Middlesex, UK

Samford Wong BSc RD
Lead Dietitian in Spinal Injuries
National Spinal Injuries Centre
Aylesbury, UK

Alison Woodall PhD RD
Senior Lecturer in Nutrition and Dietetics
University of Chester
Chester, UK

Adrienne Young PhD APD
Senior Dietitian
Royal Brisbane and Women's Hospital
Brisbane, Australia

Abbreviations

ACCP	American College of Chest Physicians	CP	chronic pancreatitis
AD	autonomic dysreflexia	CRP	C-reactive protein
ADL	activities of daily living	CT	computed tomography
AEE	activity-induced energy expenditure	CVD	cardiovascular disease
AI	adequate intake	DAFNE	Dose Adjustment for Normal Eating
AIDS	acquired immune deficiency syndrome	DEXA (DXA)	dual-energy x-ray absorptiometry
AIS	ASIA Impairment Scale	DIT	diet-induced thermogenesis
AKI	acute kidney injury	DRI	Dietary Reference Intake
ALS	amyotrophic lateral sclerosis	DRV	Dietary Reference Value
AMA	American Medical Association	DS-EF	diabetes-specific enteral formula
AN	anorexia nervosa	DSM	*Diagnostic and Statistical Manual*
AP	acute pancreatitis		
APACHE	Acute Physiological and Chronic Health Evaluation	DS-ONS	diabetes-specific oral nutritional supplement
ARR	absolute risk reduction	EAR	estimated average requirement
ASPEN	American Society for Parenteral and Enteral Nutrition	EC	European Commission
		ECF	extracellular fluid volume
BANS	British Artificial Nutrition Survey	ECG	electrocardiogram
BAPEN	British Association for Parenteral and Enteral Nutrition	EFSA	European Food Safety Authority
		EN	enteral nutrition
BCAA	branched chain amino acid	EORTC	European Organization for Research and Treatment of Cancer
BDA	British Dietetic Association		
BIA	bioelectrical impedance analysis		
BMD	bone mineral density	EPIC	European Prospective Investigation into Cancer
BMI	body mass index		
BMR	basal metabolic rate	ERAS	enhanced recovery after surgery
BW	body weight	ESKD	end-stage kidney disease
CCK	cholecystokinin	EU	European Union
CHF	chronic heart failure	FAO	Food and Agriculture Organization
CI	confidence interval		
CKD	chronic kidney disease	FFM	fat-free mass
CMV	cytomegalovirus	FFMI	fat-free mass index
COMA	Committee on the Medical Aspects of Food and Nutrition Policy	FFQ	food frequency questionnaire
		FINES	French Interdialytic Nutrition Evaluation Study
COPD	chronic obstructive pulmonary disease		
		FM	fat mass

FNB	Food and Nutrition Board	LOS	length of stay
FOOD	Feed Or Ordinary Diet trial	LRNI	lower reference nutrient intake
GFR	glomerular filtration rate	MAI	*Mycobacterium avium* complex
GI	gastrointestinal, glycaemic index	MAMC	mid-arm muscle circumference
GLP-1	glucagon-like peptide 1	MCT	medium-chain triglyceride
GRV	gastric residual volume	MD	mean difference
GSRS	Gastrointestinal Symptom Rating Scale	MDRD	Modification of Diet in Renal Disease study
HAART	highly active antiretroviral therapy	MDT	multidisciplinary team
HD	haemodialysis	MIS	Malnutrition Inflammation Score
HGS	handgrip strength	MNA	Mini Nutritional Assessment
HIV	human immunodeficiency virus	MND	motor neuron disease
HOPE	Heart Outcomes Prevention Evaluation study	MRI	magnetic resonance imaging
		MS	multiple sclerosis
HPN	home parenteral nutrition	MST	Malnutrition Screening Tool
HRQL	health-related quality of life	MTD	modified-texture diet
IBD	inflammatory bowel disease	MUAC	mid-upper arm circumference
IBW	ideal body weight	MUST	Malnutrition Universal Screening Tool
ICD	International Classification of Diseases	NaDIA	National Diabetes Inpatient Audit
		NAFLD	non-alcoholic fatty liver disease
ICU	intensive care unit	NASH	non-alcoholic steatohepatitis
IDA	iron deficiency anaemia	NB	nitrogen balance
IDDSI	International Dysphagia Diet Standardization Initiative	NBD	neurogenic bowel dysfunction
		NCPM	Nutrition Care Process and Model
IDNT	International Dietetic and Nutrition Terminology	NGT	nasogastric tube
		NHANES	National Health and Nutrition Examination Survey
IDPN	intradialytic parenteral nutrition		
IDWG	interdialytic weight gain	NHPCO	National Hospice and Palliative Care Organization
IF	intestinal failure		
IGF	insulin-like growth factor	NICE	National Institute for Health and Care Excellence
IHI	Institute for Healthcare Improvement		
IL	interleukin	NJ	nasojejunal
INR	international normalized ratio	nPCR	normalized protein catabolic rate
IOM	Institute of Medicine	nPNA	normalized protein nitrogen appearance
IU	international unit		
IV	intravenous	NRS	Nutritional Risk Screen
IVACG	International Vitamin A Consultative Group	NST	nutrition support team
		ONS	oral nutritional supplement
JBDS	Joint British Diabetes Society	OR	odds ratio
JCA	jejunocolic anastomosis	PAL	physical activity level
JRA	jejunorectal anastomosis	PCP	*Pneumocystis* pneumonia
LBM	lean body mass	PEG	percutaneous endoscopic gastrostomy
LCD	low-calorie diet	PEI	pancreatic exocrine insufficiency
LCT	long-chain triglyceride	PEPT1	peptide transporter 1
LFT	liver function test	PERT	pancreatic enzyme replacement therapy
LIDNS	Low Income Diet and Nutrition Survey		
		PG-SGA	Patient-Generated Subjective Global Assessment
LOFFLEX	LOw Fat Fibre Limited EXclusion (diet)		
		PICC	peripherally inserted central catheter

PML	progressive multifocal leucoencephalopathy
PN	parenteral nutrition
POMC	pro-opiomelanocortin
PPI	proton pump inhibitor
PTH	parathyroid hormone
PUFA	polyunsaturated fatty acid
PYY	pancreatic peptide YY
QALY	quality-adjusted life-year
RCT	randomised controlled trial
RD	registered dietitian
RDA	recommended daily allowance
RDI	recommended dietary intake
REE	resting energy expenditure
RNI	reference nutrient intake
ROS	reactive oxygen species
RR	relative risk
RRT	renal replacement therapy
RTU	ready to use
SACN	Scientific Advisory Committee on Nutrition
SBS	short bowel syndrome
SBS-QoL	short bowel syndrome quality of life questionnaire
SCI	spinal cord injury

SD	standard deviation
SES	socioeconomic status
SGA	Subjective Global Assessment
SI	small intestine, safe intake
SIRS	systemic inflammatory response syndrome
SNST	Spinal Nutrition Screening Tool
SO	sarcopenic obesity
SOFA	Sequential Organ Failure Assessment
TAG	triacylglycerol
TBSA	total body surface area
TBW	total body water
TEE	total energy expenditure
TGF	transforming growth factor
TNF	tumour necrosis factor
TSF	triceps skinfold
TSH	thyroid stimulating hormone
TUG	timed up and go (test)
UL	upper level
US	ultrasound
USG	urine specific gravity
VLCD	very low-calorie diet
VRIII	variable-rate intravenous insulin infusion
WHO	World Health Organization

SECTION 1

Background to undernutrition

Chapter 1.1

Definitions and prevalence of undernutrition

Mary Hickson[1] and Sara Smith[2]
[1]Plymouth University Institute of Health and Community, Peninsula Alllied Health Centre, Plymouth, UK
[2]Department of Dietetics, Nutrition and Biological Sciences, Queen Margaret University, Edinburgh, UK

1.1.1 Undernutrition: definition and diagnostic criteria

A universal definition for undernutrition is lacking, but it is generally accepted that malnutrition is defined as 'a state of nutrition in which a deficiency or excess (or imbalance) of energy, protein and other nutrients causes measurable adverse effects on tissue and body form (body shape, size and composition) and function and clinical outcome' [1]. Such a definition refers to both undernutrition and overnutrition; in this book, the term 'undernutrition' is used rather than 'malnutrition', to distinguish between the issues of undernutrition and overnutrition.

Global consensus work to develop universal diagnostic criteria and documentation for undernutrition is in progress and is led by the world's four largest parenteral and enteral nutrition societies [2]. The ongoing work recognises the value of unified terminology, which reflects contemporary understanding and practices, to allow global comparisons and improve clinical care [3] and ultimately aims to seek the adoption of consensus criteria by the World Health Organization and the International Classification of Disease. Early discussions have identified that consensus criteria will need to take account of differences in global practices, such as financial reimbursement and the sometimes limited availability of assessment methods in clinical practice to assess body composition, for example fat-free mass [2].

Diagnostic criteria have generally focused on dietary intake and clinically relevant changes in body mass (e.g. body mass index (BMI) and involuntary percentage weight loss) [1]. However, it is increasingly recognised that criteria should consider additional factors, such as the presence of acute or chronic inflammation and changes in muscle function [2–5]. This more aetiological approach to diagnosis would allow the recognition of important differences in the pathophysiology of undernutrition and potential response to intervention [5]. The assessment of muscle function and inflammatory markers could therefore result in earlier recognition of risk and the implementation of more effective targeted interventions [4].

The European Society of Enteral and Parenteral Nutrition [3] has proposed a more aetiological approach to the diagnosis of different categories of undernutrition (Figure 1.1.1). These categories are disease-related undernutrition with inflammation, disease-related undernutrition without inflammation and undernutrition without disease. However, further work is required to agree specific diagnostic indices for each of these categories. Furthermore, it is acknowledged that some patients may present

Advanced Nutrition and Dietetics in Nutrition Support, First Edition. Edited by Mary Hickson and Sara Smith.
© 2018 John Wiley & Sons Ltd. Published 2018 by John Wiley & Sons Ltd.

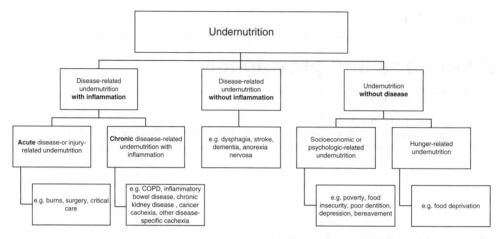

Figure 1.1.1 Diagnosis tree for undernutrition. COPD, chronic obstructive pulmonary disease. Source: Adapted with permission of Elsevier from Cederholm et al. [3].

with mixed aetiologies (e.g. disease-related undernutrition together with economic-related undernutrition). This book addresses the causes, consequences and management of undernutrition in the categories outlined in Figure 1.1.1, but the focus is on issues arising primarily in economically developed countries. The book does not attempt to explore the wide-ranging and complex issues surrounding hunger-related undernutrition in famine or conflict situations found more frequently in developing countries, particularly affecting children.

1.1.2 Prevalence of undernutrition

The reported prevalence of undernutrition in hospitals varies widely due to differences in study populations, assessment tools and settings. Interpretation of the data is also complicated by small and unrepresentative sample sizes, single-centre studies, geographical variations, the use of tools without validation and failure to screen the total population. In Europe, several large studies indicate rates in the range of 20–30%, with a higher prevalence in older adults (32–58%) and in cancer (31–39%). Asian studies show a prevalence of 27–39%, again increasing with age (88%), and higher rates in critically ill (87%), surgical (56%) and

gastrointestinal malignancy (48%) populations. Similar prevalence is found North America (37–45%) and Australia (23–42%). Prevalence of undernutrition in Latin American hospitals appears to be slightly higher with most studies indicating rates of 40–60%. Consistent with other countries, rates were higher in gastrointestinal surgery patients (55–66%) and older adults (44–71%) [6].

Over 20 years of data are available in the UK since the seminal paper by McWhirter and Pennington [7] was published, and include a national survey called 'Nutritional Screening Week' carried out by the British Association of Parenteral and Enteral Nutrition (BAPEN) over a 4-year period, controlling for the time of the year [8]. This group of datasets shows similar patterns to those described above and also suggests that there has been little change in prevalence during this time [8]. Data on hospital incidence are completely lacking but are extremely challenging to collect and are unlikely to be available unless routine screening and storing in electronic records become the norm.

One obvious factor that will affect undernutrition is food intake during hospital stay. This has been examined by the 'Nutrition Day' survey, which is an annual 1-day survey of hospital patients' food intake. These important data show that almost half of all hospital patients (n=91 245) did not eat a full meal. The factors associated with this lower intake are eating less the week before, physical immobility, female sex, old or young age, and a very low BMI [9]. This suggests that interventions to address poor food intake, targeted at those at risk, will be crucial to reduce prevalence of undernutrition in the future.

The prevalence of undernutrition in other settings has also been examined but far fewer data exist. Nursing and residential homes have reported rates of 17–71% for defined undernutrition and up to 97% for those at risk of undernutrition [10]. The UK Nutrition Screening Week data show rates of 41% with little variation across geographical regions or types of care home [11].

Overall, it is clear that undernutrition commonly occurs concurrently with disease and at particular life stages. It is important to note that the methods used to detect undernutrition in prevalence studies are designed to identify protein and energy undernutrition. The identification of micronutrient deficiencies requires different tools and tests.

Despite decades of identifying undernutrition as a prevalent and problematic condition, it remains an elusive challenge in institutional and community settings. Understanding the causes and consequences of undernutrition is essential to subsequently designing multicomponent approaches to reducing its burden.

References

1. Todorovic V, Russell CA, Elia M. The 'MUST' Explanatory Booklet. A Guide to the Malnutrition Universal Screening Tool (MUST) for Adults. Redditch: BAPEN, 2011.
2. Cederholm T, Jensen GL. To create a consensus on malnutrition diagnostic criteria: a report from the Global Leadership Initiative on Malnutrition (GLIM) meeting at the ESPEN Congress 2016. *Clin Nutr* 2017; **36**(1): 7–10.
3. Cederholm T, Barazzoni R, Austin P, Ballmer P, Biolo G, Bischoff SC, Compher C, Correia I, Higashiguchi T, Holst M, et al. ESPEN guidelines on definitions and terminology of clinical nutrition. *Clin Nutr* 2017; **36**(1): 49–64.
4. Smith S, Madden AM. Body composition and functional assessment of nutritional status in adults: a narrative review of imaging, impedance, strength and functional techniques. *J Hum Nutr Diet* 2016; **29**(6): 714–732.
5. White JV, Guenter P, Jensen G, Malone A, Schofield M, Academy of Nutrition and Dietetics Malnutrition Work Group, ASPEN Malnutrition Task Force, ASPEN Board of Directors. Consensus statement of the Academy of Nutrition and Dietetics/American Society for Parenteral and Enteral Nutrition: characteristics recommended for the identification and documentation of adult malnutrition (undernutrition). *J Acad Nutr Diet* 2012; **112**(5): 730–738.
6. Correia MI, Perman MI, Waitzberg DL. Hospital malnutrition in Latin America: a systematic review. *Clin Nutr* 2017; **36**: 958–967.
7. McWhirter JP, Pennington CR. Incidence and recognition of malnutrition in hospital. *BMJ* 1994; **308**(6934): 945–948.
8. Ray S, Laur C, Golubic R. Malnutrition in healthcare institutions: a review of the prevalence of undernutrition in hospitals and care homes since 1994 in England. *Clin Nutr* 2014; **33**(5): 829–835.
9. Schindler K, Themessl-Huber M, Hiesmayr M, Kosak S, Lainscak M, Laviano A, Ljungqvist O, Mouhieddine M, Schneider S, de van der Schueren M, et al. To eat or not to eat? Indicators for reduced food intake in 91,245 patients hospitalised on Nutrition Days 2006–2014 in 56 countries worldwide: a descriptive analysis. *Am J Clin Nutr* 2016; **104**(5): 1393–1402.
10. Bell CL, Tamura BK, Masaki KH, Amella EJ. Prevalence and measures of nutritional compromise among nursing home patients: weight loss, low body mass index, malnutrition, and feeding dependency, a systematic review of the literature. *J Am Med Dir Assoc* 2013; **14**(2): 94–100.
11. Russell CA, Elia M. Nutrition Screening Survey in the UK and Republic of Ireland in 2011. Redditch: BAPEN, 2012. www.bapen.org.uk/pdfs/nsw/nsw-2011-report.pdf

Chapter 1.2

Physiological causes of undernutrition

Pinal S. Patel[1], Katie Keetarut[1] and George Grimble[2]

[1]Department of Nutrition and Dietetics, University College London Hospital NHS Foundation Trust, London, UK
[2]Institute of Liver and Digestive Health (Bloomsbury), University College London, London, UK

1.2.1 Altered metabolism

The characteristics of the human gastrointestinal tract

The gastrointestinal (GI) tract has a high degree of latency. Luminal contents may pass the same point several times through the action of motility patterns during the absorptive phase. These intestinal responses to the presence of luminal food operate within the intradiurnal cycle of hunger and satiety. Intestinal regions of differing function follow sequentially and each processes the output of the preceding segment in turn, presenting a suitable output to the succeeding segment. As discussed later, feeding cues stimulate the cephalic phase in order to prepare all regions of the GI tract, liver and endocrine organs to receive a large input and deal with it efficiently at an optimum metabolic cost. The oral intake of food presents a challenge because of the metabolic demand of handling large peripheral substrate loads that are specific according to the nutrient involved. Water and electrolytes pose a special challenge and the primary function of the GI tract is to maintain water and electrolyte balance in concert with the kidney, lungs and sweat glands.

Humans are mixed foregut/hindgut fermenters, deriving approximately 10% of energy intake from colonic microbial metabolism of malabsorbed macronutrients [1]. Humans lie between foregut fermenters (e.g. obligate carnivores), who have a small colon and rapid whole-GI transit, and hindgut fermenters (e.g. rabbits), whose large colon and slow transit allow colonic salvage of fermented polysaccharides so that over 30% of dietary energy is absorbed as short-chain fatty acids [1]. Intestinal size across all mammalian species is matched to metabolic mass [2], all other things being equal, and the reserve capacity of the GI tract is sufficient with a safety margin. Key studies of intestinal substrate transporter capacity in rats and mice subject to 25–75% small intestinal resection, or who were kept in cold conditions to stimulate hyperphagia, demonstrated that reserve capacity was approximately 100% [3]. Therefore, efficient assimilation and the high metabolic cost of maintaining the GI tract are balanced. Adaptation to increased nutrient loads can occur. The best human example is the case of Antarctic explorers whose daily oral intake of approximately 5000 kcal comprised 57% fat, 35% carbohydrate and 8% protein [4]. Their dietary fat intake increased from 92 g/day to 320 g/day but digestive and absorptive capacity clearly adapted above the usual safety margin.

Digestive and absorptive functions are duplicated, as in the case of the parallel routes of protein digestion via exocrine pancreatic hydrolytic enzymes and enterocyte brush-border hydrolases. For example, protein digestion

Advanced Nutrition and Dietetics in Nutrition Support, First Edition. Edited by Mary Hickson and Sara Smith.
© 2018 John Wiley & Sons Ltd. Published 2018 by John Wiley & Sons Ltd.

products are absorbed by twin routes: specific amino acid transporters (several) and the peptide transporter 1 (PEPT1) that is responsible for the absorption of di- and tripeptides [5]. Another example would be the absorption of fatty acids along the length of the small intestine, by simple diffusion across the enterocyte membrane (the *'flip-flop'* model) or via fatty acid transport proteins [5].

As indicated earlier, feeding radically alters intestinal motility. Intestinal sensors change fasting peristalsis to a pattern that repeatedly moves intestinal contents proximally (by reflux) and distally. Intestinal folds, villi and the micro-villus surface increase the surface area from that of a simple tube to about the area of a tennis court. Some clinical conditions may decrease functional absorptive area either by decreasing surface area (e.g. villous atrophy in untreated coeliac disease) or by reducing latency (e.g. dumping syndrome). Transport systems may also be impaired. Alcohol abuse specifically inhibits carrier-mediated thiamine transport across the jejunal brush-border membrane and basolateral membranes via thiamine trans-porter-1 [6]. In combination with a poor diet, this can lead to B1 deficiency and development of Wernicke's encephalopathy, which is addi-tionally becoming common in patients who have undergone bariatric surgery [7]. More general injury to the GI tract such as chemotherapy-induced mucositis, impairs the transport mecha-nisms for small molecules, though not to the same extent for all nutrients. In a rat model, 5-fluorouracil treatment markedly inhibited brush-border hydrolases and amino acid and glucose transport, but left di- and tripeptide transport untouched [8]. The latter is an example of the specific inhibition of one digestive/transport system that may be masked by the large capacity of the other. In the case of pancre-atic enzyme insufficiency arising after pancrea-tectomy, it has been demonstrated in humans that absorption of intact dietary protein was impaired, whereas a peptide diet was efficiently assimilated [9]. Likewise, perfusion studies in healthy humans showed that total carbohydrate assimilation could be increased markedly by replacing some of the maltodextrin with sucrose

so that the digestion products were absorbed via all monosaccharide transporters, that is SGLT1/GLUT2 (glucose) and GLUT5 (fructose) [10]. The term 'malabsorption' is therefore a difficult diagnosis unless it can be demonstrated that the global process for a nutrient is impaired.

1.2.2 Reduced oral intake

Physiological control of appetite

In healthy adults, body weight remains relatively stable over time due to homeostatic mechanisms which ensure that energy intake and expenditure are equal. The sensory values of food associated with hedonic pleasure derived from eating ('reward pathway') have the capacity to override these homeostatic mechanisms. High fat and sug-ary foods elicit the most hedonic pleasure [11]. The inflammatory response in certain disease states such as cancer and inflammatory bowel disease (IBD) can affect the complex interplay of sensory, postingestive and postabsorptive signals [12–14]. For example, the catabolic state of reduced oral energy intake and increased energy expenditure induced by cancer cachexia causes alterations in peripheral inputs, including sensa-tion of vagal afferents, promotion of satiety and contribution to reduced oral intake [14].

The physiological interactions involved in appetite control are complex and involve signal-ling networks of hormones, neurotransmitters and glands [15]. Afferent signals regulating oral food intake can begin even before food is eaten through visual, gustatory and olfactory stimuli. The hypothalamus receives key peripheral sig-nals from the GI tract, pancreas and adipose cells in relation to nutritional stimuli [15]. The enteric nervous system within the GI tract releases neurotransmitters and hormones that relay, amplify and modulate different signals between the GI tract, pancreas and adipose cells to control appetite.

Hormonal involvement in appetite

The hormones released from adipose cells and the GI tract stimulate the arcuate nucleus within the hypothalamus that acts as a 'key controller' maintaining energy homeostasis, critical in the regulation of appetite. The two main centres within the hypothalamus are the 'feeding centre' (controls hunger sensations) and the 'satiety centre' (sends out nerve impulses that inhibit the feeding centre) [16]. The brainstem detects nutrients and co-ordinates oral food intake and satiety, producing a negative or positive effect on energy balance. Gut hormone signalling to the hypothalamus mediates both hunger and satiation through release of GI peptide hormones [17]. These hormones are either 'orexigenic' (hunger stimulating), for example ghrelin released from the stomach, or 'anorexigenic' (satiating) and released in the postprandial state from the GI tract such as PYY (pancreatic peptide YY), GLP-1 (glucagon-like peptide 1) and oxyntomodulin (15). With ageing, increased production of satiety hormones (cholecystokinin (CCK) and PYY) may cause a reduction in oral intake [18]. The vagus nerve is the main communicator and innervates most of the GI tract, sending signals between the hypothalamus and brainstem [15]. The site and mode of action of the main hormones involved in appetite regulation are presented in Table 1.2.1.

Taste changes

The sensory properties of food (specifically taste and smell) ultimately determine its reward value. In certain disease states, taste and smell alterations can occur concurrently with reduced oral intake [12]. An understanding of the potential effects of taste changes on reduced oral intake requires knowledge of normal physiology of taste perception, explained below.

The sense of taste ('gustation') refers to the five classes of taste stimuli: sweet, sour, bitter, salty and umami [16,19]. Umami is distinct from the other flavours as it defines 'savoury deliciousness', including the amino acid glutamate; the use of monosodium glutamate as a food enhancement has been found to increase oral intake [19]. Receptors in different areas of the tongue are more receptive to different primary taste sensations: the tip, back and sides of the tongue are more sensitive to sweet and salty, bitter and sour, respectively [16]. Taste thresholds

vary with each flavour sensation, with sweet and salty the highest and bitter the lowest [16]. There are four types of taste sensation: hypogeusia (taste sensation loss/increased taste threshold), dysgeusia (altered taste perception), parageusia (distorted taste sensation) and ageusia (loss of taste sensation) [20].

Causes of taste changes

The aetiology of taste changes can be attributed to up to 30 medical and treatment conditions, including, but not limited to, respiratory infections, smoking, dry mouth, dental problems, chemotherapy and zinc deficiency [19]. Up to 50% of patients undergoing chemotherapy suffer from either dysgeusia or another taste impairment, often precipitated by damage to the oral cavity (mucositis, infection) and salivary gland dysfunction [21]. In older adults and oncology patients, alterations in taste or smell have been noted to severely reduce oral intake, contributing to undernutrition [12,22]. In Crohn's disease (CD), impaired chemosensory function may contribute to reduced oral intake and undernutrition due to alterations to digestive function, consequently reducing satisfaction and motivation in eating [15,23]. Furthermore, taste and smell may be modified by several pathophysiological processes from the level of receptor cells and peripheral neurons to regions of the brain associated with taste information processing [22].

Drugs

Over 250 medications can alter taste [20]. Saliva can store traces of drugs, with some giving rise to a metallic flavour (e.g. lithium carbonate and tetracyclines) [20]. Drugs can also affect:

- the sodium channel linked to taste receptors (e.g. amiloride)
- the creation of new taste buds and saliva (e.g. antiproliferative drugs) [20]
- mouth dryness affecting taste sensation (e.g. anticholinergics (atropine, oxybutynin); antidepressants (fluoxetine or citalopram); and tricyclics (amitriptyline)) [24].

Table 1.2.1 Key hormones involved in appetite regulation with sites of release and modes of action

Hormone	Site of release	Mode of action
Glucagon-like peptide 1 (GLP-1)	• Ileum and colon • Secreted with PYY in proportion to the amount of food ingested	• Glucose homeostasis • Stimulates insulin release and inhibits glucagon • Stimulates insulin and amylin secretion • Direct appetite suppressant on the brain • Slows gastric emptying
Leptin	• Secreted by adipose cells and skeletal muscle • *Minor* orexigen	• Central regulation of food intake • Fat storage and secretion are proportionate to fat storage • Released with low energy intake and low body fat levels • Low leptin concentrations induce hunger and drive to increase food consumption • Starvation reduces leptin and increases appetite • Released after food intake, CCK and secretin or in response to satiety
Secretin	• Released when acids reach small intestine • Secreted by cells in small intestine	• Produces pancreatic fluid, inhibits gastrin release and enhances effects of CCK
Cholecystokinin (CCK)	• Duodenum and proximal jejunum • Released from duodenum when protein and fat enter the small intestine • Major mediator of satiation	• Inhibits gastric emptying and acid secretion • Stimulates release of digestive enzymes from pancreas • Inhibits gastrin • Stimulates gallbladder contraction • Appetite suppressant to the brain to limit food consumption
Pancreatic peptide-YY (PYY)	• Ileum and colon • Cosecreted with GLP-1	• Inhibits gastric emptying • Activates the ileal brake • Inhibits gastric acid, pancreatic exocrine and bile acid secretion • Inhibits pancreatic enzyme secretion • Direct appetite suppressant to the brain
Ghrelin	• Secreted mostly from cells of the stomach	• Appetite stimulant • Released in response to low food intake/fasting • Stimulates release of growth hormone to encourage eating and acts to regulate energy balance long term • Stimulates gastric emptying and gastric acid production, inhibits insulin

Source: Adapted from Camilleri [15] and Delzenne et al. [17].

Zinc deficiency and ageing

The exact role of zinc in dysgeusia is unknown, though it has been cited to be partly responsible for the repair and production of taste buds [16,25]. Zinc is an important trace element for taste perception, including the sweet taste, with reversible hypogeusia reported in individuals with subclinical deficiency [25]. Taste changes in older adults may occur due to changes in taste cell membranes involving altered function of ion channels and receptors, and these adults are especially affected by changes in taste sensation because of age-related gustatory dysfunction, polypharmacy, increased frailty, chronic disease and dietary zinc deficiency [26]. Treatment of taste changes is based on managing the symptoms that cause taste changes including use of artificial saliva, zinc supplementation and alteration to drug treatment [19].

Drug-nutrient interactions/polypharmacy

Drug-nutrient interactions are the physiological or chemical interactions of nutrients or food components with drugs, consequently impairing nutritional status by inhibiting or impairing nutrient absorption or metabolic functions. There are many drugs that can alter nutrient status. Some (digoxin, fluoxetine, levodopa, lithium, metformin and penicillin) can cause a reduction in oral intake due to inducing anorexia and subsequent weight loss [24]. The probability of nutritional problems as a consequence of polypharmacy is highest in older adults with multiple diseases, but evidence is limited to suggest an independent role of polypharmacy and reduced oral intake [27]. Polypharmacy has been shown to correlate to undernutrition of macro- and micronutrients and weight changes by causing appetite loss, GI problems and alterations in body function [27].

1.2.3 Reduced absorption

An interruption in the GI tract from disease, surgery or medical treatments may manifest as specific or global malabsorption. This section provides an overview of malabsorption at each major part of the GI system with regard to undernutrition (deficiency of any macro- or micronutrient). Table 1.2.2 provides a summary of the malabsorptive causes at each part of the GI tract.

Mouth

This is the first site of a nutrient's journey into the GI tract; food is broken down by mastication, digestion begins with salivary enzymes, and the tongue and aperture help form a bolus. While edentulous individuals may be at increased risk of undernutrition due to poor oral intake, evidence remains equivocal regarding poor mastication and absorption due to poor methodology [28]. One of saliva's several functions is that digestive enzymes with up to 15% of total amylase are produced by the salivary glands [29]. However, as the majority of amylase is produced by the pancreas, and salivary amylase is inactivated by gastric acid, salivary amylase is not considered to have a significant effect on digestion [30]. Similarly, lingual lipase solely is thought to be of little relevance in fat digestion in adults [30,31].

Stomach

Once the food bolus reaches the stomach, secretions such as acid further digest food to produce chyme, which is then transported to the small intestine, using peristalsis. While absorption tends to play a lesser role in the stomach compared to the small intestine, any disturbance in the secretory, motor, hormonal or digestive functions in the stomach may lead to maldigestion further down the GI tract. For instance, hydrogen chloride is required for the absorption of several minerals, including calcium, phosphate and zinc. Hypochlorhydria induced by the long-term administration of proton pump inhibitors (PPI) has been associated with reduced absorption of micronutrients (vitamin B12, magnesium, calcium, iron); however, there are no recommendations for their replacement in long-term PPI use [32]. Gastric lipase has been suggested to account for up to 20% of the fat digestion of a meal, though it would not be able to normalise total fat digestion in the absence of pancreatic lipase [33].

Table 1.2.2   Summary of the main causes of malabsorption by region of the gastrointestinal (GI) tract

Region of GI tract	Causes of malabsorption
Mouth*	• Poor dentition • Poor mastication • Reduced salivary enzyme activity
Oesophagus*	• Barrett's oesophagus • Oesophageal cancer • Achalasia
Stomach*	• Gastrectomy • Hypochlorhydria • Bariatric surgery
Small intestine	• Motility disorders (gastroparesis, systemic sclerosis, visceral myopathy, visceral neuropathy) • Reduction in mucosal absorptive capacity: coeliac disease, Crohn's disease • Infection enteropathy (e.g. Whipple's disease) • Radiation enteropathy • Surgical resections (short bowel syndrome, ileal resection due to Crohn's disease, cancer or surgical complications) • Small intestinal bacterial overgrowth • Parasitic infections
Accessory organs	• Reduction in pancreatic mass: chronic pancreatitis, severe acute necrotising pancreatitis, pancreatic cancer, pancreatic resections (pancreatectomy) • Extrapancreatic causes: coeliac disease, Crohn's disease, radiation enteropathy • Congenital disorders: cystic fibrosis • Acid-mediated inactivation: Zollinger–Ellison syndrome
Large intestine*	• Surgical resection (partial or total colectomy) • Motility disorders (Hirschsprung's disease) • Ulcerative colitis • Parasitic infections

* These parts of the GI tract are not associated with significant malabsorption, though may affect oral intake or absorption further down the small intestine.

Given the extensive functions of the stomach, one would expect severe undernutrition with its absence. Indeed, gastrectomy can lead to rapid transit of largely undigested food, increasing the osmotic load through the GI tract to cause 'dumping syndrome' [34]. However, in patients who have undergone total gastrectomy, several studies demonstrate that in the majority, a reduced oral intake tends to be the cause of undernutrition, rather than reduced absorption [35]. When malabsorption does occur, lipid and vitamin B12 tend to be the nutrients that are malabsorbed [36].

Motility disorders such as gastroparesis can lead to maldigestion. Normal peristalsis ensures that partially digested food mixes with gastric secretions at the optimum time for further transport and absorption. With gastroparesis, reduced oral intake is often the cause of undernutrition rather than malabsorption [37]. Small intestinal dysmotility such as systemic sclerosis affects the muscularis propria (substituting fibre muscles with tough collagen), causing small intestinal stasis that is associated with malabsorption by inducing small intestinal bacterial overgrowth or formation of blind loops [38].

Small intestine and accessory organs

The small intestine (SI) is the main absorption site of the GI tract, with approximately 90% of absorption occurring in the duodenum and proximal jejunum. Small intestinal malabsorption can occur due to a reduction in absorptive capacity (e.g. surgeries involving small intestine resection, diseases affecting the mucosa), and interruptions in other organs linked to digestive and absorptive process of the small intestine.

Reduction in absorptive capacity can occur from diseases affecting the integrity of the SI. For example, small intestinal Crohn's disease (further discussed in Chapter 5.8) can lead to villous atrophy, crypt hyperplasia, granulomas, strictures and abscesses, resulting in deficiencies of energy, protein, iron and vitamin D, though not limited to global nutrient deficiency [39]. Another condition, coeliac disease, that leads to enteropathy and villous atrophy from ingestion of gluten, has been shown to result in short stature, iron and folate deficiency, and rickets in children and adults [40]. Microbial imbalances (e.g. parasitic infections, Whipple's disease) can also affect small intestinal absorption. small intestinal dysmotility, GI tract damage (e.g. radiation enteritis) or poor gut immunity [41], may cause deconjugation of bile salts, bacterial digestion of proteins and reduced disaccharide activity leading to fat, protein and carbohydrate malabsorption, respectively [41].

Surgeries of the small intestinal (due to disease, obstruction or cancer) can result in partial or absolute loss of small intestinal absorptive tissue. Resection of >100 cm of the ileum, for example, leads to bile salt malabsorption (BAM) as >90% of bile salts are reabsorbed in the terminal ileum. Increased concentrations of bile salts and water in the colon cause watery diarrhoea and if left untreated, weight loss and fat-soluble deficiencies may result [42]. In addition, the shorter the length of small intestine remaining, the higher the probability of malabsorption (see Chapter 5.9 for further information).

The proper function of accessory organs is a prerequisite to ensure absorption of nutrients in the small intestine. For instance, reductions in pancreatic enzyme (amylase, trypsin, lipase) activity can compensate to a certain degree, as they are overproduced up to 15-fold [29]. Lipase is the enzyme most sensitive to environmental pH, rendering it inactive in the presence of acid. It is considered more important than amylase and trypsin as the latter can be compensated by extrapancreatic enzyme activity [43].

Table 1.2.3 Drug-induced malabsorption by mechanism of action

Mechanism of action	Drug examples
Drug-induced toxicity to the small intestinal mucosa	• Colchicine • Cytospastics (methotrexate, 5-fluorouracil) • Antibiotics (neomycin)

Inhibition of enzymes
    Hydrolytic enzymes
    Preintestinal enzymes
	• Carbohydrate gelling agents (guar)
	• Anti-inflammatory (sulfasalazine)
	• Antiepileptic (phenytoin)
	• α-glucosidase inhibitors (acarbose)
	• α-amylase inhibitors (tendamistate)
	• Somatostatin analogue (octreotide)

Changing physicochemical properties	• Bile acid sequestrant (cholestyramine) • Antibiotics (neomycin) • Antacids (magnesium carbonate, aluminium hydroxide)
Chelation	• Antibiotics (penicillamine, tetracycline)
Gastrointestinal motility	• Prokinetics (metoclopramide, erythromycin)

Source: Adapted with permission of Springer from Wehrmaan et al. [44].

Colon

Food matter that reaches the colon is composed of undigested food, fibre and bacteria. Microbes are responsible for synthesis of vitamin K and B and energy, with up to 10% of energy being generated from short-chain fatty acids (acetic, propionic and butyric acid) from fermented undigested carbohydrate [1]. However, the colon is not considered essential for the absorption of nutrients.

Drug-induced malabsorption

Several common mechanisms have been suggested to account for drug-induced malabsorption including:

- toxicity to the small intestinal mucosa
- inhibition of enzyme (hydrolytic and predigestive enzymes) activity
- chelation formation
- interference in physicochemical properties
- affecting GI motility [44,45].

For example, long-term use of bile acid sequestrants may be associated with fat-soluble vitamin deficiency (Table 1.2.3). In the case of polypharmacy, several drugs have been associated with vitamin B12 deficiency, with the most common mechanism being interference in binding to intrinsic factor [45].

References

1. Stevens CE, Hume ID. Contributions of microbes in vertebrate gastrointestinal tract to production and conservation of nutrients. *Physiol Rev* 1998; **78**: 393–427.
2. Martin RD, Chivers DJ, MacLarnon AM, Hladnik CM. Gastrointestinal allometry in primates and other mammals. In: Jungers WL, editor. Size and Scaling in Primate Biology. New York: Plenum Press, 1985, pp. 61–89.
3. Hammond KA, Lam M, Lloyd KC, Diamond J. Simultaneous manipulation of intestinal capacities and nutrient loads in mice. *Am J Physiol* 1996; **271**: G969–979.
4. Stroud MA, Jackson AA, Waterlow JC. Protein turnover rates of two human subjects during an unassisted crossing of Antarctica. *Br J Nutr* 1996; **76**: 165–174.
5. Grimble G. The physiology of nutrient digestion and absorption. In: Geissler C, Powers H, editors. Human Nutrition. Edinburgh: Elsevier Churchill Livingstone, 2017.

6. Subramanya SB, Subramanian VS, Kumar JS, Hoiness R, Said HM. Inhibition of intestinal biotin absorption by chronic alcohol feeding: cellular and molecular mechanisms. *Am J Physiol* 2011; **300**: G494–501.
7. Galvin R, Bråthen G, Ivashynka A, Hillbom M, Tanasescu R, Leone MA, et al. EFNS guidelines for diagnosis, therapy and prevention of Wernicke encephalopathy. *Eur J Neurol* 2010; **17**: 1408–1418.
8. Tanaka H, Miyamoto KI, Morita K, Haga H, Segawa H, Shiraga T, et al. Regulation of the PepT1 peptide transporter in the rat small intestine in response to 5-fluorouracil-induced injury. *Gastroenterology* 1998; **114**: 714–723.
9. Steinhardt HJ, Wolf A, Jakober B, Schmuelling RM, Langer K, Brandl M, et al. Nitrogen absorption in pancreatectomised patients: protein versus protein hydrolysate as substrate. *J Lab Clin Med* 1989; **113**: 162–167.
10. Spiller RC, Jones BJM, Silk DBA. Jejunal water and electrolyte absorption from two proprietary enteral feeds in man: importance of sodium content. *Gut* 1987; **28**: 681–687.
11. Rolls ET. Taste, olfactory and food texture reward processing in the brain and obesity. *Int J Obes* 2011; **3**: 550–561.
12. Hutton JL, Baracos VE, Wismer W V. Chemosensory dysfunction is a primary factor in the evolution of declining nutritional status and quality of life in patients with advanced cancer. *J Pain Symptom Manage* 2007; **33**: 156–165.
13. Bannerman E, Davidson I, Conway C, Culley D, Aldhous MC, Ghosh S. Altered subjective appetite parameters in Crohn's disease patients. *Clin Nutr* 2001; **20**: 399–405.
14. Laviano A, Inui A, Marks DL, Meguid MM, Pichard C, Rossi Fanelli F, et al. Neural control of the anorexia-cachexia syndrome. *AJP Endocrinol Metab* 2008; **295**: E1000–1008.
15. Camilleri M. Peripheral mechanisms in appetite regulation. *Gastroenterology* 2015; **148**: 1219–1233.
16. Tortora GJ, Grabowski SR. Principles of Anatomy and Physiology, 9th edn. New York: John Wiley and Sons, 2000.
17. Delzenne N, Blundell J, Brouns F, Cunningham K, de Graaf K, Erkner A, et al. Gastrointestinal targets of appetite regulation in humans. *Obes Rev* 2010; **11**: 234–250.
18. Moss C, Dhillo WS, Frost G, Hickson M. Gastrointestinal hormones: the regulation of appetite and the anorexia of ageing. *J Hum Nutr Diet* 2012; **25**: 3–15.
19. Wylie K, Nebauer M. 'The food here is tasteless!' Food taste or tasteless food? Chemosensory loss and the politics of under-nutrition. *Collegian* 2011; **18**: 27–35.

20. Samuels MA, Feske SK. Office Practice of Neurology, 2nd edn. Philadelphia: Elsevier Science, 2003.
21. Raber-Durlacher JE, Barasch A, Peterson DE, Lalla R V., Schubert MM, Fibbe WE. Oral complications and management considerations in patients treated with high-dose chemotherapy. *Support Cancer Ther* 2004; **1**: 219–229.
22. Schiffman SS. Critical illness and changes in sensory perception. *Proc Nutr Soc* 2007; **66**: 331–345.
23. Smeets PA, Erkner A, de Graaf C. Cephalic phase responses and appetite. *Nutr Rev* 2010; **68**: 643–655.
24. Boullata JI BJ. A perspective on drug-nutrient interactions. In: Boullata JI, Armenti VT, editors. Handbook of Drug-Nutrient Interactions. Totowa: Humana Press, 2004, pp. 3–25.
25. Heyneman CA. Zinc deficiency and taste disorders. *Ann Pharmacother* 1996; **30**: 186–187.
26. Mistretta CM. Aging effects on anatomy and neurophysiology of taste and smell. *Gerodontology* 1984; **3**: 131–136.
27. Jyrkkä J, Mursu J, Enlund H, Lönnroos E. Polypharmacy and nutritional status in elderly people. *Curr Opin Clin Nutr Metab Care* 2012; **15**: 1–6.
28. N'gom PI, Woda A. Influence of impaired mastication on nutrition. *J Prosthet Dent* 2002; **87**: 667–673.
29. Keller J, Layer P. The pathophysiology of malabsorption. *Viszeralmedizin* 2014; **30**: 150–154.
30. Hamosh M. Lingual and gastric lipases. *Nutrition* 1990; **6**: 421–428.
31. Pedersen AM, Bardow A, Jensen SB, Nauntofte B. Saliva and gastrointestinal functions of taste, mastication, swallowing and digestion. *Oral Dis* 2002; **8**: 117–129.
32. Heidelbaugh JJ. Proton pump inhibitors and risk of vitamin and mineral deficiency: evidence and clinical implications. *Ther Adv Drug Saf* 2013; **4**: 125–133.
33. Carrière F, Grandval P, Gregory PC, Renou C, Henniges F, Sander-Struckmeier S, et al. Does the pancreas really produce much more lipase than required for fat digestion? *JOP* 2005; **6**: 206–215.
34. van Beek AP, Emous M, Laville M, Tack J. Dumping syndrome after esophageal, gastric or bariatric surgery: pathophysiology, diagnosis, and management. *Obes Rev* 2017; **18**: 68–85.
35. Bae JM, Park JW, Yang HK, Kim JP. Nutritional status of gastric cancer patients after total gastrectomy. *World J Surg* 1998; **22**: 254–60-1.
36. Hu Y, Kim HI, Hyung WJ, Song KJ, Lee JH, Kim YM, et al. Vitamin B(12) deficiency after gastrectomy for gastric cancer: an analysis of clinical patterns and risk factors. *Ann Surg* 2013; **258**: 970–975.
37. Parkman HP, Yates KP, Hasler WL, Nguyan L, Pasricha PJ, Snape WJ, et al. Dietary intake and nutritional deficiencies in patients with diabetic or idiopathic gastroparesis. *Gastroenterology* 2011; **141**: 486–498.
38. Owens SR, Greenson JK. The pathology of malabsorption: current concepts. *Histopathology* 2007; **50**: 64–82.
39. Donnellan CF, Yann LH, Lal S. Nutritional management of Crohn's disease. *Ther Adv Gastroenterol* 2013; **6**: 231–242.
40. Tikkakoski S, Savilahti E, Kolho KL. Undiagnosed coeliac disease and nutritional deficiencies in adults screened in primary health care. *Scand J Gastroenterol* 2007; **42**: 60–65.
41. Dukowicz AC, Lacy BE, Levine GM. Small intestinal bacterial overgrowth: a comprehensive review. *Gastroenterol Hepatol* 2007; **3**: 112–122.
42. Mekjian HS, Phillips SF, Hofmann AF. Colonic secretion of water and electrolytes induced by bile acids: perfusion studies in man. *J Clin Invest* 1971; **50**: 1569–1577.
43. Domínguez-Muñoz JE. Pancreatic enzyme therapy for pancreatic exocrine insufficiency. *Curr Gastroenterol Rep* 2007; **9**: 116–122.
44. Wehrmann T, Lembcke B, Caspary WF. Drug-induced malabsorption. In: Drug-Induced Injury to the Digestive System. Milan: Springer Milan, 1993, pp. 89–109.
45. White R, Ashworth A. How drug therapy can affect, threaten and compromise nutritional status. *J Hum Nutr Diet* 2000; **13**: 119–129.

Chapter 1.3

Socioeconomic causes of undernutrition

Lynne Kennedy and Alison Woodall
Department of Clinical Sciences and Nutrition, University of Chester, Chester, UK

1.3.1 Introduction

In this chapter, we explore the role of socioeconomic factors in the development of undernutrition in high-income countries with particular reference to food access and nutrition inequality. For the purpose of this chapter, we use the term undernutrition to refer to the physiological effects of inadequate food supply resulting from the inability to access sufficient quantity and quality of food to meet recommended nutritional requirements; a situation otherwise termed food poverty or food insecurity (Box 1.3.1).

In affluent societies, hunger and undernutrition coexist alongside obesity and diet-related diseases such as coronary heart disease and diabetes. Before the food system was industrialised in the mid-20th century, people ate a basic, traditional diet of limited variety. Hunger and undernutrition were common. Today, food is both varied and widely available. Access to cheap, energy-dense and nutrient-poor food is linked with the so-called obesity epidemic and diseases of affluence. Despite this, a growing number of people in societies such as the UK experience hunger or undernutrition because of limited access to or availability of a nutritionally adequate diet [3,5]. Also, although the majority of people have access to sufficient amounts of food, undernutrition is as much of a problem now as it was in the early 20th century. Reports suggest that 'wartime' nutritional deficiency diseases are also on the increase but not for lack of food; the incidence of rickets amongst UK children has risen dramatically in the past decade or so, partly because of inadequate exposure to sunlight but mainly due to poor-quality diets (high in fat, salt and sugar and low in micronutrients) and rising levels of overweight. Moreover, certain types of undernutrition are compounded by obesity, such as the deficiency disease rickets, due to the sequestering of vitamin D in central adipose tissue.

Estimates suggest that some 3 million people in the UK (3–5% of the population) are undernourished at any one time; of these, 93% live in the community, 5% in care homes and 2% in hospital [6]. Those most vulnerable include the elderly, young children, women in the third trimester of pregnancy (when energy and protein requirements increase), families on low income and lower socioeconomic groups.

1.3.2 Socioeconomic differences in diet and nutrition

Undernutrition in individuals is directly linked to patterns of food consumption and dietary quality. There is sufficient evidence of a socioeconomic gradient in the dietary and nutritional intakes of populations from high-income countries. In the UK, the 2011 Low Income Diet and Nutrition Survey [7] revealed how the dietary patterns and corresponding nutrient profiles of low-income households are consistently poorer than those of individuals in more affluent households; diets are deficient in fresh fruit and vegetables, folate, iron and vitamin D, but

Advanced Nutrition and Dietetics in Nutrition Support, First Edition. Edited by Mary Hickson and Sara Smith.
© 2018 John Wiley & Sons Ltd. Published 2018 by John Wiley & Sons Ltd.

Box 1.3.1   Key concepts and terms regarding socioeconomic causes of undernutrition

- *Food security*: The ability to secure 'access to sufficient amounts of safe and nutritious food for normal growth and development and an active, healthy life' is referred to as food security [1]. Food security includes the accessibility, availability, distribution and utilisation of food and covers the nutrient requirements for a healthy life [2]. According to major global organisations, such as the Food and Agriculture Organization [1] and the World Health Organization, food security is unambiguously associated with health and with three important elements: food availability, food access and food use. Adequate food availability means that sufficient amounts of food are consistently available, food access means that there are adequate resources to secure proper food for a decent diet and food use implies that there is elementary knowledge on nutrition in order to use food appropriately.
- *Food insecurity:* A key reason for poor nutritional status which can affect people temporarily (acutely), chronically or seasonally. Amongst others, it may occur because food is not available, is not affordable or is unevenly distributed. This can be intrahousehold food insecurity or inappropriate use, for example resulting from inadequate storage or cooking facilities for people living in homeless shelters [2–4].
- *Food poverty*: A term with a similar meaning to food insecurity, it has many definitions. In the UK, food poverty is defined as 'the inability to afford, or to have access to, food to make up a healthy diet'. People may be affected by food poverty because other household expenses restrict money for food, their living environment and transport facilities limit the availability of food, or they are not able to prepare decent meals because of insufficient cooking knowledge, skills, equipment and facilities [4,5].

---

abundant in foods high in fat, sugar and salt. An equally comprehensive survey, involving 6800 individuals aged >1.5 years in the UK [8], concurred that dietary quality varied significantly according to socioeconomic group and is directly associated with income. Fruit and vegetable consumption showed the most striking difference, with only 3% of boys aged 11–18 years in the lowest income quintile meeting the recommendation for eating five portions of fruit and vegetables a day, compared to 26% in the highest quintile. This variation in dietary quality and nutritional status according to social class is referred to as nutrition inequality.

There is considerable evidence within the public health nutrition literature of a causal relationship between a diet low in fruit, vegetables, white meat, non-animal oils and fish and high levels of salt and increased risk of chronic disease, including certain cancers, and low socioeconomic status. The consequence of nutrition inequality is best illustrated by socioeconomic differences in the prevalence of the primary causes of morbidity and premature mortality associated with diet. In a landmark paper, James et al. [9] demonstrated how dietary patterns affect the social gradient for disease risk or health outcomes in Britain, highlighting the increased burden for lower socioeconomic groups. Problems significantly associated with

poor nutrition more common in lower socioeconomic classes included anaemia, premature delivery and low birthweight, poor oral health, eczema and asthma, diabetes, obesity, cardiovascular diseases, cancers and bone disease. The authors identified excessive consumption amongst the poorest households of energy-dense nutrient-poor foods with high sodium and low potassium, magnesium and calcium content, high sugar snacks and beverages, lower breastfeeding rates and lower levels of physical inactivity. Causes of undernutrition associated with food poverty and food insecurity are, however, complex and multiple and the primary factors are social, economic (affordability) and physical (access).

1.3.3 Food insecurity

Food insecurity is a primary factor related to undernutrition and occurs when food is unavailable, unaffordable, unevenly distributed or unsafe to eat due to inappropriate storage or preparation [2]. Globally, it is widely accepted that food insecurity is associated with hunger and poor nutrition. In high-income countries, however, the relationship with undernutrition, compared to the situation in low- to middle-income countries, is more complex due to exposure and temporality (acute versus chronic undernutrition). There is no single agreed measure of food insecurity and as such, the exact numbers affected by hunger, over time, and the impact for undernutrition due to socioeconomic factors remain unclear. Aside from the Low Income Diet and Nutrition Survey (LIDNS) [7], data on household level food security are not routinely observed in the UK [2]. However, this may change if recent efforts to quantify and explain rising hunger and food poverty in Eire and Wales are successful.

According to the 2011 LIDNS [7], a third (29%) of households surveyed reported restricted access to sufficient food at some time during the previous year and might therefore be described as food insecure. Furthermore, in the past year, 39% of the families were also concerned that 'food would run out before their next pay day', 36% stated 'they could not afford a balanced diet', 22% 'indicated regularly reducing or skipping meals' and 5% reported 'not eating any food for a whole day', all aspects considered within the literature as potential indicators of food security [10]. The 2014 all-parliamentary inquiry into hunger and malnutrition in the UK estimated that some 500 000 children are living in households unable to provide adequate amounts or quality of food for a diet that supports normal growth and development [11], with growing numbers regularly experiencing hunger.

In many high-income countries, food security is not routinely measured. Researchers have suggested that UK levels are similar to trends in other high-income countries such as the USA, Canada and Australia. We also know that the elderly, young children and individuals with limited economic or material resources are particularly vulnerable to undernutrition and they are also more likely to experience food insecurity.

1.3.4 Food security and socioeconomic factors

Research indicates that the key factors associated with food insecurity are household income, followed by low socioeconomic status (often measured as a combination of education, income

and occupation), living in highly deprived areas and living in rented accommodation [12]. In New Zealand, a study of almost 19 000 households identified that the strongest predictors of food insecurity were being female, younger to middle-aged (25–44 years), divorced, living in a sole-parent family and being unemployed or in receipt of means-tested government benefit [13]. In a study comparing food security in Australia and the UK [14], the authors suggest that despite evidence of poor diet and food insecurity being greater amongst households of lower socioeconomic status, certain sociodemographic characteristics, such as marital status, ethnic group or education, may provide protection against undernutrition linked with food insecurity. It is widely acknowledged that healthier eating patterns are associated with higher educational attainment, and adult-only households are linked to higher consumption of fruits and vegetables, rich in micronutrients and associated with reduced risk of undernutrition.

The remainder of this chapter will explore the role of socioeconomic factors – social (acceptability), economic (affordability) and environmental – on undernutrition in food-insecure households.

Social factors

The social and cultural context in which people live (structure) is as important as individual agency (autonomy and control) and material wealth in determining people's health-related behaviour and risk. Indeed, as illustrated in the widely documented schematic of the social determinants of health, health-related behaviours (such as eating) are directly influenced by the circumstances in which people are born, grow up, live, work and age. These are in turn shaped by a wider set of forces: economic, social, fiscal and political (policy) (Figure 1.3.1) [15]. The extent to which individuals or professionals can influence these factors varies between individuals, their situation and the resources (material, financial, social and cultural) at their disposal.

It is firmly established that food and eating are not only essential physiological requirements but satisfy important social and cultural

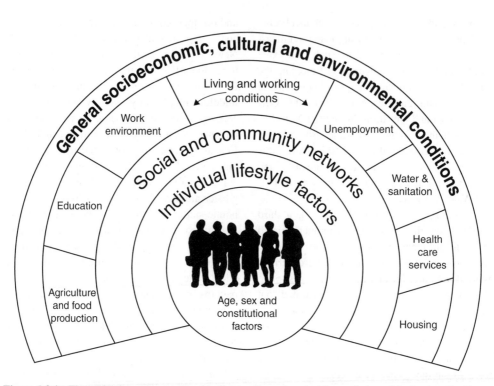

Figure 1.3.1   The social determinants of health. Source: Reproduced with permission of the Institute for Future Studies from Dahlgren and Whitehead [15]

purposes; moreover, the factors influencing food choices are, like health (see Figure 1.3.1), socially and culturally determined (Figure 1.3.2). The social function of food and eating, through religious festivals or family celebrations (weddings, for example), is well documented. Classic research studies conducted on the family unit suggest how undernutrition is influenced by adequate access to food inside the family home and the complex interpersonal negotiations whereby food is allocated, prioritised or denied according to age or gender [16–22]. In 2014, a report on behalf of the Trussel Trust [23], the UK food bank charity, reported that one in five parents (mainly women) in Britain skip a meal in order to ensure their children have sufficient food to eat. It is well documented that social and cultural factors also influence decisions on the types of foods purchased and consumed.

The Family Food survey illustrates both regional (cultural) and socioeconomic differences in food purchasing patterns for the UK [24]. For example, the South East spent the highest per person per week on all food and drink (£27.70) compared to Yorkshire and Humberside (£23.48), with people in the South East purchasing more fresh fruits, vegetables and 'healthier' fats (vegetable oils). Social and cultural factors are important determinants of individual and collective food choice, and thus dietary behaviour, because they are embedded in deep-seated attitudes, social norms or social relationships and are thus resilient to change. For a more detailed consideration of social and cultural factors influencing food choice in low income families see Kennedy and Ling [4] and Leather [25].

Economic factors

Sufficient household income is a major threat to food security and undernutrition. Food prices increased by 43.5% between 2005 and 2013, meaning many families find it difficult to afford adequate amounts and quality of food to meet

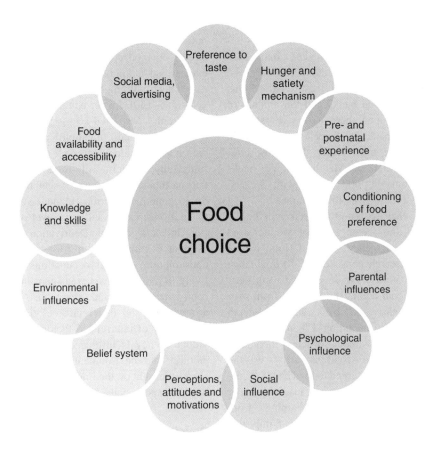

Figure 1.3.2 Range of factors influencing food choice. Source: Adapted from Kennedy and Ling [4] and Kennedy [5].

their dietary needs [2], with many people buying cheaper energy-rich, nutrition-poor foods instead of healthier options such as fruit, vegetables, unprocessed meat and fresh fish. In times of financial hardship, food expenditure is usually the most flexible and first to be cut, leading to low or irregular consumption of meals, or missed meals based on limited or lack of income to buy food. Case study data show weight loss and weight cycling as a consequence of a limited food budget [25].

Difficulties affording sufficient amounts or quality of food are consistently reported in the nutrition literature. The DEFRA Family Food survey [24] clearly demonstrates that the cost of securing a nutritionally adequate diet has increased; in the period 2007–2011, food prices rose by 12% in real terms, and the proportionate spend on food and drink by the average household rose from 10.5% in 2007 to 11.3% in 2011, but rose from 15.2% to 16.6% for low-income households. Researchers from the CEDAR Centre reported that in 2012, 1000 kcal of healthy food cost £7.49 whilst 1000 kcal of more unhealthy food cost £1.77 [26]. Thus, although, as research indicates, it is possible to construct a relatively healthy meal for a limited cost, the feasibility of this is, in terms of social justice and sustainability, fiercely contested.

Food insecurity, hunger and emergency aid

The link between food insecurity and the need for people to access emergency food aid is increasingly relevant in high-income countries. In the UK, recent welfare reforms and 'benefit sanctions', whereby you can have payment reduced if you miss or are late for an appointment at the Job Centre, are cited as a major contributor to the rising demand for emergency food aid. Data from the Trussel Trust illustrates that the number of food banks and the amount of people reliant upon them have risen steadily since the first bank was launched in the UK in 2000 [27]. The most recent data show how, between April 2013 and March 2014, food banks provided some 900 000 people with 3 days' emergency food in over 400 locations.

A comprehensive report undertaken in the UK highlighted the factors leading to increased referrals to emergency food aid (food banks) [28]. The research consisted of 40 qualitative interviews with users of seven food bank locations, additional administrative data from over 900 users of three food banks and an in-depth caseload analysis including 178 users of one food bank. Being without sufficient income to afford adequate food – food insecurity – was the main reason families turned to food banks. Acute income crisis was sometimes caused by wider life-shocks, such as loss of earnings from employment, divorce, bereavement, family difficulties, and homelessness and health problems. Moreover, this study found that food bank users were affected by wider vulnerabilities. These included living in particular areas with poor employment opportunities, limited shops and public services, struggling with physical or mental ill health, educational disadvantages, problems with housing, limited family support and debt [28]. These factors resonate with the existing literature on how socioeconomic factors influence dietary patterns and nutritional status.

Socioeconomic status

Marmot's work in the UK suggests that the association between health, including undernutrition, and income *per se* is less important than composite measures such as socioeconomic status (SES) and social deprivation [29]. Income, education and occupation (of head of household) are the primary indicators of SES and have been used to explore socioeconomic

differences in dietary consumption and undernutrition. Income and education have similar effects on food consumption and both higher educational attainment and income levels are associated with higher intakes of fruits and vegetables [30]. Lower educational attainment (of parents), restricted access to food (shops), low car ownership, unemployment and occupation are considered stronger determinants of 'unhealthy' patterns of food consumption, but particularly fruit and vegetable intakes. Socioeconomic position (manual versus nonmanual occupation) and area level of deprivation (Index of Multiple Deprivation) have been associated with levels of fruit and vegetable consumption: manual occupations and those living in most deprived areas consume significantly less fruit and vegetables. Research around SES and diet reinforces the role and complexity of interrelated factors, where individual agency is influenced by wider social, cultural and environmental factors, but has shed little light on the impact of SES on undernutrition specifically.

Physical food environment

Several studies report on the importance of the local food environment to undernutrition [31–33]; the evidence is, however, equivocal. Poor access to food is associated with undernutrition where pre-existing vulnerabilities are present, for example the elderly and infirm, or where cultural beliefs or preferences restrict food choice in an already restricted environment [32]. The evidence is less convincing for the general population despite the use of the term 'food desert', introduced in the 1990s in reference to neighbourhoods with limited shopping facilities or access to food shops; the term arose at a time when the local shopping landscape changed from predominantly small independents to the growth of out-of-town supermarkets. Despite the unequivocal evidence, campaigners and some researchers have argued that the resulting 'food deserts' are significant factors preventing low-income households, particularly those without access to a car, from accessing a healthy diet [33].

Nonetheless, the impact in terms of someone's ability to access adequate food is less conclusive. Sauveplane-Stirling et al. [34] and Harrington et al. [35] argue that car ownership significantly affects access to food shops, which increases dependency on local stores and because of their slower stock turnover, the nutritional quality of food is inferior. This is illustrated in translating the government's recommendation 'five-a-day' message into practice, where the average household would need to purchase in excess of 30 kg of fruit and vegetables per week, which is particularly challenging for those who do not own a car. People on low incomes, the elderly and other vulnerable groups are more reliant upon smaller local shops where choice, nutritional quality and affordability are all limited. Other factors associated with the food environment might include access to cooking facilities (e.g. for people living in temporary accommodation or homeless). The important role of food literacy (the knowledge and skills associated with understanding food labelling, budgeting, cooking and healthy eating) in preventing undernutrition has not been explored, but for a comprehensive account of this in relation to overnutrition and poor diet, see, for example Kennedy and Ling [4] and Hitchman et al. [36].

1.3.5 Psychology of undernutrition

Psychological factors and significant life events (such as birth of a child, marriage, death of a loved one) can influence the development of positive or negative eating behaviours and thereby contribute to undernutrition. A child's eating behaviour and dietary habits are formed early in life where foods are slowly introduced to the diet through appropriate weaning; the influence of parents is hugely influential at this stage and growing evidence highlights how certain parenting styles can negatively impact on a child's eating habits, continuing into adulthood. Parents routinely restricting children from eating specific foods (restrained eating) has been linked to increased propensity for and craving of energy-dense food, disrupting energy regulation and internal cues to hunger [37]. Although inconclusive, some researchers consider restrained eating may be linked with emotional eating, typically involving highly palatable and energy-dense food [38], with implications for energy and nutritional intake.

Psychosociological constructs may contribute to undernutrition for people living in the community with long-standing health conditions, such as cancer. People living with head and neck cancer, for example, can experience long-term psychological and sociological inhibitions arising from the cancer itself but also from the pain and discomfort from associated treatments and symptoms, difficulty in eating and swallowing [39]. Eating habits form part of personal identity and self-image so the emotional loss of satisfaction from food, often a side effect of the physiological changes accompanying cancer and its treatment, such as xerostomia (dry mouth) and odynophagia (painful swallowing), social marginalisation resulting from feeling embarrassed about eating with others, and loss of the psychological comfort derived from eating, especially eating with others, all impact negatively on food consumption, nutritional status, recovery and quality of life [39]. Education and social support are required to tackle both the undernutrition itself and the contributory psychological and sociological changes.

Psychological well-being is an important determinant of nutritional status in the elderly. In a cross-sectional study of the nutritional status of elderly people (n = 200) in the community, the authors concluded that older people 'living alone' consumed a diet lower in protein, fruit and vegetables and consequently were more likely to suffer from undernutrition [40]. The role of stress, anxiety and depression on nutritional status in otherwise healthy adults has been researched, in all populations, but evidence of any direct association is lacking. Depression, poverty and loneliness (along with other physiological factors) have been linked with anorexia of ageing [41]; estimates for the prevalence of anorexia due to ageing vary between 12% and 62% of older adults, depending on country, socioeconomic status, health and living conditions, but this issue is often overlooked because it is seen by many as a normal response to ageing. Researchers in Helsinki observed that nursing home residents with poor psychological well-being were more likely to refuse food and snacks and usually ate alone [42]. Engel et al. [43] found poor emotional well-being and depression were associated with inadequate nutritional intake as was poor ability to manage life when under stress (defined in the literature by concepts such as resilience and 'hardiness'). This is consistent with other studies [44], where undernutrition is said to be exacerbated when older adults lose autonomy and can no longer shop, choose or cook their own food. For some people who lack material or financial resources and social support, or feel socially isolated, there appears to be a continuum whereby self-neglect leads sequentially to cognitive impairment, frailty and undernutrition.

Progressive age-related physiological decline with decreased functional reserve are increasingly linked together as 'frailty', a construct used to identify risk of adverse health and social outcomes for older people [44]. When considering undernutrition (a key outcome measure for frailty), it is clear that frailty needs to be considered from physiological, functional and psychosocial dimensions in order to give a clear assessment of risk for all health and social outcomes. For example, depression, cognitive impairment, functional impairment and swallowing difficulties are all directly associated with undernutrition [44]. Similar studies illustrate the close relationship of psychosocial factors with undernutrition, along with the fact that undernutrition is often not self-perceived or recognised as a health concern in its own right. Once established, undernutrition further exacerbates the symptoms of frailty and leads to increased risk of mortality. As such, a combination of physiological, nutritional, cognitive and psychological inputs to improve well-being and quality of life are likely to be included in treatment.

Inappropriate attitudes towards eating, which encompass phobic, obsessional and hypochondriacal states, may affect the nutritional status of older people. Food anxieties, common in elderly subjects in the clinical or care setting, may be exacerbated by a tendency for obsessive or overdeveloped concerns about food and weight and can result in issues similar to eating disorders.

Finally, although there is limited literature available, undernutrition in combination with chemical exposure is becoming an important consideration in high-income societies, particularly in the context of increased trends around drug and alcohol abuse, food faddism and people receiving bariatric surgery or drug treatment for certain medical conditions, including cancers [41,45].

1.3.6 Summary

Socioeconomic circumstances of individuals and communities strongly influence the availability and consumption of adequate food and therefore nutrient quality of diets. Different social groups may be affected by socioeconomic factors in different ways, with the purchase of fruits and vegetables and non-processed foods particularly sensitive to socioeconomic circumstances. However, until recently these factors were not strongly associated with undernutrition unless additional factors such as age, health status and cultural traditions and belief systems were present.

In the current climate, historical concerns about constraints on budgeting, food purchasing and food security among lower income households have been exacerbated by changing social and structural factors, such as economic recession and affordability of nutrient-dense foods, as well as reduced income and job security. Food security is therefore strongly linked with undernutrition and is particularly concerning where pre-existing vulnerabilities exist. The consequences in terms of health problems associated with undernutrition require interventions which take socioeconomic status into consideration.

Acknowledgements

Christine A Wolfendale, MA, RD, Programme Leader BSc Nutrition and Dietetics Programme, University of Chester, for advising on the content and proof reading.

Miss Antonia Zengerer MSc, Research Intern, Department of Clinical Sciences, University of Chester, for helping to source the relevant literature.

Ms Vanisa Taylor, MSc Public Health Nutrition Student, University of Chester, for adapting and creating Figure 1.3.2.

References

1. Food and Agriculture Organization (FAO). The State of Food Insecurity in the World 2001. Rome: FAO, 2001.
2. Lambie-Mumford H, Crossley D, Jensen E, Verbeke M, Dowler E. Household Food Security in the UK: A Review of Food Aid. Warwick: Warwick University, 2014.
3. Lambie-Mumford H, O'Connell R. Food, Poverty and Policy: Evidence Base and Knowledge Gaps. Sheffield: University of Sheffield, Political Economy Research Institute, 2014.
4. Kennedy LA, Ling M. Nutrition education for low income groups – is there a role? In: Kohler BM, Feichtinger E, Barlosius E, Dowler E, editors. Poverty and Food in Welfare Societies. Berlin: Edition Sigma, 1997, pp. 349–362.
5. Kennedy LA. Hunger and Malnutrition in Affluent Societies: Influencing Policy and Practice. Inaugural Lecture, University of Chester, 10 December 2015. www.chester.ac.uk/node/32198 (accessed 25 August 2017).
6. British Association for Parenteral and Enteral Nutrition (BAPEN). Combating Malnutrition: Recommendations for Action. Redditch: BAPEN, 2009.
7. Nelson M, Erens B, Bates B, Church S, Boshier T. Low Income Diet and Nutrition Survey. London: Stationery Office, 2007.
8. Bates B, Lennox A, Prentice A, Bates C, Page P, Nicholson S, Swan G. National Diet and Nutrition Survey. Results from Years 1–4 (Combined) of the Rolling Programme (2008/2009 – 2011/12). London: Public Health England, 2014.
9. James WPT, Nelson M, Ralph A, Leather S. Socioeconomic determinants of health: the contribution of nutrition to inequalities in health. *BMJ* 1997; **314**: 1545–1549.
10. Sharpe L. Time to Count the Hungry: The Case for a Standard Measure of Household Food Insecurity in the UK. Oxford: UK Food Poverty Alliance, 2016.
11. Feeding Britain: A Strategy for Zero Hunger in England, Wales, Scotland and Northern Ireland. Report of the All-Party Parliamentary Inquiry into Hunger in the United Kingdom. London: Children's Society, 2014.
12. Carter MA, Dubois L, Tremblay MS. Place and food insecurity: a critical review and synthesis of the literature. *Public Health Nutr* 2014; **17**(1): 94–112.
13. Carter K, Lanumata T, Kruse K, Gorton D. What are the determinants of food insecurity in New Zealand and does this differ for males and females? *Aust NZ J Public Health* 2010; **34**(6): 602–608.
14. Thornton LE, Pearce JR, Ball K. Socio-demographic factors associated with healthy eating and food security in socio-economically disadvantaged groups in the UK and Victoria, Australia. *Public Health Nutr* 2014; **17**(1): 20–30.
15. Dahlgren G, Whitehead M. Policies and Strategies to Promote Social Equity in Health. Background Document to WHO – Strategy Paper for Europe. Stockholm: Institute for Future Studies, 2007.
16. Arber S. Class, paid employment and family roles: making sense of structural disadvantage, gender and health status. *Soc Sci Med* 1991; **32**: 425–436.
17. Graham H. Women, Health and the Family. Brighton: Harvester Wheatsheaf, 1984.
18. Kerr M, Charles N. Servers and providers: the distribution of food within the family. *Soc Rev* 1986; **34**(1): 115–157.
19. McKie LJ, Wood RC, Gregory S. Women defining health: food, diet and body image. *Health Educ Res* 1993; **8**(1): 35–41.
20. Charles N, Kerr M. Women, Food, and Families. Manchester: Manchester University Press, 1988.
21. Murcott A. Nutrition and inequalities. A note on sociological approaches. *Eur J Public Health* 2002; **12**: 203–207.
22. Pill R, Parry O. Making changes – women, food and families. *Health Educ J* 1989; **48**: 51–54.
23. Cooper N, Purcell S, Jackson R. Below the Breadline. The Relentless Rise of Food Poverty in Britain. London: Church Action on Poverty, Oxfam, Trussel Trust, 2014.
24. Department for Environment, Food and Rural Affairs (DEFRA). Family Food 2013. London: DEFRA, 2014.
25. Leather S. The Making of Modern Malnutrition. An Overview of Food Poverty in the UK. London: Caroline Walker Trust, 1996.
26. Jones NRV, Conklin AI, Suhrcke M, Monsivais P. The Growing Price Gap Between More and Less Healthy Foods: Analysis of a Novel Longitudinal UK Dataset. *PLOS One* 2014; **9**: e109343.
27. Trussel Trust. Stats. www.trusselltrust.org/stats (accessed 25 August 2017).
28. Perry J, Williams M, Sefton T, Haddad M. Emergency Use Only – Understanding and Reducing the Use of Food Banks in the UK. London: Oxfam, 2014.
29. The Marmot Review. Fair Society, Healthy Lives: Strategic Review of the Health Inequalities in England Post-2010. London: Institute of Health Equity, University College London, 2010.

30. Turrell G, Kavanagh AM. Socio-conomic pathways to diet: modelling the association between socio-economic position and food purchasing behaviour. *Public Health Nutr* 2006; **9**(3): 375–383.

31. Burgoine T, Alvanides S, Lake AA. Assessing the obesogenic environment of North East England. *Health Place* 2011; **17**: 738–747.

32. Schenker S. Undernutrition in the UK. *Nutrition Bulletin* 2003; **28**: 87–120.

33. Lang T, Caraher M. Access to healthy foods: part II. Food poverty and shopping deserts: what are the implications for health promotion policy and practice? *Health Educ J* 1998; **57**: 202–211.

34. Sauveplane-Stirling V, Crichton D, Tessier S, Parrett A, Garcia AL. The food retail environment and its use in a deprived, urban area of Scotland. *Public Health* 2014; **128**: 360–366.

35. Harrington J, Friel S, Thunhurst C, Kirby A, McElroy B. Obesogenic island: the financial burden of private transport on low-income households. *J Public Health* 2008; **30**(1): 38–44.

36. Hitchman C, Christie I, Harrison M, Lang T. Inconvenience Food. The Struggle to Eat Well on a Low Income. London: Demos, 2002.

37. Birch LL, Fisher JO. Development of eating behaviours among children and adolescents. *Paediatrics* 1998; **101**: 539–549.

38. Farrow CV, Haycraft E, Blissett JM. Teaching our children when to eat: how parental feeding practices inform the development of emotional eating – a longitudinal experimental design. *Am J Clin Nutr* 2015; **101**: 908–913.

39. Ganzer H, Touger-Decker R, Byham-Gray L, Murphy BA, Epstein JB. The eating experience after treatment for head and neck cancer: a review of the literature. *Oral Oncol* 2015; **51**: 634–642.

40. Ramic E, Pranjic N, Batic-Mujanovic O, Karic E, Alibasic E, Alic A. The effect of loneliness on malnutrition in elderly population. *Med Arch* 2011; **65**: 92–95.

41. Wysokinski A, Sobow T, Kloszewska I, Kostka T. Mechanisms of the anorexia of aging – a review. *AGE* 2015; **37**: 64–80.

42. Muurinen S, Savikko N, Soini H, Suominen M, Pitkälä K. Nutrition and psychological well-being among long-term care residents with dementia. *J Nutr Health Aging* 2015; **19**: 178–182.

43. Engel JH, Siewerdt F, Jackson R, Akobundu U, Wait C, Sahyoun N. Hardiness, depression, and emotional well-being and their association with appetite in older adults. *J Am Geriatr Soc* 2011; **59**: 482–487.

44. Porter Starr KN, McDonald SR, Bales CW. Nutritional vulnerability in older adults: a continuum of concerns. *Curr Nutr Rep* 2015; **4**: 176–184.

45. Spencer PS, Palmer V. Interrelationships of under nutrition and neurotoxicity: food for thought and research attention. *Neurotoxicology* 2012; **33**: 605–616.

Chapter 1.4

Institutional causes of undernutrition

Clare Corish
School of Public Health, Physiotherapy and Sports Science, University College Dublin, Ireland

1.4.1 Introduction

In developed countries, food is widely available; nonetheless, undernutrition exists in certain population groups. Those in the institutional setting have been identified as being at particular risk.

The reasons for undernutrition are multifactorial, with both physiological and non-physiological factors (e.g. social or psychological) contributing to its development [1]. Direct consequences of disease such as malabsorption, increased metabolism and catabolism also play a role. Surgery and medical treatments, such as chemotherapy and radiotherapy, may promote the development of undernutrition or further compound pre-existing undernutrition [2]. These contributors to undernutrition are prevalent among patients admitted to hospital and in older people who spend long periods in nursing homes or residential care. There is generally poor awareness of the prevalence and consequences of undernutrition among staff working in these institutions, potentially contributing to its development. Therefore, changes to the education and professional practice of those working within institutional healthcare settings are required in order to address this issue.

An accurate picture of institutional undernutrition prevalence has been hindered by the lack of a gold standard assessment and heterogeneity among those being assessed; nonetheless, recent data worldwide indicate a high prevalence, regardless of the method by which it is identified. Using the Mini Nutritional Assessment (MNA), a large multinational study which evaluated pooled data from 4507 older people in hospital, rehabilitation, nursing home and community settings in 12 countries reported a prevalence of undernutrition of 50.5% in rehabilitation, 38.7% in hospital and 13.8% in nursing home settings [3]. Spanish data on 400 hospitalised patients with a mean age of 67.5 (SD 16.1) years indicated that 31.5%, 34.5%, 35.3% and 58.5% were at risk of undernutrition using the Malnutrition Universal Screening Tool (MUST), the Nutritional Risk Screen (NRS-2002), the Subjective Global Assessment (SGA) and the MNA respectively [4]. A Dutch study using unintentional weight loss and body mass index (BMI) reported that 26% of nursing home rehabilitation patients were severely undernourished and 14% moderately undernourished [5]. Using MUST criteria, UK data on over 8500 individuals showed that 25% of patients in the acute hospital setting, 41% in the care home setting and 19% in mental health units were at risk of undernutrition on admission [6]. The Australian Nutrition Care Day Survey showed that 41% of 3122 acute hospital patients were at nutritional risk using the Malnutrition Screening Tool (MST), while 32% were undernourished when appraised using SGA [7]. The recent Canadian Malnutrition Task Force prospective cohort study of 1022 patients consecutively recruited from 18 hospitals (academic and community) showed that 51% of patients admitted to academic or community hospitals were undernourished using SGA [8].

Advanced Nutrition and Dietetics in Nutrition Support, First Edition. Edited by Mary Hickson and Sara Smith.
© 2018 John Wiley & Sons Ltd. Published 2018 by John Wiley & Sons Ltd.

1.4.2 Identification and consequences of institutional undernutrition

Identification of institutional undernutrition

The published literature suggests that identification of institutional undernutrition is improving but remains inadequate. UK data indicate that 99% of hospitals have nutrition screening policies and 97% use a nutrition screening tool [6]. Despite this, only 67% of hospitals report weighing, and 60% report recording height, on all wards. This situation is not unique to the UK. A German study of older patients highlighted that clinical judgement was predominantly used to identify undernutrition, BMI was not routinely calculated, and nutritional problems were not adequately documented [8]. In order to identify undernutrition, a definition of treatable under-/malnutrition needs to be established, and screening tools appropriate for each setting identified and used routinely [10,11]. The definition and screening tools used need to consider population trends in overweight and obesity to ensure that patients with weight loss but normal BMI are appropriately identified and managed.

Consequences of institutional undernutrition

Despite the adverse effects of institutional undernutrition being extensively documented in the literature, inadequate appreciation of its effects among healthcare staff may facilitate development of undernutrition. The primary structural and functional consequences are loss of lean and non-lean tissue which present as body weight loss. The clinical consequences of these changes can negatively affect immune function, wound healing, infection rate, risk of pressure ulcers and falls. Furthermore, undernutrition represents an independent and significant risk factor for in-hospital mortality, longer length of hospital stay (LOS) and prolonged rehabilitation [12]. A study of six different screening tools concluded that all independently predicted longer LOS in hospitalised patients despite each tool assessing different dimensions of nutritional status [13]. These negative clinical consequences have substantial cost implications. In the UK, disease-related undernutrition costs over £13 billion, equating to 10% of total UK expenditure on health and social care [14]. Timely identification and intervention for patients at risk of treatable undernutrition could prevent or reduce the manifestation of associated effects, which would in turn potentially result in cost savings.

1.4.3 Determinants of institutional undernutrition

In order to correctly identify patients who are at risk of institutional undernutrition, it is important to be aware of its main determinants. The factors that can contribute to the occurrence or development of undernutrition within institutional settings are broadly summarised in Box 1.4.1. Factors which have been recognised for over a decade include older age, type of admission/diagnosis, cognition, food service/ eating pattern and inadequate nutritional management [15,16]. Factors recently associated with risk of undernutrition in community-dwelling older adults, including inability to go outside, intestinal problems, cancer, eating fewer than three snacks daily, smoking, nausea, osteoporosis, physical inactivity and dependency in activities of daily living (ADL), need to be considered in future studies of older persons in the institutional care setting [17]. Moreover, documentation of undernutrition using a standardised care process and language is increasingly recognised as being important in achieving high-quality nutritional provision [18].

Older age

In the Netherlands, undernutrition in older people is regarded as a geriatric syndrome due to its high prevalence in older populations and the threat it poses to independence and quality of life [19]. The proposed mechanistic explanation for undernutrition as a geriatric syndrome is that the burden of chronic and acute disease multiplies

Box 1.4.1 Factors contributing to undernutrition in the institutional setting

Individual	**Institutional**
• Older age	• Poor staff education
• Loss of appetite	• Lack of awareness of clinical standards
• Poor oral health	• Inadequate staff:patient ratio
• Poor oral intake	• Inadequate nutritional management
• Tiredness/apathy	• Poor nutrition screening practices
• Dissatisfaction with food quality	• Failure to calculate nutritional requirements accurately
• Lack of consideration of patient/family preferences	• Limited or no access to nutrition support team
• Impaired physical function/immobility	• Poor dining environment
	• Poor-quality food
	• Timing of meals leading to long periods without food
Disease related	• Inappropriate portion sizes
• Diagnosis, e.g. gastrointestinal or respiratory disease, cancer	• Mealtime interruptions
	• Missed meals not replaced
• Multiple comorbidities	• Snacks not offered during the day
• Emergency admission	• Little feeding assistance
• Depression	• Fasting practices for medical/surgical tests/procedures
• Impaired cognition	• Poor advice on food fortification
• Medical/surgical treatment	• Excessive hygiene regulations
• Hospital-acquired infection	• Poor practices around oral nutritional supplement service, e.g. container, temperature
• Polypharmacy	• Poor documentation practices
• Malabsorption	
• Swallowing difficulties/dysphagia	
• Early satiety	
• Chemosensory changes	

with increasing age, which directly influences the balance of nutritional needs and intake. This is compounded by anorexia, reduced appetite and sarcopenia; each is affected by both ageing and disease and all are associated with decreased muscle mass and function. The development of numerous morbidities directly relates to the incidence of undernutrition in older people [2].

In Spanish hospitals, older patients were at greatest risk of undernutrition [4]. In the UK, patients aged more than 65 years were at greater nutrition risk compared with younger patients; 34% of those admitted to care of older adult wards were at risk [6]. Women were also at higher risk, particularly if older than 65 years, although this gender bias is not consistently shown in all studies [20].

Diagnosis and severity of medical condition

The type, severity and duration of a patient's medical condition greatly influence risk of undernutrition [21]. Risk of undernutrition on admission to hospital in the UK was estimated at 27% for emergency admissions and 20% for elective admissions [6]. Greater risk of undernutrition has been described in gastroenterology, respiratory and cancer patients [6] and these have been related to increased likelihood of clinical complications and prolonged LOS [22]. Swallowing difficulties and dysphagia are consistently noted to be associated with undernutrition [22]; dysphagia can be due to neurological, physical or psychological causes. Cachexia and precachexia involve an inflammatory response and are common in chronic diseases such as cancer, chronic obstructive airways disease, chronic heart failure, liver disease and rheumatoid arthritis. Not all undernourished patients are cachectic, but all cachectic patients are malnourished to some degree [23]. The Canadian Malnutrition Task Force study of 1022 patients examined factors associated with nutritional decline in medical and surgical patients aged 18 years and over who remained in hospital for 2 or more days [8]. Having controlled for SGA on admission, and the presence of a surgical procedure, this study showed that nutritional decline in hospital was significantly associated with cancer diagnosis, two or more diagnostic categories, illness affecting food intake in medical patients, new in-hospital infection, as well as with lower admission BMI, reduced food intake and dissatisfaction with food quality. Interestingly, for surgical patients in this study, only male sex was associated with nutritional decline.

Polypharmacy

Polypharmacy, or the use of multiple medications, is another factor which may contribute to poor nutritional status by causing impaired swallowing related to xerostomia (dry mouth), loss of appetite, gastrointestinal problems and other changes in body function, potentially resulting in reduced dietary intake, decreased absorption of essential nutrients and increased risk of drug–nutrient interactions [2] (see Chapter 1.2). One issue that is problematic in exploring the relationship between polypharmacy and nutritional status is that polypharmacy

does not have a standard definition. Although many studies have described polypharmacy as the regular use of five or more drugs, three or four and more different medications have also been used, and a separate definition of 'excessive polypharmacy', meaning the typical use of nine or more drugs concomitantly, has recently been adopted [24]. A systematic review of 44 studies indicated that up to 91%, 74% and 65% of residents in long-term care facilities take more than five, nine and 10 medications, respectively [25].

A narrative review of the limited evidence from published studies examining the relationship between polypharmacy and nutritional status noted that the studies available for inclusion were predominantly cross-sectional, often without proper adjustment for potential confounders [24]. The studies examined used different markers of nutritional status, including MNA, weight loss or reduced energy and/or nutrient intake, making direct comparisons difficult. The authors suggested that there was growing evidence to support the association between an increase in prescribed medications and undernutrition, particularly in older persons. However, they also emphasised that the prevalence of undernutrition directly attributable to polypharmacy is unknown and that longitudinal studies to elicit the relationship between polypharmacy and undernutrition which allow adjustment for diseases are required.

Furthermore, a recent editorial on the relationship between polypharmacy and frailty, commenting on six cross-sectional studies, concluded that a relationship between polypharmacy and frailty exists with more than six medicines [26]. The authors recommended that all frail older persons have their medications reviewed by a pharmacist with the principle of reducing medications to six or fewer.

The major confounding factors in examining the relationship between polypharmacy and undernutrition is that patients who take more medications may also be more medically unwell and that the eating problems related to the disease itself may be more important than the role of drugs in the development of poor nutritional status [24].

Impaired cognition

Impaired cognition is more common in older populations and is consistently documented as a determinant of nutritional risk in the institutional setting [7,27]. One Italian study of 623 hospitalised older patients who underwent comprehensive geriatric assessment to evaluate their medical, cognitive (normal, mild impairment and dementia), affective and social condition, and MNA to evaluate their nutritional status clearly demonstrated that even patients with mild cognitive impairment had poorer nutritional status than those with normal cognition [28]. This study indicated that as dementia progresses, nutrient intake deteriorates, leading to a progressive decline in nutritional status, associated with increased morbidity and mortality.

Inadequate food intake

Inadequate food intake is common in institutional care and contributes to undernutrition. The recent comprehensive Canadian Malnutrition Task Force study of over 1000 patients admitted to 18 large and small hospitals indicated that reduced food intake during the first week of hospitalisation is an independent predictor of LOS [29]. Furthermore, the common barriers to adequate dietary intake in these patients included not being given food when a meal was missed (69.2%), loss of appetite (63.9%), not wanting ordered food (58%), feeling too sick (42.7%) or tired (41.1%) to eat, and being interrupted at mealtimes (41.8%) [30].

Patients who were already undernourished, women, those with a greater number of comorbidities and those who ate less than 50% of their meal reported the occurrence of several barriers. However, those aged over 65 years compared with those under 65 were less likely to report being disturbed at meals (33.9% versus 44.6%) and to missing a meal for tests (31% versus 39%), perhaps reflecting increased awareness of undernutrition among older people in the hospital setting.

According to recommendations for food and nutritional care in European hospitals, in order to achieve adequate food intake, eating episodes should be spread throughout the day [31]. This will ensure sufficient time between each meal to allow between-meal snacks in the morning, afternoon and late evening to meet energy and nutrient requirements. In the Nordic countries, these recommendations are even more specific, stating that the overnight fast should not exceed 11 hours in older people, and that the individual should have at least four eating episodes a day [32]. A Swedish cross-sectional study of 1771 patients aged ≥65 (mean age 78) years admitted to internal medicine, surgical or orthopaedic wards that used the MNA to determine nutritional status reported that 35.5% were well nourished, 55.1% were at risk of undernutrition and 9.4% were malnourished. Overnight fasts exceeding 11 hours, fewer than four eating episodes a day and not cooking independently prior to admission to hospital were associated with both increased prevalence of undernutrition and risk of undernutrition [33]. The study showed that 78% of patients in the hospital setting exceeded an 11-hour overnight fast and 49% had fewer than four eating episodes daily.

An Australian nutrition survey that investigated the association between suboptimal food intake and undernutrition risk in over 3000 hospital patients reported that 25% of those who were undernourished were not offered snacks throughout the day [7]. Another Australian qualitative paper discussed the difficulty residents in aged care facilities experience in receiving adequate and acceptable food and fluids [34]. Unacceptable dining room experiences, poor-quality food and excessive food hygiene regulations contributed to iatrogenic undernutrition and dehydration. Meal service and even the method by which oral nutritional supplements (ONS) are served can influence food and fluid intake [35,36].

These findings have implications for staffing, clinical supervision, education of carers and the impact of negative attitudes to older people. Hospital food service (catering) is internationally recognised as a key component of good clinical care of patients and has the potential to provide a population approach to managing undernutrition. Although clinical standards have been established in many countries, audits have focused on processes being in place and not on patient outcomes. A recent study evaluating food provision and consumption over 24 hours in inpatients 65 years and older in postacute geriatric orthopaedic wards in National Health Service hospitals in Scotland, UK, showed that food provision was significantly less than standards set for energy and protein provision for 'nutritionally well' patients; patients consumed approximately three-quarters (74%) of the food provided. Higher provision of both energy and protein was associated with more adequate consumption [37].

1.4.4 Causes of undernutrition in long-term care

A systematic review of the factors most consistently associated with undernutrition in nursing home patients concluded that depression, poor oral intake, swallowing issues and eating/chewing dependency were associated with weight loss [38]. Sixteen studies met the inclusion criteria as they contained prevalence data for general nursing home populations on at least one of the following: weight loss, low BMI, MNA or other measure of undernutrition, poor oral intake or dependency for feeding. The factors most consistently associated with weight loss were depression, poor oral intake, swallowing issues and eating/chewing difficulties. The factors most consistently associated with low BMI included immobility, poor oral intake, chewing problems, dysphagia, female gender and older age. Those most consistently associated with poor nutrition included impaired function, dementia, swallowing/chewing difficulties, poor oral intake and older age. Staffing factors were associated with weight loss in most of the studies included in this systematic review, though the relationship between staffing and undernutrition is not consistently observed in all institutional settings [39].

An Australian study, carried out as part of a larger project on aged care facility residents, was undertaken with the 76 staff caring for the study residents. This study identified the barriers to promoting optimal nutrition as being insufficient time to observe residents (56%), being unaware of residents' feeding issues (46%), poor nutritional knowledge (44%) (for example, staff were unaware of the need for increased energy and protein in residents with pressure ulcers and few exhibited correct knowledge of fluid requirements) and unappetising appearance of the food served (57%) [40]. Furthermore, while nutritional assessment was considered an important part of practice by 83% of respondents, just 53% indicated that they actually carried out such assessments.

There is a need to build a comprehensive picture of the determinants of undernutrition, define treatable undernutrition and identify screening tools applicable within different settings which can characterise those who are able to positively respond to nutritional treatment in order to effectively tackle undernutrition in the institutional setting.

Acknowledgements

The author thanks Amanda Courtney, Deirdre Mullally, Lauren Power and Karla Smuts for their critical review of this chapter.

References

1. Bernstein M, Munoz N. Position of the Academy of Nutrition and Dietetics: food and nutrition for older adults: promoting health and wellness. *J Acad Nutr Diet* 2012; **112**: 1255–1277.
2. Stratton RJ, Green CJ, Elia M. Disease-Related Malnutrition. Wallingford: CABI Publishing, 2003.
3. Kaiser MJ, Bauer JM, Rämsch C, Uter W, Guigoz Y, Cederholm T et al. Frequency of malnutrition in older adults: a multinational perspective using the mini nutritional assessment. *J Am Geriatr Soc* 2010; **58**(9): 1734–1738.
4. Velasco C, García E, Rodríguez V, Frias L, Garriga R, Álvarez J et al. Comparison of four nutritional screening tools to detect nutritional risk in hospitalized patients: a multicentre study. *Eur J Clin Nutr* 2011; **65**(2): 269–274.
5. Van Zwienen-Pot JI, Visser M, Kuijpers M, Grimmerink MFA, Kruizenga HM. Undernutrition in nursing home rehabilitation patients. *Clin Nutr* 2017; **36**: 755–759.

6. Russell C, Elia M, British Association for Parenteral and Enteral Nutrition (BAPEN). Nutrition Screening Survey in the UK and Republic of Ireland in 2011. Hospitals, Care Homes and Mental Health Units. Redditch: BAPEN, 2012.

7. Agarwal E, Ferguson M, Banks M, Bauer J, Capra S, Isenring E. Nutritional status and dietary intake of acute care patients: results from the Nutrition Care Day Survey 2010. *Clin Nutr* 2012; **31**(1): 41–47.

8. Allard JP, Keller H, Teterina A, Jeejeebhoy KN, Laporte M, Duerksen DR et al. Factors associated with nutritional decline in hospitalised medical and surgical patients admitted for 7 d or more: a prospective cohort study. *Br J Nutr* 2015; **15**: 1–11.

9. Volkert D, Saeglitz C, Gueldenzoph H, Sieber CC, Stehle P. Undiagnosed malnutrition and nutrition-related problems in geriatric patients. *J Nutr Health Aging* 2010; **14**: 387–392.

10. National Institute for Health and Clinical Excellence. Nutrition Support in Adults: Oral Nutrition Support, Enteral Tube Feeding, and Parenteral Nutrition. London: National Collaborating Centre for Acute Care, 2006.

11. Cederholm T, Bosaeus I, Barazzoni R, Bauer J, van Gossum A, Klek S et al. Diagnostic criteria for malnutrition: an ESPEN consensus statement. *Clin Nutr* 2015; **34**(3): 335–340.

12. Barker LA, Gout BS, Crowe TC. Hospital malnutrition: prevalence, identification and impact on patients and the healthcare system. *Int J Environ Res Public Health* 2011; **8**(2): 514–527.

13. Guerra RS, Fonseca I, Pichel F, Restivo MT, Amaral TFJ. Usefulness of six diagnostic and screening measures for undernutrition in predicting length of hospital stay: a comparative analysis. *Acad Nutr Diet* 2015; **115**(6): 927–938.

14. Elia M, Stratton RJ. Calculating the cost of disease-related malnutrition in the UK in 2007 (public expenditure only). In: Combating Malnutrition: Recommendations for Action. Report from the Advisory Group on Malnutrition, led by BAPEN. Redditch: BAPEN, 2009.

15. Kyle UG, Kossovsky MP, Karsegarda VL, Pichard C. Comparison of tools for nutritional assessment and screening at hospital admission: a population study. *Clin Nutr* 2006; **25**(3): 409–417.

16. Corish CA, Kennedy NP. Protein-energy under nutrition in hospital in-patients. *Br J Nutr* 2000; **3**(6): 575–591.

17. van der Pols-Vijlbrief R, Wijnhoven HA, Molenaar H, Visser M. Factors associated with (risk of) undernutrition in community-dwelling older adults receiving home care: a cross-sectional study in the Netherlands. *Public Health Nutr* 2016; **19**: 2278–2289.

18. White JV, Guenter P, Jensen G, Malone A, Schofield M, Academy Malnutrition Work Group, ASPEN Malnutrition Task Force, ASPEN Board of Directors. Consensus statement of the Academy of Nutrition and Dietetics/American Society for Parenteral and Enteral Nutrition: characteristics recommended for the identification and documentation of adult malnutrition (undernutrition). *J Parenter Enteral Nutr* 2012; **36**(3): 275–283.

19. Van Asselt DZ, van Bokhorst-de van der Schueren MA, van der Cammen TJ, Disselhorst LG, Janse A, Lonterman-Monasch S et al. Assessment and treatment of malnutrition in Dutch geriatric practice: consensus through a modified delphi study. *Age Ageing* 2012; **41**(3): 399–404.

20. Banks M, Ash S, Bauer J, Gaskill D. Prevalence of malnutrition in adults in Queensland public hospitals and residential aged care facilities. *Nutr Diet* 2007; **64**(3): 172–178.

21. Van Bokhorst-de van der Schueren MA, Lonterman-Monasch S, de Vries OJ, Danner SA, Kramer MH, Muller M. Prevalence and determinants for malnutrition in geriatric outpatients. *Clin Nutr* 2013; **32**(6): 1007–1011.

22. Suominen M, Muurinen S, Routasalo P, Soini H, Suur-Uski I, Peiponen A et al. Malnutrition and associated factors among aged residents in all nursing homes in Helsinki. *Eur J Clin Nutr* 2005; **59**: 578–583.

23. Muscaritoli M, Anker SD, Argilés J, Aversa Z, Bauer JM, Biolo G et al. Consensus, definition of sarcopenia, cachexia and pre-cachexia: joint document elaborated by Special Interest Groups (SIG) "cachexia-anorexia in chronic wasting diseases" and "nutrition in geriatrics". *Clin Nutr* 2010; **29**: 154–159.

24. Jyrkkä J, Mursu J, Enlund H, Lönnroos E. Polypharmacy and nutritional status in elderly people. *Curr Opin Clin Nutr Metab Care* 2012; **15**(1): 1–6.

25. Jokanovic N, Tan ECK, Dooley MJ, Kirkpatrick KM, Bell JS. Prevalence and factors associated with polypharmacy in long-term care facilities: a systematic review. *J Am Med Dir Assoc* 2015; **16**(6): 535.e1–535.e12.

26. Rolland Y, Morley JE. Editorial: frailty and polypharmacy. *J Nutr Health Aging* 2016; **20**(6): 645–646.

27. Saka B, Kaya O, Ozturk GB, Erten N, Karan MA. Malnutrition in the elderly and its relationship with other geriatric syndromes. *Clin Nutr* 2010; **29**(6): 745–748.

28. Orsitto G, Fulvio F, Tria D, Turi V, Venezia A, Manca C. Nutritional status in hospitalized elderly patients with mild cognitive impairment. *Clin Nutr* 2009; **28**(1): 100–102.

29. Jeejeebhoy KN, Keller H, Gramlich L, Allard JP, Laporte M, Duerksen DR et al. Nutritional assessment: comparison of clinical assessment and objective variables for the prediction of length of hospital stay and readmission. *Am J Clin Nutr* 2015; **101**(5): 956–965.

30. Keller H, Allard J, Vesnaver E, Laporte M, Gramlich L, Bernier P et al. Barriers to food intake in acute care hospitals: a report of the Canadian Malnutrition Task Force. *J Hum Nutr Diet* 2015; **28**(6): 546–557.

31. Committee of Ministers, Council of Europe. Resolution ResAP(2003)3 on Food and Nutritional Care in Hospitals. 860th meeting of the Ministers' Deputies, 2003.

32. Becker W, Lyhne N, Pedersen AN, Aro A, Fogelholm M, Phorsdottir I et al. Nordic nutrition recommendations 2004: integrating nutrition and physical activity. *Scand J Nutr* 2004; **48**(4): 178–187.

33. Söderström L, Adolfsson ET, Rosenblad A, Frid H, Saletti A, Bergkvist L. Mealtime habits and meal provision are associated with malnutrition among elderly patients admitted to hospital. *Clin Nutr* 2013; **32**(2): 281–288.

34. Bernoth MA, Dietsch E, Davies C. 'Two dead frankfurts and a blob of sauce': the serendipity of receiving nutrition and hydration in Australian residential aged care. *Collegian* 2014; **21**(3): 171–177.

35. Allen VJ, Methven L, Gosney M. Impact of serving method on the consumption of nutritional supplement drinks: randomized trial in older adults with cognitive impairment. *J Adv Nurs* 2014; **70**(6): 1323–1333.

36. Gaff L, Jones J, Davidson IH, Bannerman E. A study of fluid provision and consumption in elderly patients in a long-stay rehabilitation hospital. *J Hum Nutr Diet* 2015; **28**(4): 384–389.

37. Bannerman E, Cantwell L, Gaff L, Conroy A, Davidson I, Jones J. Dietary intakes in geriatric orthopaedic rehabilitation patients: need to look at food consumption not just provision. *Clin Nutr* 2016; **35**(4): 892–899.

38. Tamura BK, Bell CL, Masaki KH, Amella EJ. Factors associated with weight loss, low BMI, and malnutrition among nursing home patients: a systematic review of the literature. *J Am Med Dir Assoc* 2013; **14**(9): 649–655.

39. Stalpers D, de Brouwer BJ, Kaljouw MJ, Schuurmans MJ. Associations between characteristics of the nurse work environment and five nurse-sensitive patient outcomes in hospitals: a systematic review of literature. *Int J Nurs Stud* 2015; **52**(4): 817–835.

40. Beattie E, O'Reilly M, Strange E, Franklin S, Isenring E. How much do residential aged care staff members know about the nutritional needs of residents? *Int J Older People Nurs* 2014; **9**(1): 54–64.

Chapter 1.5

Consequences of undernutrition

Mary Hickson[1] and Anna Julian[2]

[1]Plymouth University Institute of Health and Community, Peninsula Alllied Health Centre, Plymouth, UK
[2]Nutrition and Dietetic Research Group Department of Medicine, Imperial College London, London, UK

1.5.1 Introduction and background

Undernutrition is complex, with interacting factors that both precipitate or exacerbate each other, leading to a vicious cycle in which the patient's condition spirals downwards. This chapter aims to discuss the broad range of complications that can arise from undernutrition with or without disease.

Some of the common clinical consequences of undernutrition are shown in Box 1.5.1. However, many of these are also implicated in the causes of undernutrition. This means it is difficult to find clear evidence of causal relationships between undernutrition and these listed consequences. Most evidence is observational or epidemiological, so although associations may be established, it can be difficult to untangle which event came first. In addition, it is difficult to ascertain the effect of different nutrients from one another; vitamins and minerals play a role alongside macronutrients. To prove cause and effect, intervention trials are required, of which there are few. However, a range of studies have provided evidence of a link between poor outcomes and undernutrition.

There are several recent systematic reviews of disease-related undernutrition and nutrition support, and although nutrition interventions improve energy and protein intake, and body weight, the data remain equivocal on clinical and functional outcomes such as physical function, gastrointestinal function, wound healing, complications, length of stay and mortality [1,2]. Observational data suggest associations between undernutrition and these outcomes but the evidence is insufficient to demonstrate causality [3]. Undernutrition may simply be a marker of the severity of disease. There is a consensus that large-scale, well-designed randomised intervention studies able to clarify these issues need to be carried out. Other systematic reviews in specific patient groups (such as hip fracture and liver transplant patients) have found low-quality evidence for the use of nutrition support in reducing unfavourable outcomes such as complications and mortality [4,5].

Evidence from starvation studies quantifies the effects of undernutrition on the human body. Periods of famine and acts of hunger strike have provided further insight into the mechanisms associated with prolonged fasting. Keys' Minnesota experiments created a model of semi-starvation, allowing researchers to study the processes and consequences of weight loss in a controlled environment [6]. In Keys' study, 32 lean male participants lost an average of 25% body weight over 24 weeks, following a diet designed to produce a deficit of approximately 1 kg per week. Total abstinence from food has generated more acute weight losses, with 18% body weight loss seen over a 43-day period in eight Brazilian prisoners on hunger strike [7] and at 60 days the average weight loss was 38% in 30 Irish hunger strikers [8]. Keys proposed

---

Box 1.5.1   Consequences of undernutrition

Physical consequences

Decreased:	Weight
	Muscle function – including heart and respiratory muscles
	Appetite
	Mobility (more likely to fall or suffer injury)
	Immune function
	Wound healing
Increased:	Tiredness
	Risk of infections
	Risk of pressure sores
	Morbidity
	Mortality
	Length of hospital stay

Psychological consequences

Increased:	Depression
	Anxiety
	Irritability
	Apathy
	Sense of illness
Decreased:	Concentration
	Will for recovery
	Quality of life
	Mood
	Cognitive function

Economic consequences

	Length of stay
	Readmission to hospital
	Increased treatment costs due to complications and prolonged recovery

---

that weight loss over 18% would cause significant disruption to homeostasis, with death highly likely at weight loss of 50%.

1.5.2 Physical consequences of undernutrition

Undernutrition and mortality

A body mass index (BMI) of 13 kg/m² in men and 11 kg/m² in women is considered the lowest sustainable, after which death is highly probable [9]. Keys [6] put forward the hypothesis that a greater fat mass is advantageous in fasting conditions, with higher body fat mass providing protection in the metabolic response to starvation. In starvation, fat is the primary energy source, contributing 78% and 94% of the energy expended in lean and obese subjects respectively. Obese individuals have both a higher fat mass and fat-free mass (FFM) but despite the higher protein stores, protein oxidation provides a smaller amount of energy. This suggests a protein-sparing effect in individuals with a larger proportion of body fat, resulting in smaller protein losses and a reduced rate of protein loss over the starvation period [10].

Without food, it is estimated that a healthy adult will survive for approximately 70 days having lost approximately 40% of their body weight [8]. This is supported by data from the 30 men participating in the Irish hunger strike in 1981; after about 70 days, the group had lost a mean of 38% of their body weight and 10 had died [8]. The nature of the weight loss appears to be important to survival, with 40% body weight loss being fatal in situations of complete starvation, compared to 50% in semi-starvation.

Populations at highest risk of mortality from undernutrition include older adults, those who have been recently hospitalised or had a stroke, those with a lower grip strength and/or gait speed, and those who are unable to perform activities of daily living. Current smoking, black race, higher weight and lower waist circumference also increased mortality risk [11]. Using weight loss as an indicator of undernutrition, the large, prospective Cardiovascular Health Study (n=4714) compared older participants with weight losses of over 5% to those who gained weight over a 4-year period. They demonstrated that individuals with weight loss had a greater risk of death (hazard ratio=1.67, 95% confidence interval (CI) 1.29–2.15) [11], confirming that even a modest reduction in body weight can be an important and independent marker mortality risk in older adults. A systematic review of observational studies explored mortality in older adults following a period of rehabilitation [12]. The included studies were heterogeneous and sample size relatively small, but the authors concluded that undernutrition during rehabilitation was negatively associated with physical function and quality of life, and positively associated with risk of institutionalisation, hospitalisation and mortality [12].

Whilst death as a consequence of undernutrition is rare in children and younger adults in the developed world, data from 2011 showed that 45% of child deaths in developing countries were attributable to undernutrition [13]. A review discussed mortality in pregnant women and children, reporting a link between low mid-upper arm circumference and all-cause mortality in pregnant women [14].

Undernutrition and muscle mass and function

In the presence of undernutrition, muscle mass is depleted relative to the type and duration of the exposure. Much of the available evidence comes from the Minnesota semi-starvation experiments [6], where individuals were losing an average

1 kg total body weight per week and consuming a protein-poor diet. Results demonstrated a mean muscle loss of 18% over 168 days. In complete starvation, muscle breakdown is more rapid, with initial losses of approximately 75 g/day of protein [15]. For a 70 kg person with 10 kg of muscle, this would equate to a 15% loss in 10 days, reducing total protein stores to nothing in under 70 days. This rate of muscle utilisation is not sustained; instead, the body adapts, sparing protein in favour of mobilising fat stores for energy.

Studies in obese subjects undergoing weight loss regimens provide information about the composition of the tissues lost with weight loss. One systematic review combined 16 studies (low calorie diet (LCD); very-low calorie diet (VLCD) and pharmacological intervention) with a pre/post design, demonstrating that the level of energy restriction was positively associated with the degree of FFM loss ($r^2=0.31$, P=0.006). Median FFM losses were 14%, 23% and 38% for LCD, VLCD and pharmacological intervention respectively, with several studies exceeding the safe value of 22% weight loss from FFM [16].

Muscle tissue is essential due to the relationship between muscle mass, muscle strength and function. Whilst the pathogenesis is unclear, both undernutrition and loss of muscle have been associated with reduced muscle function, suboptimal activities of daily living scores and handgrip strength [3,6,17]. However, nutrition interventions have not shown consistent improvements to muscle mass or function in recent systematic reviews [1,2]. Due to the range of outcome measures used, heterogeneous study designs and quality of studies, further large-scale intervention studies are needed before conclusions can be drawn.

In older adults, muscle loss can be masked by a concurrent increase in fat mass. As metabolically active lean tissue is lost, energy requirements can reduce by a third (where dietary intake and exercise levels remain stable), leading to weight gains [18]. Studies have shown correlation between muscle mass and metabolic disorders such as glucose metabolism, with decreases in the ratio of skeletal muscle mass to total body weight associated an increased risk of insulin resistance and diabetes.

In addition to its roles in skeletal muscle, muscle protein is integral to the function of major organs such as the heart, liver and kidneys, and these protein stores are not immune to the effects of undernutrition. Atrophy of internal organs is a critical feature of undernutrition, affecting the cardiovascular and respiratory systems by reducing muscle size and function. Congestive heart failure is aggravated by undernutrition, with heightened risk of tricuspid regurgitation and right atrial pressure [19]. Loss of diaphragm mass has been shown to decrease respiration rate and consequentially oxygen consumption, impacting on recovery following chest infection and weaning from ventilation [20]. Individuals with chronic obstructive pulmonary disease (COPD) and poor nutritional status experience worse clinical outcomes including suboptimal respiratory function, reduced ability to expectorate and heightened fatigability. Pneumonia is a common cause of death once muscle mass is reduced to 60% of normal [20].

Undernutrition and immunity

There is a strong relationship between infection, nutritional status and mortality, with elements of non-specific and specific immunity affected by a state of suboptimal nutrition. Host defence mechanisms include physical barriers, such as skin and mucous membranes, acting as the first line of defence to protect the body from infection. Inadequate nutrient availability compromises the barrier function of the skin and tract linings so that in a state of undernutrition, the GI tract becomes more permeable and more susceptible to bacteria, increasing infection risk [21]. Immunoglobulin secretion is limited, reducing the level of protection provided to epithelial cells of the respiratory tract, small intestine and urinary tract. Ordinarily, lysozymes and complement cells work together to digest invading bacteria, and T- and B-lymphocytes form part of the adaptive immune response, produced following exposure to infection. However, in a state of undernutrition, complement activity is limited

and the number of available lysozymes and T-cells is reduced [22].

In a retrospective cohort study, patients were screened with Subjective Global Assessment on admission to one of 25 Brazilian hospitals. Multiple logistic regression was used to isolate nutritional status, concluding that undernourished participants experienced more infectious complications than well-nourished subjects, irrespective of diagnosis (27% and 17% respectively) [21].The rate of sepsis and abdominal abscess post surgery was also increased, with 3.7% versus 1.1% and 2.1% versus 0.4% for undernourished and nourished participants respectively.

Undernutrition and non-infectious complications

The incidence of non-infectious complications, such as respiratory and cardiac failure, cardiac arrest and wound dehiscence, has also been shown to differ significantly between undernourished and well-nourished individuals. A significantly higher incidence of non-infectious complications was demonstrated in undernourished patients (undernourished 20.5% versus well nourished 8.4%), with 'severe' undernutrition increasing the risk of an infectious or non-infectious complication [21].

Skin is weakened by undernutrition; with poor nutrient supply and minimal fat stores, the skin loses its integrity, becoming thin and delicate with a reduced capacity to repair. By lengthening the inflammatory phase, reducing fibroblast proliferation and collagen synthesis, undernutrition reduces wound strength and may result in chronic, non-healing wounds [23]. The loss of fat and muscle as protective cushioning leads to increased pressure from bones, causing damage to both the surface and underlying layers of the skin and allowing sores to develop spontaneously. Prevalence ranges from 3% to 66% in the hospital setting, with immobile older patients most at risk [24].

There is convincing epidemiological evidence for a relationship between undernutrition and the increased incidence and severity of pressure ulcers, but evidence from trials is limited.

Multivariate analyses show that poor nutritional status, described by low body weight, BMI and suboptimal food intake, is independently associated with pressure ulcers. In a meta-analysis that included four randomised controlled trials comparing the development of pressure ulcers in at-risk populations, there was a significantly lower incidence of pressure ulcers in participants receiving nutrition support compared to those receiving usual care (n = 1224; odds ratio (OR) 0.75, 95% CI 0.62–0.89) [24]. However, these studies were generally short term and in older adults with underlying illness, which complicates interpretation. Studies exploring the effect of nutrition support on subjects with existing pressure ulcers are limited and with a lack of randomised controlled trials, so firm conclusions on the effect of nutrition support on pressure sore healing are not possible.

Micronutrient deficiencies can also have negative effects on wound healing. The wound healing process involves clotting, blood vessels and tissue repair and specific micronutrients may affect difference stages in this pathway. Amino acids (glutamine, methionine, cysteine, lysine and proline) have been implicated in fibroblast proliferation and collagen synthesis but there is little evidence to support the use of these amino acids in healing wounds. Vitamins A and C are also important and supplements may be recommended in specific situations. Trace elements magnesium, copper and zinc are crucial to cellular metabolism and a lack may influence healing. Zinc, in particular, may be supplemented to enhance wound healing but evidence is limited [23].

1.5.3 Psychological consequences of undernutrition

Undernutrition and quality of life

The effects of undernutrition on health-related quality of life are thought to be indirect, resulting from a combination of the physical, functional and cognitive changes discussed above, raising infection risk, delaying discharge from hospital and increasing dependence [25].

Apathy and lethargy as symptoms of undernutrition have been described by Keys [6]. Keys observed depression and reduced motivation in his cohort, exemplified by participants' withdrawal from university classes as their body weight and macronutrient intakes reduced.

A systematic review exploring the relationship between nutritional status and quality of life in older adults found that quality of life was better in well-nourished individuals compared to undernourished (OR 2.85; 95% CI 2.20–3.70, P < 0.001, from 15 studies) [25]. It also showed that nutrition interventions to treat undernutrition improved both physical and mental quality of life domains (physical domain: standard mean difference 0.23, CI 0.08–0.38, P = 0.002; mental domain: standard mean difference 0.24, CI 0.11–0.36, P < 0.001). The authors included both interventional and observational data, and only used studies which employed validated techniques to measure quality of life, but found evidence of publication bias and limitations in the design of studies [25], so some caution is required when interpreting these data. However, more recent studies continue to suggest that there is a link between nutritional status and quality of life, in specific patient groups and in children as well as adults [26].

Undernutrition and depression and anxiety

The relationship between mood and nutritional status is complicated and may be reciprocal. For example, undernutrition seems to play a causal role in depression but the symptoms of depression include reduced appetite, which may lead to undernutrition. This makes studying these symptoms more difficult as it is necessary to establish that the state of undernutrition came first and that treating the undernutrition will result in improvements in mood. Two aspects of mood that are commonly studied are depression and anxiety.

A systematic review of the factors related to undernutrition in nursing home residents consistently found an association with depression [27] and suggested that since this factor was modifiable, targeting depression may help reduce weight loss and undernutrition in the population, making the assumption that depression resulted in weight loss. Yet, the data were unable to demonstrate a causal link between depression and undernutrition, only establishing an association, and it may be that undernutrition caused the depression. Similarly, a review explored the relationship between undernutrition, depression and anxiety in patients with anorexia nervosa, and concluded that evidence of undernutrition resulting in depressive symptoms or anxiety was very limited [28]. The quality of the studies available was poor, the variability in the tools to assess all three outcomes was great, and the findings were contradictory. This indicates that further work to establish the causal link between undernutrition and mood is required.

There are acknowledged mechanisms by which a lack of certain micronutrients may influence mood, including minerals and trace elements (zinc, magnesium, lithium, iron, calcium, chromium, copper, selenium, manganese, iodine and vanadium) and vitamins (B complex, C, D and E); these are comprehensively reviewed elsewhere [29–31]. They offer an explanation as to why undernutrition may result in detrimental mood changes. However, unless micronutrient deficiency is examined in populations studied for undernutrition and the treatment focus is moved from energy and protein repletion to specific nutrients, the evidence for these micronutrients is likely to remain weak.

Undernutrition and cognitive function

It has long been thought that food restriction will have some effect on cognitive function, which includes domains such as psychomotor ability, memory, processing speed, visual attention and executive function. The evidence to support a detrimental effect of semi-starvation and undernutrition is inconsistent or absent. Some studies show no effect of prolonged fasting whilst others suggest deficits in short-term memory, encoding, attention, reaction time and/or vigilance [32].

Understanding the acute effects of fasting on cognition in healthy adults may help to elucidate the unfavourable consequences of undernutrition; this has been explored in a recent systematic review [32]. The findings show no consistency in the effect on any of the cognitive functions studied. This presents an incomplete picture of what is and what is not affected by acute fasting and hunger and so consequently offers limited evidence as to how the brain may be influenced by undernutrition. The lack of consistency, however, was mainly due to the variation in study design (inconsistent fasting conditions, procedures used, test settings and populations used) and confounding variables (unreported gender, age, culture, circadian rhythm, etc.). Despite the problems with the existing literature, some important findings were that reaction time and processing speed did appear to be slower in relation to fasting, but interpretation was complicated because motivation and fatigue were not always controlled for. Memory was highly studied and data seemed to suggest that although short-term memory was not impacted by fasting, time to retrieval was. Attention capacity did appear to be affected by low blood glucose concentrations and further study of this aspect of cognition was recommended [32].

1.5.4 Economic consequences of undernutrition

Health economics is the study of how scarce resources are allocated among alternative uses for the care of sickness and the promotion, maintenance and improvement of health, including the study of how healthcare and health-related services, their costs and benefits, and health itself are distributed among individuals and groups in society [33]. This field of study has gained increasing prominence as healthcare resources become more limited and recently a subspecialism of nutrition economics has been established [34].

The economic costs arising from undernutrition are attributable to increased length of hospital stay and the treatments associated with higher complication rates and prolonged recovery. The overall costs of disease-related undernutrition (as opposed to poverty and food scarcity) are estimated to be €31 billion in Europe [35], $157 billion in the USA [36] and $66 billion in China [37]. These figures are comparable and modelled using similar assumptions with data from published studies on prevalence, morbidity and mortality, agreed healthcare costs and assessments of quality of life. There are other published figures, for example £19.6 billion in England [38] and €1.9 billion in the Netherlands [39], but these authors have used different methodologies.

Nevertheless, given that much undernutrition is preventable, there is a high cost associated with failure to prevent and treat it. These costs also place a substantial burden on health and social care systems, with the majority spent on more frequent, lengthier hospital admissions and the greater demand for social care. The healthcare cost of managing an undernourished person is estimated to be more than twice that of an adequately nourished person [40]. Nevertheless, the heterogeneity of research and varying definitions of undernutrition make cost estimate comparison difficult and precise estimates should be treated with some caution [41].

The most recent systematic review on how treatments may reduce hospital-related costs of undernutrition found surprisingly few studies (n = 3), although these were moderate or high quality. The authors concluded that this lack of evidence limits the ability of clinicians or managers to make informed decisions about what is cost-effective. The three included studies all showed cost savings ranging from €76 to €252 per patient in the treatment group. However, the methods and assumptions made were highly variable, making comparisons difficult [41]. Another systematic review with broader inclusion criteria (included eight studies) also showed consistent cost savings for the use of enteral medical nutrition [42]. Studies on specific patient groups have also demonstrated cost savings; for example, undernourished colorectal cancer patients undergoing surgery were found to have longer length of stay compared to well-nourished patients (3.4 days longer, P = 0.017) and correspondingly higher costs (€3360 higher) [43]. Similar data exist for community-dwelling populations showing

higher costs, greater use of healthcare resources (such as general practitioner consultations, nurse and dietitian visits, hospital outpatient appointments, etc.) [40,44].

1.5.5 Summary

The consequences of undernutrition are detrimental, both physical and psychological, and far-reaching, with associated costs (financial and quality of life) affecting both individuals and society. The relationship with disease is complicated since undernutrition may precipitate disease and be precipitated by disease, which makes studying the outcomes of undernutrition challenging. Other chapters in the book discuss in more detail the assessment and treatment of undernutrition, as well as particular issues relating to specific conditions or settings.

References

1. Bally MR, Blaser Yildirim PZ, Bounoure L, Gloy VL, Mueller B, Briel M, Schuetz P. Nutritional support and outcomes in malnourished medical inpatients: a systematic review and meta-analysis. *JAMA Intern Med* 2016; **176**(1): 43–53.
2. Milne AC, Potter J, Vivanti A, Avenell A. Protein and energy supplementation in elderly people at risk from malnutrition. *Cochrane Database Syst Rev* 2009; **2**: CD003288.
3. Felder S, Lechtenboehmer C, Bally M, et al. Association of nutritional risk and adverse medical outcomes across different medical inpatient populations. *Nutrition* 2015; **31**(11–12): 1385–1393.
4. Avenell A, Smith TO, Curtain JP, Mak JC, Myint PK. Nutritional supplementation for hip fracture aftercare in older people. *Cochrane Database Syst Rev* 2016; **11**: CD001880.
5. Langer G, Grossmann K, Fleischer S, Berg A, Grothues D, Wienke A, Behrens J, Fink A. Nutritional interventions for liver-transplanted patients. *Cochrane Database Syst Rev* 2012; **8**: CD007605.
6. Keys A, Brožek J, Henschel A, Mickelsen O, Taylor HL. The Biology of Human Starvation. Minnesota: University of Minnesota Press, 1950.
7. Faintuch J, Soriano FG, Ladeira JP, Janiszewski M, Velasco IT, Gama-Rodrigues JJ. Changes in body fluid and energy compartments during prolonged hunger strike. *Rev Hosp Clin Fac Med Sao Paulo* 2000; **55**(2): 47–54.

8. Allison S. The uses and limitations of nutritional support: the Arvid Wretlind Lecture given at the 14th ESPEN Congress in Vienna, 1992. *Clin Nutr* 1992; **11**(6): 319–330.

9. Henry C. Body mass index and the limits of human survival. *Eur J Clin Nutr* 1990; **44**(4): 329–335.

10. Elia M, Stubbs RJ, Henry CJK. Differences in fat, carbohydrate, and protein metabolism between lean and obese subjects undergoing total starvation. *Obes Res* 1999; **7**: 597–604.

11. Newman AB, Yanez D, Harris T, Duxbury A, Enright PL, Fried LP. Weight change in old age and its association with mortality. *J Am Geriatr Soc* 2001; **49**(10): 1309–1318.

12. Marshall S, Bauer J, Isenring E. The consequences of malnutrition following discharge from rehabilitation to the community: a systematic review of current evidence in older adults. *J Hum Nutr Diet* 2014; **27**(2): 133–141.

13. Kramer CV, Allen S. Malnutrition in developing countries. *J Paediatr Child Health* 2015; **25**(9): 422–427.

14. Black RE, Victora CG, Walker SP, et al. Maternal and child undernutrition and overweight in low-income and middle-income countries. *Lancet* 2013; **382**(9890): 427–451.

15. Brennan MF. Uncomplicated starvation versus cancer cachexia. *Cancer Res* 1977; **37**(7 Part 2): 2359–2364.

16. Chaston T, Dixon J, O'Brien P. Changes in fat-free mass during significant weight loss: a systematic review. *Int J Obes* 2007; **31**(5): 743–750.

17. Norman K, Pichard C, Lochs H, Pirlich M. Prognostic impact of disease-related malnutrition. *Clin Nutr* 2008; **27**(1): 5–15.

18. Welch AA. Nutritional influences on age-related skeletal muscle loss. *Proc Nutr Soc* 2014; **73**(1): 16–33.

19. Carr JG, Stevenson LW, Walden JA, Heber D. Prevalence and hemodynamic correlates of malnutrition in severe congestive heart failure secondary to ischemic or idiopathic dilated cardiomyopathy. *Am J Cardiol* 1989; **63**(11): 709–713.

20. Rochester DF, Esau SA. Malnutrition and the respiratory system. *Chest* 1984; **85**(3): 411–415.

21. Correia MITD, Waitzberg DL. The impact of malnutrition on morbidity, mortality, length of hospital stay and costs evaluated through a multivariate model analysis. *Clin Nutr* 2003; **22**(3): 235–239.

22. Marcos A, Nova E, Montero A. Changes in the immune system are conditioned by nutrition. *Eur J Clin Nutr* 2003; **57** Suppl 1: S66–69.

23. Stechmiller JK. Understanding the role of nutrition and wound healing. *Nutr Clin Pract* 2010; **25**(1): 61–68.

24. Stratton RJ, Ek AC, Engfer M, Moore Z, Rigby P, Wolfe R, Elia M. Enteral nutritional support in prevention and treatment of pressure ulcers: a systematic review and meta-analysis. *Ageing Res Rev* 2005; **4**(3): 422–450.

25. Rasheed S, Woods RT. Malnutrition and quality of life in older people: a systematic review and meta-analysis. *Ageing Res Rev* 2013; **12**(2): 561–566.

26. Brinksma A, Sanderman R, Roodbol PF, Sulkers E, Burgerhof JG, de Bont ES, Tissing WJ. Malnutrition is associated with worse health-related quality of life in children with cancer. *Support Care Cancer* 2015; **23**(10): 3043–3052.

27. Tamura BK, Bell CL, Masaki KH, Amella EJ. Factors associated with weight loss, low BMI, and malnutrition among nursing home patients: a systematic review of the literature. *J Am Med Dir Assoc* 2013; **14**(9): 649–655.

28. Mattar L, Huas C, Duclos J, Apfel A, Godart N. Relationship between malnutrition and depression or anxiety in Anorexia Nervosa: a critical review of the literature. *J Affect Disord* 2011; **132**(3): 311–318.

29. Kaplan BJ, Crawford SG, Field CJ, Simpson JS. Vitamins, minerals, and mood. *Psychol Bull* 2007; **133**(5): 747–760.

30. Mlyniec K, Davies CL, de Aguero Sanchez IG, Pytka K, Budziszewska B, Nowak G. Essential elements in depression and anxiety. Part I. *Pharmacol Rep* 2014; **66**(4): 534–544.

31. Mlyniec K, Gawel M, Doboszewska U, Starowicz G, Pytka K, Davies CL, Budziszewska B. Essential elements in depression and anxiety. Part II. *Pharmacol Rep* 2015; **67**(2): 187–194.

32. Benau EM, Orloff NC, Janke EA, Serpell L, Timko CA. A systematic review of the effects of experimental fasting on cognition. *Appetite* 2014; **77**: 52–61.

33. BMJ Clinical Evidence. http://clinicalevidence.bmj.com/x/set/static/ebm/toolbox/678253.html (accessed 21 Feb 2017).

34. Lenoir-Wijnkoop I, Nuijten MJC, Gutierrez-Ibarluzea I, Hutton J, Poley MJ, Segal L. Workshop report: concepts and methods in the economics of nutrition – gateways to better economic evaluation of nutrition interventions. *Br J Nutr* 2012; **108**: 1714–1720.

35. Inotai A, Nuijten MJ, Roth E, Hegazi R, Kalo Z. Modelling the burden of disease associated malnutrition. *e-SPEN J* 2012; **7**: e196–e204.

36. Snider JT, Linthicum MT, Wu Y, LaVallee C, Lakdawalla DN, Hegazi R, Matarese L. Economic burden of community-based disease-associated malnutrition in the United States. *J Parenter Enteral Nutr* 2014; **38**(2 Suppl): 77s–85s.

37. Linthicum MT, Thornton Snider J, Vaithianathan R, Wu Y, LaVallee C, Lakdawalla DN, Benner JE, Philipson TJ. Economic burden of disease-associated malnutrition in China. *Asia Pac J Public Health* 2015; **27**(4): 407–417.

38. Elia M. The Cost of Malnutrition in England and Potential Cost Savings from Nutritional Interventions (Short Version). Southampton: BAPEN, 2015.

39. Freijer K, Tan SS, Koopmanschap MA, Meijers JM, Halfens RJ, Nuijten MJ. The economic costs of disease related malnutrition. *Clin Nutr* 2013; **32**(1): 136–141.

40. Guest JF, Panca M, Baeyens JP, de Man F, Ljungqvist O, Pichard C, Wait S, Wilson L. Health economic impact of managing patients following a community-based diagnosis of malnutrition in the UK. *Clin Nutr* 2011; **30**(4): 422–429.

41. Mitchell H, Porter J. The cost-effectiveness of identifying and treating malnutrition in hospitals: a systematic review. *J Hum Nutr Diet* 2016; **29**(2): 156–164.

42. Freijer K, Bours MJ, Nuijten MJ, Poley MJ, Meijers JM, Halfens RJ, Schols JM. The economic value of enteral medical nutrition in the management of disease-related malnutrition: a systematic review. *J Am Med Dir Assoc* 2014; **15**(1): 17–29.

43. Melchior JC, Preaud E, Carles J, et al. Clinical and economic impact of malnutrition per se on the postoperative course of colorectal cancer patients. *Clin Nutr* 2012; **31**(6): 896–902.

44. Abizanda P, Sinclair A, Barcons N, Lizan L, Rodriguez-Manas L. Costs of malnutrition in institutionalized and community-dwelling older adults: a systematic review. *J Am Med Dir Assoc* 2016; **17**(1): 17–23.

SECTION 2

Identification of undernutrition

Nutritional screening

Sue M. Green
Faculty of Health Sciences, University of Southampton, Southampton, UK

2.1.1 Introduction

Is there an efficient and effective way to identify people who are undernourished or at risk of undernutrition? This is a key question for healthcare settings. People across the world experience undernutrition, with significant consequences to health and wealth at individual and population levels. Undernutrition affects all age groups, with prevalence varying within and across countries. It is a problem in both lower and higher income countries, with up to 50% patients in hospitals worldwide classified as undernourished [1]. Undernutrition is also an issue in community and long-term care settings, particularly those where older people reside [2]. Reducing the incidence of undernutrition can reduce healthcare costs, morbidity and mortality, and economic productivity [3,4].

This chapter focuses on screening for undernutrition caused by a reduction in body mass as a result of protein and energy deficiency and includes acute or chronic disease-related undernutrition [5]. Micronutrient deficiencies are common but usually determined following an assessment rather than a screening process as more invasive and costly tests are required.

2.1.2 Purpose of screening

Undertaking a nutrition assessment will identify those who are at risk of becoming, or are already malnourished but it is a complex process and requires considerable time, equipment, expertise and personnel resource. Therefore, a quick and easy screening stage can be used to screen out those in a population who are not at risk of undernutrition so that resources and care can focus on those with or at risk of undernutrition. 'Population screening' is defined as the process of identifying healthy people who may be at increased risk of a disease or condition [6], although some populations screened may not be considered 'healthy' as they require healthcare intervention. The American Society for Parenteral and Enteral Nutrition (ASPEN) defines nutritional screening as 'a process to identify an individual who is malnourished or who is at risk of malnutrition to determine if a detailed nutrition assessment is indicated' [7]. The intervention required following the screening process is determined by an assessment which enables consideration of the causes and effects of undernutrition and leads to a plan of care, care plan [8] or entry into a care pathway [9,10] or process [11].

National and international guidelines recommend that people who enter care settings are screened for undernutrition [1,12–14]. Screening is usually undertaken by healthcare professionals when patients or clients enter their care in a hospital or community setting. Screening can also be undertaken as part of a general health screen, such as the NHS Health Check [15].

Screening should be repeated regularly during a hospital stay as nutritional status can deteriorate rapidly as a result of treatment or illness. In other clinical settings, such as the community,

Advanced Nutrition and Dietetics in Nutrition Support, First Edition. Edited by Mary Hickson and Sara Smith.

it should be repeated when there is cause for clinical concern [13]. A screening process can be used to evaluate a nutrition intervention to establish effectiveness.

2.1.3 Screening methods

Screening for undernutrition can be undertaken using a single measure or can incorporate several objective and sometimes subjective measures of nutritional status and take the form of a 'screening tool'.

Single measures

Single measures, such as weight, BMI and mid-upper arm circumference (MUAC), can be used to screen for undernutrition. A single measure, interpreted using cut-off points, enables rapid screening with little equipment and is particularly valuable where there is limited staff resource. However, the problem with use of a single measure is that any measurement error will lead to misclassification as no other measures can be taken into account.

The World Health Organization recommends the use of MUAC to identify severe acute undernutrition in younger children [16]. It is less commonly used as a screening tool for adults though recent reports have suggested it can be a useful first measure [17]. The use of an armband that can indicate if MUAC is low has been promoted in some areas [18].

Weight and BMI can also be considered as single measures that can screen for undernutrition. Weight is useful where previous weight is known as it will indicate if weight has been lost but has less use as an isolated measure. BMI can be used to screen for malnutrition where height is known or can be measured, and has recently been proposed as a definitive method of assessment for undernutrition [19].

Screening tools

The earlier part of this century saw the development of numerous malnutrition screening tools with limited attention paid to validity and reliability during the development of many [8,20]. Use of a valid, reliable tool is essential otherwise people who are undernourished but not identified as at risk by a tool with poor ability to detect undernutrition may have their nutritional needs neglected. Several screening tools have demonstrated reliability and validity, such as the Nutritional Risk Screening 2002 (NRS-2002), Mini Nutritional Assessment-Short Form (MNA-SF), Malnutrition Universal Screening Tool (MUST) [12] and Malnutrition Screening Tool [21].

The choice of which tool to use should take into account the needs of the setting and the quality of the screening tool [8]. Tools developed for use in one clinical area may not demonstrate evidence of validity and reliability in another area. For example, screening tools developed for use in acute care settings may not effectively screen for undernutrition in nursing homes [22]. Whilst some screening tools have been shown to be valid and reliable and consequently demonstrate specificity and sensitivity in certain populations, there is no 'gold standard' for malnutrition screening tools [23]. A framework which can be used to facilitate screening tool selection has been developed by Elia and Stratton [23]. Figure 2.1.1 shows the key components of the framework and indicates that tool selection should be based on identified needs and the quality of the tool. The characteristics of the screening programme need to be carefully considered to enable appropriate choice of a valid tool.

Given that tools may have limited specificity and sensitivity and that there is little evidence that they can predict the outcome of nutrition interventions [23], it is important that tools are only used to guide rather than substitute for clinical decision making. Screening tools have their limitations and are generally not designed to assess functional status. In addition, the required information may not be available to complete the screening tool. Where healthcare practitioners consider a person to be at risk of undernutrition using their clinical judgement, there should be referral opportunities in place for further assessment. Criteria for referral to other healthcare practitioners should not be based purely on a positive score from a screening tool.

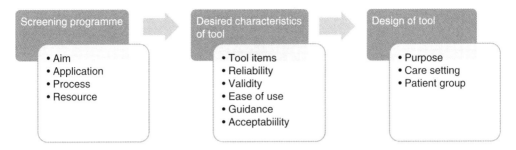

Figure 2.1.1 Summary of framework to facilitate nutritional screening tool selection

2.1.4 Process following screening

Those identified as at risk of undernutrition should undergo a nutritional assessment to determine if and why the person is malnourished or at risk of undernutrition, leading to the development of a plan of care informed by a care pathway. Whilst screening tools are now commonly used to screen for undernutrition, there is limited evidence that their use is effective in terms of improved nutritional outcomes [24]. Nutritional outcomes are only likely to improve if appropriate nutrition intervention is implemented following screening. It should also be noted that identifying those at risk of undernutrition may lead to increased levels of support to meet nutritional needs without any measurable improvement in clinical outcomes.

2.1.5 Implementing screening in healthcare settings

In many high-income countries, there is an expectation that screening for undernutrition is undertaken on admission to care [13,14,19]. Much research has been devoted to the development of screening tools but less consideration has been given to how they can be successfully implemented in clinical practice and how their use can be sustained. Some work on barriers and facilitators to the use of screening tools in high-income countries has been undertaken [25]. Figure 2.1.2 summarises some barriers and facilitators to the use of screening tools in

clinical practice [25,26]. These include organisational and personal factors and are likely to vary according to settings. In order to implement and maintain a screening process successfully in a care setting, consideration should be given to the potential or actual barriers and facilitators to screening [26].

The requirement to screen for undernutrition should be stated in organisational policy. Healthcare practitioners need to be supported to undertake the screening process by appropriate managerial expectation and resources, including time to complete the process and suitable equipment [25]. Training should be provided, and use of a screening tool or process that is easy to use and relevant to the clinical area [26]. An audit cycle can monitor use of the screening process and outcomes, such as a plan of care. The proportion of patients screened in a setting may be set by commissioners as a standard to measure quality of care.

Although tools that enable people to self-screen for undernutrition have been available for many years [8,27], recently there has been more emphasis on providing online resources that encourage self-screening in at-risk groups [28]. Online provision is one opportunity to increase accessibility of resources for self-screening. Providing facilities to self-screen in healthcare settings provides another opportunity. Self-screening using the MUST screening tool has been shown to be a reliable and acceptable method of screening for undernutrition conducted in outpatient settings [29,30]. The incorporation of self-screening into whole-community approaches to reducing undernutrition may

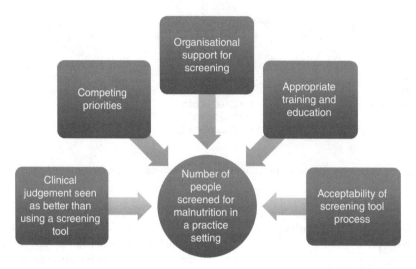

Figure 2.1.2   Summary of the factors that can influence rates of nutritional screening

result in early identification and timely management of those at risk and ensure that those who
do not access online services or visit healthcare
settings can be identified using alternative
methods [31].

Nutritional screening tools have been widely
implemented in many clinical practice areas
with the assumption that their use will improve
nutritional care as a result of identifying those at
risk of undernutrition. As screening for undernutrition is costly in terms of time and resources,
further research to evaluate the outcomes and
economic impact of screening in conjunction
with associated interventions and care pathways
is needed [32].

2.1.6 Conclusion

Screening for undernutrition can identify those
who require further nutritional assessment and a
plan of care. Screening can be undertaken using
a single measure or more commonly a tool
which has demonstrated validity and reliability.
Implementation and continued use of a tool in
practice settings require consideration of the
local context and potential barriers and facilitators. Finally, there remains a need to demonstrate that screening for undernutrition leads to
better nutritional outcomes.

References

1. Correia MITD, Hegazi RA, Higashiguchi T, Michel J,
   Reddy BR, Tappenden KA, Uyar M, Muscaritoli M.
   Evidence-based recommendations for addressing malnutrition in health care: an updated strategy from the
   feedM.E. Global Study Group. *J Am Med Dir Assoc*
   2014; **15**(8): 544–550.
2. Guyonnet S, Rolland Y. Screening for malnutrition
   in older people. *Clin Geriatr Med* 2015; **31**(3): 429–437.
3. Freijer k, Bours MJL, Nuijten MJC, Poley MJ, Meijers
   JMM, Halfens RJG, Schols JMGA. The economic
   value of enteral medical nutrition in the management
   of disease-related malnutrition: a systematic review.
   J Am Med Dir Assoc 2014; **15**(1): 17–29.
4. Black RE, Victoria CG, Walker SP, Bhutta ZA,
   Christian P, de Onis M, Ezzati M, Grantham-
   McGregor S, Katz J, Martorell R, Uauy R, Maternal
   and Child Nutrition Study Group. Maternal and child
   undernutrition and overweight in low-income and
   middle-income countries. *Lancet* 2013; **382**(9890):
   427–451.
5. Jensen GL, Mirtallo J, Compher C, Dhaliwal R,
   Forbes A, Figueredo Grijalba R, Hardy G, Kondrup J,
   Labadarios D, Nyulasi I, Castillo Pineda J, Waitzberg
   D. Adult starvation and disease-related malnutrition.
   J Acad Nutr Diet 2010; **34**(2): 156–159.
6. Public Health England. NHS population screening
   explained.   www.gov.uk/nhs-population-screening-
   explained (accessed 28 August 2017).
7. American Society for Parenteral and Enteral Nutrition
   Board of Directors and Clinical Practice Committee.
   Definition of Terms, Style, and Conventions Used.
   Silver Spring: ASPEN, 2012.

8. Green SM, Watson R. Nutritional screening and assessment tools for older adults: literature review. *J Adv Nurs* 2006; **54**(4): 477–490.

9. Keller HH, McCullough J, Davidson B, Vesnaver E, Laporte M, Gramlich L, Allard J, Bernier P, Duerksen D, Jeejeebhoy K. The integrated nutrition pathway for acute care (INPAC): building consensus with a modified Delphi. *Nutr J*; **14**(1): 63–74.

10. Correia MITD, Hegazi IA, Ignacio Diaz-Pizarro Graf J, Gomez-Morales G, Fuentes Gutiérrez C, Fernanda Goldin M, Navas A, Lucia Pinzón Espitia O, Millere Tavares G. Addressing disease-related malnutrition in healthcare. A Latin American perspective. *J Parenter Enteral Nutr* 2016; **40**: 319–325.

11. Field LB, Hand RK. Differentiating malnutrition screening and assessment: a nutrition care process perspective. *J Acad Nutr Diet* 2015; **115**(5): 824–828.

12. Kondrup J, Allison SP, Elia M, Vellas B, Plauth M. EPSEN guidelines for nutrition screening 2002. *Clin Nutr* 2003; **22**(4): 415–421.

13. National Institute for Health and Care Excellence. Nutrition Support in Adults. London: NICE, 2012.

14. Mueller C, Compher C, Ellen DM, ASPEN Board of Directors. Clinical guidelines: nutrition screening, assessment and intervention in adults. *J Parenter Enteral Nutr* 2011; **35**(1): 16–24.

15. NHS. Free NHS health check. www.healthcheck.nhs.uk/, 2015.

16. WHO. Guideline: Updates on the Management of Severe Acute Malnutrition in Infants and Children. Geneva: World Health Organization, 2013.

17. Tang AM, Dong K, Deitchler M, Chung M, Maalouf-Manasseh Z, Tumilowicz A, Wanke C. Use of Cutoffs for Mid-Upper Arm Circumference (MUAC) as an Indicator or Predictor of Nutritional and Health-Related Outcomes in Adolescents and Adults: A Systematic Review. Washington: Food and Nutrition Technical Assistance III Project, 2013.

18. Age UK. The Paperweight Nutrition Armband. Salford: Age UK, 2015. www.ageuk.org.uk/salford/paperweight/ (accessed 28 August 2017).

19. Cederholm T, Bosaeus I, Barazzoni R, Bauer J, Van Gossum A, Klek S, Muscaritoli M, Nyulasi I, Ockenga J, Schneider SM, de van der Schuerenk MAE, Singer P. Diagnostic criteria for malnutrition – an ESPEN consensus statement. *Clin Nutr* 2015; **34**(3): 335–340.

20. Jones MJ. Nutritional Screening and Assessment Tools. New York: Nova Science Publishers, 2006.

21. Skipper A, Ferguson M, Thompson K, Castellanos VH, Porcari J. Nutrition screening tools. An analysis of the evidence. *J Parenter Enteral Nutr* 2012; **36**(3): 292–298.

22. Van Bokhorst-de van der Schueren MA, Guaitoli PR, Jansma PR, de Vet HC. A systematic review of malnutrition screening tools for the nursing home setting. *J Am Med Dir Assoc* 2014; **15**(3): 171–184.

23. Elia M, Stratton RJ. An analytic appraisal of nutrition screening tools supported by original data with particular reference to age. *Nutrition* 2012; **28**(5): 477–494.

24. Omidvari A, Vali Y, Murray SM, Wonderling D, Rashidian A. Nutritional screening for improving professional practice for patient outcomes in hospital and primary care settings. *Cochrane Database Syst Rev* 2013; **6**: CD005539.

25. Green SM, James EP. Barriers and facilitators to undertaking nutritional screening of patients: a systematic review. *J Hum Nutr Diet* 2013; **26**(3): 211–221.

26. Green SM, James EP, Latter S, Sutcliffe M, Fader MJ. Barriers and facilitators to screening for malnutrition by community nurses: a qualitative study. *J Hum Nutr Diet* 2014; **27**(1): 88–95.

27. McGurk P, Jackson JM, Elia M. Rapid and reliable self-screening for nutritional risk in hospital outpatients using an electronic system. *Nutrition* 2013; **29**(4): 693–696.

28. BAPEN. New BAPEN Malnutrition Self-Screening Tool. www.bapen.org.uk/media-centre/press-releases/1st-december-bapen-launches-malnutrition-self-screening-tool (accessed 28 August 2017).

29. Cawood A, Elia M, Sharp SK, Stratton RJ. Malnutrition self-screening by using MUST in hospital outpatients: validity, reliability, and ease of use. *Am J Clin Nutr* 2012; **96**(5): 1000–1007.

30. Sandhu A, Mosli M, Yan B, Wu T, Gregor J, Chande N, Ponich T, Beaton M, Rahman A. Self-screening for malnutrition risk in outpatient inflammatory bowel disease patients using the Malnutrition Universal Screening Tool (MUST). *J Parenter Enteral Nutr* 2016; **40**(4): 507–510.

31. Malnutrition Task Force. Preventing Malnutrition in Later Life. www.malnutritiontaskforce.org.uk/prevention-programme/ (accessed 28 August 2017).

32. Hamirudin AH, Charlton K, Walton K. Outcomes related to nutrition screening in community living older adults: a systematic literature review. *Arch Gerontol Geriatr* 2016; **62**: 9–25.

Chapter 2.2

Nutritional assessment

Laura Frank
MultiCare Health System, Tacoma, United States

2.2.1 Background

Nutrition assessment was introduced in clinical medicine during the 1970s when protein and energy undernutrition of hospitalised patients was first recognised in North America [1]. In 2006, The British Dietetic Association (BDA) published the Nutrition and Dietetic Care Process, which described the knowledge and skills of the dietitian [2]. Furthermore, it provided a framework for the development of tools to support the dietetic profession in the UK. The Care Process was influenced by the American Dietetic Association's Nutrition Care Process and Model (NCPM), published in 2003 [3]. The Nutrition Care Process consists of distinct, interrelated steps including nutrition assessment, diagnosis, intervention and monitoring/evaluation and is described as a problem-solving model. The critical reasoning skills particularly required in the assessment step are demonstrated in Box 2.2.1 [4].

Nutrition assessment is the first step in the nutrition and dietetic process and is a systematic process of collecting and interpreting information in order to make decisions about the nature and cause of nutrition-related health issues that affect an individual, a group or a population [4]. It is a systematic method for obtaining, verifying and interpreting data needed to identify nutrition-related problems, the associated aetiology(ies) related to the problem, the significance of the problem, as well as the signs and symptoms manifested by the nutrition-related problem [5].

Overall, the purpose of the nutrition assessment is to obtain adequate and relevant information in order to identify nutrition-related problems and to inform the development and monitoring of the intervention [4]. The intent of the nutrition assessment is to document baseline nutrition parameters, identify nutritional risk factors and specific nutrition deficits, establish individual nutrition needs, and identify medical, psychosocial and socioeconomic factors that may influence the prescription and administration of nutrition support therapy [6]. Therefore, assessment will include reassessment and provides the baseline against which changes in health and the outcomes of the intervention are measured [4]. Historically, the objectives of nutritional assessment are to:

- accurately define the nutritional status of the patient
- define clinically relevant undernutrition
- monitor changes in nutritional status during nutrition support [7].

2.2.2 Process of nutrition assessment

Nutrition assessment should be undertaken in all patients identified as being at risk by nutritional screening and will give the basis for the diagnosis decision and the identification of further actions, including patient-centred treatment plans [8]. A nutrition assessment should also be initiated by other identifiers of need, such as a referral by a healthcare professional, self-referral,

Advanced Nutrition and Dietetics in Nutrition Support, First Edition. Edited by Mary Hickson and Sara Smith.

Box 2.2.1 Critical reasoning and specialist skills required in nutritional assessment.

- Comparison with standards.
- Determining whether dietetic care will provide benefit.
- Identifying which multidisciplinary health and care team members to consult.
- Observing for verbal and non-verbal cues to guide and prompt effective interviewing methods.
- Determining appropriate data to collect in different situations.
- Matching assessment method to the situation, with individual, group or community.
- Applying relevant assessments in valid and reliable ways.
- Distinguishing important from unimportant data.
- Validating the data.
- Organising the data.
- Problem solving.
- Identifying key partners and key workers and their role in the assessment process.
- Determining whether the problem requires consultations with or referral to another health professional.

Source: Reproduced with permission from the British Dietetic Association [4]

---

high-level public health data, epidemiological data or other similar process [4].

Nutrition assessment at the individual, group, community and hospital level forms the basis of nutrition practice and intervention and has also been described using the ABCD (Anthropometric, Biochemical, Clinical and Dietary) approach [9]. The ABCD approach has also been expanded to the ABCDE approach, where the 'E' is an abbreviation for Environmental/psychosocial [4].

The International Dietetic and Nutrition Terminology (IDNT) reference manual [5] identified and grouped the nutrition assessment into five domains:

- Food/Nutrition-Related History
- Anthropometrics
- Biochemical Data, Medical Tests and Procedures
- Nutrition-Focused Physical Findings
- Patient/Client History.

According to the American Society for Parenteral and Enteral Nutrition (ASPEN), a nutrition assessment requires the collection of information from a variety of sources because there is no single clinical or laboratory indicator of nutritional status [10]. These sources of data include historical (weight history, medical/surgical history, medication history), clinical signs/physical examination, anthropometric, laboratory, dietary and functional domains.

Box 2.2.2 Measures or components of nutritional assessment

- Medical history
- Physical examination
- Biochemical analysis
- Social and psychological history
- Nutrition history
- Energy and fluid needs
- Protein needs
- Micronutrient needs

Source: Reproduced with permission of Elsevier [8]

In an attempt to come to a consensus regarding the definitions and terminology of clinical nutrition, the European Society of Clinical Nutrition (ESPEN) recently published guidelines stating that the assessment of nutritional status comprehends information on body weight and height, body mass index (BMI), body composition and biochemical indices (strong consensus, 97% agreement) [8]. A strong consensus (94% agreement) was also found among the stakeholders that the objectives of the assessment are to evaluate the patient at nutritional risk according to several measures (Box 2.2.2).

Sources of information to support dietitians in gathering the appropriate information to complete a comprehensive nutrition assessment have been previously described [4]. Nutrition assessment indicators should be compared to criteria, relevant norms and standards for interpretation [11,12]. From this data, a determination of whether a nutrition diagnosis or nutrition problem exists can be made and used to document the presence of undernutrition [6].

Anthropometric assessment

Anthropometric measurements are widely used in the assessment of nutrition status, particularly when a chronic imbalance between intakes of protein and energy occurs [9]. Such disturbances influence the patterns of physical growth and the relative portions of body tissues including body fat, lean body mass or muscle tissue, and total body water. Anthropometric measurements include information about the patient's height, weight, weight history, BMI, growth pattern indices and percentile ranks (important for paediatric nutrition assessment) [5]. Use of comparative standards for anthropometrics is encouraged. Body composition data can also be part of anthropometric measurements.

Most anthropometric methods used to assess body composition are based on a model in which the body consists of two chemically distinct compartments: fat and fat-free mass (e.g. skeletal muscle, non-skeletal muscle and soft-lean tissues and the skeleton) [9].Therefore, variations in the amount and proportion of fat mass versus fat-free mass, including muscle, can be used as indices of nutritional status [8,9,11]. Some of these indices include skinfold thickness measures (e.g. triceps skinfold), arm muscle circumference and bioelectrical impedance analysis (BIA), and these are discussed in more detail in Chapter 2.3. More sophisticated measures of body composition include ultrasound, computed tomography (CT) and dual-energy x-ray absorptiometry (DEXA) [8–11]and these are discussed in more detail in Chapter 2.7.

Biochemical assessment

Biochemical data are important in helping to define a nutrition diagnosis or problem, including nutrient deficiencies and/or toxicities.

Biochemical assessment or laboratory assessment can also be used to detect subclinical nutrient deficiency states and can provide an objective means of assessing nutritional status [9]. Static biochemical tests measure concentrations of a nutrient or its metabolite in a preselected specimen, typically using whole blood, plasma or serum, that reflects the amount of the nutrient, the body stores of the nutrient and/or the metabolic or biochemical reflection of the impact of the amount of the nutrient. Biochemical markers, such as serum concentrations of visceral proteins, should not be used as indicators of a patient's nutritional status without concomitant evaluation of the inflammatory process [8]. A more detailed discussion of biochemical assesssment is presented in Chapter 2.4

Clinical assessment

Clinical assessment consists of medical history as well as physical assessment [9]. Patient/client history includes the personal history, medical/health/family/social history, treatments and complementary/alternative medicine use [5]. Indeed, past and present medical history is an important tool in the nutrition care process. Critical thinking skills are necessary to determine the appropriate data to collect from both objective and subjective sources. Clinical judgement is required to determine whether there is a need for additional data gathering in order to diagnose nutrition problems and generate nutrition intervention strategies accordingly. Indeed, distinguishing between relevant/important and irrelevant/unimportant data is an important skill for registered dietitians (RD) [13].

Alternative methods for identifying subclinical deficiency states, based on measurements of functional impairment, have been developed [14]. Functional tests have been defined as diagnostic tests to determine the sufficiency of host nutriture to permit cells, tissues, organs, anatomical systems or the host to perform optimally the intended, nutrient-dependent biological function. Measurable declines in strength and physical performance will be associated with clinical signs and symptoms such as loss of muscle mass and function that accompany advanced undernutrition syndromes [10]. Factors contributing to functional decline may include nutrient deficiencies and impairment of organ system functions. The most commonly used measure for routine clinical assessment is hand-grip strength [10,15,16], which has been shown to be an outcome predictor and marker of nutritional status [16]. Gait speed and chair rise tests can also be used, as well as composite functional scores like the Short Performance Physical Performance Battery, De Morton Mobility Index or the Barthel Index [8].

A nutrition-focused physical assessment can determine changes in body composition associated with loss of muscle mass, subcutaneous fat mass and fluid accumulation, which may reflect the severity of undernutrition [5,8,15]. Historically, the physical examination, as defined by Jelliffe in 1966 [17], assesses the changes in the body related to inadequate nutrition, that can be seen or felt in superficial epithelial tissue, especially in the skin, eyes, hair, buccal mucosa or in organs near the surface of the body (parotid and thyroid glands). A detailed description of the physical exam has been previously provided by the Academy of Nutrition and Dietetics [18]. Further discussion of the use of physical assessment and clinical signs and symptoms reflecting nutritional status is included in Chapter 2.5.

Dietary assessment

Dietary assessment should address food and nutrition-related history and can be used to detect inadequate or imbalanced food or nutrient intakes, which can lead to nutrient deficiencies or excesses [5,8–10]. Also included in this category are food and nutrient administration, medication, herbal supplement use, knowledge, beliefs, and attitudes to food and supplements, eating and food behaviours, factors affecting access to food and/or food/nutrition-related supplies, physical activity and function [5]. Dietary assessment is further discussed in Chapter 2.6.

Environmental/psychosocial assessment

Environmental and psychosocial history should be evaluated in order to establish potential effects of living conditions, loneliness and depression on nutritional needs, and whether input from other professional groups may be of benefit [5,8]. Furthermore, social/environmental circumstances have been identified as contexts associated with adult undernutrition [15].

2.2.3 Summary

A formal nutrition assessment provides the basis for the nutrition care plan and is a key step in the nutrition care process [2–5]. The nutrition care process guides a comprehensive nutrition therapy by defining its rationale, identifying and describing appropriate interventions, setting short- and long-term goals, and monitoring and evaluating targeted outcome measures in order to determine the need for reassessment and re-evaluation across the continuum of care. It is important for dietitians to use critical thinking skills pertaining to the specific domains associated with data gathering and interpretation of the nutrition assessment. Data collected during the nutrition assessment guide dietitians in the identification and selection of one or more appropriate nutrition-related problem(s), also known as the nutrition diagnosis, in an effort to create evidence-based, patient-centred intervention strategies designed to improve patient outcomes.

References

1. Blackburn GL, Bistran BR, Maini BS, Shlamm HT, Smith MF. Nutritional and metabolic assessment of the hospitalized patient. *J Parenter Enteral Nutr* 1977; **1**: 11–22.
2. British Dietetic Association. The Nutrition and Dietetic Care Process. Birmingham: British Dietetic Association, 2009.
3. Lacey K, Pritchett E. Nutrition care process and model: ADA adopts road map to quality care and outcomes management. *J Am Diet Assoc* 2003; **103**(8): 1061–1072.

4. British Dietetic Association. BDA Model and Process for Nutrition and Dietetic Care. Birmingham: British Dietetic Association, 2012.

5. Academy of Nutrition and Dietetics. International Dietetics and Nutrition Terminology (IDNT). Reference Manual. Standardized Language for the Nutrition Care Process, 4th edn. Chicago: Academy of Nutrition and Dietetics, 2012.

6. Ukleja A, Freeman KL, Gilbert K, et al. Standards for nutrition support: adult hospitalized patients. *Nutr Clin Pract* 2010; **25**: 403–414.

7. Bozetti F. Nutritional assessment from the perspective of the clinician. *J Parenter Enteral Nutr* 1987; **11**: 115S–121S.

8. Cederholm T, Barazzoni R, Austin P, et al. ESPEN guidelines on definitions and terminology of clinical nutrition. *Clin Nutr* 2017; **36**(1): 49–64.

9. Gibson RS, editor. Principles of Nutritional Assessment, 2nd edn. New York: Oxford University Press Inc., 2005.

10. Mueller C, editor. The A.S.P.E.N. Adult Nutrition Support Core Curriculum, 2nd edn. Silver Spring: American Society for Parenteral and Enteral Nutrition, 2012.

11. Gibson RS, editor. Principles of Nutritional Assessment. New York: Oxford University Press Inc., 1990.

12. Gandy J, editor. Assessment of nutritional status. In: Manual of Dietetic Practice. New Jersey: Wiley-Blackwell, 2014.

13. American Dietetic Association. Nutrition Diagnosis and Intervention: Standardized Language for the Nutrition Care Process. Chicago: American Dietetic Association, 2007.

14. Solomons NW, Allen LH. The functional assessment of nutritional status: principles, practice and potential. *Nutr Rev* 1983; **41**: 33–50.

15. White JV, Guenter P, Jensen G, Malone A, Schofield M, Academy Malnutrition Work Group, A.S.P.E.N. Malnutrition Task Force, A.S.P.E.N. Board of Directors. Consensus statement: Academy of Nutrition and Dietetics and American Society for Parenteral and Enteral Nutrition: characteristics recommended for the identification and documentation of adult malnutrition (undernutrition). *J Parenter Enteral Nutr* 2012; **36**: 275–283.

16. Norman K, Stobaus N, Gonzalez MC, Schulzke JD, Pirlich M. Hand grip strength: outcome predictor and marker of nutritional status. *Clin Nutr* 2011; **30**: 135–142.

17. Jelliffe DB, editor. The Assessment of the Nutritional Status of the Community. Geneva: World Health Organization, 1966.

18. Academy of Nutrition and Dietetics. www.eatrightstore.org/product/924b0333-dbf7-4cad-9fcf-a127005693e5 (accessed 25 September 2017).

Chapter 2.3

Anthropometric assessment of undernutrition

Angela Madden

School of Life and Medical Sciences, University of Hertfordshire, Hatfield, UK

2.3.1 Introduction

Anthropometry is the science of measuring physical body dimensions and in nutrition support, its application includes the evaluation of these measurements in terms of reference or cut-off values and their relationship to predicting clinical outcome. Anthropometric evaluation is often regarded as the first step of nutrition screening and assessment, that is, the 'A' in the ABCDE approach (see Chapter 2.2). Such measurements are routinely collected in clinical practice and, in most cases, no sophisticated equipment is needed. As a result, anthropometry could easily be perceived, incorrectly, as simplistic and mundane. However, careful anthropometric evaluation using standardised measurement protocols followed by judicious interpretation of results, including understanding of methodological limitations, can provide quick, meaningful and cost-effective information about an individual's nutritional status and health risk.

2.3.2 Weight

Body weight should be routinely measured in clinical healthcare and represents the sum of all body compartments, including muscle, fat and water, but does not differentiate between them. Weight change, therefore, may reflect variation in one or more compartments in response to nutritional and/or pathological factors and, in turn, this may indicate clinical risk. In order to ensure that small fluctuations in weight can be identified, a standardised procedure, reliable equipment and an understanding of confounding factors are required.

Weighing procedure

A standardised protocol is required which should include the removal of shoes, outer garments such as jackets, heavy jewellery, loose change and keys. No allowance is usually made for light indoor clothes or diurnal weight variation of up to 2 kg which is associated with food and fluid intake and bladder and bowel evacuation. However, a consistent approach to clothing and time of measurement should be undertaken and this should be recorded [1].

Scales

The type of scales used may influence measured values by up to 1.6 kg, with discrepancy increasing with weight [2]. Step-on, seat or bed scales utilising either a digital or balance mechanism are available and an appropriate standardised procedure should be used for each, for example bedding, urinary catheter bag, etc. should not be weighed when using bed scales. Most clinically available scales are capable of weighing up to

Advanced Nutrition and Dietetics in Nutrition Support, First Edition. Edited by Mary Hickson and Sara Smith.
© 2018 John Wiley & Sons Ltd. Published 2018 by John Wiley & Sons Ltd.

150–200kg but bariatric platforms with hand-rails are also available for individuals weighing up to 500kg. Regular calibration is required to ensure that reliable values are obtained and is legally required in some jurisdictions.

Factors confounding measurement of weight

Fluctuation in fluid balance may influence body weight but this is unlikely to conceal systematic changes in body weight due to loss or gain of muscle or fat mass in healthy adults. Typically, variation in body weight across the menstrual cycle is <1.2% whilst variation associated with thirst-evoking dehydration is <1.5% [1]. However, pathological changes in fluid balance, even when not clinically detectable, may be substantial and may obscure the identification of nutritional change, that is, simultaneous loss of muscle [3]. In haemodialysis, mean interdialytic weight change of 1.9±1.6kg has been observed [4], whilst large-volume paracentesis in liver disease may be accompanied by a mean weight loss of 13.8±0.5kg over 72 hours [5]. Estimates of excess fluid weight in patients with alcoholic liver disease have been made by evaluating weight gained during refeeding [6] and practice guidance includes estimates of weight gain associated with oedema [7] (Table 2.3.1).

Table 2.3.1 Estimated contribution of fluid to body weight in patients with alcoholic hepatitis and ascites [6] and with oedema [7]

Clinical description of ascites	Estimated fluid weight (kg)
Minimal	2.2
Moderate	6
Tense	14

Clinical description of oedema	Estimated fluid weight (kg)
Barely detectable	2
Severe	>10

Source: Reproduced from Madden and Smith [1], with permission from Wiley.

Whilst estimated values vary considerably, these can be informed through clinical examination, abdominal ultrasound scans and careful evaluation of serial weight measurements. Even so, estimates of fluid weight must be made cautiously, recorded clearly and their limitations recognised. Adjustment to measured body weight is also necessary following limb amputation and when an unmoveable cast is worn, and standard values for modifying weight in these situations are available [1] (Table 2.3.2).

Estimated weight

In the absence of measured weight, self-reported values can be used but these tend to underestimate measured weight with a mean discrepancy of up to 6.5kg [8]. However, self-reported weight of hospitalised patients aged ≥16years may be more accurate than estimates made by healthcare professionals, where only 53% of estimates were within 10% of measured values and with less accurate estimates made in obese individuals [9].

Table 2.3.2 Adjustment of body weight following amputation or with an immoveable cast

Amputation	Contribution to total body weight (%)	Multiplier of measured weight required for adjustment
Upper limb	4.9	1.05
Upper arm	2.7	1.03
Forearm	1.6	1.02
Hand	0.6	1.01
Lower limb	15.6	1.18
Thigh	9.7	1.11
Lower leg	4.5	1.05
Foot	1.4	1.01
Cast	Estimated cast weight	
Upper limb cast	<1kg	
Lower leg or back cast	0.9–4.5kg	

Source: Reproduced from Madden and Smith [1], with permission from Wiley.

This level of error is not acceptable in patients requiring nutrition support so self-reported or observer-estimated weights are not recommended, especially in those with cognitive impairment.

Interpreting body weight values

In nutrition support, body weight in adults is interpreted either by calculating body mass index (BMI) or by evaluating repeat measurements to ascertain weight change. Normative weight tables, which were previously used for adults, are no longer considered useful [10]. In children, body weight is interpreted using Z-scores for age or height [11] using reference population data. It is important to note that undernutrition, which impacts adversely on clinical outcome, may coexist in individuals with high body weight due to excessive adipose fat and that a single body weight measurement on its own makes a limited contribution to nutritional evaluation.

Unintentional weight loss

Weight loss is included in many nutritional screening tools [12] and unintentional weight loss is an independent risk factor for increased morbidity and mortality after elective surgery in patients with cancer and in haemodialysis [13,14]. The European Society of Parenteral and Enteral Nutrition proposes two cut-off values for defining unintentional weight loss as diagnostic criteria for undernutrition when combined with age-specific low BMI and/or sex-specific low fat-free mass index [15]:

- loss of >10% body weight over any time period, or
- loss of >5% body weight over the last 3 months.

Using these criteria based on self-reported weight loss, undernutrition was identified in 14% of acutely ill middle-aged adults and 6% of elderly hospital outpatients [16]. Recording body weight regularly to facilitate the identification of unintentional weight loss will therefore assist in the management of patients requiring nutrition support.

2.3.3 Height

Standing height in adults and height or length in children are combined with other anthropometric variables, usually weight, to assess nutritional status and estimate energy requirements.

Procedure for measuring height

A standardised technique will help reduce intra-observer error which may be ~1.3 cm for adult height [1]. This requires removal of shoes and the measured person to stand upright with arms loosely to the side, back straight and heels against a vertical measure. The position of the head should be checked to ensure it is in the Frankfort plane, that is, from a side view, the bottom of the eye socket should be level with the top of the ear canal, and then the measurement made after a deep in-breath [17].

Height measuring equipment

Free-standing or portable stadiometers or a wall-mounted measure should be used to assess standing height and all require regular calibration. Variation between measurements made using difference equipment is usually small providing that the apparatus has been assembled or positioned correctly [1].

Factors confounding measurement of height

Standing height varies throughout the day, with a ~6 mm loss in height recorded in measurements taken 7 hours apart in healthy adults. This may be partly reversed by resting supine for ~50 minutes [1]. When accurate serial values are required, the time of measurement should be recorded so that a consistent approach can be taken. Irreversible height loss occurs with ageing >40 years; this is estimated at approximately 1 mm loss per year but the rate of loss increases with age [1]. Standing straight for measurement may be difficult for some individuals, for example those with scoliosis or abnormal spinal curvature, and so the exact method of determining height should be clearly documented and the measurement evaluated carefully.

Estimating height

If height cannot be measured, for example in very old or hospitalised patients with contractures, a surrogate measure can be used. Self-reported height tends to overestimate measured values with mean differences of up to 7.5 cm [8]. Overestimates tend to increase with age and are higher in women, possibly associated with greater height loss due to osteoporosis. The clinical significance of these height differences has been explored in small studies and had little impact on nutritional screening category but did influence BMI category in older women. Estimates of height made by healthcare professionals are less accurate than self-reports [9]. Current evidence does not support routine use of self-reported or healthcare professional estimates of height.

An estimate of standing height can be calculated from other body dimensions including knee height, arm span, demi-span, ulna length and hand length [1]. Most height prediction equations have been derived in healthy young adults and, because the relationship between height and other body variables is influenced by age and ethnicity, their accuracy and precision in clinical populations are variable. Studies that have evaluated these equations have reached different conclusions about which equation is best, indicating that more useful estimates of height are provided by equations which were derived in a population comparable for age and ethnicity to the population being investigated. As a result, no recommendation for the best equation for predicting height can be made at present.

However, the practical aspects of measuring alternative body dimensions should be taken into account when assessing bed-bound or frail individuals so that undressing and participant effort are minimised. As a result, ulna length, knee height or hand length measurement may be more convenient than demi-span.

2.3.4 Body mass index

Calculation of BMI requires reliable measures of body weight and standing height:

$$BMI = \frac{weight\,(kg)}{height\,squared\;(m^2)}$$

In nutrition support, BMI can provide a quick overview of nutritional status that impacts on clinical risk, for example in assessing undernutrition and obesity, and is included in several widely used nutritional screening tools and criteria for identifying undernutrition [15,18]. Although very useful, BMI has limitations, some of which are described below.

The World Health Organization classification of BMI describes 11 principal categories ranging from severe thinness to obesity class III, with the normal range defined as $18.50–24.99\,kg/m^2$ [19]. Additional categories are provided to take account of clinical risk in diverse populations; for example, diabetes and cardiovascular disease risk in Asians are associated with lower BMI values than in other groups.

Interpreting low BMI values

Low BMI values are associated with increased risk of mortality, postsurgical complications, infection and length of hospital stay in clinical populations and usually indicate the need for nutrition support. Values $<18.5\,kg/m^2$ are defined as diagnostic for undernutrition or, when combined with unintentional weight loss, values <20 or $<22\,kg/m^2$ are considered diagnostic in those aged <70 years and ≥70 years respectively [15]. Age-related height loss may lead to apparently higher BMI values so older individuals with low-normal BMI require review.

Interpreting high BMI values

High BMI values are associated at population level with increased risk of mortality, cardiovascular disease and some cancers. Values $≥25\,kg/m^2$ and $≥30\,kg/m^2$ are used to define overweight and obesity and, in many cases, indicate excess body fat stored as adipose tissue. However, taller adults and particularly men with large muscle stores may have BMI values >25 kg/m² without excess fat. High BMI values are more difficult to interpret in patients requiring nutrition support as high fat stores may mask the depletion of lean tissue that often accompanies acute and chronic illness, especially when nutrient intake is impaired.

With increasing obesity prevalence in many populations, this presents a challenge to nutritional assessment that focuses on BMI measurement. For example, high BMI values are associated with increased clinical risk in pancreatitis and after trauma [20,21]. However, following ischaemic stroke, the relationship between BMI and mortality is U-shaped with the lowest risk associated with BMI of 35 kg/m² [22]. A similar 'protective effect' of obesity has been observed in patients with decompensated heart failure but only in those aged >75 years [23].

These diverse results indicate the complexity of assessing nutritional status in patients who need nutrition support and suggest the limitation of using BMI on its own and the need to evaluate other nutrition-responsive variables.

Fat-free mass index

Reduced skeletal muscle, which may not be detected by BMI assessment, is a major predictor of impaired physical function and mortality [24] so the fat-free mass index (FFMI) has been proposed to evaluate lean tissue [25], using a similar formula to BMI:

$$FFMI = \frac{\text{fat-free mass (kg)}}{\text{height squared (m}^2)}$$

Fat-free mass index values <15 kg/m² in women and <17 kg/m² in men, based on data from >5000 healthy Swiss adults, are proposed as cut-offs for diagnosing undernutrition when accompanied by unintentional weight loss (see Chapter 1.6) [15]. The challenge in applying this assessment to a patient population is the difficulty of obtaining accurate and precise measures of fat-free mass in a clinical population.

Waist-to-height ratio as an alternative to BMI

The ratio of waist circumference to height has been shown to be a better predictor of mortality than BMI at population level [26]. This has relevance in public health where healthy adults are advised to keep their waist circumference less than half their standing height [27]. However, there is no evidence that waist circumference is useful in the assessment of patients requiring nutrition support.

2.3.5 Mid-upper arm circumference

Mid-upper arm circumference (MUAC) is used to identify chronic energy deficiency and to predict mortality in acutely hospitalised adults [1].

Standard procedure for measuring mid-upper arm circumference

To maximise measurement reliability, a standard protocol should be followed, such as that described by the Centers for Disease Control and Prevention [28]. In summary, the measured person stands with their forearm placed across their chest with palm inwards so that the midpoint between the acromium process of the scapula and the olecranon process of the ulna can be identified. Their arm is then relaxed so that it hangs freely and the circumference of the upper arm is measured at the mid-point using a nonstretchable tape that is placed parallel to the floor and fitted snugly around the arm without compressing the skin. Typically, three measurements are taken and the mean value calculated. Protocols vary in which arm is measured [1].

Interpreting mid-upper arm circumference

Mid-upper arm circumference can be used predict BMI when height or weight is unavailable:

- Male: BMI (kg/m²) = 1.01 × MUAC (cm) – 4.7
- Female: BMI (kg/m²) = 1.10 × MUAC (cm) – 6.7

Mid-upper arm circumference values <25 and <23.5 cm are approximately equal to BMI <20 and <18.5 kg/m² respectively [1]. BMI values derived from MUAC should be interpreted with caution because although mean differences may be small (<0.1 kg/m²), the 95% confidence intervals range between -5.6 to +4.1 kg/m², potentially adding error to individual values that would lead to misclassification of nutritional status [1].

Predictive value of mid-upper arm circumference

The clinical predictive value of MUAC varies with different studies, probably as a result of diverse populations [29]. However, low MUAC values are useful in clinical practice to indicate potential nutritional concern and that more detailed assessment is needed. Combining MUAC with triceps skinfold measurement allows mid-arm muscle circumference to be calculated and this may have greater predictive importance.

2.3.6 Triceps skinfold

Measuring triceps skinfold (TSF) thickness facilitates assessment of body fat stores and allows calculation of mid-arm muscle circumference. Clearly, measurement of subcutaneous fat at a single peripheral site provides only limited information about total body fat and no insight into intra-abdominal adipose tissue.

Standard procedure for measuring triceps skinfold

As with MUAC, a standard protocol for measuring TSF should be followed [30]. After identifying the mid-arm point, and with the arm hanging loosely at the side, a skinfold running parallel with the humerus bone is picked up and held between the measurer's thumb and forefinger. Skinfold calipers are placed on the skinfold at 90° to the humerus and then released to apply pressure to the skinfold for 3 seconds and then the measurement is recorded. The measurer continues to hold the skinfold throughout the process. Typically, three measurements are taken

and the mean value calculated. Protocols vary in the arm measured and body position, that is, standing, sitting or lying [1]. It is recommended that the procedure is practised so that a skillful practitioner achieves an intraobserver technical error measurement of ≤5% [1]. Precision-engineered calipers, for example Harpenden or Holtain, should preferably be used and although disposable plastic versions are also available, their accuracy varies [1]. To facilitate the interpretation of repeated TSF measurements, the arm measured, body position and calipers used should be recorded.

Interpreting triceps skinfold

Triceps skinfold measurements can be compared with population standards but their application in disease has been questioned [31]. In addition, increasing obesity prevalence means that cut-off values used to identify depletion, which has typically been set at the 5% percentile, move upwards. For example, in adult men in the USA, the 5th percentile for TSF has increased from 4.5 mm to 6.1 mm over a 27-year period [32,33]but there is no evidence that health risk associated with undernutrition has changed during this time. To facilitate comparison of data over decades, continuing to use the earlier standards of Bishop et al. [32] seems logical. Alternatively, using repeat measurements taken at least 7 days apart should be considered for ongoing monitoring.

Predictive value of triceps skinfold

The independent prognostic value of TSF varies with study populations, reflecting gender difference and the adverse effects of both severe fat depletion and excessive fat stores. In addition, no studies have investigated whether risk is associated with low fat stores *per se*, or with depletion of fat stores during illness.

2.3.7 Mid-arm muscle circumference

Estimates of mid-arm muscle circumference (MAMC), calculated from MUAC and TSF [34], are used to assess fat-free mass and as an outcome measure to evaluate nutritional interventions:

$$MAMC(cm) = MUAC(cm) - [TSF(mm) \times 0.3142]$$

Interpreting mid-arm muscle circumference

As with TSF, MAMC can be interpreted either by comparison with population standards or by evaluating repeat measures. No international standards exist and although data from specific European populations are available [1], the large Health and Nutrition Examination Survey dataset from the USA published in 1981 [32] is mostly often used for comparison and the 5th percentile used to identify muscle depletion. Subsequent National Health and Nutrition Examination Survey (NHANES) datasets published in 2000 include 10th but not 5th percentiles [35], whilst those from 2008 do not include MAMC [33].

Comparing a single MAMC value with reference data has limitations, including the measurer's proficiency, measurement protocol (left/right arm) and participant's ethnicity. However, a value <5th percentile should raise concern, indicating that action is required. Repeat measures taken over a period of ≥7 days by an experienced practitioner with intraobserver technical error measurement of ≤5% may provide a more useful assessment and allow change in fat-free mass to be detected. If measurements are repeated more frequently, any changes detected probably indicate alteration in fluid rather than muscle [1]. As standard procedures for measuring MUAC and TSF differ, the information recorded with MAMC results should include details of how measurements were undertaken, such as on the left/right side.

Predictive value of mid-arm muscle circumference

Low MAMC values are predictive of worse clinical outcomes in a range of different health conditions, including increased risk of mortality in critical illness, haemodialysis, HIV and tuberculosis infection and people aged ≥80 years [1].

2.3.8 Calf circumference

Calf circumference reflects fat-free mass and is related to physical function. As it is straightforward to measure, it provides a quick and useful assessment of nutritional and functional status although with some limitations.

Standard procedure for measuring calf circumference

A standard protocol for measuring calf circumference should be followed [36]. This requires a non-stretch tape to be placed snugly but without causing indentations around the widest circumference of the lower leg with the tape at 90° to the tibia bone. Although the measurement is typically made on the right leg with the participant seated, if this is not possible, the left leg or a supine position can be used [1]. The details of the measurement, that is, leg and position, should be recorded to allow consistent repeat measures to be made.

Interpreting calf circumference

Calf circumference measurements can be interpreted either by comparison with published reference data or by making repeat measurements. No international data are available so NHANES percentiles derived from USA adults aged 20–80+ years [33] are most commonly used. Data from older adults in Brazil, Ireland and Sweden are also available [37–39]. A calf circumference of <31 cm in women aged ≥70 years has been proposed as a cut-off indicating risk of functional impairment [1]. Interpretation of calf circumference measurements becomes difficult in the presence of peripheral oedema, which is commonly seen in older people, as changes in calf measurements are closely associated with fluid-related weight change [1] and, therefore, alternative assessment measures may be needed.

Predictive value of calf circumference

Low values of calf circumference in older people are associated with lower physical functioning, greater disability and mobility impairment and these values are better at predicting future need for care than BMI [40]. Conversely, higher values in community-living older adults are related to a lower risk of frailty [41]. However, in an acute hospital population aged ≥18 years, calf circumference is poorly associated with physical activity and handgrip strength and not predictive of length of hospital stay or 30-day readmission [42]. This indicates that calf circumference is a useful assessment measure in older people but more evidence is needed to support its use in adults in an acute hospital setting.

2.3.9 Bioelectrical impedance analysis

Fat-free mass and total body water can be assessed using bioelectrical impedance analysis (BIA) which utilises the principle that an electrical current is not conducted by lipid and passes only through fat-free tissue [43]. Portable devices which transmit and receive painless, low-amplitude currents at single or multiple frequencies are relatively inexpensive and straightforward to use for both participant and assessor. Multifrequency BIA allows the additional assessment of intra- and extracellular water.

Procedure for bioelectrical impedance analysis

Bioelectrical impedance analysis measurement techniques vary with different BIA devices. Older models require the participant to lie supine and four electrodes are attached to the hand, wrist, ankle and foot, or other limb segments, on one side of the body and then connected to the device. More recently developed devices transmit and receive current through metal plates which the participant either stands on with bare feet and/or grasps with their hands to allow whole-body measurements to be made in the

vertical position. Cheaper devices are available and aimed at personal use rather than clinical or research purposes but some, such as hand-to-hand models, provide less accurate results [44]. As measurements are influenced by body fluid, participants should be adequately hydrated before assessment, which should be undertaken after a period of rest and emptying the bladder [43]. The effect of body position, such as standing or supine, may influence intra- and extracellular water so should be recorded.

Interpreting bioelectrical impedance analysis results

Regression equations are used to derive fat-free mass from BIA raw data, that is, resistance and reactance, and these are usually computed within the device itself. Most regression equations have been developed in healthy, lean populations and often in those with specific age and ethnic demographics [43]. The accuracy of individual results, therefore, depends on the similarity between their characteristics and those of the population in which the equation was derived, with use of dissimilar equations resulting in systematically biased results. Reference values for fat-free mass derived from BIA are available for European populations [45,46] and, in comparison with these, measurements that are <5th percentile raise possible concern but are not necessarily indicative of depletion. In clinical populations, the added confounding effects of body fluid perturbation mean that fat-free mass derived using BIA may be significantly under- or overestimated, for example in patients with ascites, oedema or dehydration [43].

In order to reduce the errors introduced by regression equations, raw BIA data have been explored with interest focused on phase angle. Reference values for phase angle, derived in European and USA populations [47,48], are available and low values are associated with depletion but because studies vary, it is not possible to identify a single cut-off value that identifies undernutrition. It is, therefore, advisable to undertake repeat measurements and use falling phase angle values to identify patients with increasing clinical risk.

Predictive value of bioelectrical impedance analysis

There is no evidence in patient populations that fat-free mass index determined using single-frequency BIA is any better at predicting clinical outcomes, including mortality and length of stay, than anthropometry alone [43]. However, many studies have identified the prognostic value of phase angle in clinical populations including cancer, sepsis, cirrhosis, dialysis and pulmonary disease [49].

References

1. Madden AM, Smith S. Body composition and morphological assessment of nutritional status in adults: a review of anthropometric variables. *J Hum Nutr Diet* 2016; **29**: 7–25.
2. Byrd J, Langford A, Paden SJ, et al. Scale consistency study: how accurate are inpatient hospital scales? *Nursing* 2011; **41**: 21–24.
3. Morgan MY, Madden AM, Jennings G, Elia M, Fuller NJ. Two-component models are of limited value for the assessment of body composition in patients with cirrhosis. *Am J Clin Nutr* 2006; **84**: 1151–1162.
4. Chan C, Smith D, Spanel P, McIntyre CW, Davies SJ. A non-invasive, on-line deuterium dilution technique for the measurement of total body water in haemodialysis patients. *Nephrol Dial Transplant* 2008; **23**: 2064–2070.
5. Van Thiel DH, Moore CM, Garcia M, George M, Nadir A. Continuous peritoneal drainage of large-volume ascites. *Dig Dis Sci* 2011; **56**: 2723–2727.
6. Mendenhall CL. Protein-calorie malnutrition in alcoholic liver disease. In: Watson RR, Watzl B, editors. Nutrition and Alcohol. Florida: CRC Press, 1992, pp. 363–384.
7. Todorovic V, Russell C, Elia M. The MUST Explanatory Booklet. Redditch: BAPEN. www.bapen.org.uk/pdfs/must/must_explan.pdf (accessed 29 August 2017).
8. Connor Gorber S, Tremblay M, Moher D, Gorber B. A comparison of direct vs self-report measures for assessing height, weight and body mass index: a systematic review. *Obes Rev* 2007; **8**: 307–326.
9. Hendershot KM, Robinson L, Roland J, Vaziri K, Rizzo AG, Fakhry SM. Estimating height, weight and body mass index: implications for research and patient safety. *J Am Coll Surg* 2006; **203**: 887–893.
10. Kushner RF. Body weight and mortality. *Nutr Rev* 1993; **51**: 127–136.
11. Becker PJ, Nieman Carney L, Corkins MR, et al. Consensus statement of the Academy of Nutrition and Dietetics/American Society for Parenteral and Enteral Nutrition: indicators recommended for the identification and documentation of pediatric malnutrition (undernutrition). *J Acad Nutr Diet* 2015; **114**: 1988–2000.
12. Mueller C, Compher C, Ellen DM, American Society of Parenteral and Enteral Nutrition (ASPEN) Board of Directors. ASPEN clinical guidelines: nutrition screening, assessment and intervention in adults. *J Parenter Enteral Nutr* 2011; **35**: 16–24.
13. Campbell KL, MacLaughlin HL. Unintentional weight loss is an independent predictor of mortality in a hemodialysis population. *J Ren Nutr* 2010; **20**: 414–418.
14. Thirunavukarasu P, Sanghera S, Singla S, Attwood K, Nurkin S. Pre-operative unintentional weight loss as a risk factor for surgical outcomes after elective surgery in patients with disseminated cancer. *Int J Surg* 2015; **18**: 7–13.
15. Cederholm T, Bosaeus I, Barazzoni R, et al. Diagnostic criteria for malnutrition – an ESPEN consensus statement. *Clin Nutr* 2015; **34**: 335–340.
16. Rojer AG, Kruizenga HM, Trappenburg MC, et al. The prevalence of malnutrition according to the new ESPEN definition in four diverse populations. *Clin Nutr* 2016; **35**(3): 758–762.
17. Department of Health. National Diet and Nutrition Survey: Headline Results from Years 1, 2 and 3 (Combined) of the Rolling Programme 2008/9–2010/11. www.gov.uk/government/statistics/national-diet-and-nutrition-survey-headline-results-from-years-1-2-and-3-combined-of-the-rolling-programme-200809-201011 (accessed 29 August 2017).
18. Skipper A, Ferguson M, Thompson K, Castellanos VH, Porcari J. Nutrition screening tools: an analysis of the evidence. *J Parenter Enteral Nutr* 2012; **36**: 292–298.
19. World Health Organization. BMI Classification. www.euro.who.int/en/health-topics/disease-prevention/nutrition/a-healthy-lifestyle/body-mass-index-bmi (accessed 25 September 2017).
20. Glance LG, Li Y, Osler TM, Mukamel DB, Dick AW. Impact of obesity on mortality and complications in trauma patients. *Ann Surg* 2014; **259**: 576–581.
21. Sawalhi S, Al-Muramhy H, Abdelrahman AI, Allah SE, Al-Jubori S. Does the presence of obesity and/or metabolic syndrome affect the course of acute pancreatitis? A prospective study. *Pancreas* 2014; **43**: 565–570.
22. Skolarus LE, Sanchez BN, Levine DA, et al. Association of body mass index and mortality after acute ischemic stroke. *Circ Cardiovasc Qual Outcomes* 2014; **7**: 64–69.
23. Shah R, Gayat E, Januzzi JL, et al. Body mass index and mortality in acutely decompensated heart failure across the world: a global obesity paradox. *J Am Coll Cardiol* 2014; **63**: 778–785.

24. Bosy-Westphal A, Müller MJ. Identification of skeletal muscle mass depletion across age and BMI groups in health and disease-there is need for a unified definition. *Int J Obes* 2014; **39**: 379–386.

25. Schutz Y, Kyle UU, Pichard C. Fat-free mass index and fat mass index percentiles in Caucasians aged 18-98 y. *Int J Obes Relat Metab Disord* 2002; **26**: 953–960.

26. Ashwell M, Mayhew L, Richardson J, Rickayzen B. Waist-to-height ratio is more predictive of years of life lost than body mass index. *PLoS One* 2014; **9**: e103483.

27. Ashwell M, Gibson S. A proposal for a primary screening tool: 'keep your waist circumference to less than half your height'. *BMC Med* 2014; **12**: 207.

28. Centers for Disease Control and Prevention. National Health and Nutrition Examination Survey Anthropometry Procedures Manual. www.cdc.gov/nchs/data/nhanes/nhanes_13_14/2013_Anthropometry.pdf (accessed 29 August 2017).

29. De Hollander EL, Bemelmans WJ, de Groot LC. Associations between changes in anthropometric measures and mortality in old age: a role for mid-upper arm circumference? *J Am Med Dir Assoc* 2013; **14**: 187–193.

30. Centers for Disease Control and Prevention. National Health and Nutrition Examination Survey Anthropometry Procedures Manual. www.cdc.gov/nchs/data/nhanes/nhanes_09_10/BodyMeasures_09.pdf (accessed 29 August 2017).

31. Thuluvath PJ, Triger DR. How valid are our reference standards of nutrition? *Nutrition* 1995; **11**: 731–733.

32. Bishop CW, Bowen PE, Ritchey SJ. Norms for nutritional assessment of American adults by upper arm anthropometry. *Am J Clin Nutr* 1981; **34**: 2530–2539.

33. McDowell MA, Fryar CD, Ogden CL, Flegal KM. Anthropometric Reference Data for Children and Adults: United States, 2003–2006. www.cdc.gov/nchs/data/nhsr/nhsr010.pdf (accessed 29 August 2017).

34. Frisancho AR. Triceps skinfold and upper arm muscle size norms for assessment of nutritional status. *Am J Clin Nutr* 1974; **27**: 1052–1057.

35. Kuczmarski MF, Kuczmarski RJ, Najjer M. Descriptive anthropometric reference data for older Americans. *J Am Diet Assoc* 2000; **100**: 59–66.

36. Centers for Disease Control and Prevention. National Health and Nutrition Examination Survey Anthropometry and Physical Activity Monitor Procedures Manual. www.cdc.gov/nchs/data/nhanes/nhanes_05_06/BM.pdf (accessed 29 August 2017).

37. Silva Rodrigues RA, Martinez Espinosa M, Duarte Melo C, Rodrigues Perracini M, Rezende Fett WC, Fett CA. New values anthropometry for classification of nutritional status in the elderly. *J Nutr Health Aging* 2014; **18**: 655–661.

38. Corish CA, Kennedy NP. Anthropometric measurements from a cross sectional survey of Irish free living elderly subjects with smoothed centile curves. *Br J Nutr* 2003; **89**: 137–145.

39. Gavriilidou NN, Pihlsgård M, Elmståhl S. Anthropometric reference data for elderly Swedes and its disease-related pattern. *Eur J Clin Nutr* 2015; **69**: 1066–1075.

40. Hsu WC, Tsai AC, Wang JY. Calf circumference is more effective than body mass index in predicting emerging care-need of older adults – results of a national cohort study. *Clin Nutr* 2016; **35**(3): 735–740.

41. Landi F, Onder G, Russo A, et al. Calf circumference, frailty and physical performance among older adults living in the community. *Clin Nutr* 2014; **33**: 539–544.

42. Jeejeebhoy KN, Keller H, Gramlich L, et al. Nutritional assessment: comparison of clinical assessment and objective variables for the prediction of length of hospital stay and readmission. *Am J Clin Nutr* 2015; **101**: 956–965.

43. Smith S, Madden AM. Body composition and functional assessment of nutritional status in adults: a narrative review of imaging, impedance, strength and functional techniques. *J Hum Nutr Diet* 2016; **29**(6): 714–732.

44. Esco MR, Olson MS, Williford HN, Lizana SN, Russell AR. The accuracy of hand-to-hand bioelectrical impedance analysis in predicting body composition in college-age female athletes. *J Strength Cond Res* 2011; **25**: 1040–1045.

45. Pichard C, Kyle UG, Bracco D, Slosman DO, Morabia A, Schutz Y. Reference values of fat-free and fat masses by bioelectrical impedance analysis in 3393 healthy subjects. *Nutrition* 2000; **16**: 245–254.

46. Franssen FM, Rutten EP, Groenen MT, Vanfleteren LE, Wouters EF, Spruit MA. New reference values for body composition by bioelectrical impedance analysis in the general population: results from the UK Biobank. *J Am Med Dir Assoc* 2014; **15**: 448.e1–6.

47. Barbosa-Silva MC, Barros AJ, Wang J, Heymsfield SB, Pierson RN Jr. Bioelectrical impedance analysis: population reference values for phase angle by age and sex. *Am J Clin Nutr* 2005; **82**: 49–52.

48. Bosy-Westphal A, Danielzik S, Dörhöfer RP, Later W, Wiese S, Müller MJ. Phase angle from bioelectrical impedance analysis: population reference values by age, sex, and body mass index. *J Parenter Enteral Nutr* 2006; **30**: 309–316.

49. Grundmann O, Yoon SL, Williams JJ. The value of bioelectrical impedance analysis and phase angle in the evaluation of malnutrition and quality of life in cancer patients – a comprehensive review. *Eur J Clin Nutr* 2015; **69**(12): 1290–1297.

Chapter 2.4

Biochemical assessment in undernutrition

Alan Torrance
Royal Victoria Infirmary, Newcastle upon Tyne, UK

2.4.1 Introduction

The assessment of biochemical parameters is part of a series of investigations used in the assessment of nutritional status. It contributes to determining nutrient deficiency, adequacy and excess and in diagnosing nutrition-related factors relevant to causation and treatment of disease states. Regular re-evaluation (monitoring) is necessary to provide an accurate indication of disease progression and the adequacy of interventions [1]. Individual results taken in isolation are rarely of value and should be interpreted with caution. Laboratory tests are expensive to undertake and report and so should be selected carefully to yield useful results [2]. The type and frequency of tests will be based on the nature and severity of disease, the type of nutrition support being provided, results of previous tests and the setting where care is being provided (for example, primary or secondary care) and agreed local protocols. In general, the tests undertaken to monitor the provision of enteral or parenteral nutrition are the same.

2.4.2 Baseline biochemical tests

Sodium, potassium, urea and creatinine

Disorders of serum sodium concentrations (usually in association with water balance) commonly occur in clinical practice and result in the development of either hyponatraemia or hypernatraemia. In both conditions the additional measurement of urinary Na+ (mmol/L) can aid the diagnosis. The diagnosis and management of hyponatraemia should be considered by means of a structured protocol with consideration of the factors outlined in Box 2.4.1 [3–5].

Hypernatraemia, less common than hyponatraemia, is frequently encountered in the critical care setting. The usual cause is water loss, but the diagnosis should be confirmed following a similar approach to that of hyponatraemia with consideration of the factors outlined in Box 2.4.1 [3–5].

Hypokalaemia occurs with or without a K^+ deficit. Alkalosis or insulin excess are the usual causes. Poor dietary intake, for example in alcoholism or anorexia nervosa, increased cellular uptake, gastrointestinal (GI) loss (e.g. vomiting/diarrhoea) or increased urinary loss (urinary K^+ >20 mmol/L), usually as a result of mineralocorticoid excess, renal tubular acidosis or diuretic therapy, all occur in association with a K^+ deficit. Hyperkalaemia can occur in a wide range of clinical settings. The principal causes are outlined in Box 2.4.2 [6].

Serum urea concentration can increase post-surgically or as a result of trauma/stress due to the release of catabolic hormones such as adrenaline which enhance protein breakdown. If renal function is adequate, an increased urea load can be excreted. However, where there is renal impairment, urea (and creatinine) serum concentrations will rise. When urea increases without a concomitant rise in creatinine, the cause is

Box 2.4.1 Factors to consider in hyponatraemia and hypernatraemia

Hyponatraemia

A deficit of Na^+ and (predominantly) water, resulting in a reduced extracellular fluid volume (ECF). This is caused by renal losses such as those precipitated by diuretics, Addison's disease, excess sodium or bicarbonate excretion or ketonuria (urinary Na^+ >20) or extrarenal losses such as vomiting or diarrhoea (urinary Na^+ <20).

Excess body water, which has little effect on the ECF volume, is normally the result of endocrine factors, for example glucocorticoid deficiency, hypothyroidism, syndrome of inappropriate ADH secretion or pain/stress/drugs (urinary Na^+ >20).

Excess of Na^+ (predominantly) and water results in increased ECF volume due to nephrotic syndrome, cardiac failure, liver cirrhosis (urinary Na^+ <20) or acute kidney injury/chronic kidney disease (urinary Na^+ >20).

Hypernatraemia

Na^+ and water loss resulting in reduced total body sodium. This is caused by increased renal losses due to, for example, osmotic diuretics or raised serum glucose/urea concentrations (urinary Na^+ >20) or extrarenal losses, for example, excess sweating or diarrhoea (urinary Na^+ <20).

Water losses only, without affecting total body Na^+, via the kidneys as a result of, for example, central diabetes insipidus, nephrogenic diabetes insipidus or hypodipsia or extrarenal losses such as increased respiratory or skin water loss.

Note that for both cases, the urinary sodium concentration is likely to be variable.

Excess Na^+ intake/administration which over time increases the total body Na^+ concentration and is often due to endocrine factors such as primary hyperaldosteronism (Conn's syndrome), Cushing's disease or the intravenous infusion of sodium containing solutions such as $NaHCO_3$. In each case, the urinary sodium concentration will be >20 mmol/L.

Box 2.4.2 Principal causes of hyperkalaemia

'Pseudo-hyperkalaemia', for example, a haemolysed blood sample, thrombocytosis/leucocytosis.

Redistribution of K^+ between cells and plasma, for example, during acidosis, glucose loading (in diabetics) or the use of β-blockers (which prevent the entry of K^+ into cells).

K^+ excess due to reduced excretion of potassium, usually as a result of renal disease, the use of K^+-sparing diuretics, a mineralocorticoid deficiency such as Addison's disease or as excess dietary intake or cellular release of K^+ (e.g. haemolysis/rhabdomyolysis/burn injury).

usually dehydration. An increase in urea concentration of 6 mmol/day (or more) can suggest renal failure together with an increased level of catabolism. Raised urea concentrations can also be the result of a high-protein diet, tissue destruction, such as GI bleeding, severe infection, cellular necrosis, autoimmune disease or drugs such as corticosteroids. Reduced urea concentrations can occur as a result of a prolonged period of low protein intake, diabetes insipidus where there is an excessive fluid intake and consequent dilute urinary output. Since urea is synthesised in the liver, hepatic diseases such as hepatitis or cirrhosis may compromise urea synthesis and ultimately result in lower serum concentrations [7,8].

Serum creatinine concentration provides a direct and accurate indicator of renal function since creatinine is excreted by glomerular filtration and is produced at a constant rate so plasma concentrations are inversely proportional to the glomerular filtration rate. Serum creatinine concentrations will rise when renal function is impaired. Because creatinine is a byproduct of muscle metabolism, serum concentrations can depend on muscle mass, increasing where there is higher proportion of muscle tissue to body weight and falling where there is a reduced level. The influence of dietary intake on serum creatinine concentration is generally insignificant [9].

Serum albumin and C-reactive protein

Serum albumin, although used as a biochemical marker of nutrition status, is a poor indicator of nutrition status. Changes in serum albumin concentrations are frequently the result of over- and underhydration and liver disease. Hospital patients with low serum concentrations have an increased incidence of clinical complications and mortality, usually because they are more seriously ill, often with associated undernutrition. A low serum albumin concentration may identify an 'at-risk' patient who would benefit from a detailed assessment of their nutritional requirements. In the short term (1–2 weeks), low protein intakes result in reduced synthesis and catabolic rate of albumin with a concomitant reduction in the extravascular albumin concentration. This minimises the effect on serum albumin concentration. The rate of synthesis rapidly returns to normal when protein intake is increased to meet individual calculated requirements. Serum albumin is thus an unreliable marker of nutritional status [10,11].

Plasma C-reactive protein (CRP) is an acute phase protein whose plasma concentration increases in response to inflammation (of which it is a marker), usually due to the secretion of the cytokines interleukin (IL)-1, IL-6, IL-8 and TNF-α. CRP should be routinely measured at initial assessment, then 2–3 times weekly until stable [12]. It aids interpretation of protein, trace element and vitamin status and indicates the presence of an acute phase response, which is characterised by fever, leucocytosis, reduced serum iron and zinc concentrations and the mobilisation of amino acids from muscles, followed by their uptake by the liver for synthesis of acute phase proteins such as CRP itself. The incorporation of amino acids into plasma proteins may increase 2–10-fold during the acute phase response and the normal concentration of CRP (1 mg/L) may peak at 100–1000 times higher than basal concentrations (although in practice, values >500 mg/L are unusual). CRP has a short half-life (6 hours) and increases are apparent within 4–6 hours, peaking within 24–48 hours, thus making it a sensitive measure of the acute phase response [12].

Calcium, phosphate and magnesium

Hypocalcaemia in an acute clinical setting is often due to a low serum albumin concentration (approximately 40% of total plasma Ca^{++} is bound to albumin, and so decreases in serum albumin concentrations will directly affect total measured Ca^{++}). True hypocalcaemia is most frequently due to vitamin D deficiency (either dietary or as a result of malabsorption) or abnormal metabolism (e.g. renal impairment). Hypoparathyroidism can lead to hypocalcaemia but is uncommon. Associated hypomagnesaemia can precipitate hypocalcaemia by reducing parathyroid hormone (PTH) secretion and impairing the skeletal responsiveness to PTH [13]. The main causes of hypercalcaemia are primary hyperparathyroidism and malignant disease. Thiazide diuretic and vitamin D (and its analogues) therapy, endocrine and granulomatous disorders such as thyrotoxicosis and sarcoidosis respectively may also lead to hypercalcaemia. Where hypoalbuminaemia is present, most laboratories can provide an estimate of the 'corrected' serum Ca^{++} (adjusted Ca^{++}). This takes into account changes in ionised Ca^{++} induced by changes in pH (as well as any reduction in albumin). At a constant pH, total serum Ca^{++} falls by about 0.025 mmol/L for every 1 g/L drop in serum albumin below 40 g/L [14].

Hypophosphataemia can be the result of hyperparathyroidism, renal loss, alcoholism and cellular redistribution, for example during insulin/glucose administration or acute respiratory alkalosis. Inadequate intake is a common cause in clinical settings, often as a result of insufficient provision of phosphate during nutrition support, especially where parenteral nutrition is being used [15]. Hyperphosphataemia is most commonly due to renal impairment. Excess PO_4^{--} concentrations can interfere with vitamin D metabolism and combine with Ca^{++} to form insoluble precipitates of calcium phosphate leading to subsequent hypocalcaemia [16].

Hypomagnesaemia is normally the result of diuretic therapy, chronic alcoholism and cirrhosis, reduced intake or reduced intestinal absorption, for example due to malabsorption or

Table 2.4.1 Other biochemical parameters used in the assessment of a patient for nutrition support [1]

Parameter	Frequency	Comment
Plasma glucose	At initial assessment, 4–6 hourly until stable then 1–2 times weekly	Hyperglycaemia common in PN and poorly managed EN. Glycaemic control advised to avoid morbidity [18,19]. Lab analysis or hand-held glucometers at ward level or at home
Full blood count (red, white blood cells and platelets)	At initial assessment then 1–2 times weekly until stable	In particular, monitor haemoglobin and white cell count. Anaemia due to iron or folate deficiency common. Likely to be affected by sepsis
Selenium	If considered at risk of depletion (<1 μmol/L) at initial assessment then every 2–4 weeks	Deficiency likely in severe illness and sepsis and long-term nutrition support. Acute phase response lowers serum concentrations
Zinc and copper	If considered at risk of depletion (<9 μmol/L and <11 μmol/L respectively) at initial assessment then every 2–4 weeks	Deficiency is common with increased losses. Acute phase response lowers zinc and raises copper concentration [1,20]
Iron and ferritin	If considered at risk of depletion (<10 μmol/L and <25 μmol/L respectively) at initial assessment otherwise every 3–6 months if long-term nutrition support is being administered	Acute phase response lowers iron and raises ferritin concentrations [1,20]
Folate and vitamin B12	Folate deficiency (<5 nmol/L) is common and so should be considered for assessment purposes within 1–2 weeks	Often included as part of full blood count [1,20]
Manganese and vitamin D	Every 3–6 months where long-term nutrition support is being administered, e.g. home PN	Excess provision of manganese should be avoided, particularly in liver disease [1,20]

EN, enteral nutrition; PN, parenteral nutrition.

small bowel resection [17]. Hypermagnesaemia principally occurs in renal impairment – acute kidney injury or chronic kidney disease [17].

There are a number of other parameters (Table 2.4.1) which can influence nutritional status, either directly or indirectly, and may form part of the overall assessment process. The frequency and extent of these measurements will be dependent on individual patient circumstances or disease states.

2.4.3 Biochemical interpretation and application

Dehydration

Dehydration occurs as a result of body (cellular) water loss which is usually associated with a raised serum sodium concentration and can result in volume depletion (loss of water as well as other osmolytes such as electrolytes, glucose and urea).

Box 2.4.3 Calculation of water deficit

Method 1

$$\text{Water deficit} = \text{normal}(\text{or previous})\,\text{total body water} \times \left(1 - \frac{\text{actual serum Na}^+}{\text{desired serum Na}^+}\right)$$

Example: body weight 70 kg, actual serum Na$^+$ = 160 mmol/L, desired serum Na$^+$ = 140 mmol/L
Assuming 60% total body weight is water:

$$70 \times 0.6 = 42\,\text{L}$$

Then,

$$42 \times \left(1 - \frac{160}{140}\right) = -6\,\text{L}$$

Method 2
Administration of 3–4 mL/kg of electrolyte free water lowers serum sodium by approximately 1 mmol/L

$$\text{Water deficit} = \text{weight}(\text{kg}) \times \text{mL required}(3 - 4\,\text{mL}) \times (\text{difference between actual and desired serum Na}^+)$$

Example: if 4 mL/kg is administered to a 70 kg person to reduce serum Na$^+$ from 160 to 140 mmol/L:

$$\text{Water deficit} = 70 \times 4 \times -20 = -5600\,\text{mL or} -5.6\,\text{L}$$

As volume contraction develops, further sodium and water losses occur from the extracellular fluid and more pronounced changes in blood pressure and pulse rate occur. In practice, it is difficult to distinguish between dehydration and volume depletion and as a result, the terms are often used interchangeably, but treatment of the two conditions differs [21].

Dehydration should be treated with free (pure) water if the patient is able to take fluids orally or with 5% glucose (dextrose) intravenously. Where the serum sodium is excessively raised (>160 mmol/L), the aim should be to lower this by no more than 6–8 mmol/L/day. In order to achieve this, the water deficit (the amount of water to be replaced) needs to be estimated. This can be calculated in two different ways (Box 2.4.3) [22]. Volume depletion should be treated with isotonic (normal) saline (0.9%) to expand the intravascular volume. Fluid replacement is administered more rapidly, for example 150–200 mL/h to improve blood pressure and glomerular filtration rate [21].

Overhydration

Overhydration or hypervolaemia occurs as a result of excess accumulation of isotonic fluid (water and sodium) in the interstitial and intravascular compartments (Box 2.4.4). In the initial stages of overhydration, serum osmolality usually remains within a normal range because fluids and solutes are assimilated in equal proportions. If overhydration is prolonged, severe water intoxication can occur (where excess fluid moves from the extracellular to intracellular fluid compartment). Hypervolaemia can also result due to acute kidney injury or chronic kidney disease (with reduced urine output), nephrotic syndrome, heart failure and liver cirrhosis. Peripheral oedema is the main clinical symptom (usually in association with hyponatraemia). Pulmonary oedema may also be present. Treatment focuses on restriction of fluid and sodium intake and drug administration to resolve any pre-existing complications such as heart failure (digoxin) and pulmonary oedema (morphine and glyceryl trinitrate). The cause of the overhydration should also be addressed [23]. In cases of renal failure, renal replacement therapy (RRT) may be required. Generally, in adults, fluid is restricted to 1 L/24 h but is best determined on the basis of a 24-hour urine output measurement. A negative fluid balance of 500 mL raises the serum sodium concentration by 1 mmol/L.

Box 2.4.4 Calculation of water excess

Water excess (and therefore the fluid volume deficit to be attained) can be estimated using the following formula:

$$\text{Water excess} = \text{normal (or previous) total body water} \times \left(1 - \frac{\text{actual serum Na}^+}{\text{desired serum Na}^+}\right)$$

Example: body weight 70 kg, actual serum $Na^+ = 125$ mmol/L, desired serum $Na^+ = 140$ mmol/L
Assuming 60% total body weight is water:

$$70 \times 0.6 = 42\,L$$

Then

$$42 \times \left(1 - \frac{125}{140}\right) = 4.5\,L$$

Systemic inflammatory response and sepsis

Systemic inflammatory response syndrome (SIRS), sepsis and septic shock are common complications in postsurgical and critically ill patients. The definitions for these conditions have recently been reviewed and are outlined in Table 2.4.2 [24].

The systemic inflammatory response syndrome is characterised by a host inflammatory response in organs remote from the initial insult. The inflammatory response involves the activation of leucocytes and endothelial cells with a concurrent release of inflammatory mediators and (toxic) oxygen free radicals from both intracellular and extracellular fluid compartments. In turn, abnormalities occur in tissue perfusion and tissue hypoxia that ultimately lead to

Table 2.4.2 Definition of systemic inflammatory response syndrome (SIRS), sepsis, severe sepsis and septic shock [24]

SIRS	The presence of two or more of the following: abnormal body temperature, increased respiratory rate, change in level of consciousness, low blood pressure
Sepsis	SIRS in response to an infective process
Severe sepsis	Sepsis with sepsis-induced organ dysfunction or tissue hypoperfusion (presenting as hypotension, raised serum lactate or decreased urine output)
Septic shock	Severe sepsis in addition to persistently low blood pressure despite administration of intravenous fluids

---

Box 2.4.5 Key features of SIRS and sepsis

- Raised lactate >2 mmol/L – inadequate cellular oxygenation results in anaerobic metabolism and increased lactate concentration. The severity and duration of hyperlactaemia are both predictive of morbidity and mortality and appropriate management of lactate concentration is effective in improving clinical outcomes.
- Urine output <0.5 mL/kg/h for more than 2–3 hours despite adequate fluid administration.
- Arterial base deficit reflects tissue acidosis (>–2 to –4 mmol/L) which can be useful to assess the severity of shock usually associated with low bicarbonate concentration (<20 mmol/L).
- Measurements of central (via a central venous catheter) or mixed (via a pulmonary artery catheter) oxygen saturation assess the balance of oxygen delivery, consumption and extraction and act as a predictor of mortality. The greater the oxygen requirement, the more acutely ill a patient is.
- Raised creatinine >175 μmol/L.
- Bilirubin >35 μmol/L.
- Platelet count $<100 \times 10^9$/L.
- Coagulopathy (international normalised ratio >1.5)

1. Identify 'at-risk' patients

Patient has one of the following:

- BMI <16 kg/m^2
- Unintentional weight loss >15% within last 3–6 months
- Negligible or no nutritional intake for >7–10 days
- Low serum concentrations of phosphate or magnesium prior to feeding

OR has two or more of the following:

- BMI <18.5 kg/m^2
- Unintentional weight loss of >10% within last 3–6 months
- Negligible or no nutritional intake for >5–10 days
- Drugs including insulin, chemotherapy, antacids or diuretics, history of alcohol excess
- Low serum potassium

2. Initiate treatment

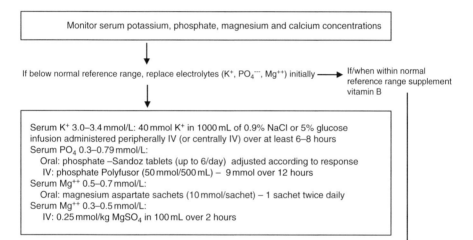

Monitor serum potassium, phosphate, magnesium and calcium concentrations

If below normal reference range, replace electrolytes (K$^+$, PO$_4$$^{---}$, Mg^{++}) initially ⟶ If/when within normal reference range supplement vitamin B

Serum K$^+$ 3.0–3.4 mmol/L: 40 mmol K$^+$ in 1000 mL of 0.9% NaCl or 5% glucose infusion administered peripherally IV (or centrally IV) over at least 6–8 hours
Serum PO$_4$ 0.3–0.79 mmol/L:
   Oral: phosphate –Sandoz tablets (up to 6/day) adjusted according to response
   IV: phosphate Polyfusor (50 mmol/500 mL) – 9 mmol over 12 hours
Serum Mg^{++} 0.5–0.7 mmol/L:
   Oral: magnesium aspartate sachets (10 mmol/sachet) – 1 sachet twice daily
Serum Mg^{++} 0.3–0.5 mmol/L:
   IV: 0.25 mmol/kg MgSO$_4$ in 100 mL over 2 hours

For oral and enterally fed patients, prior to and for 10 days after commencing feeding, give thiamine 100 mg twice daily and vitamin B co strong – 1 tablet three times a day + a standard multivitamin supplement (once daily) (dispersible/soluble versions are available for tube feeding).
For IV infusion: Pabrinex® 1 pair of ampoules numbers 1 & 2 daily for 72 hours (dilute in 100 mL 5% glucose or isotonic saline 0.9% and give over 30 minutes).

Commence feeding/diet immediately, initially at 10 mL/kg/24 h and increase in 5–10 kcal/kg/24 h increments over 1–2 days until an energy level of 30 kcal/kg/24 h is achieved (usually within 7 days).

Monitor serum glucose, potassium, phosphate, magnesium and calcium daily until stable, then twice weekly and correct any deficiencies or excesses as necessary.

3. Assessment
Accurate food/feed intake records and fluid balance charts should be completed and a detailed dietetic assessment carried out (where available) to advise on ongoing management.

4. Step-down
When full nutritional requirements are being provided and a patient's serum electrolyte concentrations have normalised and are stable, the refeeding protocol can be discontinued. This should be a multidisciplinary decision and documented in the medical case notes. If at any point a patient meets the refeeding criteria again, they should be treated as a new patient and the treatment process (as outlined above) repeated.

Figure 2.4.1 Protocol for the avoidance of the refeeding syndrome in patients on enteral or parenteral nutrition (adults only). Source: Newcastle upon Tyne Hospitals NHS Trust (2012), modified with permission

necrosis, multiorgan failure and eventual death if not corrected (Box 2.4.5 outlines the key features of SIRS and sepsis). Disturbances in liver function and blood clotting are also common features [25].

Initial haematological and biochemical testing aims to locate the source of infection and identify evidence of organ dysfunction. It is usual to include a whole blood count, specifically haemoglobin, haematocrit, platelets and white blood cell subtypes. Standard biochemical measurements should normally include serum electrolytes, bicarbonate (HCO_3^-), creatinine and glucose, liver enzymes and either arterial (or venous) blood gas analysis and serum lactate.

Sepsis occurs when micro-organisms (such as Gram-negative and Gram-positive aerobes, anaerobes, fungi and viruses) invade the body and initiate a systemic inflammatory response. This host response frequently leads to perfusion abnormalities with associated organ dysfunction (severe sepsis) and eventually hypotension as a result of vasodilation secondary to the release of inflammatory mediators such as endotoxins, tissue necrosis factor and IL-6 (septic shock) [26]. Gram-positive organisms are the predominant cause of sepsis, with the respiratory system being the most common site of infection. Cardiovascular function is often compromised and management involves a careful balance of vasoconstriction and fluid resuscitation [27,28]. Additionally, it is common for patients with septic shock to develop deficiencies in potassium, phosphate and magnesium as a consequence of increases in resting energy expenditure, protein turnover rate and fluid requirements and these should be corrected based on individual clinical assessment.

Refeeding syndrome

Refeeding syndrome is a potentially serious (but avoidable) complication of nutrition support, particularly in at-risk patients receiving enteral nutrition or parenteral nutrition. The prevalence of refeeding syndrome is reported as being in the region of 2% of hospital patients commenced on artificial nutrition support, but any patient who has been nil by mouth or given hypocaloric feeding for periods >5 days may be at risk [29–31].

Refeeding syndrome occurs when nutrients are administered disproportionately during the repletion of malnourished patients, leading to a sudden rise in serum insulin concentrations. This in turn can result in the rapid movement of phosphate, potassium and magnesium from the extracellular to intracellular fluid compartments as well as the possibility of glucose intolerance, abnormalities in liver function and hyper- or hypocalcaemia. Additionally, there is often fluid retention, reduction in salt and water excretion and a risk of thiamine deficiency [1,32–34]. Complications include delirium, central pontine myelinosis, axonal polyneuropathy and respiratory failure, which are largely mediated through the severe and sudden onset of hypophosphataemia. Cardiac sequelae are common as a result of hypokalaemia and hypomagnesaemia. Biochemical monitoring should include daily assessment of serum potassium, calcium, phosphate and magnesium concentrations in addition to the recording of accurate daily fluid balance [1,35].

An example of a refeeding syndrome management protocol is provided in Figure 2.4.1.

2.4.4 Summary

Biochemical assessment is an essential component of the assessment and management of all patients receiving nutrition support. With practice and experience, the most appropriate tests (and their interpretation) can be confidently selected. The basis for this is best achieved through a multidisciplinary approach to determine relevant protocols which in turn are likely to facilitate the best patient care outcomes.

References

1. National Institute for Clinical Excellence. Nutrition Support in Adults: Oral Nutrition Support, Enteral Tube Feeding and Parenteral Nutrition. NICE Clinical Guideline No. 32. London: NICE, 2006.
2. Gidden F, Shenkin A. Laboratory support of the clinical nutrition service. *Clin Chem Lab Med* 2000; **38**(8): 693–714.
3. Overgaard-Steensen C, Ring T. Clinical review: practical approach to hyponatraemia and hypernatraemia in critically ill patients. *Crit Care* 2013; **17**(1): 206–220.

4. Bagshaw SM, Townsend DR, McDermid RC. Disorders of sodium and water balance in hospitalized patients. *Can J Anaesth* 2009; **56**(2): 151–167.

5. Stelfox HT, Ahmed SB, Khandwala F, Zygan D, Shahpori R, Laupland K. The epidemiology of intensive care unit – acquired hyponatraemia and hypernatraemia in medical-surgical intensive care units. *Crit Care* 2008; **12**(6): R162.

6. Lehnhardt A, Kemper MJ. Pathogenesis, diagnosis and management of hyperkalemia. *Pediatr Nephrol* 2011; **26**(3): 377–384.

7. Beier K, Eppanapally S, Bazick HS, et al. Elevation of blood urea nitrogen is predictive of long Term mortality in critically ill patients independent of 'normal' creatinine. *Crit Care Med* 2011; **39**: 305–313.

8. Meyer TW, Hotstetter TH. Uremia. *N Engl J Med* 2007; **357**(13): 1316–1325.

9. Stark J. Interpretation of BUN and serum creatinine. An interactive exercise. *Crit Care Nurs Clin North Am* 1998; **10**(4): 491–496.

10. Alp Ikizler T. The use and misuse of serum albumin as a nutritional marker in kidney disease. *Clin J Am Soc Nephrol* 2012; **7**: 1375–1377.

11. Banh L. Serum proteins as markers of nutrition: what are we testing? *Pract Gastroenterol* 2006; 46–64.

12. Jain S, Gautam V, Naseem S. Acute-phase proteins: as diagnostic tool. *J Pharm Bioallied Sci* 2011; **3**(1): 118–127.

13. Cooper MS, Gittoes NJL. Diagnosis and management of hypocalcaemia. *BMJ* 2008; **336**: 1298–1302.

14. Maier JD, Levine SN. Hypercalcemia in the intensive care unit: a review of pathophysiology, diagnosis and modern therapy. *J Intens Care Med* 2015; **30**(5): 235–252.

15. Amanzadeh J, Reilly RF. Hypophosphatemia: an evidence-based approach to its clinical consequences and management. *Nat Clin Pract Nephrol* 2006; **2**(3): 136–148.

16. Hruska KA, Mathew S, Lund R, Qiu P, Pratt R. Hyperphosphatemia of chronic kidney disease. *Kidney Int* 2008; **74**(2): 148–157.

17. Swaminathan R. Magnesium and its disorders. *Clin Biochem Rev* 2003; **24**(2): 47–66.

18. Niven DJ, Rubenfeld GD, Kramer AA, Stelfox MD. Effect of published scientific evidence on glycaemic control in adult intensive care units. *JAMA Intern Med* 2015; **175**(5): 801–809.

19. Gardner AJ. The benefits of tight glycaemic control in critical illness: sweeter than assumed? *Indian J Crit Care Med* 2014; **18**(12): 807–813.

20. National Institute for Clinical Excellence. Monitoring Nutrition Support: Nutrition Support in Adults Pathway. London: NICE, 2016.

21. Bhave G, Neilson EG. Volume depletion versus dehydration: how understanding the difference can guide therapy. *Am J Kidney Disease* 2011; **58**(2): 302–309.

22. Sterns RH, Silver SM. Salt and water: read the package insert. *QJM* 2003; **96**: 549–552.

23. Spasovski G, Vanholder R, Allolio B, et al. Clinical practice guideline on diagnosis and treatment of hyponatraemia. *Eur J Endocrinol* 2014; **170**: G1–G47.

24. Singer M, Deutschman CS, Seymour CW, et al. The third international consensus definitions for sepsis and septic shock (sepsis-3). *JAMA* 2016; **315**(8): 801–810.

25. Kleinpell R, Aitken L, Schorr CA. Implications of the new international sepsis guidelines for nursing care. *Am J Crit Care* 2013; **22**(3): 212–222.

26. Duque GA, Descoteaux A. Macrophage cytokines: involvement in immunity and infectious disease. *Front Immunol* 2014; **5**(491): 1–12.

27. Dellinger RP, Levy MM, Rhodes A, et al. Surviving sepsis campaign: international guidelines for management of severe sepsis and septic shock. *Crit Care Med* 2013; **41**(2): 580–637.

28. Schmidt GA, Mandel J. Evaluation and management of severe sepsis and septic shock in adults. www.uptodate.com/contents/evaluation-and-management-of-suspected-sepsis-and-septic-shock-in-adults (accessed 29 August 2017).

29. Rio A, Whelan K, Goff L, Reidlinger DP, Smeeton N. Occurrence of refeeding syndrome in adults started on artificial nutrition support: prospective cohort study. *BMJ Open* 2013; **3**: e002173.

30. Husein B, Iqbal J, Mohammed A, Shorrock C. Too much, too soon. *Gut* 2009; **58**(12): 1575.

31. Mehanna M, Hankivell PC, Moledina J, Travis J. Refeeding syndrome: awareness, prevention and management. *Head Neck Oncol* 2009; **26**(1): 1–5.

32. Presier JC, van Zanten ARH, Berger MM, et al. Metabolic and nutritional support of critically ill patients: consensus and controversies. *Crit Care* 2015; **19**(35): 1–11.

33. Doig GS, Simpson F, Heighes PT, et al. Refeeding syndrome trial investigators group 2015. Restricted versus continued standard caloric intake during the management of refeeding syndrome in critically ill adults: a randomised, parallel-group, multicentre, single-blind controlled trial. *Lancet Respir Med* 2015; **3**(12): 943–952.

34. Coutaz M, Gay N. Refeeding syndrome: unrecognised in geriatric medicine. *JAMDA* 2014; **15**(11): 848–849.

35. Bankhead R, Boullata J, Brantley S, et al. ASPEN enteral nutrition practice recommendations. *J Parenter Enteral Nutr* 2009; **33**: 122–167.

Chapter 2.5

Clinical assessment of undernutrition

Mary Krystofiak Russell
Baxter Healthcare Corporation, Deerfield, USA

2.5.1 Introduction

Anthropometry, biochemistry and dietary intake are common components included in the nutritional assessment of a patient at risk of undernutrition. However, clinical assessment that covers both the effect of undernutrition on a person's ability to function (i.e. functional assessment) and the presence and severity of clinical features likely to exacerbate undernutrition (clinical status assessment) is also important, but often overlooked.

2.5.2 Functional assessment of nutritional status

Functional assessment has been a critical, if arguably underappreciated, part of nutrition assessment for decades [1]. Understanding of the components of functional assessment has recaptured the attention of the nutrition community, as a consequence of several pivotal papers published over the last few years [2–4].

Assessment of physical function is critical as reductions in function are associated with reduced quality of life, increased healthcare costs and increased risk of falls, fractures and depression [5]. Tomey and Sowers note that several authors have commented: '*the degree to which individuals can and do deal with diminished abilities and environmental challenges determines how well they function in their real-life setting*' [5]. Physical function is closely linked to muscle strength and low muscle strength is known to increase mobility limitations and mortality [6]. Thus both sarcopenia (loss of muscle tissue with ageing) and dynapenia (age-associated loss of muscle strength not caused by neurological or muscular diseases) predispose individuals to functional limitations and mortality [6].

Where interventions such as oral nutrition supplements or enteral nutrition are initiated, the effect of these on the ability of the patient to function is of great importance and therefore should be routinely measured where possible. A number of approaches to functional assessment have been described in the literature, some of which are applicable to the hospital setting, although none of these lend themselves to use in the intensive care environment. The most commonly used functional assessment tools are discussed below.

Handgrip strength

Handgrip strength (HGS) is a surrogate measure of voluntary muscle strength and is increasingly employed as an outcome variable in nutrition intervention studies [3]. HGS correlates well with measures of muscle function such as peak forced expiratory volume and knee extensor strength. HGS alone does not take into account the full spectrum of functional status including lower body strength, activities of daily living (ADLs) and/or walking speed [3]. It has, however, been suggested that, in healthy individuals,

Advanced Nutrition and Dietetics in Nutrition Support, First Edition. Edited by Mary Hickson and Sara Smith.
© 2018 John Wiley & Sons Ltd. Published 2018 by John Wiley & Sons Ltd.

HGS and knee extensor strength share a common construct and either could be used to determine muscle strength [3].

At present, there is a lack of consensus on specific protocols used to assess HGS and an absence of proposed and validated cut-off values to assess differing levels of function. A typical protocol for measuring HGS is to measure hand-grip strength on the non-dominant hand with a Jamar dynamometer (Sammons Preston Rolyan, Chicago,USA) [7]. Patients perform the test while sitting comfortably with shoulder adducted and forearm neutrally rotated, elbow flexed to 90° and forearm and wrist in neutral position. Patients are instructed to perform a maximal isometric contraction which is repeated within 30 seconds, with the highest value of three tests used for the analysis [7]. However, other protocols have utilised a different approach where HGS (measured using a Jamar dynamometer; model BK-7498, Fred Sammons Inc., Brookfield, IL) has been measured in a supine position on the dominant hand with patients being encouraged to exhibit the greatest possible force and the best value of three assessments of the dominant hand used for analysis [8]. The assessment of grip strength using a hand-held dynamometer has been shown to be reliable and valid among hospitalised older patients, with no difference between the sitting and supine positions [8].

Reference values by Bohannon et al. [9] have commonly been used to characterise grip strength. However, practitioners must review the reference values used and confirm their applicability to the target population. In various studies, HGS <85% of the standard value has been correlated with 87% of predicted complications of abdominal surgery, 74% of complications of general surgery and significantly greater postoperative complications of oral and maxillofacial cancer surgery. In elderly patients, grip strength <10 kg has been correlated with greater odds of discharge to home and death within 30 days of discharge in elderly individuals with pneumonia. In epidemiological studies, the lowest tertile of HGS has been shown to predict increased risk of functional limitations and disability in healthy men aged 45–68 years, among other findings [3].

Whilst the Jamar dynamometer is considered by the American Society of Hand Therapists as the 'gold standard' [10], it may not be ideal for use in some individuals who are older or frail [11]. The Takei (Takei Scientific Instruments, Tokyo Japan) or pneumatic squeeze dynamometers may therefore be more suitable for use with these populations [12].

Chair stand (sit to stand) test

The sit to stand test is designed to test lower extremity strength, transitional movements and balance and fall risk. There are several variations of the test, such as the 30-second sit to stand and the 60-second sit to stand. In both versions, the person is directed to cross arms across the chest, then rise from a seated position in a chair and return to a seated position, repeating as quickly as possible for 30 seconds. The test scores can be compared with test-specific and age-specific norms (25th to 75th centiles) expressed as the total number of stands [13–15]. Values lower than the 25th centile are considered to predict a higher risk of falls. The five time sit to stand test is another variation, suited to older adults, where individuals are asked to sit in a chair and cross arms across the chest, then stand up straight five times, as quickly as possible, without stopping in between. The time taken to complete five sit to stands is recorded. Currently, there appears to be no significant evidence that this test correlates specifically with nutritional status.

Timed up and go test

The Timed up and go (TUG) test was initially intended to assess fall risk and measure of function in older persons; its use has been expanded to include individuals with Parkinson's disease, hip fracture, multiple sclerosis and dementia, among other indications [15]. The person is seated and, upon the command of the tester, is asked to rise from the chair, walk 3 metres, return to the chair and be seated again. The process is timed and the time compared to reference data. The individual is allowed to use an assistive device (with documentation of the device used) and a practice round is allowed prior to the official test.

Typical values for the TUG test, as reported in a meta-analysis of 21 diverse studies for various age groupings (expressed as mean measurement in seconds), are [16]:

- 60–69 years: 8.1 seconds
- 70–79 years: 9.2 seconds
- 80–99 years: 11.3 seconds.

Currently, data specifically correlating the results of TUG tests to nutritional status do not appear to exist, although it would be reasonable to assume that a better nourished, healthier individual without physical limitations would perform better at any age than someone who is less well nourished and/or physically challenged.

Walking/gait speed assessment

A walking/gait speed assessment is a simple and increasingly recognised indicator of functional status in older adults. Walking requires some co-ordination and energy expenditure and slower gait speed indicates reduced energy availability and impairments in the integration of body systems [17]. Reduced gait speed has been shown to predict risk of falling, future health status and hospitalisation [10,17,18]. A change in gait speed has been suggested as a useful outcome measure for assessing effect of various clinical and nutrition interventions [10]. It has also been used to assess function in individuals in the late stage following a stroke and in individuals with chronic obstructive pulmonary disease [11]. The assessment may be incorporated into the timed up and go test; the measurement is the time that the person takes to walk the distance, independently of rising from the chair and being seated.

The walking speed/gait assessment test procedure suffers from the same challenges as other functional assessment tests, including lack of comprehensive reference ranges/'cut-off' points for individuals of specific ages (rather than within an age range) and/or who are ethnically diverse. Reference ranges are typically cited in metres/second for individuals and range from 1.36 for males of 20–29 years to 0.56 for females of 80–99 years [10].

Stair climb test

The stair climb test is one of a battery of tests used to assess not only the outcomes of individuals in studies of nutritional status but also the clinical status of people with osteoarthritis [19,20]. Variations of this test include a timed (in seconds) ascent with or without descent of a number of stairs ranging from five to 27. Values obtained increase with age and are also affected by any physical issues. Normative values are insufficient for any group, except possibly those over 65, per the comprehensive systematic review of Nightingale et al. [20]. Dobson et al. [19] offer a highly detailed assessment of recommended performance tests to assess physical function in individuals with osteoarthritis; the paper is a useful reference for discussion of many physical function tests.

Self-reporting questionnaires of physical function

Physical function assessment may be carried out directly (with observation of an individual performing specific physical activities) or indirectly, via use of a questionnaire or diary. Prince et al. conducted a systematic review of the value of direct versus self-report measures [21]. The purpose of the review was to determine the extent of agreement between subjectively (questionnaire reports) and objectively (direct performance measures, such as those described) assessed physical activities in adults. The review suggested that correlations between self-reported and direct measures were low to moderate, with no clear differentiation between objective/performance measures and subjective/self-reported measures of physical activity. More than one-third of the studies reviewed had lower quality scores. The authors called for valid, accurate and reliable measures of physical activity for several important reasons, including the important relationships between physical activity and health outcomes [21]. Other studies [22] have also found differences between subjective/self-report and objective/performance measures, with disability and mental health playing important roles in

Table 2.5.1 Summary of common quality of life and functional measurement tools

Measurement tool	Remarks
Katz Index of Activities of Daily Living [24]	Assesses a person's ability to perform six activities: toileting, eating, bathing, dressing, continence and transferring. A score of 6 suggests independence and 0 suggests total dependence. This index is sensitive to declines in health status but is not useful for assessing small, incremental changes
Lawton Instrumental Activities of Daily Living Scale [25]	Used to assess an individual's current independent living skills. After an initial evaluation, the tool may be repeatedly used to assess deterioration or improvements in function following interventions and/or the passage of time. This tool includes eight assessments with graded scale characteristics within each, and evaluates tasks such as ability to prepare food, do laundry, drive, take medications and handle finances [25]. An individual receives a score of 1 for most items for which he or she demonstrates minimal level competence at least. Total score ranges from 0 to 8, with a lower score associated with a higher level of dependence. There is no direct correlation of this score to nutritional status
Barthel Index [26]	Similar to the Lawton Scale, this measures a person's ability to function, in particular the activities of daily living (ADL) and mobility [26]. The 10 items assessed are feeding, transfers from bed to wheelchair and to and from a toilet, grooming, walking on a level surface, going up and down stairs, dressing, continence of bowels and bladder. The criteria are assessed based on the individual's ability to accomplish them independently, with assistance, or not at all (depending on the specific criterion). This index may also be used to determine a baseline level of functioning and to monitor improvements in ability to perform ADLs over time. It is not specifically correlated with nutritional status
Medical Outcomes Scale SF-36 [27]	Constructed to survey both quality of life and health status across eight health concepts, including limitation in social and 'usual role' activities, bodily pain, mental health, vitality and general health perceptions. Individuals are asked to rate these various perceptions over the previous week, on a Likert scale. The tool has been widely used and is noted to have excellent psychometric validity
EQ-5D [28]	A 'preference-based' measure of health in which 'full health' is rated at 1 and death at 0. These measures are used to calculate quality-adjusted life-years (QALYS) and often are used to complement data from clinical trials to assess the perceived value of one or more healthcare interventions. The EQ-5D assesses five dimensions of life: mobility, usual activities, self-care, pain/discomfort and anxiety/depression. Each has three levels (no problems, some problems, unable or extremely) and overall defines 243 separate 'health states'. It may be used as a generic measure of health and has a valuable economic evaluation component; it is not correlated specifically to measures of nutritional status [29]

the differentiation [23]. This suggests that the most effective evaluation will probably be a combination of both approaches.

Quality of life and functional assessment

There are a number of questionnaires that aim to assess quality of life and functional status and

a summary of commonly used tools is provided in Table 2.5.1.

2.5.3 Clinical status

Disease can have a significant impact on the nutritional status of a patient, affecting nutritional requirements (e.g. hypermetabolism), nutritional intake (e.g. disease-related anorexia) and nutritional losses (e.g. malabsorption). Therefore, determining the presence and severity of disease is essential.

Clinical status scoring tools

Clinical scoring tools are often used in inpatient and outpatient settings to aid in clinical decision making, classify disease or severity and predict outcomes. These serve as a guide for the clinician in assessing the severity of the disease or condition which indirectly leads to a decision about need for nutrition intervention. Selected examples of tools are provided in Table 2.5.2 using examples that can be applied generically (e.g. MMSE) and those that are specific to a particular disorder (e.g. Child–Pugh, CDAI). It is imperative to consult a comprehensive reference document (preferably the primary literature) to fully understand the breadth of scoring tools available and their complexity.

In addition to clinical scoring tools, nutrition-focused physical assessment of a patient or client is a critical part of any nutrition evaluation. This comprehensive assessment includes many evaluations which go beyond the scope of this chapter. Two important components, assessment of gastrointestinal tract function as it relates to stool output, and pressure ulcer risk evaluation, will be discussed here.

Gastrointestinal function

The assessment and monitoring of gastrointestinal (GI) function is a key component of any nutrition support regimen. Medications, inactivity, disease states and procedures, among many others, affect GI tract motility. The clinician must look for and follow progression of signs and symptoms such as unintentional weight loss, nausea, vomiting, diarrhoea, constipation and abdominal distension and/or cramping. A thorough history and physical examination are typically performed by a physician or mid-level practitioner. Other clinicians, such as registered nurses and registered dietitians, may assess initial presence of some or all of the symptoms noted above, follow their progression and

(within their scope of practice) suggest or recommend interventions to manage the signs and symptoms.

Assessment of stool output is a key component of clinical nutrition monitoring that may affect nutrient and fluid balance. Researchers have developed several tools which assist clinicians and patients/clients in evaluation of bowel function. The Bristol Stool Form Scale may be used by clinicians and patients to assess stool form. This scale has undergone some validity and reliability testing [37]. The scale is ordinal, rating stool from hardest (type 1) to softest (type 7). Stool types 3–5 are considered 'normal'; stools types 1–2 are consistent with constipation and stool types 6–7 consistent with diarrhoea [37]. The tool, originally developed with written descriptors only, was later revised to include pictures. The scale helps healthcare professionals communicate with individuals about the type and frequency of stool and thus assess a typical or 'normal' pattern for the individual. This tool is probably of most value when assessing the nutrition regimen for an individual who is eating by mouth, as this is in whom validation studies have been performed. There are no validation studies of its use in enteral or parenteral nutrition, critical illness or short bowel syndrome.

The King's Stool Chart may be used for characterising stool output in patients receiving enteral nutrition [38]. The chart may be used by healthcare providers and individuals who are not providers and includes written directions and pictures. The evaluator considers the stool consistency (hard and formed, soft and formed, loose and unformed, liquid), stool weight ($<100\,g$, $100–200\,g$, $>200\,g$) and stool frequency by comparing the stool with written and pictorial descriptors [38]. The King's Stool Chart has been validated for content, construct and concurrent validity and reliability in numerous studies in which stool output of patients receiving enteral nutrition was monitored [39].

In addition to measuring stool output (consistency, frequency, volume), the measurement of gastrointestinal symptoms is of great importance in nutritional assessment due to their impact on nutrient intake (e.g. nausea, abdominal pain) and the potential impact of nutrition intervention

Table 2.5.2 Summary of selected clinical scoring tools

Name	Purpose	Description	Selected criteria	Scoring
Mini Mental Status Examination (MMSE)	Cognitive impairment [30]	Sensitive and reliable 30-point questionnaire	• What is the year, season and date? • Count backwards from 100 by 7 • Remember three things shown earlier • Repeat a phrase • Read a sentence and perform the command	A score of <24 demonstrates impairment
Acute Physiology and Chronic Health Examination (APACHE) Scale, versions I–IV	Severity of illness and prognosis of critically ill adults [31]	Measures typically collected during an intensive care unit (ICU) admission via an electronic medical record	• Age • Temperature • Respiratory rate • Concentrations of various lab values • Chronic health conditions • ICU admission data	Higher scores correspond to greater severity of severe disease and a higher risk of mortality
Child–Pugh Score	Estimates severity of cirrhosis in an individual patient [32]		• Concentrations of serum bilirubin and albumin • International normalised ratio (INR) • Presence of ascites and encephalopathy	Score of 5–6: Class A Score of 7–9: Class B Score of 10–15: Class C
MELD Score (Model for End-Stage Liver Disease)	Quantitates the degree of end-stage liver disease to assist the clinical team with planning for potential liver transplant [33]	Values should be no older than 48 hours	• Presence of twice-weekly dialysis • Serum albumin, sodium, bilirubin • Assessment of INR $MELD = 0.78 \times \ln[\text{serum bilirubin (mg/dL)}] + 11.2 \times \ln[INR] + 9.57 \times \ln[\text{serum creatinine (mg/dL)}] + 6.43$	0 or more: 71.3% mortality 30–39: 52.6% mortality 20–29: 19.6% mortality 10–19: 6.0% mortality <9: 1.9% mortality
Crohn's Disease Activity Index [34]	Quantitates the severity of symptoms and activity of disease remission/relapse	Extraintestinal complications such as arthritis/arthralgia, erythema nodosum, aphthous stomatitis, fissure/fistula/ abscess, fever >37.8°C	• Number of liquid stools • Abdominal pain • General well-being • Extraintestinal complications • Antidiarrhoeal drugs • Abdominal mass • Haematocrit • Body weight	<150 disease remission >150 active disease
Lung Injury Score [35,36]	Differentiates between adult respiratory distress syndrome (ARDS) and acute lung injury (ALI)		• Acute onset of bilateral pulmonary infiltrates consistent with oedema • Partial pressure of oxygen in blood/fraction of inspired oxygen • Pulmonary artery wedge pressure • No clinical evidence of fluid overload	≤200 ARDS ≤300 ALI

on GI symptoms (e.g. flatulence, bloating). A common method for measuring GI symptoms is the Gastrointestinal Symptom Rating Scale (GSRS), consisting of 15 questions with a four-point (absent, mild, moderate, severe) or seven-point Likert scale response set, thus measuring the frequency (presence/absence) and severity of symptoms including acid reflux, nausea, vomiting and abdominal pain [40].

Pressure ulcers

Assessment of risk for and progression of existing pressure ulcers is important in community settings, as well as acute and long-term care. In 2006, Pancorbo-Hidalgo and colleagues published a systematic review of 33 studies of pressure ulcer assessment tools, only some of which had been validated [41]. They found no reduction in incidence of pressure ulcers which could be attributed to use of an assessment tool, yet noted that use of a tool increases the intensity and effectiveness of prevention interventions. The Braden Scale had the best sensitivity/specificity balance; the Norton Scale had reasonable scores for sensitivity, specificity and risk prediction, and the Waterlow Scale had high sensitivity, but low specificity and a good risk prediction score [41].

2.5.4 Conclusion

Clinical nutrition assessment of a patient requires a comprehensive approach not only to established nutrition indicators such as weight loss, dietary intake and presence of cachexia or sarcopenia, but also to physical function parameters and specific criteria relevant to clinical status. This chapter provides only an overview of important testing and scoring procedures that should become familiar to clinicians at all levels of practice.

References

1. Russell MK. Functional assessment of nutritional status. *Nutr Clin Pract* 2015; **30**: 211–218.
2. White JV, Guenter P, Jensen J, et al. Consensus statement of the Academy of Nutrition and Dietetics/American Society for Parenteral and Enteral Nutrition: characteristics recommended for identification and documentation of adult malnutrition (undernutrition). *J Acad Nutr Diet* 2012; **112**: 730–738.
3. Norman K, Stobäus N, Gonzalez MC, Schulske JD, Pirlich M. Hand grip strength: outcome predictor and marker of nutritional status. *Clin Nutr* 2011; **30**: 135–142.
4. Jensen GL, Hsiao P, Wheeler D. Adult nutrition assessment tutorial. *J Parenter Enteral Nutr* 2012; **36**: 267–274.
5. Tomey M, Sowers M. Assessment of physical functioning: a conceptual model encompassing environmental factors and individual compensation strategies. *Phys Ther* 2009; **89**: 705–714.
6. Clark B, Manini T. What is dynapenia? *Nutrition* 2012; **28**: 495–503.
7. Norman K, Stobäus N, Smoliner C, et al. Determinants of hand grip strength, knee extension strength and functional status in cancer patients. *Clin Nutr* 2010; **29**: 586–591.
8. Savino E, Martini E, Lauretani F, et al. Handgrip strength predicts persistent walking recovery after hip fracture surgery. *Am J Med* 2013; **126**: 1068–1075.
9. Bohannon RW, Peolsson A, Massy-Westropp N, et al. Reference values for adult grip strength measured with a Jamar dynamometer: a descriptive meta-analysis. *Physiotherapy* 2006; **92**: 11–15.
10. Smith S, Madden AM. Body composition and functional assessment of nutritional status in adults: a narrative review of imaging, impedance, strength and functional techniques. *J Hum Nutr Diet* 2016; **29**: 714–732.
11. Roberts HC, Denison HJ, Martin HJ. A review of the measurement of grip strength in clinical and epidemiological studies: towards a standardised approach. *Age Ageing* 2011; **40**: 423–429.
12. Dodds RM, Sydall HE, Cooper R, et al. Grip strength across the life course: normative data from twelve British studies. *PLoS One* 2014; **9**: e113637.
13. Rikli RE, Jones CJ. Functional fitness normative scores doe community residing older adults ages 60–94. *J Aging Phys Ther* 1999; **7**: 160–179.
14. Strassmann A, Steurer-Stey C, Lana K, et al. Population-based reference values for the 1-min sit-to-stand test. *Int J Public Health* 2013; **58**: 949–953.
15. Bennell K, Dobson F, Hinman R. Measures of physical performance assessments. *Arthritis Care Res* 2011; **63**: S350–S370.
16. Bohannan RW. Reference values for the five-repetition sit-to-stand test: a descriptive analysis of data from elders. *Percept Mot Skills* 2006; **103**: 215–222.
17. Beavers K, Beavers D, Houston D, et al. Associations between body composition and gait-speed decline: results from the health, aging and body composition study. *Am J Clin Nutr* 2013; **97**: 552–560.

18. Fritz S, Lusardi M. White paper: 'walking speed – the 6th vital sign'. *J Geriatr Phys Ther* 2009; **32**: 2–5.

19. Dobson F, Hinman RS, Roos EM, et al. OARSI recommended performance-based tests to assess physical function in people diagnosed with hip or knee osteoarthritis. *Osteoarthritis Cartilage* 2013; **21**: 1042–1052.

20. Nightingale EJ, Pourkazemi F, Hiller C. Systematic review of times stair tests. *J Rehabil Res Dev* 2014; **51**: 335–350.

21. Prince SA, Adamo KB, Hamel ME, et al. A comparison of direct versus self-report measures for assessing physical activity in adults: a systematic review. *Int J Behav Nutr Phys Act* 2008; **5**: 56.

22. Wittink H, Rogers W, Sukiennik A, Carr DB. Physical functioning: self-report and performance measures are related but distinct. *Spine* 2003; **28**: 2407–2413.

23. Norman K, Stobäus N, Smoliner C, et al. Determinants of hand grip strength, knee extension and functional status in cancer patients. *Clin Nutr* 2010; **29**: 586–591.

24. Katz S, Ford AB, Moskowitz RW, Jackson BA, Jaffe MW. Studies of illness in the aged: the index of ADL: a standardized measure of biologic and physical function. *JAMA* 1963; **185**: 914–919.

25. Lawton MP, Moss MA, Fulcomer M, Kleban M. A research and service oriented multilevel assessment instrument. *J Gerontol* 1982; **37**: 91–99.

26. Mahoney FI, Barthel D. Functional evaluation: the Barthel Index. *Md State Med J* 1965; **14**: 56–61.

27. Jordan-Marsh MA. The SF-36 quality-of-life instrument: updates and strategies for critical care research. *Crit Care Nurse* 2002; **22**: 35–43.

28. Brazier J, Roberts J, Tsuchiya A, Busschbach J. A comparison of the EQ-5D and SF-6D across seven patient groups. *Health Econ* 2004; **13**: 873–884.

29. Kondrup J, Elia M. Basic concepts in nutrition. In: Sobotka L, editor. *Basics in Clinical Nutrition*, 4th edn. Prague: Galen, 2011, pp. 25–26.

30. Marshal F, Folstein MD, Lee N, et al. The minimental state examination. *Arch Gen Psychiatr* 1983; **40**: 812.

31. Zimmerman JE, Kramer AA, McNair DS, Manila FM. Acute physiology and chronic health evaluation (APACHE) IV: hospital mortality assessment for today's critically ill patients. *Crit Care Med* 2006; **34**: 1297–1310.

32. Pugh RHN, Murray-Lyon IM, Dawson JL, et al. Transection of the oesophagus for bleeding oesophageal varices. *Br J Surg* 1973; **60**: 646–649.

33. Peng Y, Qi A, Guo X. Child–Pugh versus MELD score for the assessment of prognosis in liver cirrhosis: a systematic review and meta-analysis of observational studies. *Medicine (Baltimore)* 2016; **95**(8): e2877.

34. Beld WR, Becktel JM, Singleton JW, et al. Development of a Crohn's disease activity index. *Gastroenterology* 1967; **70**: 439–444.

35. Artigas A, Bernard GR, Carlet J, et al. The American-European consensus conference on ARDS, part 2: ventilatory, pharmacologic, supportive therapy, study design strategies, and issues related to recovery and remodeling. Acute respiratory distress syndrome. *Am J Respir Crit Care Med* 1998; **157**(4 Pt 1): 1332–1347.

36. Bouch DC, Thompson JP. Severity scoring systems in the critically ill. *Contin Educ Anaesth Crit Care Pain* 2008; **8**: 181–185.

37. Blake MR, Raker JM, Whelan K. Validity and reliability of the Bristol Stool Form Scale in healthy adults and patients with diarrhoea-predominant irritable bowel syndrome. *Aliment Pharmacol Ther* 2016; **44**: 693–703.

38. King's Stool Chart. www.kcl.ac.uk/stoolchart (accessed 29 August 2017).

39. Whelan K, Judd PA, Taylor MA. Assessment of fecal output in patients receiving enteral tube feeding: validation of a novel chart. *Eur J Clin Nutr* 2004; **58**: 1030–1037.

40. Svedlund J, Sjodin I, Dotevall G. GSRS – a clinical rating scale for gastrointestinal symptoms in patients with irritable bowel syndrome and peptic-ulcer disease. *Dig Dis Sci* 1988; **33**: 129–134.

41. Pancorbo-Hidalgo P, Garcia-Fernandez F, Lopez-Medina I, Alvarez-Nieto C. Risk assessment scales for pressure ulcer prevention: a systematic review. *J Adv Nurs* 2006; **54**: 94–110.

Chapter 2.6

Dietary assessment in undernutrition

Claire E. Robertson
Department of Life Sciences, University of Westminster, London, UK

2.6.1 Introduction

The principal aim of dietary assessment is to capture a true record of food intake. The rationale for its inclusion in a research study or clinical case review will vary in complexity but ultimately, this is motivated by the potential offered through dietary adjustment. For example, the World Cancer Research Fund and American Institute for Cancer Research estimate that dietary change holds the potential to prevent 25% of all cancers [1]. Similarly, intake of probiotics has been conclusively linked to prevention of acute upper respiratory tract infections [2]. While clinical and anthropometric measures enable clinicians to determine a patient's nutritional status, to gain any perspective of how the plethora of 'food-related' factors can affect health outcomes, dietary assessment is required. Diet is seldom the principal focus of any study, yet understanding how it affects health outcomes enables tailoring of dietetic advice and public health recommendations, to improve health and minimise costs associated with treatment of conditions where nutrition plays a key role in the aetiology. To enable this, carefully planned assessments of intake are required.

As outlined within this book, multiple causes for undernutrition are known, including physiological, psychological, socioeconomic and institutional. Many causal factors can directly or indirectly influence dietary choices. For example, biological satiation signals may be affected differently by macronutrients or food energy content [3]; palatability triggers (e.g. food texture, sight stimuli, taste or olfaction) can negatively affect food intake and appetite [4]; while social (e.g. level of autonomy, environmental/family support and access to food) and psychological (e.g. stress, depression) factors interplay to determine how individuals approach their diet [5]. These features combine to mean that dietary assessment is an inherently complex data collection tool. Considerable time and financial resources are required, irrespective of the method(s) chosen or the population studied.

2.6.2 Determining the 'ideal' dietary assessment tool

When choosing a dietary assessment method, the greatest emphasis is typically placed on *what* researchers and/or clinicians want to know. The Diet and Physical Activity Measurement Toolkit [6] advises consideration of the following questions prior to making that decision.

- What are the objectives of the research or clinical question?
- What dietary outcome measures are central to the aims and outcome measures of the study (or clinical case review)?
- What specific kinds of information are needed (i.e. should this encompass nutrients, foods, eating patterns, taste perception, self-efficacy, etc.)?
- What resources are available (i.e. time, money, staff – skilled/non-skilled, etc.)?
- Do special subject characteristics need to be considered, such as memory or literacy?

Advanced Nutrition and Dietetics in Nutrition Support, First Edition. Edited by Mary Hickson and Sara Smith.
© 2018 John Wiley & Sons Ltd. Published 2018 by John Wiley & Sons Ltd.

- What analysis methods are required for the data collected?
- What resources or experiences are required to complete this process?

When reviewing each of these questions, acknowledging the challenges imposed by the characteristics of the respondent is an integral requirement. As shown elsewhere in this book, undernutrition does not apply to only one population demographic. The British Association for Parenteral and Enteral Nutrition outline this diversity, noting that individuals at increased risk include (but are not limited to) the elderly (particularly those living in care and nursing homes and those who have been hospitalised); those with physical impairments (e.g. sensory, mobility or fine motor skill), chronic progressive conditions (e.g. cancer or dementia) or sociocultural constraints (e.g. poverty, social isolation) [7]. Within each of these population sectors, both the capacity of individuals to share information on their dietary intake and their personal food habits will vary. Reasons as diverse as religio-cultural food practices [8], illness, anxiety and avoidant restrictive food intake disorder [9] and lack of economic stability (yet the desire to demonstrate this [10]) are known to alter eating habits and reports of consumption. Similarly, variance in the perception of and actual support provided to individuals by close family and friends can have both positive and adverse impacts on eating habits [5]. Such diversity on an individual level makes selection of dietary assessment methods for use at the group level extremely problematic.

2.6.3 The utility of traditional dietary assessment methods

There is no gold standard method of dietary assessment. All are expensive, time-consuming to complete and subject to errors. A variety of methods, both paper and software, can be used, each requiring differing amounts of time and skill for data capture and processing of collected information.

The burden of data capture alters with the aims of the dietary assessment method, the skills and experience of the interviewer or researcher, and the capacity of the respondent to provide the details required. We must also acknowledge that even a complete, accurate record of food consumption will not correspond to utilisation of the contained nutrients. Undernourished individuals with reduced intestinal function (e.g. patients in intensive care, with active Crohn's disease or refractory coeliac disease) may present with dehydration, energy, protein and micronutrient deficiencies and thus reduced quality of life, and yet have apparently sufficient dietary intakes when intake is assessed [11]. Determining the utility of each dietary assessment method must be considered in the context of the undernourished individual's capacity to complete the method, and any existing knowledge of what factors contribute to this.

2.6.4 Retrospective methods of dietary assessment

Methods which require subjects to report on past intake typically utilise frequency, recall, history and/or checklist methods.

Food frequency questionnaires

Food frequency questionnaires (FFQ) gather reports of intake consumed over the previous 12 months (although this can be shortened or lengthened according to the needs of the assessment), aiming to quantify 'habitual' intake. Where intake is relatively consistent, the FFQ offers a low-burden, time-saving and comprehensive method for assessment of dietary intake (for both the interviewer and respondent), making it a method of choice for large-scale longitudinal cohort studies (e.g. European Prospective Investigation into Cancer (EPIC) [12] and National Health and Nutrition Examination Survey (NHANES) [13]). The perceived utility of this method is not without compromise, however.

Food frequency questionnaires can be designed for a specific purpose (e.g. quantification of n3 fatty acid intakes [14]), yet this limits the capacity to learn about aspects not hypothesised to be important at the outset of investigations, yet indicated to be so during them. They can also be more comprehensive, including 200 or more questions about intakes of different groups of food, as is the case in EPIC [12], enabling capture of 'whole diet' information. Where this 'whole diet' approach is used, it requires inclusion of multiple foods within single questions, for example: *How often did you eat pork (including chops, roasts, and in mixed dishes)? (Please do not include ham, ham steak, or sausage).* Such intricacy in question wording complicates interpretation for the respondent, particularly when they may already have reduced capacity to answer correctly without direction. Further disparities incurred through the researchers' attempts to match 'usual' portion sizes to a diverse food and consumer group to enable nutrient intake conversion add further complexity. For individuals completing such extensive questionnaires, this can translate as survey fatigue, leading to drop-out or guesswork. For some population groups (e.g. children, the elderly, patients with cognitive impairment or poor literacy skills), self-completion is unlikely, increasing the researcher burden and potentially reducing the capacity for collection of information from the ideal sample size.

In addition to this, the FFQ method is not exempt from the typical imprecisions reported across the dietary assessment literature, for example underreporting of energy and negatively perceived dietary components (e.g. alcohol, fats) and overreporting of socially acceptable foods (e.g. fruits and vegetables) [15,16].

Diet history

Another retrospective method of data collection, the diet history technique, is used traditionally within clinical settings, by trained dietitians. Burke originally described this method using three phases [17]. First, a face-to-face interview using either a checklist of 'commonly eaten foods' or a 24-hour recall method (described later) which is then cross-checked against a frequency checklist before being validated using a prospective record of intake (e.g. a 3-day diary). Researchers or clinicians require careful training

to ensure they can probe for details meal by meal, day by day and over seasons to capture a picture of typical eating habits (and deviations from these).

The benefits of the dietary history method in case appraisals are well acknowledged. It limits participant burden, has no requirement for literacy and can be tailored to capture additional data on foods and/or nutrients identified to be of concern. The integration of aspects from several dietary assessment methods also increases the utility of data captured in this way, for example preventing errors imposed by poor respondent memory or recall through use of an interviewer-led format and food models, quantifying 'usual' intakes in a more personalised way than FFQ methods allow [18,19]. However, like all methods of dietary assessment, it is subject to errors including memory, conceptualisation (e.g. of portion sizes) and interviewer bias. It is also known to exaggerate the regularity of dietary habits. Resultant estimates of the repeatability, reliability and robustness of the diet history method [5,19,20] rationalise why it is not a researcher's method of choice, yet its ability to capture seasonal variation in intakes and to assess nutrient interactions and/or confounding at an individual level while offering a means to capture details on usual foods consumed, portion sizes, recipes and frequency of food consumption in the recent past means that it is unlikely to be overlooked in clinical care settings [19].

Dietary screeners

Screener tools such as the example published by the National Institutes of Health [21] offer a fast and targeted appraisal of intake, requiring respondents to tick food categories on each eating occasion over a 24-hour period. This prospective method does not rely on memory, has a relatively low respondent and investigator burden and has not been associated with alteration of eating behaviours [19]. Despite this, design of screener tools must be reactive to the population under study if they are to be considered a useful means of assessing intake. For the Low Income Diet Methods Study (LIDMS), a 4-day weighed diary, 4-day semi-weighed diary, four repeat 24-hour recalls and a 4-day dietary checklist were compared by respondents (for ease of completion) and researchers (for value of data obtained). Reactive to difficulties including lower literacy, numeracy and English language skills (particularly within ethnic minority groups), dietary checklists were the preferred method of dietary assessment for respondents but these were not found to capture the level of detail targeted by researchers [10,22].

While these methods could be considered to hold an advantage through capture of dietary intake data over a longer period, this benefit is typically offset by lower reliability of findings. Several of the problems identified above are shared with prospective methods, and like all methods, these are associated with their own problems. One of the leading considerations is the period of data capture to be included. It is well understood that day-to-day variability in dietary intakes *within person* can be 4–6 times as large as that seen *between person* [20], and this varies considerably with nutrient type studied [12,20].

Twenty-four hour recall

When a 24-hour recall method is used, repeat collection is needed to correct for this. Dennis et al. [23] report on the complexity of using a multiple-pass, 24-hour recall method of assessment in what is generally regarded to be the most comprehensive epidemiological study to date focused on the effects of dietary intake on cardiovascular health outcomes. In the INTERMAP study, dietary (and other) data were collected from 4680 men and women (ages 40–59 years) located in in 17 centres across China, Japan, United Kingdom and United States. Recalls were collected by trained staff on four occasions using an interviewer-led, multiple-pass 24-hour recall method. Extensive local (senior nutritionists on site), national (senior country nutritionists) and international checks were completed to ensure the precision of data collection (interviews were taped and evaluated [24]) and processing (coded recalls were recoded blind [25]) and comparability of results from all participants (e.g. to standardise coding of

carbohydrate intake data internationally, using monosaccharide equivalent data [26]). Within interviews alone, checks are needed to ensure disturbances do not hinder participant recall; the interviewer is interested in what the participant is reporting (thus encouraging accurate rather than fast reports of intake); information is documented as it was reported; questions are not rushed or biased; and probing is used to ensure all information collected is complete [24].

Even with such comprehensive checks, errors can and do enter all methods of dietary data collection and processing. This study illustrates just one example of the efforts which can be (and often are) made to identify the principal sources of error likely to affect dietary assessment, to explore their potential impact on results and design use of methods which can prevent or control for as many of these errors as possible [23].

2.6.5 Prospective methods of dietary assessment

Where prospective methods of data collection are preferred, diary methods (weighed or estimated) or dietary observation are typically used.

Dietary records

With dietary records, subjects are taught to describe the food they eat (in paper or recorded logs), ideally immediately prior to consumption, and also to record any leftovers. Reactive to the within- and between-person variance limitations described earlier, collection of information in this way typically spans 3–7 days. This method places one of the highest burdens on the respondent (particularly when portion sizes are weighed) and consequently, it is typically the least favoured method of screening for respondents (e.g. in the LIDMS [10]). Errors of omission and commission [15,16,20] are highly likely and therefore, like all methods of assessment, validation using urinary biomarkers or similar is necessary [12,19,23].

Despite these limitations, the use of data captured in this way can allow evaluation of whether other dietary components (e.g. non-nutritive substances) consumed in an attempt to reach

Table 2.6.1 Steps for consideration of the utility of dietary assessment methods for appraisal of undernourished patients

Consideration	Example questions for consideration	Possible methods for dietary assessment to capture this detail		
		Goal	Method(s)?	Researchers to note:
Objectives of the research or clinical question	• Has a change in typical dietary habits led to dietary inadequacy, and increased risk of undernutrition? • Is [*insert physiological or psychological factor here*] responsible for decline in nutritional status?	Assessment of 'habitual' intake needed Change from 'past' to current intakes needed	• FFQ • Diet history • Diet history	• Is the respondent capable of self-completion of questionnaires? • Validation of intake (e.g. biomarker) needed • Requires a tailored assessment, and appraisal of 'reaction' to questions • Where diet history questionnaires are used, multiple visits may be needed to gain respondents' confidence
Dietary outcome measures central to aims	• Food intake • Patterns of consumption • Nutrient bioavailability • Nutrient intake	Clear evidence-based review of 'what' is of interest, and detailed synopsis of this prior to dietary assessment method design	• Frequency checklist (specific foods) • Questionnaire (where bioavailability of nutrients is of concern)	• It is vital that the 'question' to be asked is clear prior to the design of the dietary assessment method • Where targeted questions are known, tailor FFQ or diet history to address this. Where question is less certain, ensure scope to determine impact of wider dietary determinants (including all examples listed here)
Specific information needed	• As points above • Self-efficacy (i.e. who is preparing food, observation of respondent while eating?) • Taste perception (alterations) • Personal reflections of intake • Portion sizes • Respondent capacity	Detailed overall synopsis of diet needed, including social aspects of eating and personal perceptions of experiences (to enable appraisal of psychological impacts)	• Interview based • Diet history/ FFQ • Recall/ diary, i.e. current intake overview also needed	• Research or clinical question must remain central to design, but methods chosen should be reactive to likelihood of needing more information to fully understand associations • Consider tiered assessment protocol, with expansion of 'basic' detail reactive to early results • Careful review of respondent capacity needed • Do any validated estimates of 'usual' intake for the study population exist?

Resources available	• Skilled/unskilled interviewers • Financial • Time • Portion size estimates	Review of published literature to determine whether tools exist that can be used or amended for use. The capacity of respondents (and/ or their carers) will be pivotal to determination of the most appropriate method for appraisal of intake	• n/a	• Interviewers will require good knowledge of nutrition and dietary habits within population being reviewed (particularly when ethnic groups involved) • Research budgets will require review of all aspects covered previously in this table, and capacity of respondents to enable data capture at required sample size • Where portion size estimates typical for study population are not available, methods are likely to require determination of this
Special characteristics of subjects	• Age • Ethnicity • Social support networks • Physiological health • Psychological health	Guide collection of information with reference to 'known' influences on intake within the sociodemographic characteristics of the respondent group. In doing this, encourage involvement in food decisions, aiming to determine how and/or why situations encountered have arisen	• n/a	• Any method chosen must be reactive to the characteristics of the respondent, and to how this will affect food choices and capacity to prepare food independently • Clinical review of physiological and psychological health should be carried out where possible • Involvement of those in social support networks ideally in data capture

Source: Adapted with reference to the DAPA Toolkit [6], with permission from the Medical Research Council. FFQ, food frequency questionnaire; n/a, not applicable.

Table 2.6.2 Basic review of the likely capacity of undernourished individuals to complete traditional dietary assessment methods

Method of assessment	Measures variation of diet with time?	Estimates portion sizes?	Typical error sources reported in the dietary assessment literature				Training of interviewer[†] needed?
			Reporting errors (e.g., memory, bias)?	Modified eating pattern (caused by data capture)?	Literacy requirements?[*]	Tailoring by socio-demographic needed?	
Food Frequency Questionnaire	No	Yes	Yes	No	Yes	Yes	No
24 hour recall	Yes	Yes	Yes	No	No	Yes	Yes
Weighed food record	Yes	Yes	Yes	Yes	Yes	Yes	N/a
Estimated food record	Yes	Yes	Yes	Yes	Yes	Yes	N/a
Diet history	No	Yes	Yes	No	No	Yes	Yes
Food checklist	No	n/a	Yes	No	No	Yes	Yes

* Assumes interviewer led where necessitated by the respondent group.

† Where interviewers are needed for data collection, diary methods are unlikely to be a good choice for undernourished groups.

satiation may be causing problems with absorption of nutrients, for example, through physiological blockages to intestinal absorption. Similarly, it may be possible to explore whether sporadic consumption of affordable or donated foods is addressing the most urgent needs of the recipients. This means that dietary records (and the repeat 24-hour recall method) are the method of choice for small cohort and/or intervention studies [27,28].

2.6.6 Summary

Table 2.6.1 summarises the considerations described above for each dietary assessment method using the DAPA toolkit question framework [6], while Table 2.6.2 summarises the likely capacity for undernourished individuals to complete traditional dietary assessment methods. Both tables have been compiled in response to the seven key data collection considerations detailed by Adamson et al. [29] in the context of undernutrition:

- training and skill of data collectors
- collection time and quality of interaction
- complexity of task
- memory and recall
- portion size assessment
- data preparation (for nutritional analysis)
- validity and quality of data.

Understanding and tackling undernutrition globally is clearly vital, and much can be learnt from international efforts in the developed world [30,31], where learning from aspects of household food security through management of literacy issues (which may limit ability to self-record intakes) is the norm rather than the exception. Challenges imposed by data collection of dietary information are additive and multidirectional, and their effects are not always small. A vital first step to determining whether a correctable dietary inadequacy is evident requires accurate empirical assessment of intake. Food and its consumption have effects in the short term (currency of life, means to satisfy hunger, pleasure), yet effects are also long term.

No basic model exists to outline how best to assess the cause or effects of dietary intake on health outcomes, yet where linked to a preventable condition, that is, where an inadequacy is implicated in causation of disease and/or demise to health, the potential for positive impact is considerable. Impacts can be quantified both economically (linked to decreased lengths of stay in hospital, costs of treating illnesses, improved speed of return to work [32]) and through consideration of their effects on quality of life (increased enjoyment of food, decreased impact of disease symptoms). As no single presentation of undernutrition is straightforward, the condition no longer being confined to developing populations or specific population subgroups, flexibility in application of dietary assessment methodologies is necessary. Without data on eating habits, causation for undernutrition may be hard to explain, and harder to correct.

References

1. World Cancer Research Fund, American Institute for Cancer Research. Food, Nutrition, Physical Activity, and the Prevention of Cancer: A Global Perspective. Washington: AICR, 2007.
2. King S, Glanville J, Sanders ME, Fitzgerald A, Varley D. Effectiveness of probiotics on the duration of illness in healthy children and adults who develop common acute respiratory infectious conditions: a systematic review and meta-analysis. *Br J Nutr* 2014; **112**(1): 41–54.
3. Donini L, Poggiogalle E, Piredda M, et al. Anorexia and eating patterns in the elderly. *PLoS One* 2013; **8**(5): e63539.
4. Payette H, Shatenstein B. Determinants of healthy eating in community-dwelling elderly people. *Can J Public Health* 2005; **96**: S27–S31.
5. Schilp J, Wijnhoven HAH, Deeg DJH, Visser M. Early determinants for the development of undernutrition in an older general population: longitudinal aging study amsterdam. *Br J Nutr* 2011; **106**(5): 708–717.
6. Medical Research Council. The Diet and Physical Activity Measurement Toolkit. www.dapa-toolkit.mrc.ac.uk/ (accessed 29 August 2017).
7. BAPEN. Introduction to Malnutrition. www.bapen.org.uk/malnutrition-undernutrition/introduction-to-malnutrition?tmpl=component&print=1&page= (accessed 29 August 2017).

8. Johnson KA, White AE, Boyd BM, Cohen AB. Matzah, meat, milk, and mana: psychological influences on religio-cultural food practices. *J Cross Cult Psychol* 2011; **42**(8): 1421–1436.

9. King LA, Urbach JR, Stewart KE. Illness anxiety and avoidant/restrictive food intake disorder: cognitive-behavioral conceptualization and treatment. *Eating Behav* 2015; **19**: 106–109.

10. Holmes B, Dick K, Nelson M. A comparison of four dietary assessment methods in materially deprived households in england. *Public Health Nutr* 2008; **11**(5): 444–456.

11. Wierdsma NJ, Peters JHC, Bokhorst-de Van DS, Mulder CJJ, Metgod I, Bodegraven AA. Bomb calorimetry, the gold standard for assessment of intestinal absorption capacity: normative values in healthy ambulant adults. *J Hum Nutr Diet* 2014; **27**: 57–64.

12. Bingham SA, Gill C, Welch A, et al. Validation of dietary assessment methods in the UK arm of EPIC using weighed records, and 24-hour urinary nitrogen and potassium and serum vitamin C and carotenoids as biomarkers. *Int J Epidemiol* 1997; **26**: S137–S151.

13. Carriquiry AL. Estimation of usual intake distributions of nutrients and foods. *Nutr J* 2003; **133**(2): 601S–608S.

14. Dahl L, Kringen C, Bjørkkjær T. A short food frequency questionnaire to assess intake of seafood and n-3 supplements: validation with biomarkers. *Nutr J* 2011; **10**: 127.

15. Becker W, Welten D. Under-reporting in dietary surveys – implications for development of food-based dietary guidelines. *Public Health Nutr* 2001; **4**(2): 683–687.

16. Macdiarmid J, Blundell J. Assessing dietary intake: who, what and why of under-reporting. *Nutr Res Rev* 1998; **11**(2): 231–253.

17. Burke BS. The dietary history as a tool in research. *J Am Diet Assoc* 1947; **23**: 1041–1046.

18. Gonzalez C. Relative validity and reproducibility of a diet history questionnaire in Spain 3. Biochemical markers. Int J Epidemiol 1997; **26**: S110–S117.

19. Margetts BM, Nelson M. Design Concepts in Nutritional Epidemiology, 2nd edn. Oxford: Oxford University Press, 1997.

20. Basiotis PP, Welsh SO, Cronin FJ, Kelsay JL, Mertz W. Number of days of food intake records required to estimate individual and group nutrient intakes with defined confidence. *J Nutr* 1987; **117**(9): 1638–1641.

21. National Institute of Health. Dietary Screener Questionnaire. http://epi.grants.cancer.gov/nhanes/dietscreen/dsq_english.pdf (accessed 29 August 2017).

22. Hughes J, Bates C, Bingham SA, Kelly S, Lowe C. British national diet and nutrition survey of people aged >=65y: feasibility study of the dietary assessment method. *Am J Clin Nutr* 1997; **65**(4): 1338–1339.

23. Dennis B, Stamler J, Buzzard M, et al. INTERMAP: the dietary data – process and quality control. *J Hum Hypertens* 2003; **17**(9): 609–622.

24. Robertson C, Conway R, Dennis B, Yarnell J, Stamler J, Elliott P. Attainment of precision in implementation of 24h dietary recalls: INTERMAP UK. *Br J Nutr* 2005; **94**(4): 588–594.

25. Conway R, Robertson C, Dennis B, Stamler J, Elliott P. Standardised coding of diet records: experiences from INTERMAP UK. *Br J Nutr* 2004; **91**(5): 765–771.

26. Schakel SF, Dennis BH, Wold AC, et al. Enhancing data on nutrient composition of foods eaten by participants in the INTERMAP study in China, Japan, the United Kingdom, and the United States. *J Food Compost Anal* 2003; **16**(3): 395–408.

27. Zujko ME, Witkowska AM, Waśkiewicz A, Mirończuk-Chodakowska I. Dietary antioxidant and flavonoid intakes are reduced in the elderly. *Oxid Med Cell Longev* 2015: e843173.

28. Feart C, Lorrain S, Ginder Coupez V, et al. Adherence to a Mediterranean diet and risk of fractures in French older persons. *Osteoporos Int* 2013; **24**(12): 3031–3041.

29. Adamson AJ, Collerton J, Davies K, et al. Nutrition in advanced age: dietary assessment in the Newcastle 85+ study. *Eur J Clin Nutr* 2009; **63**(Suppl 1): S6–S18.

30. Black RE, Victora CG, Walker SP, et al. Maternal and child undernutrition and overweight in low-income and middle-income countries. *Lancet* 2013; **382**(9890): 427–451.

31. Hoddinott J, Maluccio JA, Behrman JR, Flores R, Martorell R. Effect of a nutrition intervention during early childhood on economic productivity in Guatemalan adults. *Lancet* 2008; **371**(9610): 411–416.

32. Walzer S, Droeschel D, Nuijten M, Chevrou-Séverac H. Health economic analyses in medical nutrition: a systematic literature review. *Clinicoecon Outcomes Res* 2014; **6**: 109–124.

Chapter 2.7

Advanced imaging techniques for assessment of undernutrition

Carla M. Prado[1], Sarah A. Elliott[1] and Joao F. Mota[2]
[1]Division of Human Nutrition, University of Alberta, Edmonton, Canada
[2]Federal University of Goiás, Goiânia, Brazil

2.7.1 Introduction

Accurate assessment of body composition can be useful to monitor disease progress as well as a guide to nutrition support. Weight loss and body mass index (BMI) lack the sensitivity to detect changes in body composition, specifically in populations in which perturbations in body composition are apparent. Additionally, monitoring changes in the fat mass (FM) and fat-free mass (FFM) compartments may help health professionals understand energy metabolism in various disease states, which could lead to the development of preventive and interventional nutritional strategies that counteract the loss of FFM.

The use of new techniques has allowed the assessment of body composition to emerge as a fundamental part of nutritional assessment in clinical populations, as distinct body tissues are associated with specific health outcomes. Malnutrition, characterised by either over- or undernutrition, frequently coexists in patients with chronic diseases, and is associated with adverse outcomes such as increased mortality, impaired quality of life and worse overall health profile [1].

Historically, body composition techniques have not been used as a frontline tool for healthcare providers but new developments in the field, coupled with the value of the obtained information, have increased their use as an important physiological marker of nutritional status. Of particular interest is the use of imaging techniques, most of which are available in the clinical setting.

Body composition assessment

While the science behind body composition assessment techniques dates back to their early use in the 1930s and 1950s, it has only been in recent years that technological advances, coupled with their routine use in some diagnostic care settings, have allowed imaging techniques to become a part of routine body composition assessment in clinical practice.

The history, categorisation and development of body composition models have been extensively documented elsewhere [2]. The five-level model, in which body mass is considered as the sum of all components at each of the five levels: atomic, molecular, cellular, tissue organ and whole body, is central to body composition research. Inherent in this model are rules which underpin all body composition models, and collectively encompass the field of body composition research. It is important to understand that different techniques measure different compartments of the body, a difference that may have important implications for the interpretation of body composition measurements. The technique of choice will also determine the nomenclature of body compartments, which is often (incorrectly) used interchangeably [3].

An overview of available body composition techniques, their strengths and limitations is shown in Table 2.7.1. This table also includes considerations related to the use of each technique in the clinical setting (if applicable). Ideally, body composition techniques for clinical practice need to be quick, non-invasive and acceptable for repeated measures.

Methods such as hydrodensitometry, total body potassium counting, isotopic dilution, air displacement plethysmography, neutron activation analysis and magnetic resonance imaging (MRI) are often reserved for scientific use and referred to as 'reference' methods from which the validity of newer body composition techniques is assessed [2]. Bioelectrical impedance analysis (BIA), dual-energy x-ray absorptiometry (DXA) and, more recently, computed tomography (CT) and ultrasound (US) imaging appear to be the most convenient for use in clinical practice, the three latter being imaging methods, and the focus of this chapter.

2.7.2 Advances in imaging techniques

Imaging methods for the assessment of body composition include DXA, CT, MRI and US, and three-dimensional (3D) (photonic) imaging (Figure 2.7.1) (see Table 2.7.1).These methods can measure body composition at the molecular (DXA) tissue organ (CT, MRI, US) or whole-body (3D imaging, MRI) level. With the exception of US and 3D imaging, imaging techniques are now considered to be the most accurate tools for measuring adipose tissue and organs in clinical research [4] and are also gold-standard methods against which others are validated. The use of these techniques has revolutionised the capacity to assess body composition and aid in the diagnosis and monitoring of a multitude of disease states and treatment regimes.

Dual-energy x-ray absorptiometry

Dual-energy x-ray absorptiometry is a low-dose x-ray instrument that was primarily developed for the diagnosis of bone disease. However, advances and improvements in x-ray generation and detection technology, data acquisition protocols and image analysis algorithms (allowing the differentiation between bone mineral, fat mass and lean soft tissue) have contributed to its emergence as a criterion measure for the assessment of body composition. This technique not only allows for regional analysis (limb, trunk) but it also quantifies body fat distribution (android:gynoid ratio). Similarly to osteoporosis, sarcopenia is a condition that can be identified by DXA when measures of muscle mass are used. Sarcopenia, a term used to depict low skeletal muscle mass, has been most commonly identified using DXA-derived gender-specific cut-off values of appendicular skeletal muscle mass [5]. The assessment of appendicular skeletal muscle mass (lean soft tissue from arms and legs, which is mostly skeletal muscle) is an important advantage of the DXA technique.

Dual-energy x-ray absorptiometry analysis is considered a gold standard, simple, reproducible, precise and accurate technique which offers greater convenience, safety (low radiation dose) and comfort. It is therefore safe for longitudinal studies (including interventional studies) when repeated measures of body composition are required. As different disease processes may affect bone mineral density and/or lean soft tissue, having a comprehensive view of body composition such as that obtained by whole-body DXA is beneficial for a variety of clinical research and practice applications.

The potential role of DXA in the assessment of body composition has been documented in many clinical cohorts [6]. Its ability to measure bone mineral density (BMD) at the spine and hip has considerably advanced the diagnosis and treatment of bone health. Using DXA, internationally accepted cut-off values for the diagnosis of osteopenia and osteoporosis were developed, not only facilitating the recognition of osteoporosis as a disease, but also improving its diagnosis, prevention and treatment.

Table 2.7.1 Overview of available body composition techniques and relevance for clinical practice

Modality	Overview of technique/ principles	Strengths	Limitations	Value in clinical/ research application
Impedance Bioelectrical impedance analysis	• Measures resistance and reactance of electrical current passed through the body; water content of different body compartments determines the conductibility of the electrical current • Measures TBW, intra- and extracellular water, which is then used to estimate FFM and FM • Measures phase angle	• Quick and non-invasive • Most are portable • Safe, reproducible and low cost	• Does not differentiate among components of FM and FFM compartments • Precision affected by hydration status leading to overestimation of FFM and underestimation of FM • Internal regression equations for calculating FFM from BIA resistance are not released by the manufacturer • Regression equations among machines can vary, producing large differences in FFM calculation • Not a precise method in subjects with BMI >35 kg/m²	• Previously used in several groups, e.g. children and adolescents, elderly, overweight individuals, malnourished, patients with eating disorders, cancer, cystic fibrosis, receiving dialysis • Phase angle can be used as a prognostic marker in patients with critical illness
Body volume/density Underwater weighing or hydrodensitometry	• BD is calculated from body volume measured by water displacement in underwater weighing	• Reliable and valid for measuring body volume and determining body fat %	• Time-consuming and high patient burden • Relies on assumed densities of FFM and FM • Does not differentiate among components of FM and FFM compartments • Requires water adaptation • Limited application to highly specialised laboratories and/or research settings • Precision affected by subject hydration	• More used in athletes and overweight subjects (but not in severely obese) • Not appropriate for elderly and disabled patients

(Continued)

Table 2.7.1 (*Continued*)

Modality	Overview of technique/ principles	Strengths	Limitations	Value in clinical/ research application
Air displacement plethysmography	• BD is calculated from body volume measured by air displacement	• Relatively fast and non-invasive • Capacity: patients up to 250 kg; accommodates obese and very tall individuals • Excellent precision and accuracy for measurement of volume • Safely used in all age groups (infants to elderly)	• Relies on assumed densities of FFM and FM compartments • Does not differentiate among the FM and FFM components • Mostly used in research settings but has potential to be accessible in the clinical setting • Overestimates thoracic gas volume in obese/ overweight patients • Some studies reported poor validity compared with hydrodensitometry	• Provides a quick and safe body composition assessment which can be used in a variety of subjects, e.g. elderly, children, obese individuals • Good method for longitudinal assessment in clinical setting
Imaging/x-ray attenuation				
Dual-energy X-ray absorptiometry	• Measures BMD, BMC and FM, FFM using very low-radiation x-ray emission of two beams of energy. The generation of a high- and low-energy emission by an x-ray source is used to differentiate between soft tissue (LST) and bone	• Fast and non-invasive • High precision and accuracy • Low radiation exposure • Total and regional measures of body composition can be obtained • Option to assess visceral fat at L3 lumbar site • Ability to use hemi-scans for obese patients • Measurement of appendicular LST (surrogate for skeletal muscle mass) • Short scan time (5– 15 min)	• Differences within and between manufacturers and software versions • Inability to differentiate compartments within fat and LST • Measurements are influenced by thickness of tissue and LST hydration • Unsafe for pregnant women, individuals using pacemakers or undergoing procedures with iodine, barium or isotopes over a period of 7 days prior to the test	• Widely used technique throughout age spectrum; children, elderly and in several clinical conditions for cross-sectional and regional assessment • Diagnostic criteria for osteopenia/osteoporosis
Computed tomography	• Different Hounsfield unit attenuations among tissues allow for the differentiation of the detected bidimensional image created through the use of attenuated x-rays	• High resolution cross- sectional images • Most accurate quantitative and qualitative measure of body composition at the tissue-organ level, particularly total and regional adipose and skeletal muscle tissue	• Limited application to highly specialised clinical and/or research settings • High radiation exposure, which limits its use as secondary analysis Costly, and requires specialised skills to operate	• Extensively used in oncology. Potential use to predict prognosis including chemotherapy toxicity • Other cohorts in which these images are readily

Method	Principle	Advantages	Limitations	Applications
		• Adipose tissue, skeletal muscle, bone, visceral organs and brain tissue can be identified • Consistent image attenuation values within and between scans • Useful in clinical settings where these images are acquired for medical diagnosis/follow-up purposes		available include patients with cirrhosis, respiratory failure, kidney stones, traumatic injuries, transcatheter aortic valve replacement
Magnetic resonance imaging	• Protons aligned in a magnetic field are activated by a radiofrequency wave, absorbing energy. The generated signal is then used for body composition differentiation • Quantifies adipose tissue, skeletal muscle, oedema and visceral organs	• Most accurate method of quantification of internal organs or tissue volumes as well as a range of dynamic, functional and qualitative measurements • Best method for multiple-image protocols for whole-body and serial measurements • Determine body composition at the tissue-organ level, specifically whole-body and regional adipose tissue • Safe across age range and groups and for repeated measurements • No exposure to ionising radiation	• Limited application to highly specialised laboratories and/or research settings • Costly, and requires specialised skills to operate • Cannot accommodate very large subjects • Images are more varied and require comprehensive analysis • Fewer options for automated analysis; strict protocols must be followed in order to reduce individual analyst bias • Longer scan time (~30 min)	• In research settings, this technique has been primarily used in healthy, elderly and obese individuals. Use in clinical cohorts of patients with hepatic steatosis and cardiovascular diseases has been reported
Ultrasound	• Acoustic waves are transmitted through the skin, which are partially reflected back to the transducer when in contact with a tissue. The amount of echo returning to the transducer is different among body composition compartments	• Safe, portable and fast, inexpensive • Provides an accurate measurement of adipose tissue • No radiation exposure	• Lack of standardised measurement techniques, protocol standardisation • Subjective differentiation of LST from muscle may lead to technical errors • Provides more qualitative than quantitative results • Results are highly dependent on the skills of trained operator	• Has been used in elderly subjects, obese, critically ill, stroke survivals, patients with cystic fibrosis, among others

(Continued)

Table 2.7.1 (Continued)

Modality	Overview of technique/ principles	Strengths	Limitations	Value in clinical/ research application
3D body surface imaging	• A 3D image is generated by optical measurement (densitometry)	• Easy to use, low cost, safe • Provides total and regional measures of circumferences, lengths and percent body fat can be calculated • Additional anthropometric parameters can be calculated: waist and hip circumferences, sagittal abdominal diameter, segmental volumes and body weight • Accommodates severely obese individuals	• Limited availability of the technique • For accurate percentage body fat estimation, subjects must follow specific protocol including type of clothing, positioning and breathing, which may not be feasible in patients with certain clinical conditions	• Applicable to obesity research (paediatric, adult and elderly), large studies, patients with scoliosis, growth defects. Also for monitoring fitness and diet, obesity and diabetes
Total body water or hydrometry				
Labelled water-isotope dilution techniques	• TBW is determined as administered tracer/ tracer concentration • Estimates FM and FFM	• Practical for field research and repeated measurements • Safety and low patient burden	• Limited application to highly specialised laboratories and/or research settings • Costly, and requires specialised skills to operate • Several assumptions are made with regard to tracer distribution and effect in the body • Relies on assumed hydration of the FFM compartment (73.2%)	• In research settings, this technique has been used in healthy subjects, lactating women, elderly and obese individuals. It is often used for building multi-compartment models
Major body elements				
Neutron activation analysis	• Neutron activation produces isotopic atoms that have measurable unique emissions and decay paths, which can be used to estimate FM, TBW, BMM and protein content	• High precision and accuracy • Capable of quantifying all the main atomic elements found *in vivo* • Estimates bone mineral content, FFM and FM	• Limited application to highly specialised laboratories and/or research settings • High cost, including set-up and maintenance; and high technical skills are required to operate • Involves neutron radiation exposure, which poses potential danger during childhood and pregnancy	• Mostly used for building multi-compartment models in research settings, especially body composition validation studies

| Whole-body counting (potassium, K) | • Amount of intracellular ^{40}K is constant in the BCM and FFM and can be quantified | • High precision and accuracy for the assessment of BCM
• Safe and applicable across age groups
• Not affected by altered hydration status | • Limited application to highly specialised laboratories and/or research settings
• High technical skills and costly | • In research settings, the technique has been used in children, elderly, normal-weight and obese individuals. It is of special interest for the analysis of body composition in patients with altered hydration status such as patients with ovarian cancer, cirrhosis |

For references regarding each specific technique, please refer to the following key papers: Prado et al. [3] and Heymsfield et al. [42].
BCM, body cell mass; BD, body density; BIA, bioimpedance analysis; BMD; bone mineral density; BMI, body mass index; BMM, bone mineral mass; FFM, fat free mass; FM, fat mass; LST, lean soft tissue; TBW, total body water.

(a)

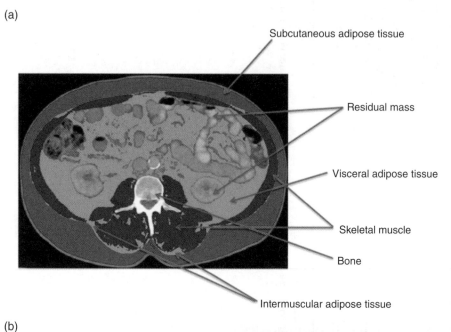

Subcutaneous adipose tissue

Residual mass

Visceral adipose tissue

Skeletal muscle

Bone

Intermuscular adipose tissue

(b)

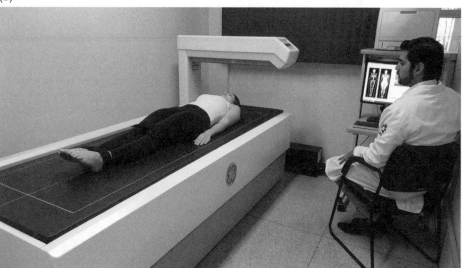

Figure 2.7.1 Imaging techniques available for the assessment of body composition. (a) CT/MRI image. (b) Dual-energy X-ray absorptiometry (DXA) examination. (c) Ultrasound imaging examination. (d) 3-D imaging output. Source: (c) Courtesy of Dr Thiago Gonzalez Barbosa-Silva, Universidade Católica de Pelotas School of Medicine and Postgraduate Program in Epidemiology, Universidade Federal de Pelotas School of Medicine. (d) shows stages in generation of 3D outputs from reconstruction to creation of raw image, and measurement of key body landmarks. Open access images extracted from: Wells JCK, Stocks J, Bonner R, et al. Acceptability, precision and accuracy of 3D photonic scanning for measurement of body shape in a multi-ethnic sample of children aged 5–11 years: the SLIC Study. *PloS One* 2015; **10**(4): e0124193.

(c)

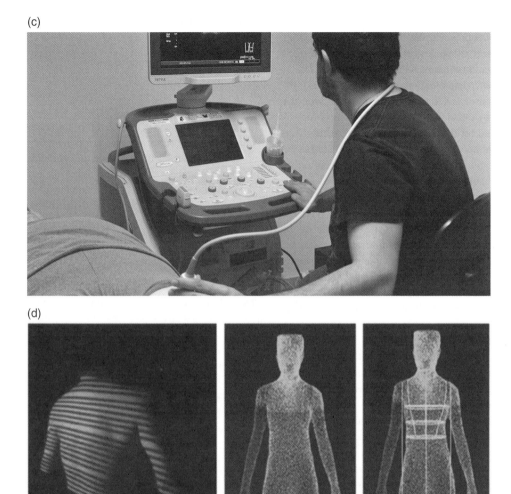

(d)

Figure 2.7.1 (Continued)

DXA has also been extensively used for the study of sarcopenia and its consequences in older adults and in patients with clinical conditions such as cirrhosis and renal problems, cancer, human immunodeficiency syndrome (HIV), type 2 diabetes and chronic obstructive pulmonary disease, among others [6].

Dual-energy x-ray absorptiometry has been used to monitor unfavourable changes in body composition that occur with disease-specific treatment, such as glucocorticoid use affecting bone mineral content and muscle mass [7] and adrenocortical steroids leading to redistribution of fat from peripheral to central regions in individuals with Cushing's disease [8]. An additional example is the use of DXA to monitor lean soft tissue loss occurring with androgen deprivation therapy for prostate cancer [9] and adjuvant chemotherapy for breast cancer [10]. Therefore, DXA can be used to monitor the impact of treatment regimens on body composition and for the development of interventions to prevent and treat these unfavourable changes.

The main factors influencing the accuracy of DXA include subject size and thickness, instrument company make and model, x-ray beam settings and software versions used. Whilst a major drawback of DXA is the inability to differentiate between the different types of fat and non-fat tissues (e.g. subcutaneous versus visceral and lean soft tissue versus muscle and organ mass), a major advantage is its low radiation exposure which allows body composition to be assessed in subjects of all age ranges, as well as longitudinally.

Early studies documented that DXA made no assumptions regarding the hydration of soft tissue in the estimation of fat mass components. However, more recent reports have suggested that the underlying principles and models which DXA relies on could be influenced by hydration status. The influence of hydration on DXA soft tissue estimates has been discussed in depth by Pietrobelli et al. [11]. Errors in estimating fat tissue at various soft tissue hydration levels were small (<1%), when compared in the context of the physiological range compatible with human life. Clinically, there is the potential for larger estimation errors when soft tissue overhydration is severe (20–25%) which is rare; however, large local accumulations can occur in some clinical cases (oedema or ascites).

Dual-energy x-ray absorptiometry also allows for the assessment of 'hemi-scans' for individuals who may not be able to fit entirely within the borders of the DXA bed. Additionally, the introduction of scanners with a wider bed platform and higher weight limit now allows DXA to be performed in individuals up to 450 lb (rather than 300 lb, the limit of old machines) and also taller individuals, with higher resolution images and improved precision. For these reasons, DXA is an indispensable clinical and research tool.

Computed tomography

Combining the physics of x-rays, computer technology and reconstructive mathematics, CT can produce diagnostic-quality cross-sectional images. CT images provide an accurate, reliable and highly differentiated assessment of body composition [12]. Due to its high radiation exposure, CT imaging is not a routine body composition assessment technique and is therefore only routinely used when images are already available in the medical records, conducted for medical purposes. In this case, the use of CT scanning as an indicator of nutritional status is clinically and practically relevant.

Computed tomography images can provide a cross-sectional assessment of skeletal muscle, adipose tissue and organ mass cross-sectional areas, which allows for the differentiation of adipose tissue (subcutaneous, visceral and intramuscular) as well as muscle attenuation (a measure of intra- and extramyocellular lipid) [13].

The premise of CT scans for body composition assessment has been widely documented, with several recent studies suggesting CT imaging at the third lumbar vertebra could strongly predict whole-body adiposity, muscularity and FFM in a range of clinical patients [3]. However, while single-slice images are often used in research to reduce costs and limit radiation exposure, their use in longitudinal studies may not be as valid in comparison to total body images, particularly in the case of adipose tissue assessment. Overtime, soft tissue structures move and, subsequently, the quantity of visceral fat in the landmark slice may have moved, which could reduce the accuracy of single-slice images for the determination of longitudinal changes.

While CT imaging assessment of body composition is mainly documented in cancer patients due to its routine clinical use during diagnosis and treatment follow-up [14], it has also been used to assess nutritional status and treatment outcomes in patients with chronic obstructive pulmonary disease (COPD) [15], chronic back pain [16], Cushing's syndrome [17], HIV [18], schizophrenia [19], stroke [20], intensive care unit (ICU) patients [21], patients undergoing Roux-en-Y gastric bypass and laparotomy surgery [22,23] and transcatheter aortic valve replacement [24]. Collectively, these studies demonstrate that abnormal CT-assessed body composition manifest as low muscle and/or high adipose tissue independently predicts poor prognosis and overall health status. Muscle attenuation is also an important prognostic marker as evidenced by recently conducted studies [25].

Advances in CT imaging such as quicker scan times (resulting in lower radiation exposure), improved image resolution and the introduction of helical methods that allow for regional analysis with rapid tissue and organ reconstructions, have cemented CT as a leading method for quantifying visceral adipose tissue in both clinical and research settings.

Magnetic resonance imaging

Several groups have demonstrated the feasibility of measuring total (whole-body) and regional adipose tissue and skeletal muscle mass using multiple MRI protocols in various clinical cohorts. Unlike CT, MRI does not use ionising radiation and while the estimation of total and regional body composition components is similar, the techniques differ in the way the images are acquired. The feasibility of MRI in human body composition studies is expanded by comparison to CT, as a result of differences in data acquisition, which affect the applicability, cost and practicality of the method [4].

While the principal application of MRI in human body composition assessment has been to characterise the quantity and distribution of adipose tissues and skeletal muscle, several studies have correlated the results from MRI fat distribution analysis with medical indices such as cardiovascular risk factors [26] and diabetes [27]. The acquisition of whole-body MRI data offers distinct advantages in assessing the influence of weight change on body composition. Weight change may induce regional changes in adipose tissue or muscle; MRI can detect if an increase in skeletal muscle in one anatomical region is masked by a loss of skeletal muscle in another, an important feature for clinical interventional studies.

The latest developments in the field of whole-body MRI (acceleration of data acquisition, introduction of moving-table scanning) have led to reduced imaging times and increased patient comfort, and therefore also increased acceptance. MRI allows for the quantification of specific high metabolic rate organs in order to improve understanding of resting energy expenditure, and the influence malignant disease may have on specific tissue sites. Notwithstanding, this method is highly sophisticated.

Ultrasound imaging

The biomedical diagnostic application of US is well known, but its use to measure adipose tissue and muscle thicknesses in humans is less understood. Acoustic waves (ultrasound) are reflected from tissue in the path of the ultrasound beam transmitted through the skin, which is partially reflected back to the transducer when in contact with a tissue. The amount of 'sound' reflected is dependent on the changes in acoustic impedance, which is different in air, fat, muscle and bone.

Ultrasound imaging has been used to quantify subcutaneous and visceral adiposity, showing a strong correlation to CT and MRI measurements in overweight [28], healthy [29] and obese [30] subjects. Recent research has shown that both visceral and subcutaneous adiposity can be estimated with adequate intra- and interobserver reproducibility, suggesting that US is a reliable, valid and fast method for assessing body composition.

Measurements of muscle and bone thickness are currently being studied with promising results. The use of US for the assessment of muscle layer thickness is of particular interest as it provides an index of lean tissue and its change throughout clinical conditions, as recently reviewed by Mourtzakis and Wischmeyer [31]. More recently, the echo intensity of an ultrasound image has been used to indicate changes in muscle quality, including increases in intramuscular fibrous and adipose tissues [32]. Additionally, the link between muscle quality assessed via echo intensity and muscle strength of a person has also been suggested as a useful tool to assess body composition in clinical cohorts. Studies have found echo intensity to be significantly correlated with muscle strength [33], which could lead the way for this non-invasive technique to be routinely used in clinical practice to monitor and assess the development of sarcopenia. As this technology is refined, a number of studies on this unique measure of muscle quality will be published over the coming years.

Clinical conditions in which US measurement has been utilised include older adults and critically ill patients [34], multiple organ failure, COPD [35] and HIV-infected patients [36], among others. This technique could be particularly useful in populations, such as spinal cord injury, that present special challenges for traditional body composition techniques due to reduced mobility [37]. Collectively, the evidence suggests that US is a potential method to evaluate lean tissue status in hospital settings and to assess the effects of nutrition and exercise-based interventions on muscle wasting.

There are several emerging US devices of interest to body composition researchers and clinicians. A small, portable, hand-held US transducer designed specifically for body composition assessment (BodyMetrix, BX2000, IntelaMetrix, Inc., Livermore, CA) has arrived on the market. Nevertheless, standard measurement procedures for the assessment of body composition using US are not clearly defined, with considerable variability in US frequencies and measurement sites. In spite of these limitations, US use is emerging as an important clinical tool because it is a safe, portable, fast and low-cost technique.

Three-dimensional imaging

Three-dimensional body surface scanners are transforming our ability to accurately measure a person's body size, shape and skin surface area. Due to the low cost, non-invasive character and ease of use, this technique is appealing for widespread clinical applications. This digitalised technique uses an optical measurement to create a 3D body image along with total and regional body volumes and dimensions, such as body circumferences, lengths, widths, thicknesses and percentage body fat [38].

Three-dimensional imaging may be used by clinicians to estimate skin surface area measurements for burn treatments and to calculate drug and chemotherapy doses for use in many circumstances. It is also the preferred criterion for indexing the glomerular filtration rate [39]. Additionally, it has applications in treating eating disorders such as anorexia nervosa, where distorted body image is a defining characteristic [40]. Additionally, Wells et al. [41] suggested that 3D body surface scanning could benefit obesity research, and act as a mainstream medical tool to asses surface area for drug dosage calculations. Despite this, further work exploring associations between body shape and risk of morbidity and mortality is required before 3D scanning is implemented in clinical practice. Additionally, research surrounding the validity of this technique in different clinical cohorts is warranted before its use can be evaluated in clinical practice.

One study validated first-generation 3D scanners by using underwater weighing and plethysmography techniques, finding no significant differences with respect to absolute total-body volume [36]. Wang et al. [38] reported that 3D scanning accurately and rapidly predicted body volume, circumferences and length although for the measurement of percent body fat and total body volume, a specific protocol should be followed: use of close-fitting, minimal clothing and standing motionless while holding the breath.

The main limitation of this technique is the software, which is becoming more sophisticated, mainly for the quantification of percentage body fat. Compared to other body composition imaging techniques, its use in clinical practice is hindered by its inability to assess differences in adipose tissue subdivisions and the lack of documented use in clinical settings.

2.7.3 Summary

A variety of methods are now available for the assessment of body composition and choice should take into account criteria such as the body compartment of interest, validity/reliability, degree of training required for the examiner, cost and patient burden. The past few decades have seen major conceptual and technological advances in the assessment of body composition and its independent value for predicting patient health and prognosis. Once thought to be too unmanageable, time-consuming and burdensome to the patient, body composition was rarely measured in the clinical setting.

The use of imaging techniques is of particular interest since these are collectively the most reliable and (in most cases) readily available, providing dietitians and other health professionals with a unique opportunity to assess the impact of different body compartments on physiological roles. In addition to its diagnostic value, body composition assessment can be used to monitor the efficacy of nutrition support during treatment and follow-up. Its assessment should therefore be included in routine clinical practice in many clinical conditions in which abnormalities in body composition are likely to occur undetected by alterations in body weight alone. This includes surgery, liver transplant patients, COPD, intensive care patients, Crohn's disease, Duchenne muscular dystrophy, cancer, diabetes and HIV, among others.

Guidelines for the use of body composition assessment in the clinical setting are currently being developed by the American Society of Parenteral and Enteral Nutrition. It is anticipated that this will be an important document endorsing the use of imaging techniques in the assessment of nutritional status.

References

1. Norman K, Pichard C, Lochs H, Pirlich M. Prognostic impact of disease-related malnutrition. *Clin Nutr* 2008; **27**(1): 5–15.
2. Duren DL, Sherwood RJ, Czerwinski SA, Lee M, Choh AC, Siervogel RM, Cameron Chumlea W. Body composition methods: comparisons and interpretation. *J Diabetes Sci Technol* 2008; **2**(6): 1139–1146.
3. Prado CM, Heymsfield SB. Lean tissue imaging: a new era for nutritional assessment and intervention. *J Parenter Enteral Nutr* 2014; **38**(8): 940–953.
4. Ross R. Advances in the application of imaging methods in applied and clinical physiology. *Acta Diabetol* 2003; **40** (Suppl 1): S45–50.
5. Baumgartner RN, Koehler KM, Gallagher D, Romero L, Heymsfield SB, Ross RR, Garry PJ, Lindeman RD. Epidemiology of sarcopenia among the elderly in New Mexico. *Am J Epidemiol* 1998; **147**(8): 755–763.
6. Albanese CV, Diessel E, Genant HK. Clinical applications of body composition measurements using DXA. *J Clin Densitom* 2003; **6**(2): 75–85.
7. Vuillerot C, Braillon P, Fontaine-Carbonnel S, Rippert P, André E, Iwaz J, Poirot I, Bérard C. Influence of a two-year steroid treatment on body composition as measured by dual X-ray absorptiometry in boys with Duchenne muscular dystrophy. *Neuromuscul Disord* 2014; **24**(6): 467–473.
8. Ragnarsson O, Glad CA, Bergthorsdottir R, Almqvist EG, Ekerstad E, Widell H, Wangberg B, Johannsson G. Body composition and bone mineral density in women with Cushing's syndrome in remission and the association with common genetic variants influencing glucocorticoid sensitivity. *Eur J Endocrinol* 2015; **172**(1): 1–10.
9. Smith MR, Saad F, Egerdie B, Sieber PR, Tammela TL, Ke C, Leder BZ, Goessl C. Sarcopenia during androgen-deprivation therapy for prostate cancer. *J Clin Oncol* 2012; **30**(26): 3271–3276.
10. Demark-Wahnefried W, Kenyon AJ, Eberle P, Skye A, Kraus WE. Preventing sarcopenic obesity among breast cancer patients who receive adjuvant chemotherapy: results of a feasibility study. *Clin Exerc Physiol* 2002; **4**(1): 44–49.
11. Pietrobelli A, Wang Z, Formica C, Heymsfield SB. Dual-energy X-ray absorptiometry: fat estimation errors due to variation in soft tissue hydration. *Am J Physiol* 1998; **274**(5 Pt 1): E808–816.
12. Prado CM. Body composition in chemotherapy: the promising role of CT scans. *Curr Opin Clin Nutr Metab Care* 2013; **16**(5): 525–533.
13. Shen W, Wang Z, Punyanita M, Lei J, Sinav A, Kral JG, Imielinska C, Ross R, Heymsfield SB. Adipose tissue quantification by imaging methods: a proposed classification. *Obes Res* 2003; **11**(1): 5–16.
14. Prado C, Cushen S, Orsso C, Ryan A. Sarcopenia and cachexia in the era of obesity: clinical and nutritional impact. *Proc Nutr Soc* 2016; **75**(2): 188–198.
15. Marquis K, Debigare R, Lacasse Y, LeBlanc P, Jobin J, Carrier G, Maltais F. Midthigh muscle cross-sectional area is a better predictor of mortality than body mass index in patients with chronic obstructive pulmonary disease. *Am J Respir Crit Care Med* 2002; **166**(6): 809–813.
16. Danneels LA, Vanderstraeten GG, Cambier DC, Witvrouw EE, De Cuyper HJ. CT imaging of trunk muscles in chronic low back pain patients and healthy control subjects. *Eur Spine J* 2000; **9**(4): 266–272.
17. Sahdev A, Reznek RH, Evanson J, Grossman AB. Imaging in Cushing's syndrome. *Arq Bras Endocrinol Metabol* 2007; **51**: 1319–1328.

18. Tong Q, Sankalé JL, Hadigan CM, Tan G, Rosenberg ES, Kanki PJ, Grinspoon SK, Hotamisligil GS. Regulation of adiponectin in human immunodeficiency virus-infected patients: relationship to body composition and metabolic indices. *J Clin Endocrinol Metab* 2003; **88**(4): 1559–1564.

19. Thakore JH, Mann JN, Vlahos I, Martin A, Reznek R. Increased visceral fat distribution in drug-naive and drug-free patients with schizophrenia. *Int J Obes Relat Metab Disord* 2002; **26**(1): 137–141.

20. Ryan AS, Dobrovolny CL, Smith GV, Silver KH, Macko RF. Hemiparetic muscle atrophy and increased intramuscular fat in stroke patients. *Arch Phys Med Rehabil* 2002; **83**(12): 1703–1707.

21. Braunschweig CA, Sheean PM, Peterson SJ, Perez SG, Freels S, Troy KL, Ajanaku FC, Patel A, Sclamberg JS, Wang Z. Exploitation of diagnostic computed tomography scans to assess the impact of nutrition support on body composition changes in respiratory failure patients. *J Parenter Enteral Nutr* 2014; **38**(7): 880–885.

22. Olbers T, Björkman S, Lindroos A, Maleckas A, Lönn L, Sjöström L, Lönroth H. Body composition, dietary intake, and energy expenditure after laparoscopic Roux-en-Y gastric bypass and laparoscopic vertical banded gastroplasty: a randomized clinical trial. *Ann Surg* 2006; **244**(5): 715.

23. Lee JS, Terjimanian MN, Tishberg LM, Alawieh AZ, Harbaugh CM, Sheetz KH, Holcombe SA, Wang SC, Sonnenday CJ, Englesbe MJ. Surgical site infection and analytic morphometric assessment of body composition in patients undergoing midline laparotomy. *J Am Coll Surg* 2011; **213**(2): 236–244.

24. Dahya V, Xiao J, Prado MM, Chagas da Silva A, Burroughs P, Noel T, Batchelor W. Body composition assessed by computed tomography predicts length of stay after TAVR. *Catheter Cardiovasc Interv* 2015; **85**(S2): S147.

25. Martin L, Birdsell L, Macdonald N, Reiman T, Clandinin MT, McCargar LJ, Murphy R, Ghosh S, Sawyer MB, Baracos VE. Cancer cachexia in the age of obesity: skeletal muscle depletion is a powerful prognostic factor, independent of body mass index. *J Clin Oncol* 2013; **31**(12): 1539–1547.

26. Després JP. Body fat distribution and risk of cardiovascular disease: an update. *Circulation* 2012; **126**(10): 1301–1313.

27. Katergari SA, Milousis A, Mantatzis M, Gioka T, Tripsianis G, Passadakis P, Prassopoulos P, Papachristou DN. Body fat distribution by anthropometric and MRI-based techniques in relation to insulin secretion and action in men with diabetes. *Minerva Endocrinol* 2014; **39**(2): 107–117.

28. Guldiken S, Tuncbilek N, Okten O, Arikan E, Tugrul A. Visceral fat thickness determined using ultrasonography is associated with anthropometric and clinical parameters of metabolic syndrome. *Int J Clin Pract* 2006; **60**(12 Suppl): 1576–1581.

29. Hirooka M, Kumagi T, Kurose K, Nakanishi S, Michitaka K, Matsuura B, Horiike N, Onji M. A technique for the measurement of visceral fat by ultrasonography: comparison of measurements by ultrasonography and computed tomography. *Intern Med* 2005; **44**(8): 794–799.

30. Ribeiro-Filho FF, Faria AN, Azjen S, Zanella MT, Ferreira SRG. Methods of estimation of visceral fat: advantages of ultrasonography. *Obes Res* 2003; **11**(12): 1488–1494.

31. Mourtzakis M, Wischmeyer P. Bedside ultrasound measurement of skeletal muscle. *Curr Opin Clin Nutr Metab Care* 2014; **17**(5): 389–395.

32. Cadore EL, Izquierdo M, Conceicao M, et al. Echo intensity is associated with skeletal muscle power and cardiovascular performance in elderly men. *Exp Gerontol* 2012; **47**(6): 473–478.

33. Fukumoto Y, Ikezoe T, Yamada Y, Tsukagoshi R, Nakamura M, Mori N, Kimura M, Ichihashi N. Skeletal muscle quality assessed from echo intensity is associated with muscle strength of middle-aged and elderly persons. *Eur J Appl Physiol* 2012; **112**(4): 1519–1525.

34. Campbell IT, Watt T, Withers D, England R, Sukumar S, Keegan MA, Faragher B, Martin DF. Muscle thickness, measured with ultrasound, may be an indicator of lean tissue wasting in multiple organ failure in the presence of edema. *Am J Clin Nutr* 1995; **62**(3): 533–539.

35. Menon MK, Houchen L, Harrison S, Singh SJ, Morgan MD, Steiner MC. Ultrasound assessment of lower limb muscle mass in response to resistance training in COPD. *Respir Res* 2012; **13**: 119.

36. Wells JC, Douros I, Fuller NJ, Elia M, Dekker L. Assessment of body volume using three-dimensional photonic scanning. *Ann N Y Acad Sci* 2000; **904**: 247–254.

37. Emmons RR, Garber CE, Cirnigliaro CM, Kirshblum SC, Spungen AM, Bauman WA. Assessment of measures for abdominal adiposity in persons with spinal cord injury. *Ultrasound Med Biol* 2011; **37**(5): 734–741.

38. Wang J, Gallagher D, Thornton JC, Yu W, Horlick M, Pi-Sunyer FX. Validation of a 3-dimensional photonic scanner for the measurement of body volumes, dimensions, and percentage body fat. *Am J Clin Nutr* 2006; **83**(4): 809–816.

39. Yu CY, Lo YH, Chiou WK. The 3D scanner for measuring body surface area: a simplified

calculation in the Chinese adult. *Appl Ergon* 2003; **34**(3): 273–278.

40. Keizer A, Smeets MAM, Dijkerman HC, van den Hout M, Klugkist I, van Elburg A, Postma A. Tactile body image disturbance in anorexia nervosa. *Psychiatry Res* 2011; **190**(1): 115–120.

41. Wells J, Ruto A, Treleaven P. Whole-body three-dimensional photonic scanning: a new technique for obesity research and clinical practice. *Int J Obes* 2008; **32**(2): 232–238.

42. Heymsfield SB, Ebbeling CB, Zheng J, Pietrobelli A, Strauss BJ, Silva AM, Ludwig DS. Multi-component molecular-level body composition reference methods: evolving concepts and future directions. *Obes Rev* 2015; **16**(4): 282–294.

SECTION 3

Nutritional requirements in nutrition support

Chapter 3.1

Fluid requirements and assessment in nutrition support

Stephanie Baron[1], Gérard Friedlander[1], Eve M. Lepicard[2] and Marie Courbebaisse[1]

[1]European Hospital Georges-Pompidou, Paris, France
[2]Institute for European Expertise in Physiology, Paris, France

3.1.1 Hydration status: physiopathology

Definition and regulation of hydration status

Water is the main constituent of the body; water accounts for 75% of body weight in newborns and 60% in adults. Seven percent of total body water is extracellular fluid, such as plasma, 28% is interstitial fluid and the remaining 65% is intracellular fluid. The physiological functions of water are numerous. It is responsible for vascular volume maintenance and nutrient transport, as well as excretion as urine removes plasma solutes. Moreover, intracellular water is indispensable to biochemical reactions as it traps heat production; thus, water is necessary for thermoregulation.

The balance between water output and input defines hydration status. Water output is mainly due to excretion via the kidneys. Sweating, the respiratory tract and faeces water losses account for less volume and are not regulated, whereas water excretion via the kidney is tightly regulated and removes solutes from the blood. Water output must be counterbalanced by water intake to maintain a neutral hydration balance. Most of our water intake comes from drinking water in beverages (around 60% of total daily water intake). The rest comes from food and metabolism; the latter accounts for around 250 mL/day [1].

Excess loss of water or insufficient water intake induces a state of dehydration. This dehydration is hypertonic when water loss exceeds electrolyte loss, leading to a higher electrolyte blood concentration and thus an increased plasma osmolality. This increase implies an intracellular dehydration and a decrease in cellular volume [2]. Thus, kidney water excretion and water intake are mainly controlled by plasma osmolality changes. Increased plasma osmolality through hypothalamic osmoreceptor activation is responsible for vasopressin (AVP or antidiuretic hormone) release and thirst, two main effectors of water balance regulation. AVP is released from the postpituitary gland and is responsible for renal water reabsorption. A small increase in plasma osmolality elicits thirst and thus water intake.

Dehydration consequences and related disorders

Dehydration may result from acute or chronic processes. Acute dehydration results mainly from an excess of water loss due to pathological conditions, such as diarrhoea or pyrexia, or to physical exercise. It must be kept in mind that severe acute dehydration with a fluid deficit exceeding 8% can lead to death [3]. Chronic dehydration seems to be mainly linked to a lack of water intake and is often less serious and clinically more difficult to diagnose. Mild dehydration is associated with altered cognitive performance, degraded mood and impaired physical performance. Although nephrolithiasis (renal stone formation) is the only disorder that has been consistently associated with chronic low daily water intake [4], many other pathological conditions, such as constipation, asthma, cardiovascular disease and chronic kidney disease, are linked to insufficient fluid intake [5].

Daily fluid intake requirement

To fulfil water requirements, the scientific and medical community have made recommendations about daily water intake for infants, children and adults of both genders [6–11]. Recommendations in basal conditions (moderate environmental conditions and physical activity) are summarised in Table 3.1.1. Daily water intake recommendations are based on three factors: water intakes recorded in population subgroups, desirable urine osmolalities and theoretical water requirements. The European Food Safety Authority (EFSA) indicates that 1 litre is necessary to excrete 1000 kcal of osmolar charge. Discrepancies among recommendations from different sources, especially regarding intake during pregnancy and lactation, are due to difficulties in accurately assessing these three factors. Recommendations are based on total water intake and take into account water from beverages and food. In general, in adults, 70–80% of total water comes from beverages and the rest from food.

In patients with a previous history of nephrolithiasis, the majority of experts recommend a fluid intake higher than 2 L per day to maintain a diuresis of at least 2 L per day in order to optimise urine dilution [12]. Environmental temperature, altitude, humidity level, physical activity, diet and pathophysiological conditions can affect water needs. There are also seasonal variations in hydration status, and it is well known that dehydration secondary to heat waves is potentially very harmful, particularly among susceptible subpopulations such as the elderly, and for particularly fragile patients. Indeed, young children, non-autonomous persons and the elderly are at higher risk of dehydration than the general population, because of difficulties in accessing water and a decreased perception of thirst.

Studies in diverse populations show that fluid requirement recommendations are not met in many children and adults and that the elderly are even less likely than other adult age groups to ingest enough fluid [13,14]. Actually, the scientific basis for water intake recommendations for the elderly is scarce; consequently, the recommendations from different nutrition societies are not as consistent as the recommendations that have been made for children or young adults.

3.1.2 Assessment of hydration status

Several means are available to assess hydration status. The main characteristics of each are summarised in Table 3.1.2.

Body weight change

Body weight change is probably the simplest way of assessing water loss for a short period of time. Total body water corresponds to around 60% of body weight [2], and an acute change in body water levels can be monitored through measurement of body mass. This parameter is sensitive enough to detect acute, moderate fluid losses of 2–3% of body mass [15]. Thus, body mass change is commonly used to evaluate dehydration severity. In physiological conditions, intraindividual body mass variation is very low, but because of the important interindividual variations, a precise personal baseline is absolutely fundamental [16].

Isotope dilution

Isotope dilution methods are considered the gold standard to assess body water. These methods are based on the distribution of a tracer substance after oral or intravenous administration [17]. Use of deuterium oxide or tritiated water as tracer enables measurement of total body water (TBW), since these tracers distribute to all body fluid compartments. Other tracers that distribute only

Table 3.1.1 Recommendations for adequate water intake expressed as volume in litres/day except Belgium (including fluid from food and beverages)

Age	Europe, including UK (EFSA) 2010	Belgium 2009	Germany, Austria, Switzerland 2008	Australia and New Zealand (nutrient reference values) 2006	United States (Institute of Medicine and USDA) 2005	World Health Organization 2005
0–4 months		130–150 mL/kg	0.68 L			
0–6 months	0.7 L			0.7 L	0.7 L	0.7 L
4–8 months		120–130 mL/kg	1.0 L			
7–12 months	0.8–1.0 L	100–110 mL/kg	1.0 L	0.8 L	0.8 L	0.8 L
8–12 months						
1–3 years	1.1–1.2 L	75–100 mL/kg	1.3 L	1.4 L	1.3 L	1.3 L
3–4 years			1.3 L			
4–6 years		75–100 mL/kg				
4–7 years			1.6 L			
4–8 years	1.6 L			1.6 L	1.7 L	1.7 L
6–11 years		65–80 mL/kg				
7–10 years			1.8 L			
9–13 years	M 2.1 L F 1.9 L			M 2.2 L F 1.9 L	M 2.4 L F 2.1 L	M 2.4 L F 2.1 L
10–13 years			2.15 L			
11–14 years		65–70 mL/kg				
13–15 years			2.45 L			
14–18 years	M 2.5 L F 2.0 L	45–60 mL/kg		M 2.7 L F 2.2 L	M 3.3 L F 2.3 L	M 3.3 L F 2.3 L
15–19 years			2.8 L			
19–25 years			2.7 L			
19–70 years	M 2.5 L F 2.0 L	2.5 L		M 3.4 L F 2.8 L	M 3.7 L F 2.7 L	M 3.7 L F 2.7 L
25–50 years			2.6 L			
Elderly (>70 years)	M 2.5 L F 2.0 L		2.25 L	M 3.4v F 2.8 L	M 3.7 L F 2.7 L	M 3.7 L F 2.7 L
Pregnancy	2.3 L		2.7 L	3.1 L	3.0 L	
Lactation	2.7 L		3.1 L	3.5 L	3.8 L	

M, male; F, female.

Table 3.1.2 Advantages and disadvantages of methods available for assessing hydration status

Techniques	Fluids involved	Practicability	Accuracy	Risk for subjects	Intraindividual variability	Interindividual variability
Body mass change (acute context only)	All (extra- and intracellular fluid)	Not expensive, quick, low technical expertise	Moderate	Non-invasive	1.1%	26.6%
Isotope dilution	All (extra- and intracellular and total body water)	Expensive, technical expertise	High	Non-invasive	–	–
Bioelectrical impedance	Uncertain	Moderate cost, time-consuming, technical expertise required	Moderate	Non-invasive	–	–
Plasma osmolality	Extracellular fluid	Not expensive, quick, middle technical expertise	Moderate	Invasive (venous puncture)	1.3%	1.5%
Urine osmolality	Excreted urine	Not expensive, quick, middle technical expertise	Moderate	Non-invasive	28.3%	57.9%
Urine specific gravity	Excreted urine	Not expensive, quick, low technical expertise	Moderate	Non-invasive	0.4%	1.0%
Urine colour	Excreted urine	Low cost, quick, low technical expertise	Moderate	Non-invasive	30.9%	47.4%
Saliva osmolality	Fluids involved	Not expensive, quick, middle technical expertise	Moderate	Non-invasive	9.5%	35.8%

Data from Cheuvront et al. [16].

in extracellular volume (radioactively labelled bromide, sodium or chloride) are used to measure extracellular water [18]. The difference between total and extracellular water provides intracellular water levels.

Bioelectrical impedance analysis

Bioelectrical impedance analysis (BIA) relies on the electrical properties of tissues. Electrical current conduction of tissues differs depending on water and electrolyte content. Thus, formulae have been developed to predict total, extra- and intracellular water using body resistance to the electrical current. Several variations of BIA have been proposed since the 1970s using single and multiple frequencies [19], different equations, mathematical modelling and specific segment exploration. The main advantage is the rapid feedback, but caution is required in their use since they exhibit significant variability, both intra- and inter-individuals and between different BIA methods [20,21]. Finally, multiple-frequency BIA methods are probably more relevant than single-frequency BIA.

Plasma osmolality

The most important regulated variable in the central nervous system that controls human fluid–electrolyte balance is intracellular osmolality. Because plasma osmolality reflects intracellular osmolality, it has historically been considered as a good marker of hydration status [22]. Osmolality of a solution is defined as the number of osmoles of solutes per 1 kg of solvent (water in the case of plasma). Neuroendocrine regulation of osmolality is such that normal plasma values rarely deviate by more than 1–2% from a basal value of 287 mOsm/kg in healthy well-hydrated individuals. Plasma osmolality exhibits low intraindividual and interindividual variations in normal physiological conditions (no excess water loss and free access to water). Because of this small deviation window, a cut-off of 290 mOsm/kg is commonly used to define the limit between euhydration and dehydration [23,24]. Plasma osmolality is measured using either a freezing point depression osmometer

(temperature freezing point depends on solute concentration) or, more rarely, a vapour pressure depression osmometer (vapour pressure is related to particle concentration). These two methods have a high reproducibility [16].

Even though plasma sodium concentration is the most important factor driving plasma osmolality (with its matched anions, urea and glucose), plasma osmolality measurement cannot be replaced by sodium concentration. Indeed, 'false hyponatraemia' could happen especially in some pathophysiological conditions such as diabetic hyperglycaemia or hyperuraemia, or when any osmotic substance is present in plasma (e.g. alcohol, mannitol). If a false hyponatraemia has been discounted (by concomitantly measuring plasma osmolality and sodium concentration, both low in the case of hypo-osmotic hyponatraemia), plasma sodium concentration is well correlated to plasma osmolality [25] and could be used to estimate plasma osmolality using the following calculation: $2 \times [Na+]$ (plasma osmolality corresponds to the number of osmoles per 1 L of solvent). Plasma glucose and/or urea concentrations should be added only in cases of hyperglycaemia and/or hyperuraemia because these two molecules have no osmotic properties otherwise.

In case of acute changes, especially during physical exercise, plasma osmolality may change, whereas in a chronic dehydration context, such as insufficient water intake, plasma osmolality is preserved while only urine indices change because of kidney adaptation [26]. Consequently, plasma osmolality cannot be used to monitor chronic hypohydration.

Urinary indices

The kidneys are the main regulator of water balance. Renal adaptation to dehydration leads to decreased urine output and increased urine concentration. Thus it is relevant to assess hydration status with urine indices. Three methods are widely used: osmolality, specific gravity and colour.

Urine osmolality

Urine osmolality depends on the intake of solutes and on the volume of urine excreted. The most important particles are sodium, potassium and urea. In physiological conditions, their concentrations depend mainly on the diet, and daily osmole elimination in urine is closely related to daily osmole intake.

Urine osmolality ranges from 60 to 1200 mOsm/kg in humans. One unit variation of plasma osmolality can lead to a 100 unit variation of urine osmolality, demonstrating the strong adaptation of urine to hydration status [27]. Intraindividual and interindividual variations are large, with mean 24-hour urine osmolality ranging from 360 mOsm/kg to 860 mOsm/kg depending on the study, dietary fluid intake and osmole intake. Thus, setting a cut-off value to define dehydration is difficult. However, in line with results of Manz and Wentz and EFSA conclusions, an osmolality over 800 mOsm/kg is a reasonable limit between a euhydrated and a slightly dehydrated status [6,27].

Urine specific gravity

Urine specific gravity (USG) is defined as the weight of urine solution compared to that of an equal volume of distilled water. USG can be rapidly and easily measured by a refractometer. In normal physiological conditions, USG intra- and interindividual variations are negligible, making this measurement very robust and reliable [16]. USG in euhydrated subjects usually ranges from 1.013 to 1.029. In contrast to definitions based on urine osmolality, there is consensus for the cut-off value: a USG of 1.029 or more defines dehydration.

Single gravity test strips could partially replace refractometers in measurement of USG. Patients can use these test strips themselves, making it a useful method even though it has low analytical performance (interference with glucosuria, proteinuria, bacteruria, leucocyturia, alkaline urine pH).

Finally, the only disadvantage of USG is that both the number and the size of the particles in the solution affect its measurement. USG can vary when unusual quantities of larger molecules such as glucose, proteins and urea are found in the urine, generating falsely elevated values that wrongly suggest high urine concentration.

Nonetheless, in most situations USG is probably the most specific of urine markers with negligible analytical variation [16].

Urine colour

A urine colour chart has been developed to assess urine concentration in healthy humans. The scale ranges from 1, which is pale yellow (diluted urine), to 8, which is dark brown (concentrated urine) [28]. The cut-off value to distinguish euhydration and dehydration is 4 units [29]. The main disadvantage of the urine colour chart is its lack of sensitivity (81% with a 5.5 cut-off value) [16]. Moreover, urine colour can be affected by dietary factors, illness or medications, leading to important intra- and interindividual variability [16].

Validity of urinary indices to assess hydration status

A few rare pathological conditions disturb kidney concentration capacity. This makes the use of urine indices inappropriate for patients who have diseases such as diabetes insipidus, syndrome of inappropriate antidiuresis or preterminal stage of chronic kidney disease.

Urine can be collected at different time points. Usually, it is either collected in the morning after fasting or all urine is collected over a 24-hour period. Different collection times do not lead to the same information. Spot urine gives information about a single time point, whereas 24-hour urine collection reflects the body water balance over a day [30]. Moreover, urine is stored in the bladder before excretion. Thereby, urinary measurements should be interpreted relative to the timing of urine collection performed.

The majority of researchers consider 24-hour urine collection as the gold standard for urine hydration markers in daily life [30]. Nevertheless, collecting 24-hour urine is difficult. Afternoon urine collection could be a good representation of the whole day and has become an alternative to 24-hour urine collection [31].

The ratio between urine osmolality and creatinine concentration appears to be informative. This ratio takes into account hydration status (urine osmolality) without interference from water volume output (creatinine concentration). Even though it seems to be reproducible in individuals over 5 years of age [32], further studies are needed to validate this ratio and to determine its correlation with other accurate hydration markers.

Finally, urinary indices provide an accurate assessment of hydration status during mild dehydration. However, these measurements may be less accurate in some situations such as during a rehydration period, during isotonic dehydration (loss of water and sodium in the same concentration as plasma), or during hypotonic dehydration (loss of sodium).

What about other fluids?

Saliva is easily accessible, and its flow rate may be an informative parameter. In physiological unstimulated situations, saliva flow rate is between 0.3 and 0.5 mL/min. This rate decreases in dehydration conditions and saliva osmolality increases. Nonetheless, this increase occurs later than other hydration marker changes, exhibiting poor sensitivity. In addition, the large intra- and interindividual variability, highlighted by several clinical studies, leads to poor specificity [16].

Recently, tear osmolality has been suggested as a marker for hydration status. Tear osmolality has good correlation with plasma osmolality but further studies are needed to validate its use [33,34].

3.1.3 Summary

Water is an indispensable element necessary for organism functions. Despite environmental conditions and physical activity, water intake must be high enough to maintain an optimal hydration status. To check this hydration status, many tools are available. The method must be chosen with caution in accordance with the context.

References

1. Perrier E, Rondeau P, Poupin M, et al. Relation between urinary hydration biomarkers and total fluid intake in healthy adults. *Eur J Clin Nutr* 2013; **67**(9): 939–943.

2. Cheuvront SN, Kenefick RW, Charkoudian N, Sawka MN. Physiologic basis for understanding quantitative dehydration assessment. *Am J Clin Nutr* 2013; **97**(3): 455–462.

3. Grandjean AC, Reimers KJ, Buyckx ME. Hydration: issues for the 21st century. *Nutr Rev* 2003; **61**(8): 261–271.

4. Armstrong LE. Challenges of linking chronic dehydration and fluid consumption to health outcomes. *Nutr Rev* 2012; **70**(Suppl 2): S121–127.

5. Popkin BM, d'Anci KE, Rosenberg IH. Water, hydration, and health. *Nutr Rev* 2010; **68**(8): 439–458.

6. EFSA Panel on Dietetic Products. Scientific opinion on dietary reference values for water. *EFSA J* 2010; **8**(3): 1459–1507.

7. Institute of Medicine of National Academies (IMNA). Dietary References Intakes: The Essential Guide to Nutrient Requirements. Washington: National Academies Press, 2006.

8. Australian National Health and Medical Research Council (NHMRC) and the New Zealand Ministry of Health (MoH). Nutrient Reference Values for Australia and New Zealand including Recommended Dietary Intakes. 2006. www.nhmrc.gov.au/guidelines-publications/n35-n36-n37 (accessed 29 August 2017).

9. Institute of Medicine. Dietary Reference Intakes for Water, Potassium, Sodium, Chloride, and Sulfate. 2004. http://insanemedicine.com/wp-content/uploads/2016/07/water-potassium-intake-Institue-of-Medicine.pdf (accessed 30 August 2017).

10. World Health Organization. Water Requirements, Impinging Factors, and Recommended Intakes. 2005. www.who.int/water_sanitation_health/dwq/nutrientschap3.pdf (accessed 30 August 2017).

11. German Nutrition Society, Austrian Nutrition Society, Society for Nutrition Research, Swiss Nutrition Association. Referenzwerte für die Nährstoffzufuhr. Frankfurt am Main: Umschau Braus, 2008.

12. Meschi T, Nouvenne A, Borghi L. Lifestyle recommendations to reduce the risk of kidney stones. *Urol Clin North Am* 2011; **38**(3): 313–320.

13. Decher NR, Casa DJ, Yeargin SW, et al. Hydration status, knowledge, and behavior in youths at summer sports camps. *Int J Sports Physiol Perform* 2008; **3**(3): 262–278.

14. Kaushik A, Mullee MA, Bryant TN, Hill CM. A study of the association between children's access to drinking water in primary schools and their fluid intake: can water be 'cool' in school? *Child Care Health Dev* 2007; **33**(4): 409–415.

15. Armstrong LE, Costill DL, Fink WJ. Influence of diuretic-induced dehydration on competitive running performance. *Med Sci Sports Ex* 1985; **17**(4): 456–461.

16. Cheuvront SN, Ely BR, Kenefick RW, Sawka MN. Biological variation and diagnostic accuracy of dehydration assessment markers. *Am J Clin Nutr* 2010; **92**(3): 565–573.

17. Armstrong LE. Hydration assessment techniques. *Nutr Rev* 2005; **63**(6 Pt 2): S40–54.

18. Lukaski HC. Methods for the assessment of human body composition: traditional and new. *Am J Clin Nutr* 1987; **46**(4): 537–556.

19. Gudivaka R, Schoeller DA, Kushner RF, Bolt MJ. Single- and multifrequency models for bioelectrical impedance analysis of body water compartments. *J Appl Physiol* 1999; **87**(3): 1087–1096.

20. Olde Rikkert MG, Deurenberg P, Jansen RW, van't Hof MA, Hoefnagels WH. Validation of multifrequency bioelectrical impedance analysis in detecting changes in fluid balance of geriatric patients. *J Am Geriatr Soc* 1997; **45**(11): 1345–1351.

21. Ward LC, Elia M, Cornish BH. Potential errors in the application of mixture theory to multifrequency bioelectrical impedance analysis. *Physiol Meas* 1998; **19**(1): 53–60.

22. Grant MM, Kubo WM. Assessing a patient's hydration status. *Am J Nurs* 1975; **75**(8): 1307–1311.

23. Gaebelein CJ, Senay LC Jr. Influence of exercise type, hydration, and heat on plasma volume shifts in men. *J Appl Physiol* 1980; **49**(1): 119–123.

24. Cheuvront SN, Sawka MN. Hydration assessments of athletes. *Sports Sci Exchange* 2005; **18**: 1–6.

25. Costa RJ, Teixeira A, Rama L, et al. Water and sodium intake habits and status of ultra-endurance runners during a multi-stage ultra-marathon conducted in a hot ambient environment: an observational field based study. *Nutr J* 2013; **12**: 13.

26. Perrier E, Vergne S, Klein A, et al. Hydration biomarkers in free-living adults with different levels of habitual fluid consumption. *Br J Nutr* 2013; **109**(9): 1678–1687.

27. Manz F, Wentz A. 24-h hydration status: parameters, epidemiology and recommendations. *Eur J Clin Nutr* 2003; **57**(Suppl 2): S10–18.

28. Armstrong LE, Soto JA, Hacker FT Jr, Casa DJ, Kavouras SA, Maresh CM. Urinary indices during dehydration, exercise, and rehydration. *Int J Sport Nutr* 1998; **8**(4): 345–355.

29. Cleary MA, Hetzler RK, Wasson D, Wages JJ, Stickley C, Kimura IF. Hydration behaviors before and after an educational and prescribed hydration intervention in adolescent athletes. *J Athl Train* 2012; **47**(3): 273–281.

30. Armstrong LE, Johnson EC, McKenzie AL, Munoz CX. Interpreting common hydration biomarkers on the basis of solute and water excretion. *Eur J Clin Nutr* 2013; **67**(3): 249–253.

31. Perrier E, Demazieres A, Girard N, et al. Circadian variation and responsiveness of hydration biomarkers to changes in daily water intake. *Eur J Appl Physiol* 2013; **113**(8): 2143–2151.

32. Godevithanage S, Kanankearachchi PP, Dissanayake MP, et al. Spot urine osmolality/creatinine ratio in healthy humans. *Kidney Blood Press Res* 2010; **33**(4): 291–296.

33. Fortes MB, Diment BC, di Felice U, et al. Tear fluid osmolarity as a potential marker of hydration status. *Med Sci Sports Exerc* 2011; **43**(8): 1590–1597.

34. Santos MT, Batista R, Guare RO, et al. Salivary osmolality and hydration status in children with cerebral palsy. *J Oral Pathol Med* 2011; **40**(7): 582–586.

Chapter 3.2

Energy requirements in nutrition support

C. Jeyakumar Henry[1,2,3] and Stefan G.J.A. Camps[1,2]

[1] Clinical Nutrition Research Centre (CNRC), National University of Singapore, Singapore

[2] Singapore Institute for Clinical Sciences (SICS), Agency for Science, Technology and Research (A*STAR), Singapore

[3] Department of Biochemistry, Yong Loo Lin School of Medicine, National University of Singapore, Singapore

3.2.1 Introduction

During most periods of our lives, humans are in energy balance, when energy intake matches expenditure. Under this equilibrium status, energy expenditure determines energy requirements and energy requirement is met by energy intake:

Energy balance: energy intake = energy expenditure

In the case of undernutrition, when energy intake is too low to meet energy expenditure, there is a negative energy balance resulting in weight loss. In many clinical settings, where food intake is limited and energy expenditure is increased, negative energy balance is the norm. Under such circumstances, it is important to increase energy intake in order to restore energy balance. Being in positive energy balance, when energy intake exceeds energy expenditure, will lead to weight gain. The accurate measurement or prediction of energy expenditure is essential for targeted nutrition support to avoid negative consequences associated with over- or underfeeding [1,2].

For several decades, it was routine to measure food intake to estimate energy requirements. Since the measurement of energy (food) intake is prone to considerable experimental errors, novel methods to estimate energy requirements have evolved. The advent of doubly labelled water to estimate total energy expenditure (TEE) and the publication in 1985 of the Food and Agriculture Organisation, World Health Organisation and United Nations University (FAO/WHO/UNU) report on protein and energy requirements stimulated considerable interest in the measurement of energy expenditure rather than food intake to predict human energy needs [3]. The FAO report also emphasised the application of basal metabolic rate (BMR) as the template for estimating energy requirements. The measurement or prediction of BMR and the energy cost of various physical activities formed the basis for estimating energy requirements. The estimation of total energy expenditure from BMR is based on the factorial method where the basal metabolic rate is multiplied by an individual's physical activity level (PAL). BMR can represent up to 70% of total energy expenditure, and is the largest component of energy expenditure.

The term 'basal' was initially used to differentiate energy expended at rest from that expended during physical activity. Basal metabolic rate represents the integration of oxygen consumption by all the tissues in the body. A lucid definition of BMR was that by Mitchell who said, 'Basal metabolism of an animal is the minimal rate of energy expenditure compatible with life' (4).

3.2.2 Measurement of energy expenditure

Energy expenditure may be measured either directly or indirectly. Direct calorimetry enables the measurements of heat production by the

Advanced Nutrition and Dietetics in Nutrition Support, First Edition. Edited by Mary Hickson and Sara Smith.
© 2018 John Wiley & Sons Ltd. Published 2018 by John Wiley & Sons Ltd.

body. Subjects are enclosed in a specially built chamber that precisely measures heat lost over a finite period. In view of the sophisticated nature of precisely measuring heat lost from the body, this method is rarely used today.

Indirect calorimetry, as the term implies, measures oxygen consumption and carbon dioxide produced as a proxy or indirect indicator of energy expenditure. The concepts we use today were laid down by Lavoisier nearly 200 years ago. The equation below simplifies the process of heat production, the moles of glucose oxidised, the consumption of O_2 and the production of CO_2.

$$C_6H_{12}O_6 + 6O_2 \rightarrow 6CO_2 + 6H_2O + Heat$$
$$(180g)\,(6\times22.41)\,(6\times22.31)\,(6\times18g)\,(2.78MJ)$$

From the above, it is apparent that oxidation of 1 g of glucose will yield 15.4 kJ (2780/180). Similarly, 1 L of oxygen consumed will be equivalent to the production of 20.7 kJ (2780/6×22.4). These two principles are now used to estimate energy expenditure in humans. Once we can compute the amount of oxygen consumed, we can estimate heat production and hence energy expenditure. Since glucose is not the only source of fuel utilisation by the human body, Table 3.2.1 provides substrate oxidation variables in relation to energy expenditure from fat, protein and carbohydrate [5].

Estimation of energy expenditure using doubly labelled water

In 1955, Lifson proposed the use of stable isotopes to estimate energy expenditure [6]. If two isotopes of water (H_2O^{18} and ^2H_2O) are administered and the rate of disappearance, as detected from saliva or urine, is evaluated, the disappearance rate of ^2H_2O will reflect water flux and the disappearance rate of H_2O^{18} will reflect water flux and carbon dioxide production. The difference between these two rates of disappearance will give us the rate of carbon dioxide production. Once the rate of carbon dioxide production is known, we can calculate total energy expenditure.

Energy content of foods consumed

The energy needs of the human body are ultimately met from the foods we consume or, in the context of nutrition support, the enteral or parenteral nutrition delivered. In general, foods are composed of proteins, fats and carbohydrates in varying proportions. When macronutrients are combusted in a bomb calorimeter, they will yield 9.4 kcal/g (fats), 5.65 kcal/g (protein) and 4.1 kcal/g (carbohydrates) gross energy. Since all of the macromolecules are not completely digested, some of these nutrients will be lost in the faeces. Energy content corrected for faecal losses is called digestible energy. Similarly, during protein metabolism, some of the proteins are broken down and lost as nitrogen in the urine. Energy content corrected for urinary losses is called the metabolisable energy content of food. Metabolisable energy is the potential energy available for the human body for metabolic activities. It is common to use the Atwater factors to calculate the energy content of foods using the following energy values: 17 kJ/g (4 kcal/g) for protein and carbohydrate and 37 kJ/g (9 kcal/g) for fat. Moreover, a value of 29 kJ/g (7 kcal/g) is used for alcohol [7].

Conditions to be met whilst measuring energy expenditure

The term 'basal' metabolic rate implies that the measurements are performed under standardised conditions. Thus BMR measurements must meet the following conditions [8].

• The subject should be at rest before and during the measurements. They should be in supine position, but awake.
• The subject should have fasted for at least 10–12 hours before the measurements.
• The environmental temperature during the measurements should be in the thermo-neutral range of 22–26 °C.
• The subject should be familiar with the equipment used and be free of emotional stress.
• The subject should not have been involved in any intense physical activity the day before the BMR measurement.

Table 3.2.1 Substrate oxidation variables, VO_2, CO_2 and energy expenditure during fat, protein and carbohydrate oxidation

Oxidation of 1 g	O_2 required (L)	CO_2 produced (L)	Respiratory quotient	Energy expended kJ (kcal)/g	Energy equivalent L O_2 kJ (kcal)/L
Carbohydrate	827.7	827.7	1.000	17.5 (4.18)	21.1 (5.048)
Protein	1010.3	843.6	0.835	19.7 (4.70)	19.48 (4.655)
Fat	2018.9	1435.4	0.710	39.5 (9.45)	19.6 (5.682)
Ethanol	1459.4	977.8	0.670	29.7 (7.09)	20.3 (4.86)

Fat, carbohydrate and protein are assumed to be derived from a mixed meal.
Source: Adapted from Livesey and Elia [5].

Given the time-consuming, invasive and expensive nature of measuring BMR, predictive equations have been developed to estimate BMR.

Harris–Benedict equations

The earliest predictive equations to estimate BMR are the Harris–Benedict equations. In 1919, Harris and Benedict presented a biometric analysis of BMR [9]. They measured a very small number of subjects, 136 males and 103 females, and developed the following equations:

Males : $\quad h = 66.4730 + 13.7516 W + 5.0033 S - 6.7750 A$
Females : $h = 665.0955 + 9.5634 W + 1.8496 S - 4.6756 A$

where h = kcal per day; W = weight in kilograms; S = stature in centimetres; A = age in years.

Due to the simplicity of these equations, they have been widely used in the estimation of BMR for nearly 100 years.

FAO/WHO/UNU and Schofield equations

In 1981, the FAO/WHO/UNU Expert Committee on Energy and Protein Requirements suggested that estimation of energy requirements be based on energy expenditure, rather than food intake. It also proposed that energy expenditure be expressed as multiples of BMR. The FAO/WHO/UNU requested Schofield et al. to conduct an analysis and produce a series of predictive equations for BMR. Schofield et al.

reviewed the literature and produced predictive equations for both sexes for the following ages: 0–3, 3–10, 10–18, 18–30, 30–60 and >60 years [10]. The Schofield database comprised 114 published studies of BMR, totalling 7173 data points. Although their database comprised almost 11 000 BMR values (including group mean values), most of the results were obtained from European and North American subjects. These equations formed the basis of the 1985 FAO/WHO/UNU document Energy and Protein Requirements [3].

Issues surrounding the FAO/WHO/UNU and Schofield equations

In the intervening period (1985–2010), several investigators reported that the FAO equation overestimated BMR in different ethnic groups (11–15). Henry and Rees reviewed the BMR data and reported that the FAO/WHO/UNU equations systematically overestimated the BMR in some ethnic groups [12]. They showed that in addition to Indian subjects, BMR was lower in a range of residents in the tropics, including Philippines, India, Japan, Brazil, China, Malaya and Java, by up to 8–10% (Table 3.2.2).

A significant feature of the Schofield database was that for males aged between 10 and 60 years, over 3000 (50%) data points came from Italian subjects. The Italian group appeared to have a higher BMR per kilogram than any other Caucasian group. The database also contained very few subjects from the tropics.

Table 3.2.2 The percentage by which the FAO/WHO/UNU equations overestimate (+) or underestimate (–) BMR in different ethnic groups by sex, all ages 3–60 years

	Male		Female	
Ethnicity	Mean %	Sample size	Mean %	Sample size
African	+6.5	20	No data	
Chinese	+7.6	274	+3.8	190
Ceylonese	+22.4	125	+12.5	100
Hawaiian	+7.2	19	+4.5	62
Indian	+12.8	50	+12.9	7
Japanese	+5.8	202	+4.6	152
Javanese	+5.0	86	No data	
Malayan	+9.3	62	No data	
Mayan	+1.5	76	No data	
Philippino	+9.5	172	+1.1	31
Samoan	+3.3	21	No data	
South American	+9.4	941	+4.8	227
All	+9.0	2053	+5.4	769

Source: Adapted from Henry and Rees [12].

Henry equations

In 2005, Henry developed a new series of BMR equations that were based on a dataset of 10 552 BMR values that excluded all the Italian subjects and also included a much larger number (4018) of subjects from tropical regions. The database used to derive the Henry equations contained 13 910 measurements of BMR collected from men, women and children. These data were from 174 papers published between 1914 and 2001. The database included information about ethnicity, gender, age, weight and height of each subject and the publication year of the paper. Analysis of this information led to the development of the present set of prediction equations for BMR which can be applied to individuals worldwide [8].

The age range of the subjects in the Henry database was 0–106 years. The Henry equations were based on the most comprehensive and inclusive database of BMR to date. Moreover, the number of subjects included in both the younger (children) and older age groups was much larger than reported in the Schofield equations. Although estimates of BMR made by the Schofield or Henry prediction equations differ only slightly in children or adults (i.e. the Henry equations are 3–4% lower), an assessment of the validity of different predictive equations for BMR in adults found the Henry prediction equations to be the more accurate [16].

Table 3.2.3 shows the linear equation to predict BMR in MJ/day for various age groups and both genders. In 2011, the UK Scientific Advisory Committee on Nutrition (SACN) adopted the Henry equations for estimating BMR in UK subjects. Two years later, the European Food Safety Authority (EFSA) recommended the use of the Henry equations to predict BMR in all 27 countries of the European Union [17].

The inclusion of height improved the accuracy of predicting BMR. Table 3.2.3 illustrates the weight and height coefficients to predict BMR. In the SACN report on dietary reference values for energy [16], it was recommended that both weight and height be used to estimate BMR. The Henry equations were cross-validated using a set of Dutch and US subjects [16,18]. Further evidence of the validity of the Henry equations to predict BMR is afforded by comparing the values computed with observed values, using the Dietary Reference Intake (DRI) [19]. The Henry equations predicted within ±10% of the measured value in 73% of the subjects in both cases (Table 3.2.4).

Table 3.2.3 Henry prediction equations for BMR based on weight, and weight and height

Gender	Age (years)	BMR (MJ/day) based on weight alone	BMR (MJ/day) based on weight and height
Males			
	<3	0.255 w − 0.141	0.118 w + 3.59 h − 1.55
	3–10	0.0937 w + 2.15	0.0632 w + 1.31 h + 1.28
	10–18	0.0769 w + 2.43	0.0651 w + 1.11 h + 1.25
	18–30	0.0669 w + 2.28	0.0600 w + 1.31 h + 0.473
	30–60	0.0592 w + 2.48	0.0476 w + 2.26 h − 0.574
	>60	0.0563 w + 2.15	0.0478 w + 2.26 h − 1.070
	60–70	0.0543 w + 2.37	
	>70	0.0573 w + 2.01	
Females			
	<3	0.246 w − 0.0965	0.127 w + 2.94 h − 1.2
	3–10	0.0842 w + 2.12	0.0666 w + 0.878 h + 1.46
	10–18	0.0465 w + 3.18	0.0393 w + 1.04 h + 1.93
	18–30	0.0546 w + 2.33	0.0433 w + 2.57 h − 1.180
	30–60	0.0407 w + 2.90	0.0342 w + 2.1 h − 0.0486
	>60	0.0424 w + 2.38	0.0356 w + 1.76 h + 0.0448
	60–70	0.0429 w + 2.39	
	>70	0.0417 w + 2.41	

Coefficients and constants shown for equations of the forms:
BMR = weight coefficient × weight (kg) + constant
BMR = weight coefficient × weight (kg) + height coefficient × height (m) + constant
Source: Adapted from Henry [8].

Table 3.2.4 Comparison of BMR prediction equations against the US Dietary Reference Intake (DRI) dataset

	BMR (kcal/day)		PAL		Accuracy	Bias %	
	Mean	SD	Mean	SD	%	Min.	Max.
Reported (DRI intake data)	1524	300	1.71	0.29			
Predicted values							
Henry weight and height	1514	273	1.71	0.29	73	−33	35
Henry weight	1509	292	1.72	0.30	70	−33	35
Schofield/FAO	1531	278	1.69	0.28	69	−36	43

Source: Adapted from SACN [16]. Crown Copyright.

Recent validation studies in Asian, South American and African populations, including the aforementioned equations of Harris–Benedict, Schofield, FAO/WHO/UNU and Henry, confirmed the overestimation of BMR by most prediction equations. However, when all equations were compared, overestimation was the lowest and accuracy the highest when using the Henry equations [13,15,20–22]. Additionally, Deurenberg et al. concluded that generally, for the same body mass index (BMI), fat percentage in Asians was 3–5% higher compared with Caucasians which can explain the overestimation of prediction equations in Asian subjects [23].

After adjustment for body weight, BMR was still lower in Asians compared to Caucasians but after adjustment for body composition, the difference was no longer present [24]. Furthermore, Adzika Nsatimba et al. showed that sub-Saharan African individuals are characterised by lower BMR and a higher respiratory quotient compared to Caucasians [25] while Luke et al. showed that African-American individuals have lower BMR than Caucasian individuals [26]. Much of this discrepancy may be attributed to a smaller mass of highly metabolically active organs (such as heart, liver, kidney and GI tract) in these populations.

3.2.3 Estimation of total energy requirements

Total energy expenditure may be divided into four components as follows:

Total energy expenditure (TEE) = basal metabolic rate (BMR) + diet-induced thermogenesis (DIT) + activity-induced energy expenditure (AEE) + growth

Of the four components, BMR can represent up to 70% of TEE, AEE up to 25–40% and DIT between 8% and 10%. In adults, growth is negligible. Growth is a major component only in infants aged 0–3 months where it can represent up to 30% of energy expenditure. In fact, growth represents a very small fraction (5–8%) of total energy expenditure even in infants between 1–5 years. It is apparent from the above that, next to BMR, the greatest variability in energy expenditure is due to physical activity. Since TEE is a function of body weight, body composition, gender, age and lifestyle, it may be expressed as a multiple of BMR. The physical activity level (PAL) enables the prediction of TEE using the following relationship:

$$TEE = BMR \times PAL$$

Energy requirement for adults

The factorial method for estimating energy requirements is based on multiplying BMR with PAL values. Given the considerable variability

in physical activity between people, PAL values used to estimate energy requirements can be nothing more than estimates. Listed below are the PAL values to estimate energy requirements for light, moderate and vigorous physical activity. The FAO/WHO/UNU in 1985 described the lower limit of PAL as 1.27, denoting a survival value of TEE for people with a minimal physical activity. The PAL values for the minimum, 10th, 25th, median, 75th, 90th and maximum are 1.27, 1.4, 1.49, 1.63, 1.78, 1.96 and 2.5 respectively. The minimum, 10th and 25th centiles represent light physical activity, median and moderate physical activity and 75th and 90th centiles represent heavy physical activity.

Energy requirement during pregnancy and lactation

The energy requirements for pregnancy and lactation are estimated as an additional energy requirement on top of the mother's normal energy requirements. On average during pregnancy, a woman will gain approximately 12.5 kg. This weight gain is not linear but exponential, with the greatest weight gain during the second and third trimesters. The total energy cost of pregnancy will therefore be an integration of the energy cost for fetal development, maternal body fat and body weight gain in the mother. The estimated energy cost of pregnancy is approximately 321 MJ or 77 000 kcal. The additional intake is recommended on top of the mother's normal energy requirement. This is divided into 0.35 MJ/day (85 kcal/day) for the first trimester, 1.2 MJ/day (285 kcal/day) for the second trimester and 2.0 MJ/day (475 kcal/day) for the third trimester.

The energy requirements for lactation are calculated based on the energy density of milk, volume of milk produced, energy cost of milk synthesis and the potential mobilisation of fat tissues from the mother. The average milk production is approximately 800 g/day with an energy density of 2.8 kJ/g (0.67 kcal/g). If we assume an energetic efficiency of 0.8 for milk production, we can use these values to compute the additional energy requirements per day for lactation. The additional energy requirement for lactation is the sum of TEE of the mother, plus

Table 3.2.5 Revised estimated average requirements (EAR) for infants aged 1–12 months

	EAR					
	Breastfed		Breast milk substitute fed		Mixed feeding or unknown	
Age (months)	MJ/kg per day (kcal/kg per day)	MJ/day (kcal/day)	MJ/kg per day (kcal/kg per day)	MJ/day (kcal/day)	MJ/kg per day (kcal/kg per day)	MJ/day (kcal/ day)
Boys						
1–2	0.4 (96)	2.2 (526)	0.5 (120)	2.5 (598)	0.5 (120)	2.4 (574)
3–4	0.4 (96)	2.4 (574)	0.4 (96)	2.6 (622)	0.4 (96)	2.5 (598)
5–6	0.3 (72)	2.5 {598)	0.4 (96)	2.7 (646)	0.3 (72)	2.6 (622)
7–12	0.3 (72)	2.9 (694)	0.3 (72)	3.1 (742)	0.3 (72)	3.0 (718)
Girls						
1–2	0.4 (96)	2.0 (478)	0.5 (120)	2.3 (550)	0.5 (120)	2.1 (502)
3–4	0.4 (96)	2.2 (526)	0.4 (96)	2.5 (598)	0.4 (96)	2.3 (550)
5–6	0.3 (72)	2.3 (550)	0.4 (96)	2.6 (622)	0.3 (72)	2.4 (574)
7–12	0.3 (72)	2.7 (646)	0.3 (72)	2.8 (670)	0.3 (72)	2.7 (646)

Source: Adapted from SACN [16]. Crown Copyright.

the energy cost of milk production and the energy value of milk. Since considerable energy is also mobilized from fat tissue deposits of the mother for milk synthesis, the energy requirement for lactation is therefore approximately 2.1 MJ/day or 505 kcal/day. This is in addition to the mother's energy requirements.

Energy requirement in infants and children

Energy requirements in infants aged 0–12 months now use TEE estimates and add on the energy cost of tissue deposition (Table 3.2.5). This is in contrast to previous reports where breast milk intake was used to estimate energy requirements in infants.

Energy requirements in children aged 1–18 years also use TEE and add on the energy cost of tissue deposition for growth (Table 3.2.6).

Energy requirement during disease

Apart from changes in body composition and age, there are other factors associated with chronic illness that have an impact on a patient's BMR. Such factors include inflammation,

Table 3.2.6 Revised estimated average requirements (EAR) for children aged 1–18 years

EAR MJ /day (kcal/day)			
Age (years)	PAL	Boys	Girls
1	1.40	3.2 (765)	3.0 (717)
2	1.40	4.2 (1004)	3.9 (932)
3	1.40	4.9 (1171)	4.5 (1076)
4	1.58	5.8 (1386)	5.4 (1291)
5	1.58	6.2 (1482)	5.7 (1362)
6	1.58	6.6 (1577)	6.2 (1482)
7	1.58	6.9 (1649)	6.4 (1530)
8	1.58	7.3 (1745)	6.8 (1625)
9	1.58	7.7 (1840)	7.2 (1721)
10	1.75	8.5 (2032)	8.1 (1936)
11	1.75	8.9 (2127)	8.5 (2032)
12	1.75	9.4 (2247)	8.8 (2103)
13	1.75	10.1(2414)	9.3 (2223)
14	1.75	11.0 (2629)	9.8 (2342)
15	1.75	11.8 (2820)	10.0 (2390)
16	1.75	12.4 (2964)	10.1 (2414)
17	1.75	12.9 (3083)	10.3 (2462)
18	1.75	13.2 (3155)	10.3 (2462)

Calculated from BMR × PAL. BMR values are calculated from the Henry equations, using weights and height.

Table 3.2.7 Stress factors for some clinical conditions

Condition	Stress factor (% BMR)
Brain injury:	
acute (ventilated and sedated)	0–30
recovery	5–50
Cerebral haemorrhage	30
Cerebrovascular accident	5
Chronic obstructive pulmonary disorder	15–20
Infection	25–45
Inflammatory bowel disease	0–10
Intensive care:	
ventilated	0–10
septic	20–60
Leukaemia	25–34
Lymphoma	0–25
Pancreatitis:	
chronic:	3
acute:	10
Sepsis/abscess	20
Solid tumours	0–20
Transplantation	20
Surgery:	
uncomplicated	5–20
complicated	25–40

Source: Todorovic and Micklewright [29], with permission of the British Dietetic Association.

Table 3.2.8 Physical activity level (PAL) of hospitalised patients

	PAL
Bed-bound, immobile	1.10
Bed-bound, mobile or sitting	1.15–1.20
Mobile, on ward	1.25
Light activity	1.27–1.49
Moderate activity	1.63

malignancies, neurological impairment and medications. In the majority of chronic conditions, BMR is usually normal or may be slightly increased, while critically ill patients show a raised BMR which is related to the severity of disease [27,28]. Table 3.2.7 represents some stress factors that can be applied for clinical conditions [29].

Since any metabolic stress-induced increase in BMR is often accompanied by a decrease in physical activity, TEE in chronically ill individuals is usually normal or decreased [16,30]. This can be seen in people with HIV who show a 10% increase in resting energy expenditure (REE) but no change in TEE [31,32]. REE is closely related to BMR; typically, REE measurement does not meet all the required conditions for BMR measurement but is more feasible in the outpatient setting. Table 3.2.8

shows the PAL values for hospitalised patients with different degrees of mobility.

In 2007, Boullata et al. concluded that no prediction equation was able to accurately predict REE in hospitalised patients and that only indirect calorimetry will provide accurate assessment of energy needs [1]. Among the tested equations was Harris–Benedict and Mifflin–St Jeor but not the FAO/WHO/UNU or Henry equations [33]. Zuconi et al. showed that REE of women with breast cancer was similar to that of healthy women and the Mifflin equation showed an accuracy of 65% which was better than Harris–Benedict [34]. On the other hand, Wu et al. showed that patients with newly diagnosed oesophageal cancer have impaired nutrition status, elevated energy expenditure and higher inflammation status [35].

Jesus et al. aimed to evaluate which predictive equations were a good alternative to BMR measurements according to the BMI and examined 28 equations in 1726 subjects [36]. They concluded that usual predictive equations of BMR are not suitable for predicting BMR in subjects with extreme BMI (BMI <16 kg/m² and >40 kg/m²). Especially, for people with an extreme low BMI, only 40% of the BMR predictions would be accurate within 10% of actual BMR. Indeed, patients with anorexia nervosa have low or very low BMR which is overestimated by Harris–Benedict [37]. Derivation of accurate predictive equations for use during the early refeeding period is needed to optimise nutritional treatments and avoid medical complications due to refeeding syndrome in the first phase of nutritional treatment.

In a clinical setting, it appears that none of the commonly used predictive equations is able to accurately predict BMR. Therefore, it is important to use the stress factors to adjust calculated BMR. Additionally, energy intake and patient outcomes, such as weight and nutritional status, should be monitored regularly to ensure appropriate nutritional management of patients and to determine whether patients' energy requirements are being met.

3.2.4 Summary

Since the development of the Harris–Benedict equations to predict BMR nearly a century ago, numerous BMR equations have been developed, with varying degrees of accuracy. Since BMR represents the largest component of energy expenditure in adults, its estimation is of the utmost importance. The recognition of BMR as the metabolic basis for the estimation of energy (and hence food requirements) has placed BMR as a central metabolic parameter. BMR prediction equations will not provide consistently accurate estimations in all populations despite pooling by age, gender, BMI and in some instances ethnicity. In the clinical setting, BMR predictions are difficult to make since BMR is also determined by disease state and medical interventions.

Of the available equations, the Henry equations may prove to be the most accurate and generalisable, considering the number of BMR measurements used to develop them and the wide spectrum of populations and geographical origins they represent. The Henry equations will enable people living in all regions of the world to predict BMR with an accuracy hitherto not available. Hence, their application in domestic, hospital and professional settings is to be encouraged.

References

1. Boullata J, Williams J, Cottrell F, Hudson L, Compher C. Accurate determination of energy needs in hospitalized patients. *J Am Diet Assoc* 2007; **107**(3): 393–401.
2. Reeves MM, Capra S. Variation in the application of methods used for predicting energy requirements in acutely ill adult patients: a survey of practice. *Eur J Clin Nutr* 2003; **57**(12): 1530–1535.
3. Report of a Joint FAO/WHO/UNU Expert Consultation. Energy and protein requirements. World Health Organ Tech Rep Ser 1985; **724**: 1–206.
4. Mitchell HH, editor. Comparative Nutrition of Man and Domestic Animals. New York: Academic Press, 1962, pp. 3–90.
5. Livesey G, Elia M. Estimation of energy expenditure, net carbohydrate utilization, and net fat oxidation and synthesis by indirect calorimetry: evaluation of errors with special reference to the detailed composition of fuels. *Am J Clin Nutr* 1988; **47**(4): 608–628.
6. Lifson N, Gordon GB, Mc CR. Measurement of total carbon dioxide production by means of D2O18. *J Appl Physiol* 1955; **7**(6): 704–710.
7. Atwater WO. Principles of nutrition and Nutritive Value of Food. Washington: US Department of Agriculture. 1910. https://archive.org/details/principlesofnutr00atwa (accessed 30 August 2017).
8. Henry CJ. Basal metabolic rate studies in humans: measurement and development of new equations. *Public Health Nutr* 2005; **8**(7A): 1133–1152.
9. Harris JA, Benedict FG. A biometric study of human basal metabolism. *Proc Natl Acad Sci USA* 1918; **4**(12): 370–373.
10. Schofield WN. Predicting basal metabolic rate, new standards and review of previous work. *Hum Nutr Clin Nutr* 1985; **39**(Suppl 1): 5–41.
11. Case KO, Brahler CJ, Heiss C. Resting energy expenditures in Asian women measured by indirect calorimetry are lower than expenditures calculated from prediction equations. *J Am Diet Assoc* 1997; **97**(11): 1288–1292.
12. Henry CJ, Rees DG. New predictive equations for the estimation of basal metabolic rate in tropical peoples. *Eur J Clin Nutr* 1991; **45**(4): 177–185.
13. Vander Weg MW, Watson JM, Klesges RC, Eck Clemens LH, Slawson DL, McClanahan BS. Development and cross-validation of a prediction equation for estimating resting energy expenditure in healthy African-American and European-American women. *Eur J Clin Nutr* 2004; **58**(3): 474–480.
14. Wahrlich V, Anjos LA, Going SB, Lohman TG. Basal metabolic rate of Brazilians living in the Southwestern United States. *Eur J Clin Nutr* 2007; **61**(2): 289–293.
15. Yang X, Li M, Mao D, et al. Basal energy expenditure in southern Chinese healthy adults: measurement and development of a new equation. *Br J Nutr* 2010; **104**(12): 1817–1823.
16. Scientific Advisory Committee on Nutrition (SACN). Dietary Reference Values for Energy. London: Scientific Advisory Committee on Nutrition, 2011.
17. EFSA Panel on Dietetic Products. Scientific Opinion on Dietary Reference Values for Energy. Parma: European Food Safety Authority, 2013.

18. Weijs PJ. Validity of predictive equations for resting energy expenditure in US and Dutch overweight and obese class I and II adults aged 18–65 y. *Am J Clin Nutr* 2008; **88**(4): 959–970.

19. Institute of Medicine. Panel on Macronutrients. Panel on the Definition of Dietary Fiber, Subcommittee on Upper Reference Levels of Nutrients, Subcommittee on Interpretation and Uses of Dietary Reference Intakes, and the Standing Committee on the Scientific Evaluation of Dietary Reference Intakes, Food and Nutrition Board. Dietary Reference Intakes for Energy, Carbohydrate, Fiber, Fat, Fatty Acids, Cholesterol, Protein and Amino Acids. Washington: National Academies Press, 2005.

20. Anjos LA, Wahrlich V, Vasconcellos MT. BMR in a Brazilian adult probability sample: the nutrition, physical activity and health survey. *Public Health Nutr* 2014; **17**(4): 853–860.

21. Rao ZY, Wu XT, Liang BM, Wang MY, Hu W. Comparison of five equations for estimating resting energy expenditure in Chinese young, normal weight healthy adults. *Eur J Med Res* 2012; **17**: 26.

22. Song T, Venkataraman K, Gluckman P, et al. Validation of prediction equations for resting energy expenditure in Singaporean Chinese men. *Obes Res Clin Pract* 2014; **8**(3): e201–298.

23. Deurenberg P, Deurenberg-Yap M, Guricci S. Asians are different from Caucasians and from each other in their body mass index/body fat per cent relationship. *Obes Rev* 2002; **3**(3): 141–146.

24. Wouters-Adriaens MP, Westerterp KR. Low resting energy expenditure in Asians can be attributed to body composition. *Obesity* 2008; **16**(10): 2212–2216.

25. Adzika Nsatimba PA, Pathak K, Soares MJ. Ethnic differences in resting metabolic rate, respiratory quotient and body temperature: a comparison of Africans and European Australians. *Eur J Nutr* 2016; **55**(5): 1831–1838.

26. Luke A, Dugas L, Kramer H. Ethnicity, energy expenditure and obesity: are the observed black/white differences meaningful? *Curr Opin Endocrinol Diabetes Obes* 2007; **14**(5): 370–373.

27. Frankenfield D, Roth-Yousey L, Compher C. Comparison of predictive equations for resting metabolic rate in healthy nonobese and obese adults: a systematic review. *J Am Diet Assoc* 2005; **105**(5): 775–789.

28. Hwang TL, Huang SL, Chen MF. The use of indirect calorimetry in critically ill patients – the relationship of measured energy expenditure to Injury Severity Score, Septic Severity Score, and APACHE II Score. *J Trauma* 1993; **34**(2): 247–251.

29. Todorovic VE, Micklewright A. A Pocket Guide to Clinical Nutrition. Birmingham: British Dietetic Association, 2004, pp. 1–12.

30. Kulstad R, Schoeller DA. The energetics of wasting diseases. *Curr Opin Clin Nutr Metab Care* 2007; **10**(4): 488–493.

31. Chang E, Sekhar R, Patel S, Balasubramanyam A. Dysregulated energy expenditure in HIV-infected patients: a mechanistic review. *Clin Infect Dis* 2007; **44**(11): 1509–1517.

32. Kosmiski L. Energy expenditure in HIV infection. *Am J Clin Nutr* 2011; **94**(6): 1677S–1682S.

33. Mifflin MD, St Jeor ST, Hill LA, Scott BJ, Daugherty SA, Koh YO. A new predictive equation for resting energy expenditure in healthy individuals. *Am J Clin Nutr* 1990; **51**(2): 241–247.

34. Zuconi CP, Ceolin Alves AL, Toulson Davisson Correia MI. Energy expenditure in women with breast cancer. *Nutrition* 2015; **31**(4): 556–559.

35. Wu J, Huang C, Xiao H, Tang Q, Cai W. Weight loss and resting energy expenditure in male patients with newly diagnosed esophageal cancer. *Nutrition* 2013; **29**(11–12): 1310–1314.

36. Jesus P, Achamrah N, Grigioni S, et al. Validity of predictive equations for resting energy expenditure according to the body mass index in a population of 1726 patients followed in a Nutrition Unit. *Clin Nutr* 2015; **34**(3): 529–535.

37. El Ghoch M, Alberti M, Capelli C, Calugi S, Dalle Grave R. Resting energy expenditure in anorexia nervosa: measured versus estimated. *J Nutr Metab* 2012; **2012**: 652932.

Chapter 3.3

Protein requirements in nutrition support

Peter W. Emery

Department of Nutritional Sciences, King's College London, London, UK

3.3.1 Metabolic requirement for protein

Protein makes up approximately 15% of the human body. There are at least 25 000 different types of protein within the body, all of which play key roles in maintaining the body's structure or performing myriad different functions. Protein is needed in the diet to provide substrates for the synthesis of these body proteins. More specifically, dietary protein is required to provide nitrogen in the form of amino acids, from which the body can synthesise tissue proteins. Hence, it is conventional to quantify the requirement for dietary protein in terms of the amount of nitrogen required [1].

Tissue proteins are constantly being synthesised and broken down, a process known as protein turnover. While some of the substrates for the synthesis of tissue proteins can come from recycling of amino acids produced by protein breakdown, there is a constant drain on the amino acid pool as amino acids are oxidised to urea or utilised to synthesise other small molecules such as purines, pyrimidines, creatine and haem. It is also the case that some amino acids undergo posttranslational modification (for example, methylation or phosphorylation), so that they cannot be reutilised for protein synthesis when they are released from tissue proteins.

Thus the main reason why protein needs to be supplied in the diet is to resupply the amino acid pool from which tissue proteins are synthesised. Dietary protein must be supplied at a rate which matches the rate at which amino acids are irreversibly lost from that pool. This is the main determinant of the dietary protein requirement for maintenance, along with a requirement to synthesise enough extra protein in tissues such as skin, hair and GI tract epithelium to replace the whole proteins that are shed from these tissues [1].

In growing children, there is a requirement for additional dietary protein to allow the net deposition of additional tissue protein (see Chapter 5.1). The same applies during pregnancy and lactation and the replacement of protein that may have been lost during illness or injury.

In addition to meeting the overall requirement for amino acid nitrogen, the diet needs to supply enough of each of the essential (indispensable) amino acids to replace their irreversible losses. Amino acid requirements vary slightly with age, since part of the requirement in growing children relates to the needs for net synthesis of new tissue. The relative amounts of the different essential amino acids needed for growth will reflect the composition of the tissue proteins being synthesised, whereas the requirement for maintenance will reflect the oxidation rates of the different amino acids [2].

The ability of a diet to meet protein requirements must thus be considered not only in quantitative terms, by considering the amount of nitrogen supplied, but also in qualitative terms. Protein quality can be measured by determining the net protein utilisation value of the diet or it can be predicted from *in vitro* measurements of digestibility and the essential amino acid content

Advanced Nutrition and Dietetics in Nutrition Support, First Edition. Edited by Mary Hickson and Sara Smith.
© 2018 John Wiley & Sons Ltd. Published 2018 by John Wiley & Sons Ltd.

of the dietary proteins. The method currently recommended for predicting protein quality is called the digestible indispensable amino acid score [3]. Protein requirements and recommendations are traditionally expressed in terms of amounts of high-quality protein, with the proviso that a correction for protein quality needs to be made when evaluating the adequacy of a given diet [4].

3.3.2 Assessment of protein requirements

Nitrogen balance

It follows from the foregoing that inadequate intake of dietary protein would lead to the net loss of tissue protein in adults and inadequate growth in children. Direct measurement of body protein content would be too insensitive to detect the small changes that might result from inadequate intake over a short period of time, so the much more sensitive measurement on nitrogen balance is used in practice to detect the adequacy of a diet and hence to define protein requirements.

In theory, it is straightforward to measure the nitrogen content of the diet fed to subjects on a nitrogen balance study, together with the major routes of nitrogen excretion, that is, the urine and faeces. It is much more challenging to measure all the minor routes by which nitrogen can be lost from the body, including skin, sweat, hair, fingernails and toenails and various bodily secretions, so that in practice this has rarely been done. Instead, an arbitrary value has often been assigned to these cutaneous and miscellaneous losses, typically 5 mg N/kg body weight/day, although there is some evidence that these losses vary slightly with protein intake and the level of activity [5,6]. In clinical situations, the challenge would be even greater, as there may be additional losses to measure, such as the exudate from a wound.

Since nitrogen balance is calculated as the small difference between two much larger quantities, nitrogen intake and excretion, the accumulation of experimental errors associated with the measurement of dietary, urinary and faecal nitrogen will result in a relatively large overall experimental error when measuring nitrogen balance. Moreover, dietary intake will tend to be overesti-mated, as the measurement of food wastage may be incomplete, while excretion will tend to be underestimated because of incomplete collection, so there may be a systematic bias in the direction of overestimating nitrogen balance [7].

The current international recommendations for protein intakes for healthy adults [4] are based on a meta-analysis of 19 published studies in which nitrogen balance had been measured in 235 individuals (males and females, mostly aged 18–30 years), each fed at least three different levels of protein intake [8]. This analysis showed that the intake required to maintain nitrogen balance varied over an extremely wide range, approximately 50–150 mg N/kg/day, which is more than would be expected from normal biological variation between individuals plus experimental error (Figure 3.3.1).

The analysis also appeared to show that balance continues to increase linearly with intake, at intakes above the requirement level, whereas theoretical considerations would suggest that nitrogen balance should remain at or only slightly above zero at higher intakes. For these reasons, there has been increasing dissatisfaction with the use of nitrogen balance for assessing protein requirements. However, no suitable alternative method has yet been identified. Methods based on measuring aspects of protein turnover, including amino acid oxidation, have been developed to estimate the requirements for specific essential amino acids (see below), but these methods have not yet been adapted satisfactorily for measuring overall protein requirements.

One of the main reasons for the apparent anomalies in the results of the nitrogen balance studies is likely to be the length of time required for the body to adapt to a given level of intake. The rate of amino acid oxidation (and hence urinary nitrogen excretion) appears to adapt over time to the customary level of intake, so that when a person changes from a high- to a low-protein diet they will be in negative nitrogen balance for several days as the urinary nitrogen excretion rate gradually decreases to a new steady state. Similarly, people switching to a high-protein diet will be in positive nitrogen balance until the rate of amino acid oxidation has increased to match the new intake.

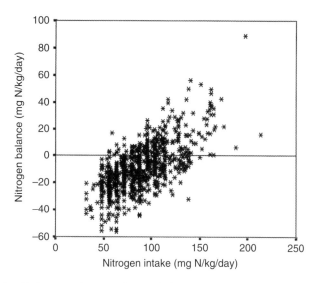

Figure 3.3.1 Relationship between nitrogen balance and nitrogen intake. Results of a meta-analysis of 19 studies involving 235 individuals. Each point represents an individual subject's observed response to a specific intake. Source: Reproduced from Rand et al. [8] with permission from *The American Journal of Clinical Nutrition*

The meta-analysis mentioned previously [8] was based on studies where a diet containing protein at around the maintenance level was fed for 10–14 days, with nitrogen balance being measured for the last 5 days. Thus these studies allowed a period of 5–9 days for subjects to adapt from their customary diet to one containing about half as much protein. However, several studies have shown that adaptation may take considerably longer [9–11]. For example, in one study subjects switching from a high- to a moderate-protein diet (36 g N/day to 12 g N/day) exhibited their most extreme erroneously low nitrogen balance when measured 12–17 days after changing diet, and a steady state of nitrogen balance was not reached until at least 42 days after the change in diet [9]. It should be noted that this issue of lengthy adaptation affects all methods used to estimate protein requirements. Moreover, it is a particularly significant problem when trying to investigate the effects of relatively short-term stimuli, such as acute illness, on protein requirements.

Factorial method

Most studies estimating protein requirements have been carried out on healthy young adult

men. The so-called factorial approach has been developed in order to be able to predict the protein requirements of other age groups, women and people in different physiological states without having to perform numerous nitrogen balance studies, which are expensive, time-consuming and technically challenging.

Obligatory losses are quantified by measuring nitrogen excretion in the urine, faeces, through the skin and by other miscellaneous routes in subjects fed a protein-free diet. However, when experimental subjects are fed a diet containing just enough protein to match the sum of these obligatory losses (47 mg N/kg/day), it is found that they are in negative nitrogen balance. In order to match the estimated average protein requirement based on nitrogen balance studies (105 mg N/kg/day, equivalent to 0.66 g protein/kg/day) [4], the sum of obligatory losses needs to be multiplied by a factor that is assumed to represent the inefficiency of utilisation of dietary protein to meet physiological requirements. The most likely reason for this apparent inefficiency is that when protein is present in the diet, it stimulates amino acid oxidation, and the rate of amino acid oxidation goes up as protein intake increases. This is why the relationship between dietary protein intake and nitrogen balance may not be linear, even at intakes below the requirement level. This in turn contributes to the difficulty in defining the intake at which nitrogen balance can just be maintained, since the slope of a line relating nitrogen balance to protein intake may become quite small as intake reaches the requirement level.

Less than a quarter of the nitrogen balance studies on which current estimates of protein requirements are based [8] were carried out on women. From these studies, it can be calculated that the median protein requirement for women is slightly lower than that for men, when expressed per unit body weight (91 mg N/kg/day for women versus 109 mg N/kg/day for men). This is probably due to the differences in body composition between women and men.

3.3.3 Amino acid requirements

The nitrogen balance method can also be used to assess the requirements for individual essential amino acids. However, there are alternative methods which are based on measurement of the rate of amino acid oxidation. This is achieved by administering an amino acid labelled with a stable isotope, ^{13}C, and collecting expired air. This allows calculation of the rate of excretion of $^{13}CO_2$, which is produced when the labelled amino acid is oxidised.

There are broadly two approaches to using this method, known as the carbon balance technique and the indicator amino acid oxidation technique. In the carbon balance technique, carboxyl-labelled leucine is infused in subjects who are adapted to consume different levels of leucine in the diet. The aim is to identify the level of leucine intake that matches the measured rate of leucine oxidation. Various protocols have been developed to account for the different rates of leucine oxidation that normally occur over a 24-hour period in response to feeding and fasting. In the indicator amino acid oxidation technique, an amount of carboxyl-labelled phenylalanine that is greater than its requirement is administered orally to subjects who are consuming different amounts of the test amino acid in the form of hourly meals. As the intake of the test amino acid increases, the rate of oxidation of the indicator amino acid, phenylalanine, decreases. The requirement for the test amino acid is identified as the point at which the phenylalanine oxidation rate ceases to decline [4].

Although the amount of data currently available from these stable isotope studies is limited, the internationally agreed estimates of essential amino acid requirements have been revised upwards from the older figures, which were based largely on nitrogen balance data [12]. Both sets of values are shown in Table 3.3.1.

Table 3.3.1 Estimated requirements for essential amino acids in adults

Amino acid	Current estimate*	1985 estimate[†]
	(mg/g protein)	(mg/g protein)
Histidine	15	15
Isoleucine	30	15
Leucine	59	21
Methionine + cysteine	22	20
Phenylalanine + tyrosine	38	21
Threonine	23	11
Tryptophan	6	5
Valine	39	15

* Values taken from World Health Organization/Food and Agriculture Organization/United Nations University [4].
[†] Values taken from Food and Agriculture Organization/World Health Organization/United Nations University [12].

3.3.4 Protein requirements of older adults

One area of current controversy is whether protein requirements increase in older adults. There is concern that inadequate protein intake may be a factor that contributes to age-related sarcopenia, although there is no direct evidence for this. Certainly there is evidence from observational studies that low protein intakes are associated with loss of muscle protein and a range of adverse health outcomes in older people [13,14]. But this does not demonstrate a causal relationship since the low protein intake is likely to be simply a marker for a range of adverse social, demographic and lifestyle factors that are more likely to be causative. Moreover, it is generally not possible to separate the effects of low protein intake from other aspects of dietary adequacy.

Only one of the studies included in the meta-analysis of nitrogen balance studies in healthy adults [8] was carried out on older subjects (aged 68–84) [15] and this provided no evidence of a significantly higher protein requirement. Only two papers have reported nitrogen balance measurements on both young and older adults at more than one level of protein intake [16,17]. Neither paper reported any significant difference between the two age groups in nitrogen balance at any intake or in their estimates of protein requirements.

A further area of controversy relates to the suggestion that recommended intakes for older people should include a specified minimum amount of protein to be consumed at each meal. This is because muscle protein mass is maintained in a cyclic fashion, with a small net deposition of protein after each meal followed by loss of this extra protein over the subsequent postprandial period. There is evidence that older people may not store sufficient extra protein in the postprandial period to maintain muscle mass, a phenomenon known as 'anabolic resistance' [18]. This anabolic resistance can be overcome by increasing the amount of protein in the meal [19], leading to the proposal that older people should be advised to consume 25–30 g high-quality protein at each of three meals every day in order to maintain muscle mass [18]. However, this work is based largely on measurements of the rate of protein synthesis rather than net protein deposition. In fact, protein deposition depends on the balance between the rates of synthesis and breakdown of protein, but measuring the rate of protein breakdown is much harder than measuring the rate of protein synthesis, because of amino acid recycling. Moreover, there is some evidence that when muscle protein synthesis rate increases in response to an anabolic stimulus, there is a concomitant increase in the rate of protein breakdown [20].

Hence, it would be premature to adopt a recommendation of 25–30 g high-quality protein three times per day until there is evidence that it actually improves nitrogen balance or muscle mass when compared with more conventional eating patterns. Indeed, the opposite recommendation has also been made, since studies in older people have shown that consuming 70–80% of the day's protein intake at a single meal (so-called pulse feeding) leads to more positive nitrogen balance [21] and increased lean tissue mass [22], compared with consuming the same amount of protein spread evenly over four meals.

An alternative approach to overcoming anabolic resistance in older people could involve supplementation with the essential amino acid leucine [18], since leucine is believed to activate the signalling pathway which leads to increased muscle protein synthesis in the postprandial period. This approach has been shown to increase the rate of muscle protein synthesis in older people [23], but again, the effect on protein breakdown has not been measured and there is no net effect on lean tissue mass [24] or muscle mass or strength [25].

It is well known that the most effective way to stimulate muscle protein deposition is through exercise. Resistance exercise in particular has been shown to increase muscle mass and strength in older people [26]. However, combining protein supplementation with resistance training does not appear to produce any further gains in muscle mass or strength [27].

3.3.5 Protein requirements in acute illness

One of the best known features of the metabolic response to both injury and severe infection is an increase in urinary nitrogen excretion, leading to negative nitrogen balance [28]. This appears to reflect increased breakdown of protein in several tissues, particularly skeletal muscle. Prolonged negative nitrogen balance and muscle wasting are associated with detrimental clinical outcomes [29], so it appears logical to recommend an increase in protein intake in such situations. However, there is little direct evidence that protein requirement can be considered to have increased.

Most of the evidence supporting the use of increased protein allowances for feeding patients who are severely ill comes from observational studies. For example, one widely quoted study is a retrospective review of changes in body protein content in critically ill patients who had been fed enterally or parenterally on different amounts of protein [30]. Results showed that loss of body protein was decreased by increasing protein intake up to 1.0 g/kg/day, with no further benefit of higher protein intakes. However, this result is likely to reflect the fact that the patients with the lowest intakes would have been those who were most severely ill, rather than any effect of different protein intakes *per se*.

A recent systematic review identified 13 controlled trials in which critically ill patients had been fed at different levels of protein intake and nutritionally relevant outcomes were measured [31]. Inevitably, these trials were of relatively short duration and so were limited by a lack of adaptation to the diets being fed, as well as being conducted on a clinically heterogeneous group of subjects. Not all trials reported nitrogen balance data, but those that did mostly showed that nitrogen balance tended to improve as protein intake increased, at least when intakes were low. In four trials [32–35], there were groups with positive and negative nitrogen balance, allowing protein requirement to be estimated by interpolation. Such estimates from these studies span a range from 1.6 to 2.4 g protein/kg/day. However, in three other studies [36–38], no consistent positive balance was achieved at any level of intake, and in each case there appeared to be a threshold intake above which no significant improvement in nitrogen balance could be observed. The thresholds in these studies covered a range from 0.63 to 1.25 g protein/kg/day.

Clinical guidelines from various bodies around the world recommend protein intakes for critically ill patients in the range 1.25–2.0 g protein/kg/day [39–41], in all cases greater than the current international recommendation for healthy adults – 0.83 g protein/kg/day. The authors of the systematic review cited above [31] interpret it as supporting an even higher recommendation, 2.0–2.5 g protein/kg/day. However, an alternative interpretation is that although protein feeding can minimise the magnitude of the negative nitrogen balance, in many cases positive balance cannot be achieved in the most acute stage of illness. The amount of dietary protein needed to minimise the negative nitrogen balance may be no greater than the amount required by healthy adults.

Perhaps the most important conclusion from this analysis is that nutritional indices such as nitrogen balance are not the most appropriate way to evaluate the optimal intake of protein for acutely ill patients. Well-designed studies using homogeneous groups of patients and measuring relevant clinical outcomes are needed, but so far no such study of different amounts of dietary protein has been performed.

References

1. Sanders TAB, Emery PW. Molecular Basis of Human Nutrition. London: Taylor & Francis, 2003.
2. Reeds PJ, Garlick PJ. Protein and amino acid requirements and the composition of complementary foods. *J Nutr* 2003; **133**: 2953S–2961S.
3. Food and Agriculture Organization of the United Nations. Dietary Protein Quality Evaluation in Human Nutrition: Report of an FAO Expert Consultation, 31 March–2 April, 2011, Auckland, New Zealand. Rome: Food and Agriculture Organization of the United Nations, 2013.
4. World Health Organization/Food and Agriculture Organization/United Nations University. Protein and Amino Acid Requirements in Human Nutrition: Report of a Joint WHO/FAO/UNU Expert Consultation. Geneva: World Health Organization, 2007.
5. Calloway DH, Odell ACF, Margen S. Sweat and miscellaneous nitrogen losses in human balance studies. *J Nutr* 1971; **101**: 775–786.
6. Ashworth A, Harrower AD. Protein requirements in tropical countries: nitrogen losses in sweat and their relation to nitrogen balance. *Br J Nutr* 1967; **21**: 833–843.

7. Wallace WM. Nitrogen content of the body and its relation to retention and loss of nitrogen. *Fed Proc* 1976; **18**: 1125–1130.

8. Rand WM, Pellett PL, Young VR. Meta-analysis of nitrogen balance studies for estimating protein requirements in healthy adults. *Am J Clin Nutr* 2003; **77**: 109–127.

9. Oddoye EA, Margen S. Nitrogen balance studies in humans: long term effect of high nitrogen intake on nitrogen accretion. *J Nutr* 1979; **109**: 363–377.

10. Gersovitz M, Motil K, Munro HN, Scrimshaw NS, Young VR. Human protein requirements: assessment of the adequacy of the current recommended dietary allowance for dietary protein in elderly men and women. *Am J Clin Nutr* 1982; **35**: 6–14.

11. Morse MH, Haub MD, Evans WJ, Campbell WW. Protein requirement of elderly women: nitrogen balance responses to three levels of protein intake. *J Gerontol A Biol Sci Med Sci* 2001; **56**: M724–730.

12. Food and Agriculture Organization/World Health Organization /United Nations University. Energy and Protein Requirements. Report of a Joint FAO/WHO/UNU Expert Cconsultation. Geneva: World Health Organization, 1985.

13. Beasley JM, Wertheim BC, La Croix AZ, et al. Biomarker-calibrated protein intake and physical function in the women's health initiative. *J Am Geriatr Soc* 2013; **61**: 1863–1871.

14. Deutz NE, Bauer JM, Barazzoni R, et al. Protein intake and exercise for optimal muscle function with aging: recommendations from the ESPEN expert group. *Clin Nutr* 2014; **33**: 929–936.

15. Uauy R, Scrimshaw NS, Young VR. Human protein requirements: nitrogen balance response to graded levels of egg protein in elderly men and women. *Am J Clin Nutr* 1978; **31**: 779–785.

16. Cheng AH, Gomez A, Bergan JG, Lee TC, Monckeberg F, Chichester CO. Comparative nitrogen balance study between young and aged adults using three levels of protein intake from a combination wheat-soy-milk mixture. *Am J Clin Nutr* 1978; **31**: 12–22.

17. Campbell WW, Johnson CA, McCabe GP, Carnell NS. Dietary protein requirements of younger and older adults. *Am J Clin Nutr* 2008; **88**: 1322–1329.

18. Paddon-Jones D, Rasmussen BB. Dietary protein recommendations and the prevention of sarcopenia: protein, amino acid metabolism and therapy. *Curr Opin Clin Nutr Metab Care* 2009; **12**: 86–90.

19. Symons TB, Sheffield-Moore M, Wolfe RR, Paddon-Jones D. A moderate serving of high-quality protein maximally stimulates skeletal muscle protein synthesis in young and elderly subjects. *J Am Diet Assoc* 2009; **109**: 1582–1586.

20. Millward DJ, Brown JG, Odedra B. Protein turnover in individual tissues with special emphasis on muscle. In: Waterlow JC, Stephen JML, editors. Nitrogen Metabolism in Man. London: Applied Science Publishers, 1981, pp. 475–494.

21. Arnal MA, Mosoni L, Boirie Y, Houlier ML, Morin L, Verdier E, Ritz P, Antoine JM, Prugnaud J, Beaufrère B, Mirand PP. Protein pulse feeding improves protein retention in elderly women. *Am J Clin Nutr* 1999; **69**: 1202–1208.

22. Bouillanne O, Curis E, Hamon-Vilcot B, Nicolis I, Chrétien P, Schauer N, Vincent JP, Cynober L, Aussel C. Impact of protein pulse feeding on lean mass in malnourished and at-risk hospitalized elderly patients: a randomized controlled trial. *Clin Nutr* 2013; **32**: 186–192.

23. Rieu I, Balage M, Sornet C, Giraudet C, Pujos E, Grizard J, Mosoni L, Dardevet D. Leucine supplementation improves muscle protein synthesis in elderly men independently of hyperaminoacidaemia. *J Physiol* 2006; **575**: 305–315.

24. Leenders M, Verdijk LB, van der Hoeven L, van Kranenburg J, Hartgens F, Wodzig WK, Saris WH, van Loon LJ. Prolonged leucine supplementation does not augment muscle mass or affect glycemic control in elderly type 2 diabetic men. *J Nutr* 2011; **141**: 1070–1076.

25. Verhoeven S, Vanschoonbeek K, Verdijk LB, Koopman R, Wodzig WK, Dendale P, van Loon LJ. Long-term leucine supplementation does not increase muscle mass or strength in healthy elderly men. *Am J Clin Nutr* 2009; **89**: 1468–1475.

26. Frontera WR, Meredith CN, O'Reilly KP, Knuttgen HG, Evans WJ. Strength conditioning in older men: skeletal muscle hypertrophy and improved function. *J Appl Physiol* 1988; **64**: 1038–1044.

27. Finger D, Goltz FR, Umpierre D, Meyer E, Telles Rosa LH, Schneider CD. Effects of protein supplementation in older adults undergoing resistance training: a systematic review and meta-analysis. *Sports Med* 2015; **45**: 245–255.

28. Cuthbertson DP. Effect of injury on metabolism. *Br J Surg* 1936; **23**: 505.

29. Weijs PJM, Looijaard WGPM, Dekker IM, Stapel SS, Girbes AR, Oudemans-van Straaten HM, Beishuizen A. Low skeletal muscle area is a risk factor for mortality in mechanically ventilated critically ill patients. *Crit Care* 2014; **18**: R12.

30. Ishibashi N, Plank LD, Sando K, Hill GL. Optimal protein requirements during the first 2 weeks after the onset of critical illness. *Crit Care Med* 1998; **26**: 1529–1535.

31. Hoffer LJ, Bistrian BR. Appropriate protein provision in critical illness: a systematic and narrative review. *Am J Clin Nutr* 2012; **96**: 591–600.

32. Long CL, Crosby F, Geiger JW, Kinney JM. Parenteral nutrition in the septic patient: nitrogen balance, limiting plasma amino acids, and calorie to nitrogen ratios. *Am J Clin Nutr* 1976; **29**: 380–391.

33. Twyman D, Young AB, Ott L, Norton JA, Bivins BA. High protein enteral feedings: a means of achieving positive nitrogen balance in head injured patients. *J Parenter Enteral Nutr* 1985; **9**: 679–684.

34. Scheinkestel CD, Adams F, Mahony L, et al. Impact of increasing parenteral protein loads on amino acid levels and balance in critically ill anuric patients on continuous renal replacement therapy. *Nutrition* 2003; **19**: 733–740.

35. Singer P. High-dose amino acid infusion preserves diuresis and improves nitrogen balance in non-oliguric acute renal failure. *Wien Klin Wochenschr* 2007; **119**: 218–222.

36. Greig PD, Elwyn DH, Askanazi J, Kinney JM. Parenteral nutrition in septic patients: effect of increasing nitrogen intake. *Am J Clin Nutr* 1987; **46**: 1040–1047.

37. Larsson J, Lennmarken C, Mårtensson J, Sandstedt S, Vinnars E. Nitrogen requirements in severely injured patients. *Br J Surg* 1990; **77**: 413–416.

38. Pitkänen O, Takala J, Pöyhönen M, Kari A. Nitrogen and energy balance in septic and injured intensive care patients: response to parenteral nutrition. *Clin Nutr* 1991; **10**: 258–265.

39. National Institute for Health and Clinical Excellence. Nutrition Support in Adults. London: NICE, 2006.

40. Singer P, Berger MM, van den Berghe G, et al. ESPEN guidelines on parenteral nutrition: intensive care. *Clin Nutr* 2009; **28**: 387–400.

41. McClave SA, Martindale RG, Vanek VW, et al. Guidelines for the provision and assessment of nutrition support therapy in the adult critically ill patient: Society of Critical Care Medicine (SCCM) and American Society for Parenteral and Enteral Nutrition (A.S.P.E.N.). *J Parenter Enteral Nutr* 2009; **33**: 277–316.

Chapter 3.4

Water-soluble vitamins in nutrition support

Alastair Forbes[1] and Emily Player[2]

[1] Norwich Medical School, University of East Anglia, Norwich, UK
[2] Norfolk and Norwich University Hospital, Norwich, UK

3.4.1 Introduction

Water-soluble vitamins are essential elements of the normal human diet. The exact amount of a specific vitamin an individual will require can vary. This chapter aims to cover the current international recommendations for vitamin intake and the research underpinning the recommendations. Furthermore, it will focus not only on the recommendations in healthy individuals, but also those in individuals predisposed to undernutrition those who are undernourished and on the nutriceutical application of vitamins.

3.4.2 Vitamin recommendations

The normal diet

In the UK, dietary reference values (DRVs) were published in the Committee on the Medical Aspects of Food Policy (COMA) report in 1991 [1]. The report provided reference values including the estimated average requirements (EARs), safe intake (SI), lower reference nutrient intake (LRNI) and the reference nutrient intake (RNI). At the time, values were produced in alignment with the most current research techniques and findings. However, in the last two decades the techniques on which some of the DRVs are based have changed. For example, the DRVs for energy were based on an estimation of total energy expenditure (TEE), but the techniques in assessing TEE have since developed [1].

The COMA group has now been replaced by the Scientific Advisory Committee on Nutrition (SACN), which is slowly updating the recommendations, and in 2011 published its DRVs for energy [1]. However, the recommendations for vitamins are currently unchanged in the UK. The recommended values can be seen in Table 3.4.1, which also highlights the fact that in the UK not all vitamins have a recommended DRV. Values recommended by the World Health Organization (WHO) are shown in Table 3.4.2.

The RNI, which provides guidance on nutrient intake, should meet the requirements of 97.5% of the population, but for 2.5% of the population it will be insufficient [2]. The RNI values are more useful in the well population than in those with known undernutrition or who are predisposed to undernutrition.

The European Society for Clinical Nutrition and Metabolism (ESPEN) summarises an alternative set of recommendations in its guidance on how much of the vitamins should be included in enteral formulas [3]. This guidance is based on a European Commission (EC) directive from 1999 [3]. The directive was designed to unify the regulations surrounding the composition and use of the so-called 'foods for special medical purposes'; these are intended for individuals who are unable to meet their needs by food alone and therefore require additional feeding. The directive was based on advice from the EC's scientific advisory board on food, with advice and discussion from member states [4] and includes information on vitamin safety in food

Advanced Nutrition and Dietetics in Nutrition Support, First Edition. Edited by Mary Hickson and Sara Smith.
© 2018 John Wiley & Sons Ltd. Published 2018 by John Wiley & Sons Ltd.

Table 3.4.1 UK and SACN recommendations in the healthy population [2]

Vitamin	Unit	Children (age in years)				Males (age in years)				Females (age in years)				Pregnancy (any age)
		<1	1–3	4–6	7–10	11–14	15–18	19–50	50+	11–14	15–18	19–50	50+	
Vitamin B1 Thiamine	mg/day	0.2	0.5	0.7	0.7	0.9	1.1	1.0	0.9	0.7	0.8	0.8	0.8	0.9
Vitamin B2 Riboflavin	mg/day	0.4	0.6	0.8	1.0	1.2	1.3	1.3	1.3	1.1	1.1	1.1	1.1	1.4
Vitamin B3 Niacin	mg/day	4	8	11	12	15	18	17	16	12	14	13	12	13
Vitamin B6	mg/day	0.3	0.7	0.9	1.0	1.2	1.5	1.4	1.4	1.0	1.2	1.2	1.2	1.2
Vitamin B9 Folate	µg/day	50	70	100	150	200	200	200	200	200	200	200	200	300
Vitamin B12	µg/day	0.3	0.5	0.8	1.0	1.2	1.5	1.5	1.5	1.2	1.5	1.5	1.5	1.5
Vitamin C	mg/day	25	30	30	30	35	40	40	40	35	40	40	40	50

Table 3.4.2 WHO recommendations for the healthy population

Vitamin	Unit	Adult males	Adult females	Pregnancy	Lactation
Vitamin B1 Thiamine	mg/day	1.2	1.1	1.4	1.5
Vitamin B2 Riboflavin	mg/day	1.3	1.1	1.4	1.6
Vitamin B3 Niacin	mg/day	16	14	18	17
Vitamin B5 Pantothenic acid	mg/day	5	5	6	7
Vitamin B6	mg/day	1.3–1.7	1.1–1.5	1.9	2.0
Vitamin B7 Biotin	µg/day	30	30	30	30
Vitamin B9 Folate	µg/day	400	400	600	500
Vitamin B12	µg/day	2.4	2.4	2.6	2.8
Vitamin C	mg/day	45	45	45	70

and the requirements for labelling. The minimum and maximum doses for vitamin supplementation in foodstuffs and enteral formulas are depicted in Table 3.4.3 [5]. For artificial formula to be designated 'complete' there must, by definition, be a full day's provision of all the vitamins in the amount of enteral formula that yields 1500 kcal. The directive does not directly address tolerable upper limits, but these have been considered by the European Food Safety Agency (EFSA) and the Scientific Committee of Food (SCF) [5]. In 2005, the Commission requested the EFSA to review the SCF recommendations on population reference intakes (PRIs) for micronutrients [5]. At the time of writing, this is yet to be achieved.

Somewhat different nomenclatures from European reference sources are used in North American vitamin reference ranges, but the USA now appears to have the most complete guidelines. The National Academy Press produced a booklet containing dietary reference intakes (DRIs) in 2006, published within the US Department of Health guidelines on diet [6,7] (Table 3.4.4). The guidance was based on work produced by the Institute of Medicine and the Food and Nutrition Board [6]. The term and values of DRIs now replace the recommended daily allowances (RDAs) and recommended nutrient intakes (RNIs) from the US and Canada respectively [7]. The DRIs are formed from up to four main criteria: vitamins usually have an EAR, from which the RDA is calculated [7]. If it is not possible to derive the EAR then an adequate intake (AI) is proposed. Similar to the EU guidance, the US has provided a tolerable upper intake level (UL) for many micronutrients [7,8]. The DRIs guide normal dietary intake and planning, and potentially may help to judge the requirements in disease prevention [7].

All the reference ranges developed internationally and discussed above are based on assessments in the general healthy population.

Table 3.4.3 ESPEN and European recommendations for the healthy population [4,5]

Vitamin	Units	Minimum	Maximum
Vitamin B1 Thiamine	mg/day	1.2	10
Vitamin B2 Riboflavin	mg/day	1.6	10
Vitamin B3 Niacin	mg/day	18	60
Vitamin B6 Pyridoxine	mg/day	1.6	10
Vitamin B7 Biotin	µg/day	15	150
Vitamin B9 Folate	µg/day	200	1000
Vitamin B12	µg/day	1.4	14
Vitamin C Ascorbic acid	mg/day	45	440

Table 3.4.4 US recommendations for dietary reference intakes [7]

Vitamin	Unit	Males, years			Females, years			Pregnancy, years	
		9–13	14–18	19+	9–13	14–18	19+	14–18	19+
Vitamin B1 Thiamine	mg/day	0.9	1.2	1.2	0.9	1.0	1.1	1.4	1.4
Vitamin B2 Riboflavin	mg/day	0.9	1.3	1.3	0.9	1.0	1.1	1.4	1.4
Vitamin B3 Niacin	mg/day	12	16	16	12	14	14	18	18
Vitamin B5 Pantothenic acid	mg/day	4	5	5	4	5	5	6	6
Vitamin B7 Biotin	µg/day	20	25	30	20	25	30	30	30
Vitamin B9 Folate	µg/day	300	400	400	300	400	400	600	600
Vitamin B12	µg/day	1.8	2.4	2.4	1.8	2.4	2.4	2.6	2.6
Vitamin C	mg/day	45	75	90	45	65	75	80	85

Undernutrition

Risk of nutritional deficiency can be identified in those who have experienced periods of anorexia, inadequate digestion or malabsorption of nutrients [3]. Causes for this may include pre-existing illness, surgery to the GI tract or any surgery resulting in periods of anorexia and increased gastrointestinal losses. Pre-existing illnesses particularly prone to cause micronutrient undernutrition include inflammatory bowel disease, alcoholism and all causes of intestinal villous atrophy. There is also a degree of specificity between micronutrient and disease, such that, for example, water-soluble vitamin deficiency is relatively unusual in cystic fibrosis, despite often considerable deficiency in macronutrients and the fat-soluble vitamins.

Pregnant and lactating women

Pregnancy presents a special risk of vitamin undernutrition due to the increased demands from the fetus, and the UK NICE guidelines (*inter alia*) accordingly consider vitamin supplementations [9].

Supplementation with folic acid in the pre-conception phase and in the first trimester of pregnancy has been shown to reduce the rate of neonatal neural tube defects such as spina bifida [9]. In the UK it is currently recommended that all women trying to conceive and those in the first 12 weeks of pregnancy should take 400 μg daily [9]. If there is a perceived increased risk of neural tube defect (e.g. positive family or personal history, or the mother is diabetic), a dose of 5 mg is recommended [9]. The key evidence for establishing these recommendations was the British Medical Research Council Vitamin Study carried out in the early 1990s [10]. In the USA a dose of 400–800 μg is recommended for all women between the ages of 15 and 45 years [11]. The Centers for Disease Control and Prevention suggest even that a higher dose of 4 mg may be recommended [11]. Less controversial is the WHO recommendation that not only pregnant women but also those in the 3 months after delivery should receive a daily supplement of 400 μg folic acid [12].

Folate in pregnancy remains one of the most well-established examples of a need for increased micronutrient intake because of increased demand. Furthermore, in the UK and elsewhere, approximately half of pregnancies are unplanned which means that many women are unaware of advice on folate until too late for useful benefit to the new infant. It has therefore been suggested by the SACN that flour should be fortified with 300 μg folate per 100 g flour; this practice has been adopted elsewhere, most notably in North America, but not to date in Europe [13].

The use of folic acid supplementation in other disease states has been studied, namely, in cardiovascular disease and cancer. The Heart Outcomes Prevention Evaluation (HOPE) study hypothesised that folate could reduce rates of coronary artery disease and stroke through reducing homocysteine. However, neither benefit nor harm was identified from supplementation with folate, and vitamins B6 and B12 [14].

The role of folate in the pathology of cancer has also been considered. In the case of gastric carcinogenesis, genetic mutations in the enzymes responsible for folate metabolism have been studied. There are many identified polymorphisms of the MTHFR gene which codes for the methylene-tetrahydrofolate reductase enzyme involved in the metabolism of folate [15]. This prompted a major review looking at this and more generally at the role of folate in carcinogenesis. Meta-analysis revealed an increased risk of gastric cancer in the genotype MTHFR 677 TT and, furthermore, individuals with this genotype were found to have lower circulating folate concentrations, suggesting a possible causal link [15].

It is understandable from the above examples that almost ubiquitous folate supplementation has been promoted, but the practice is not without risk. Hirsch et al. explored colorectal cancer diagnosis before and after the flour fortification programme designed to reduce neural tube defects in Chile [16]. Flour was fortified with 2.1 mg synthetic folate to every kilogram. The incidence of colorectal cancer after the fortification programme was introduced increased significantly in those aged 45–79 although it is not

Table 3.4.5   Comparison of recommendations for folate intake [2,4,5,7,9,12,13]

Folate recommendations	Europe, minimum and maximum values only	USA	United Kingdom	World Health Organization
Adult males	200–1000 µg/day	400 µg/day	200 µg/day	–
Adult females	200–1000 µg/day	400 µg/day	200 µg/day	–
Pregnant females	200–1000 µg/day	600 µg/day	300–400 µg/day	400 µg/day
Pregnant females at risk of neural tube defects	200–1000 µg/day	Up to 4 mg/day	5 mg/day	–

possible to draw conclusions regarding causal associations.

It may thus be fundamental to discriminate between dietary folate and folate (especially in synthetic form) given as an isolated nutriceutical supplement, and to make a clear distinction between populations with relatively low folate levels and individuals with frank deficiency states. To date, the only population group in whom folate supplementation, additional to basal requirements, can be justified is the pregnant and about-to-be pregnant female. This conclusion is not transparent in current international recommendations (Table 3.4.5).

3.4.3 Water-soluble vitamins

The term 'antioxidant' refers to a substance which can act against reactive oxygen species and free radicals [17,18]. There are several micronutrients with antioxidant functions including vitamins A, C and E [17]. Studies have often considered them as a group, and interventions have typically included multiple agents. This section aims to concentrate on the impact of the key water-soluble vitamins amongst the antioxidants, but its separation from the effects of the other agents involved is incomplete.

Vitamin C

Vitamin C is required in the maintenance of collagen, it can regenerate vitamin E (another antioxidant) and it promotes iron absorption, but it also has a direct scavenger effect on free radicals. Its supplementation in disease states where oxidant concentrations are high has accordingly been studied.

Higher doses of vitamin C are known to be required in smokers as well as those at special risk of deficiency such as patients with impaired absorption, young children and those with a limited diet such as alcoholics [19]. Additional potentially protective functions are being explored as yet without definitive conclusions, in cancer and ischaemic heart disease [17,20,21], including a possible effect on myocardial infarct size after percutaneous angioplasty [22].

Vitamin C excess also requires consideration when recommending supplementation. The most common adverse effects of high-dose vitamin C are self-limiting diarrhoea and non-specific gastrointestinal upset [8], but its impact on circulating urate permits high-dose vitamin C to contribute to kidney stone formation. Moreover, in patients with haemochromatosis, high vitamin C intake can exacerbate already high concentrations of iron in the body [8].

Consideration of the evidence for benefit and potential toxicity from vitamin C has influenced the various international guidelines (Table 3.4.6). The UK Department of Health recommends a daily upper limit of 1000 mg to avoid adverse effects, with a generally recommended dose of only 40 mg/day [23]. The USA has a higher upper limit of 2000 mg in adults [24]. The suggested EU tolerable upper limit is 1000 mg/day on the basis that although doses above this have negligible positive effects and that side effects are more likely, hazard really comes into play only at daily doses of 3 or 4 g [8]. Some ambiguity remains in respect of recommendations for individuals who would most likely benefit from the higher doses, such as smokers, those at risk of undernutrition and those with a vitamin C-deficient diet.

Table 3.4.6 Comparison of recommendations for vitamin C intake [2,4,5,7,23,24]

Vitamin C recommendation	Europe	USA	United Kingdom
Adult males	45–440 mg/day	90 mg/day	40 mg/day
Adult females	45–440 mg/day	75 mg/day	40 mg/day
Those at risk of deficiency (such as smokers)	Up to 1000 mg/day	Up to 2000 mg/day	Up to 1000 mg/day

The use of therapeutic-dose antioxidant cocktails including vitamin C has been considered in two large meta-analyses. The first, published in 2012, considered more than 20 randomised controlled trials which investigated therapeutic doses of vitamins C and E and selenium in the intensive care setting [25]. The results were promising, highlighting reduced ventilation days, decreased infection rates and decreased mortality in those prescribed the active agents. However, in 2013, a major randomised controlled trial that gave therapeutic doses of selenium, zinc, β-carotene, vitamin C and vitamin E found that there was no significant improvement in mortality in those receiving the active treatments [26]. It is unclear whether conclusions from these studies, conducted in parenterally fed critically ill patients, can be extrapolated to other clinical settings.

Thiamine

There is sufficient evidence to recommend supplementation with thiamine in those at risk of Wernicke–Korsakov's syndrome as it is directly involved in neural function [17]. Worldwide, this includes populations such as those of Japan and Thailand who have a high dietary consumption of raw fish and polished rice, which contain the anti-thiamine compound thiaminase [3]. In Europe and the US, alcohol abuse is the leading cause of thiamine deficiency [3]. There are three active mechanisms for thiamine deficiency in patients with the alcohol dependency syndrome. First, intake of thiamine is often reduced due to a poor appetite and limited diet. Second, absorption may be reduced by the gastritis and enteritis which are overrepresented in heavy drinkers. Finally, and probably most importantly, thiamine is required as a coenzyme in the metabolism of

alcohol, and demands are therefore greater in the very patients in whom background concentrations are most parlous.

Rarely, patients are seen with thiamine deficiency because of a genetic abnormality in the production of transketolase, itself a thiamine-dependent enzyme [3].

Currently there is no evidence to suggest toxic effects from high levels of thiamine supplementation [27]. The US has no recommended upper limit for supplementation with thiamine, but further research in this area is advised to confirm this [27]. The ESPEN guidelines for enteral nutrition recommend a maximum of 10 mg/day in an individual without deficiency [3]. In the UK, the amount of thiamine advised in a healthy adult male is 1 mg/day with no quoted upper limit [2].

Recommendations on thiamine intake in the general population take account of age, sex and pregnancy and lactation status (Table 3.4.7). Thiamine-deficient individuals are recommended much higher doses, such as 300 mg/day in three divided doses, at least for the first few days of treatment [28]. Given concerns about possible malabsorption, it is common to administer a combination of B group vitamins intravenously [28].

Vitamin B12

The role of vitamin B12 in preventing neurological disorders (particularly neuropathy and dementing conditions) and more generally in macrocytic anaemia is of course well rehearsed. Deficiency of vitamin B12 is broadly seen in three cohorts of patients. First, those who have a reduced intake, particularly individuals eating a vegan diet; second, those with gastric disease or pernicious anaemia who lack the parietal

Table 3.4.7 Comparison of recommendations for thiamine intake [2,4,5,7]

Thiamine recommendation	Europe	USA	United Kingdom
Adult males	1.2–10 mg/day	1.2 mg/day	1.0 mg/day
Adult females	1.2–10 mg/day	1.1 mg/day	0.8 mg/day
Those at risk of deficiency (especially alcohol dependency)	Up to 300 mg/day	Up to 300 mg/day	Up to 300 mg/day

cell-derived intrinsic factor essential for its absorption; and third, those with incapacitated terminal ileum (especially in active Crohn's disease or where this part of the small intestine has been resected). In all such patients, it is recommended that vitamin B12 is supplemented to prevent adverse haematological and neurological consequences [3]. Traditionally, it has been held that this should be by an intramuscular approach (usually 1 mg every 3 months given indefinitely), but several recent reports indicate that a very high oral dose (e.g. 1 mg per day) can be effective even in those with resection of the ileum [29].

Other B vitamins

There is limited evidence from research surrounding the supplementation of other B group vitamins. One area of topical interest concerns vitamin B6 with suggestions that supplementation may yield some protection against Alzheimer's disease and more generally against cognitive decline. However, studies thus far have not provided sufficient evidence that supplementation can be generally advocated, nor indeed in combination with vitamin B12 [30].

Pellagra from niacin (vitamin B3) deficiency is rare in nutritional practice but can be seen in those with severe undernutrition and if nutrition support is introduced without appropriate vitamin provision. The classic triad of dermatological features, diarrhoea and memory loss (dementia) [3] is not often seen, but if any of these elements occur during refeeding, extra supplementation should be given with an initial bolus given parenterally to ensure its availability to key cells. Milder forms of a pellagra-like condition occur with deficiency of vitamin B2 but this is vanishingly rare in clinical practice. This

vitamin's main claim to fame may lie in its colour as it is predominantly riboflavin that gives vitamin solutions their characteristic yellow hue.

More than 15 years ago, Bender concluded that we do not have adequate knowledge of the requirements for, nor satisfactory indices of biochemical repletion of, pantothenic acid (vitamin B5) [31]; sadly, this still appears to be the case.

Biotin (vitamin B7) has been neglected in artificial nutrition and it was not long ago that it was absent from the vitamin supplements available for parenteral use. To this day (like vitamin B5), it fails to appear in recommended intake listings for the UK population (see Table 3.4.1). Few situations exist where it has a unique contribution, although a very rare inborn error of metabolism responsible for a basal ganglia syndrome is corrected by the coadministration of biotin and thiamine [32].

3.4.4 Summary

There is overall unity between the US, UK and EU recommendations for water-soluble vitamin doses in the healthy population. The US has the most complete guidance on this, with values stated for age, gender and pregnancy status. There are some incomplete data so not all water-soluble vitamins have a recommended value in all cases. For example, pantothenic acid is not included in the EU or UK recommendations, but it is in the US data. There is also a need to update some of the UK recommendations, which are based on data from 1999.

The use of water-soluble vitamins for patients with known deficiency or at risk of deficiency is best supported by evidence in the cases of thiamine and folate. The recommendations vary slightly but are comparable across the world (see Table 3.3.4). The use of folate in reducing cardiovascular disease or cancer is not conclusive and therefore cannot be recommended at this stage. Thiamine is recommended at higher levels particularly in those at risk of deficiency, which in the UK, US and Europe is commonly caused by high alcohol intake. Supplementation with thiamine can reduce the risk of Wernicke–Korsakov's syndrome. Vitamin C supplementation is thought to be beneficial in those at risk of deficiency such as smokers, but only the use of high-dose antioxidant cocktails containing vitamin C has much supportive evidence to date.

References

1. Scientific Advisory Committee for Nutrition. Dietary Reference Values for Energy. 2011. www.gov.uk/government/publications/sacn-dietary-reference-values-for-energy (accessed 31 August 2017).
2. Department for Environment, Food and Rural Affairs. Family Food Statistics. 2017. www.gov.uk/government/collections/family-food-statistics (accessed 31 August 2017).
3. Shenkin A. Metabolism of Vitamins and Metabolism of Minerals and Trace Elements. ESPEN Lifelong Learning Programme, Topics 2.2–2.3. http://lllnutrition.com/tlll2/mod/resource/view.php?id=213 (accessed 31 August 2017).
4. European Commission. Food for Special Medical Purposes. 2016. http://ec.europa.eu/food/food/labellingnutrition/medical/index_en.htm (accessed 31 August 2017).
5. European Commission. Discussion Paper on the Setting of Maximum and Minimum Amounts for Vitamins and Minerals in Foodstuffs. 2016. http://ec.europa.eu/food/safety/docs/labelling_nutrition-vitamins_minerals-discus_paper_amount_vitamins_en.pdf (accessed 31 August 2017).
6. US Department of Agriculture and US Department of Health and Human Services. Dietary Guidelines for Americans. 2010. www.health.gov/dietaryguidelines/dga2010/DietaryGuidelines2010.pdf (accessed 31 August 2017).
7. Otten JJ, Hellwig JP, Meyers LD. Dietary Reference Intakes: The Essential Guide to Nutrient Requirements. Washington: National Academies Press, 2006.
8. Scientific Committee on Food, European Food Safety Authority. Tolerable Upper Intake Levels for Vitamins and Minerals. 2016. www.efsa.europa.eu/en/ndatopics/docs/ndatolerableuil.pdf (accessed 31 August 2017).
9. National Institute for Health and Care Excellence. Maternal and Child Nutrition: Overview. 2015. https://pathways.nice.org.uk/pathways/maternal-and-child-nutrition (accessed 31 August 2017).
10. [No authors listed] Prevention of neural tube defects: results of the Medical Research Council vitamin study. *Lancet* 1991; **338**(8760): 131–137.
11. Centers for Disease Control and Prevention. Folic Acid: Recommendations. 2016. www.cdc.gov/ncbddd/folicacid/recommendations.html (accessed 31 August 2017).
12. World Health Organization, Western Pacific Region. Weekly Iron and Folic Acid Supplementation Programmes for Women of Reproductive Age. An Analysis of Best Programme Practices. 2016. www.wpro.who.int/publications/docs/FORwebPDFFullVersionWIFS.pdf?ua=1 (accessed 31 August 2017).
13. Scientific Advisory Committee on Nutrition. Folate and Disease Prevention. London: Stationery Office, 2006.
14. Lonn E, Yusuf S, Arnold MJ, et al. Heart Outcomes Prevention Evaluation (HOPE) 2 Investigators. Homocysteine lowering with folic acid and B vitamins in vascular disease. *N Engl J Med* 2006; **354**: 1567–1577.
15. Boccia S, Hung R, Ricciardi G, et al. Meta- and pooled analyses of the methylenetetrahydrofolate reductase *C677T* and *A1298C* polymorphisms and gastric cancer risk: a huge-GSEC review. *Am J Epidemiol* 2008; **167**(5): 505–516.
16. Hirsch S, Sanchez H, Albala C, de la Maza MP, Barrera G, Leiva L, Bunout D. Colon cancer in Chile before and after the start of the flour fortification programme with folic acid. *Eur J Gastroenterol Hepatol* 2009; **21**(4): 436–439.
17. ESPEN Lifelong Learning Programme. Vitamin and Trace Element Antioxidants, Module 1. http://lllnutrition.com/tlll2/mod/resource/view.php?id=213 (accessed 31 August 2017).
18. Reddell L, Cotton BA. Antioxidant and micronutrient supplementation in critically ill trauma patients. *Curr Opin Clin Nutr Metab Care* 2012; **15**(2): 181–187.
19. Kaur B, Rowe BH, Stovold E. Vitamin C supplementation for asthma. *Cochrane Database Syst Rev* 2009; **1**: CD000993.
20. Coulter I, Hardy M, Shekelle P, et al. Effect of the Supplemental Use of Antioxidants Vitamin C, Vitamin E, and Coenzyme Q10 for the Prevention and Treatment of Cancer. Rockville: Agency for Healthcare Research and Quality, 2003.
21. Institute of Medicine (US) Panel on Dietary Antioxidants and Related Compounds. Vitamin C, Vitamin E, Selenium, and β-Carotene and Other

Carotenoids: Overview, Antioxidant Definition, and Relationship to Chronic Disease. Dietary Reference Intakes for Vitamin C, Vitamin E, Selenium, and Carotenoids. Washington: National Academies Press, 2000.

22. Rodrigo R, Hasson D, Prieto JC, et al. The effectiveness of antioxidant vitamins C and E in reducing myocardial infarct size in patients subjected to percutaneous coronary angioplasty (PREVEC Trial): study protocol for a pilot randomized double-blind controlled trial. *Trials* 2014; **15**: 192.

23. UK Department of Health. Food Supplements. Label Advisory Statements and Suggested Reformulations. 2011. www.gov.uk/government/uploads/system/uploads/attachment_data/file/204323/Advisory_Statements_DH_FINAL.pdf (accessed 31 August 2017).

24. National Institutes of Health, Office of Dietary Supplements. Vitamin C: Fact Sheet for Health Professionals. 2016. https://ods.od.nih.gov/pdf/factsheets/VitaminC-HealthProfessional.pdf (accessed 31 August 2017).

25. Manzanares W, Dhaliwal R, Jiang X, Murch L, Heyland DK. Antioxidant micronutrients in the critically ill: a systematic review and meta-analysis. *Crit Care* 2012; **16**(2): R66.

26. Heyland D, Muscedere J, Wischmeyer PE, et al. A randomised control trial of glutamine and antioxidants in critically ill patients. *N Engl J Med* 2013; **368**: 1489–1497.

27. Dietary Reference Intakes for Thiamine, Riboflavin, Niacin, Vitamin B6, Folate, Vitamin B12, Pantothenic Acid, Biotin, and Choline. A Report of the Standing Committee on the Scientific Evaluation of Dietary Reference Intakes and its Panel on Folate, Other B Vitamins, and Choline and Subcommittee on Upper Reference Levels of Nutrients. Washington: National Academy Press, 1998, 2000.

28. Thompson AD, Cook CCH, Touquet R, Henry JA. The Royal College of Physicians' report on alcohol: guidelines for managing Wernicke's encephalopathy in the accident and emergency department. *Alcohol Alcohol* 2002; **37**(6): 513–521.

29. Butler CC, Vidal-Alaball J, Cannings-John R, McCaddon A, Hood K, Papaioannou A, Mcdowell I, Goringe A. Oral vitamin B12 versus intramuscular vitamin B12 for vitamin B12 deficiency: a systematic review of randomized controlled trials. *Fam Pract* 2006; **23**(3): 279–285.

30. Clarke RJ, Bennett DA. B vitamins for prevention of cognitive decline. Insufficient evidence to justify treatment. *JAMA* 2008; **300**(15): 1819–1821.

31. Bender DA. Optimum nutrition: thiamin, biotin and pantothenate. *Proc Nutr Soc* 1999; **58**(2): 427–433.

32. Alfadhel M, Almuntashri M, Jadah RH, et al. Biotin-responsive basal ganglia disease should be renamed biotin-thiamine-responsive basal ganglia disease: a retrospective review of the clinical, radiological and molecular findings of 18 new cases. *Orphanet J Rare Dis* 2013; **8**: 83.

Chapter 3.5

Fat-soluble vitamins in nutrition support

Callum Livingstone
Clinical Biochemistry Department, Royal Surrey County Hospital NHS Foundation Trust, Guildford, UK

3.5.1 Introduction

Patients with undernutrition are often acutely ill so it is therefore necessary to consider the effect of illness on absorption and metabolism of fat-soluble vitamins and to examine the impact of deficiency on clinical outcome. This chapter reviews fat-soluble vitamin requirements in health and in patients with undernutrition, including those requiring nutrition support. Recent research findings on requirements for these vitamins in acute illness are discussed. For convenience, the vitamins are considered individually but it should be remembered that they function together in physiology and are generally provided together in nutrition support.

3.5.2 The normal diet

In order to place the discussion of undernutrition in context, it is appropriate to start by summarising current recommendations for fat-soluble vitamin intake in the healthy population.

United Kingdom

In 1991, the Committee on Medical Aspects of Food Policy (COMA) published reference nutrient intakes (RNI) for the fat-soluble vitamins, except for vitamins E and K for which there was insufficient information available [1].

COMA has been replaced by the Scientific Advisory Committee on Nutrition (SACN) which is currently updating these recommendations following recent research findings. For example, RNIs for vitamin D were originally set for population groups considered at risk of deficiency. These did not include people with exposure to sunlight, for whom dietary intake was considered unnecessary. However, it is now known that exposure to sunlight may be insufficient to meet vitamin D requirements. Consequently, the updated guidance will probably recommend vitamin D intake more widely in the population. At present the recommendations remain unchanged (Table 3.5.1).

Europe

In 1993, the Scientific Committee on Food (SCF) published population reference intakes (PRI) for nutrients including vitamins A, D and E, those for vitamins D and E being confined to adults (Table 3.5.2) [2]. The PRI for vitamin E was expressed per gram of polyunsaturated fatty acid (PUFA) because disproportionately high dietary PUFA depletes vitamin E [3]. In 2005, the European Commission (EC) asked the European Food Safety Authority (EFSA) to review the recommendations. This review is still under way. As part of the process, the EFSA is also establishing tolerable upper limits (UL) for nutrient intake [4]. Once completed, the EFSA

Advanced Nutrition and Dietetics in Nutrition Support, First Edition. Edited by Mary Hickson and Sara Smith.
© 2018 John Wiley & Sons Ltd. Published 2018 by John Wiley & Sons Ltd.

Table 3.5.1 SACN recommendations (reference nutrient intakes) for fat-soluble vitamins in the healthy population [1]

Vitamin	Unit	Children (age in years)				Males (age in years)					Females (age in years)					
		<1	1–3	4–6	7–10	11–14	15–18	19–50	>50	>65	11–14	15–18	19–50	>50	>65	Pregnancy (any age)
A	µgRAE/day	350	400	500	500	600	700	700	700	700	600	600	600	600	600	700
D	µg/day	*	7	NR	NR	NR	NR	NR	NR	10	NR	NR	NR	10	10	10

NR, no recommendation; RAE, retinol activity equivalent.
* RNI values were set for infants 0–6 months (8.5 µg/day) and infants and children 7–12 months (7 µ/day).

Table 3.5.2 Population reference intakes for fat-soluble vitamins published by the Scientific Committee for Food [2]

Vitamin	Unit	Children				Males (age in years)			Females (age in years)			Pregnancy (any age)	Lactation (any age)
		6–11 months	1–3 years	4–6 years	7–10 years	11–14	15–17	>18	11–14	15–17	>18		
A	µg/day	350	400	400	500	600	700	700	600	600	600	700	950
D	µg/day	NR	NR	NR	NR	NR	NR	0–10*	NR	NR	0–10*	NR	NR
E	mg/day†	NR	NR	NR	NR	NR	NR	0.4/g PUFA	NR	NR	0.4/g PUFA	NR	NR

NR, no recommendation; PUFA, polyunsaturated fatty acids.
* Acceptable intake (AI).
† α-tocopherol equivalents.

aims to translate the recommendations into food-based dietary guidelines. Regarding vitamin D, a conference was held in 2013 as a step towards harmonisation of reference intakes across Europe [5].

United States

Guidelines published in the US in 2006 are the most extensive available (Tables 3.5.3 and 3.5.4). These were based on work by the Institute of Medicine (IOM) and the Food and Nutrition Board (FNB) published in 2001 [6]. The term dietary reference intake (DRI) encompasses the recommended daily allowance (RDA), adequate intake (AI) and tolerable upper intake level (UL). The RDA meets the nutrient requirements of 97–98% of healthy people. In cases where there was insufficient evidence for an RDA, an AI was established instead. DRIs are useful in guiding dietary intake for health and for preventing disease. The recommendations for vitamin D were updated in 2010 based on the amount required for bone health [7].

World Health Organization

In 2004, the World Health Organization (WHO) published updated guidance on vitamin requirements in human nutrition [8]. The RNIs are shown in Table 3.5.5. In the case of vitamin E, there was insufficient evidence available to establish an RNI. Mean requirements for vitamin A were derived from subjects receiving intakes which were adequate to prevent features of deficiency. Of note, vitamin D intake was recommended for all population groups.

3.5.3 Effects of disease on absorption and metabolism of fat-soluble vitamins

Malabsorption of fat decreases the absorption of vitamin A. This can occur in coeliac disease, cystic fibrosis, cholestatic liver disease, inflammatory bowel disease or pancreatic exocrine insufficiency. During acute illness, oxidative stress increases utilisation of vitamin A by the antioxidant system,

resulting in a deficit [9], to which disease-related undernutrition and increased urinary losses may contribute [10]. During dietary deficiency, serum retinol is initially replenished from hepatic stores but these are eventually exhausted, resulting in overt deficiency.

Vitamin D absorption decreases during small bowel disease, pancreatic exocrine insufficiency and treatment with high-dose glucocorticoids. Liver disease impairs formation and storage of 25-hydroxyvitamin D (25(OH)D) and chronic renal disease impairs generation of active 1,25-dihydroxyvitamin D. Acute illness also results in vitamin D deficiency. The mechanism is complex but includes a decrease in vitamin D binding proteins caused by decreased synthesis and inflammation-induced fluid shifts. There is also increased urinary loss of vitamin D [11]. Vitamin D deficiency is more common in the elderly, in part because hepatic and renal activation decrease with age.

Vitamin E deficiency is uncommon but can occur in patients with severe pancreatic insufficiency or cholestatic liver disease, especially primary biliary cirrhosis [12]. The hyperlipidaemia which occurs in cholestasis tends to cause misleadingly high serum vitamin E levels. Consequently, vitamin E status should be assessed by measuring the vitamin E:cholesterol ratio. During acute illness, increased activity of the antioxidant system results in increased utilisation of vitamin E.

Vitamin K, in common with the other fat-soluble vitamins, can become deficient in patients with fat malabsorption of any cause. Again, this may result from gastrointestinal disease or cholestatic liver disease. It can also occur in the newborn because of a lack of GI microbiota producing vitamin K. Medications such as antibiotics, anticoagulants and excessive vitamin A provision can predispose to vitamin K deficiency.

3.5.4 Undernutrition and acute illness

During undernutrition, deficiency of the fat-soluble vitamins tends to develop later than that of the water-soluble vitamins because of more

Table 3.5.3 Dietary reference intakes for fat-soluble vitamins in males [6]

Vitamin	Unit	Age									
		0–6 months	7–12 months	1–3 y	4–8 y	9–13 years	14–18 years	19–30 years	31–50 years	51–70 years	>70 years
A	μgRAE/day	400*	500*	300	400	600	900	900	900	900	900
D	μg/day	10*	10*	15	15	15	15	15	15	15	20
E	mg/day	4*	5*	6	7	11	15	15	15	15	15
K	μg/day	2.0*	2.5*	30*	55*	60*	75*	120*	120*	120*	120*

Values are RDA except where marked.

* Adequate intake (AI).

Vitamin E recommendations are for α-tocopherol.

Source: Reproduced with permission of the Institute of Medicine.

Table 3.5.4 Dietary reference intakes for fat-soluble vitamins in females [6]

Vitamin	Unit	Age										Pregnancy		Lactation	
		0–6 months	7–12 months	1–3 years	4–8 years	9–13 years	14–18 years	19–30 years	31–50 years	51–70 years	>70 years	≤18 years	19–50 years	≤18 years	19–50 years
A	μgRAE/day	400*	500*	300	400	600	700	700	700	700	700	750	770	1200	1300
D	μg/day	10*	10*	15	15	15	15	15	15	15	20	15	15	15	15
E	mg/day	4*	5*	6	7	11	15	15	15	15	15	15	15	19	19
K	μg/day	2.0*	2.5*	30*	55*	60*	75*	90*	90*	90*	90*	75*	90*	75*	90*

RAE, retinol activity equivalent.

Values are RDA except where marked.

* Adequate intake (AI).

Vitamin E recommendations are for α-tocopherol.

Source: Reproduced with permission of the Institute of Medicine.

Table 3.5.5 WHO recommended nutrient intakes for fat-soluble vitamins [8]

Vitamin	Unit	Children						Males			Females				
		0–6 months	7–12 months	1–3 years	4–6 years	7–9 years	10–18 years	19–50 years	51–65 years	>65 years	19–50 years	51–65 years	>65 years	Pregnancy	Lactation
A	μgRAE/day	180*	190*	200*	200*	250*	330–400*	300*	300*	300*	270*	270*	300*	370*	450*
D	μg/day	5	5	5	5	5	5	5	10	15	5	10	15	5	5
K	μg/day	5†	10	15	20	25	35–55	65	65	65	65	65	65	55	55

RAE, retinol activity equivalent.

* Mean requirement.

† This intake cannot be met by breastfeeding alone. Infants should be supplemented with vitamin K at birth in accordance with national guidelines.

Source: Reproduced with permission of the World Health Organization.

abundant stores of the former. Overt deficiency is uncommon in hospitalised patients referred for nutrition support. However, sublinical deficiency is common and can adversely affect clinical outcome. Its presence cannot be confirmed objectively because of the absence of clinical signs and the low diagnostic sensitivity of laboratory tests but its likely presence should be borne in mind when providing vitamins. Vitamins A and D are potentially toxic at high doses. Caution is therefore necessary when providing them in doses higher than standard recommendations. This makes the provision of fat-soluble vitamins more problematic than that of the water-soluble ones.

Oral and enteral nutrition support

Recommendations on provision of fat-soluble vitamins in oral and enteral nutrition (EN) support have been based on the RDA or AI. Although these values apply primarily to healthy individuals taking a normal diet, they are a useful basis for planning nutrient provision in sick patients. The most recent recommendations were published by the American Society for Parenteral and Enteral Nutrition (ASPEN) in 2012 and are identical to the RDA (see Tables 3.5.3 and 3.5.4) [13]. Commercially produced EN products, although nutritionally complete, usually only deliver the RDA of a given vitamin when meeting a patient's full energy requirement.

Parenteral nutrition

The most recent recommendations for fat-soluble vitamin provision in parenteral nutrition (PN) are shown in Table 3.5.6 [13]. The recommendations for adults were originally published by the Task Force for the Revision of Safe Practices for PN [14] and, those for infants and children by the American Society for Clinical Nutrition [15]. The bioavailability of fat-soluble vitamins delivered parenterally is considerably higher than their enteral bioavailability. However, requirements also tend to be higher in patients treated with PN. This is because these patients are in general sicker than those receiving EN. There is a combination of more severe undernutrition, pre-existing deficiency and metabolic changes resulting from illness. Consequently, the daily doses recommended in PN are similar to the RDA. There is a consensus amongst guidelines that, in patients requiring total PN, fat-soluble vitamins should be supplemented on a daily basis [14,16].

Individualisation of requirements

All guidelines on micronutrient provision in nutrition support state that standard recommendations will not meet the needs of all patients and, as such, should be considered only a starting point for deciding on individual requirements. Nutrition support teams (NSTs) therefore need to be alert to the presence of factors that influence requirements. The most important of these is the underlying disease but requirements of individual patients with the same disease may differ significantly. Requirements increase during acute illness, especially if the illness is prolonged or severe. In the critically ill, requirements are likely to exceed the RDA. Physiological factors such as age, weight, pregnancy and lactation should also be considered.

Laboratory tests of fat-soluble vitamin status are an important part of determining individual requirements but all the available tests have limitations. As well as limited sensitivity for detection of deficiency, there is ongoing debate about

Table 3.5.6   Parenteral requirements for fat-soluble vitamins in infants, children and adults [13,15]

Vitamin	Infants	Children	Adults
A	150–300 μg/kg/day	150 μg/day	990 μg/day
D	0.8 μg/kg/day	10 μg/day	5 μg/day
E	2.8–3.5 mg/kg/d	7 mg/day	10 mg/day
K	10 μg/kg/day	200 μg/day	150 μg/day

the extent to which serum concentrations of the vitamins reflect their tissue status and the true requirement, especially during acute illness. There are also logistical limitations. For example, testing for vitamins A and E is costly and not widely available in clinical laboratories.

3.5.5 Vitamin A

Impact of deficiency on outcome

Overt vitamin A deficiency causes night blindness which, if untreated, leads to xerophthalmia and blindness. Deficiency, whether overt or sublinical, causes immunodeficiency. This predisposes to infection [17,18], the severity and mortality of which correlate with vitamin A status [19]. Patients can potentially enter a vicious cycle of worsening infection and vitamin A deficiency. Vitamin A deficiency also predisposes to pressure ulcers and poor wound healing, especially in patients treated with corticosteroids. During PN, the bioavailability of vitamin A can decrease because of degradation and adsorption on to plastic. Excessive degradation resulting from delays in administering PN has resulted in overt deficiency [20]. This can be avoided by ensuring that PN is infused as soon as possible after the addition of fat-soluble vitamins.

Impact of supplementation on outcome

There is extensive evidence that vitamin A supplementation improves clinical outcome in people at risk of deficiency. A meta-analysis of 43 randomised controlled trials (RCTs) in developing countries showed that vitamin A supplementation in children decreased eye disease, all-cause mortality and diarrhoea-associated mortality [21]. Vitamin A supplementation also has a beneficial effect on wound healing [22], especially in patients treated with corticosteroids, because it opposes the inhibitory effect of these drugs on wound healing [23]. The physiological requirement for vitamin A by the antioxidant and immune systems suggests that acutely ill patients may benefit from supplementation. This awaits investigation by suitably designed studies.

Requirements in undernutrition and acute illness

The WHO has made age-specific dose recommendations for vitamin A supplementation in children with severe undernutrition, diarrhoea, measles or respiratory disease who are at risk of deficiency [24]. More recent guidance is available from the International Vitamin A Consultative Group (IVACG) [25]. Patients with diseases causing malabsorption may require doses well above the RDA. For example, doses of 1500–1700 μg have been used in patients with cholestatic liver disease [26]. In patients with poor wound healing, a 10–14-day course of 6.0–7.5 mg (20 000–25 000 IU/d) has been recommended [23]. Hospitalised patients with pressure ulcers should receive sufficient vitamin A [13].

Although vitamin A requirements are likely to exceed the RDA during critical illness, data on dosing are limited because of a lack of outcome studies of supplementation. In a review of micronutrient supplementation in critical illness, it was recommended that vitamin A is supplemented over and above standard provision at doses of 3.5 mg in PN and 8.6 mg in EN [27]. In critically ill patients with sepsis, vitamin A doses as high as three times the RDA were insufficient to restore serum retinol concentration [28]. High-dose vitamin A provision should be monitored closely because of the narrow therapeutic margin between deficiency and toxicity. Excessive vitamin A provision is also teratogenic. Doses should be kept within safe limits in women of reproductive age.

3.5.6 Vitamin D

Impact of deficiency on outcome

Vitamin D deficiency results in hypocalcaemia, muscle weakness and pain, rickets in children and osteomalacia in adults [29]. It is also increasingly implicated in the development of cancer, diabetes and cognitive decline, although the evidence linking it with these conditions is largely from observational studies [5]. Until recently, it received little attention in the context of acute illness. However, vitamin D deficiency (serum 25(OH)D <20 ng/mL) is present in up to 90% of critically ill patients [30]. Given that the immune system requires vitamin D, deficiency could be anticipated to adversely affect clinical outcome, especially in patients with sepsis [31]. Indeed, evidence is accumulating that vitamin D deficiency is associated with a poor outcome in the critically ill, patients with the lowest 25(OH)D concentrations having the greatest mortality [32]. It also predisposes to bone loss [11].

Impact of supplementation on outcome

Vitamin D supplementation is effective in decreasing fracture risk [33] but no RCT-based data are available for outcomes other than bone health. Thus far, studies have demonstrated improved vitamin D status in response to supplementation of the vitamin in the critically ill, but have been underpowered to assess outcome. It is therefore unclear whether the decreased serum 25(OH)D observed in critical illness is a causal factor in poor outcome or simply a biomarker of survival [34].

Requirements in undernutrition and acute illness

Vitamin D dosing in the treatment of deficiency has recently been reviewed [33]. Approaches described in the literature vary widely, in part because of the lack of consensus on target 25(OH)D values and the definition of deficiency. In addition, requirements vary widely between individuals. The loading dose required to achieve normal serum 25(OH)D concentrations in adults can be estimated from the baseline serum 25(OH)D and body weight [35]. The loading dose should be followed by a standard maintenance dose. No loading dose protocols have been described in children (<18 years). Instead, a dose of 1 µg/d vitamin D has been recommended for every 1 nmol/L increase in serum 25(OH)D required to reach optimal concentrations [33].

There is little information available on vitamin D supplementation in the critically ill but guidelines will probably become available following appropriately designed outcome studies. A recent review recommended ergocalciferol 2000 IU daily combined with calcitriol 0.25 µg/d

[11]. When the enteral route is unavailable, vitamin D deficiency can be treated by intramuscular injection of ergocalciferol 7.5 mg [36]. When monitoring vitamin D provision in the critically ill, serum 25(OH)D results should be interpreted with caution because they are affected by the decrease in binding proteins.

Both oral and parenteral delivery of vitamin D bypass physiological control of its synthesis in the skin, leading to the potential for toxicity if provision is excessive. Toxicity can result in hypercalcaemia and the consequences thereof [33]. Vitamin D and calcium should therefore be monitored during supplementation.

3.5.7 Vitamin E

Impact of deficiency on outcome

Severe vitamin E deficiency can cause neuropathy, myopathy and haemolytic anaemia [37,38]. Milder deficiency, whilst not causing overt features, may still adversely affect clinical outcome. Insufficient intake of vitamin E, along with other micronutrients, is implicated in the development of pressure ulcers [39]. Serum vitamin E concentrations decrease during the postoperative acute phase response, though the functional consequences of this and whether it affects clinical outcome are unclear [40].

Impact of supplementation on outcome

Supplementation studies using vitamin E have observed improved clinical outcome, though these studies have generally combined the vitamin with other antioxidants such as vitamin C and selenium. In 2005, a systematic review of 11 studies of antioxidant supplementation in critically ill patients observed that antioxidants delivered parenterally were associated with a reduction in mortality [41]. More recently, a meta-analysis of 20 studies investigated the therapeutic use of vitamin E, vitamin C and selenium in the critically ill [42]. It showed lower mortality in the treatment groups and a trend towards fewer infectious complications and fewer days of artificial ventilation. Vitamin E supplementation in acutely ill patients also results in favourable biochemical changes, including decreased inflammatory markers, decreased oxidative stress and increased antibody production [43].

Requirements in undernutrition and acute illness

Vitamin E deficiency has been treated with oral supplementation of α-tocopherol at doses of 25–50 mg/kg/day [44]. During acute illness, vitamin E requirements are likely to increase in common with those of other antioxidants, but limited data are available. A study which measured total plasma antioxidant status observed that standard micronutrient supplementation in PN did not restore the deficit which occurred postoperatively [45]. Although this study did not measure vitamin E specifically, the finding suggests that standard antioxidant provision is insufficient.

Currently, there is no consensus on vitamin E dosing in critical illness but intravenous doses of 50–150 mg/day were used in the outcome studies [41]. A recent review of micronutrient supplementation in nutrition support recommended that acutely ill patients should be given vitamin E, additional to standard requirements, at doses of 400 mg/day in PN and 40–1000 mg/day in EN [28]. The ESPEN guidelines on PN in intensive care [46] recognise that requirements are likely to be increased but recommend that supplementation is not generally neccessary, on the basis that vitamin E is already present in lipid emulsions, albeit in different amounts depending on the type of lipid [47].

Vitamin E doses of 100–400 mg are safe for most patients but higher doses may have unwanted effects. A meta-analysis of 19 RCTs of long-term vitamin E supplementation observed that doses of 400 mg/day or higher were associated with a significantly increased risk of all-cause mortality [48]. This finding is not directly applicable to critical illness because the patients in these studies were not acutely ill. Nevertheless, it does suggest that caution is advisable when prescribing vitamin E at high doses over long periods. Further studies are required to determine the optimal vitamin E supplementation in acute illness.

3.5.8 Vitamin K

Impact of deficiency on outcome

Vitamin K deficiency can result in impaired coagulation, easy bruisability and bleeding. It is not known to impair functioning of the immune or antioxidant systems.

Requirements in undernutrition and acute illness

The only indication for high-dose vitamin K supplementation is the reversal of bleeding resulting from vitamin K deficiency. In patients receiving nutrition support, vitamin K should generally be supplemented as per standard recommendations [13], which should meet the requirements for both coagulation and maintenance of carboxylation status of non-coagulant Gla proteins. Parenteral lipid emulsions already contain vitamin K, the amount depending on the type of lipid.

In patients treated with warfarin, standard provision of vitamin K should help to achieve the desired level of anticoagulation. However, higher doses could inhibit the antithrombotic effect of the drug, resulting in erratic control of the international normalised ratio (INR). In anticoagulated patients receiving vitamin K, the INR should be monitored closely, to ensure that optimal anticoagulation is maintained.

3.5.9 Summary

There is a need for studies to examine clinical outcome in acutely ill patients following supplementation of the fat-soluble vitamins. The findings will facilitate development of guidelines on provision of fat-soluble vitamins for hospitalised patients. It is likely that development of new laboratory tests of the status of these vitamins will help to remove some of the uncertainty around supplementation and enable progress towards individualised provision.

References

1. Department of Health. Report 41: Dietary Reference Values for Food Energy and Nutrients for the United Kingdom. London: HMSO, 1991.

2. Commission of the European Communities. Nutrient and Energy Intakes for the European Community. Reports of the Scientific Committee for Food. 1993. www.worldcat.org/title/reports-of-the-scientific-committee-for-food-nutrient-and-energy-intakes-for-the-european-community/oclc/614442395?referer=di&ht=edition (accessed 31 August 2017).

3. Bunnell RH, de Rittter E, Rubin SH. Effect of feeding polyunsaturated fatty acids with low vitamin E diet on blood levels of tocopheral in men performing hard physical labor. *Am J Clin Nutr* 1975; **28**: 706–711.

4. Scientific Committee on Food, Scientific Panel on Dietetic Products, Nutrition and Allergies. European Food Safety Authority. Tolerable Upper Intake Levels for Vitamins and Minerals. 2006. www.efsa.europa.eu/sites/default/files/efsa_rep/blobserver_assets/ndatolerableuil.pdf (accessed 31 August 2017).

5. Brouwer-Brolsma EM, Bischoff-Ferrari HA, Bouillon R, et al. Vitamin D: do we get enough? A discussion between vitamin D experts in order to make a step towards the harmonisation of dietary reference intakes for vitamin D across Europe. *Osteoporosis Int* 2013; **24**: 1567–1577.

6. Institute of Medicine of the National Academies. Dietary Reference Intakes (DRI) Reports. 2001. www.nap.edu/collection/57/dietary-reference-intakes (accessed 17 September 2017).

7. Ross AC, Taylor CL, Yaktine AL, del Valle HB, editors. Dietary Reference Intakes for Vitamin D and Calcium. Washington: National Academies Press, 2010.

8. World Health Organization. Vitamin and Mineral Requirements in Human Nutrition, 2nd edn. 2004. www.who.int/nutrition/publications/micronutrients/9241546123/en/ (accessed 31 August 2017).

9. Goode HF, Cowley HC, Walker BE, Howdle PD, Webster NR. Decreased antioxidant status and increased lipid peroxidation in patients with septic shock and secondary organ dysfunction. *Crit Care Med* 1995; **23**: 646–651.

10. Stephenson D, Alvarez JO, Kohatsu J. Vitamin A is excreted in the urine during acute infection. *Am J Clin Nutr* 1994; **60**: 388–392.

11. Schulman RC, Mechanick JI. Metabolic and nutrition support in the chronic critical illness syndrome. *Resp Care* 2012; **57**: 958–978.

12. Kowdley KV. Lipids and lipid activated vitamins in chronic cholestatic disease. *Clin Liv Dis* 1998; **2**: 373–389.

13. Vanek VW, Borum P, Buchman A, et al. ASPEN position paper: recommendations for changes in commercially available parenteral multivitamin and multi-trace element products. *Nutr Clin Pract* 2012; **27**: 440–491.

14. Mirtallo J, Canada T, Johnson D, et al. Task force for the revision of safe practices for parenteral nutrition. Safe practices for parenteral nutrition. *J Parenter Enteral Nutr* 2004; **28**: S39–S70.

15. Greene HL, Hambidge M, Schanler R, Tsang R. Guidelines for the use of vitamins, trace elements, calcium, magnesium, and phosphorus in infant and children receiving total parenteral nutrition: report of the Subcommittee on Pediatric Parenteral Nutrient Requirements from the Committee on Clinical Practice Issues of the American Society for Clinical Nutrition. *Am J Clin Nutr* 1988; **48**: 1324–1342.

16. Braga M, Ljungqvist O, Soeters P, Fearon K, Weimann A, Bozzetti F. ESPEN guidelines on PN: Surgery. *Clin Nutr* 2009; **28**: 378–386.

17. World Health Organization. Indicators for Assessing Vitamin A Deficiency and Their Application in Monitoring and Evaluating Intervention Programmes. Micronutrient Series WHO/NUT.10. Geneva: World Health Organization, 1996.

18. Field CJ, Johnson IR, Scley PD. Nutrients and their role in host resistance to infection. *J Leukoc Biol* 2002; **71**: 16–32.

19. Russell RM. The vitamin A spectrum: from deficiency to toxicity. *Am J Clin Nutr* 2000; **71**: 878–884.

20. Howard L, Chu R, Feman S, Mintz H, Ovesen L, Wolf B. Vitamin A deficiency from long-term parenteral nutrition. *Ann Intern Med* 1980; **93**: 576–577.

21. Mayo-Wilson E, Imdad A, Herzer K, Yakoob MY, Bhutta ZA. Vitamin A supplements for preventing mortality, illness and blindness in children aged under 5: systematic review and meta-analysis. *BMJ* 2011; **343**: d5094.

22. Molnar JA, Underdown MJ, Clark WA. Nutrition and chronic wounds. *Adv Wound Care* 2014; **3**: 663–681.

23. Stechmiller JK. Understanding the role of nutrition and wound healing. *Nutr Clin Pract* 2010; **25**: 61–68.

24. World Health Organization. Vitamin A Supplements: A Guide to Their Use in the Treatment and Prevention of Vitamin A Deficiency and Xerophthalmia, 2nd edn. 1997. www.who.int/nutrition/publications/micronutrients/vitamin_a_deficiency/9241545062/en/ (accessed 31 August 2017).

25. Sommer A, Davidson FR. Assessment and control of vitamin A deficiency: the Annecy Accords. *J Nutr* 2002; **132**: 2845S–2850S.

26. Feranchak AP, Gralla J, King R, et al. Comparison of indices of vitamin A status in children with chronic liver disease. *Hepatology* 2005; **42**: 782–792.

27. Sriram K, Lonchyna VA. Micronutrient supplementation in adult nutrition therapy: practical considerations. *J Parenter Enteral Nutr* 2009; **33**: 548–562.

28. Ribeiro Nogueira C, Ramalho A, Lameu E, da Silva Franca CA, David C, Accioly E. Serum concentrations of vitamin A and oxidative stress in critically ill patients with sepsis. *Nutr Hosp* 2009; **24**: 312–317.

29. Rosenberg IH, Miller JW. Nutritional factors in physical and cognitive functions of elderly people. *Am J Clin Nutr* 1992; **55**: 1237S–1243S.

30. Nierman DM, Mechanick JI. Bone hyperresorption is prevalent in chronically critically ill patients. *Chest* 1998; **114**: 1122–1128.

31. Aranow C. Vitamin D and the immune system. *J Invest Med* 2011; **59**: 881–886.

32. Quraishi SA, Camargo CA. Vitamin D in acute stress and critical illness. *Curr Opin Clin Nutr Metab Care* 2012; **15**: 625–634.

33. Balvers MGJ, Brouwer-Brolsma EM, Endenburg S, de Groot LCPGM, Kok FJ, Gunnewirk JK. Recommended intakes of vitamin D to optimise health, associated circulating 25-hydroxyvitamin D concentrations and dosing regimens to treat deficiency: workshop report and overview of current literature. *J Nutr Sci* 2015; **4**: 1–8.

34. Arnson Y, Gringauz I, Itzhaky D, Amital H. Vitamin D deficiency is associated with poor outcomes and increased mortality in severely ill patients. *QJM* 2012; **105**: 633–639.

35. Van Groningen L, Opdenoordt S, van Sorge A, et al. Cholecalciferol loading dose guideline for vitamin D deficient adults. *Eur J Endocrinol* 2010; **162**: 805–811.

36. British National Formulary 68. September 2014–March 2015. Royal Pharmaceutical Society.

37. Kumar N. Nutritional neuropathies. *Neurol Clin* 2007; **25**: 209–255.

38. Oski FA, Barness LA. Vitamin E deficiency: a previously unrecognised cause of haemolytic anaemia in the premature infant. *J Pediatr* 1967; **70**: 211–220.

39. Rojas AI, Phillips TJ. Patients with chronic leg ulcers show diminished levels of vitamins A and E, carotenes and zinc. *Dermatol Surg* 1999; **25**: 601–604.

40. Louw JA, Werbeck A, Louw ME, Kotze TJ, Cooper R, Labadarios D. Blood vitamin concentrations during the acute phase response. *Crit Care Med* 1992; **20**: 934–941.

41. Heyland DK, Dhaliwal R, Suchner U, Berger MM. Antioxidant nutrients: a systematic review of trace elements and vitamins in the critically ill patients. *Int Care Med* 2005; **31**: 327–337.

42. Manzanares WR, Dhaliwal R, Jiang X, Murch L, Heyland DK. Antioxidant micronutrients in the critically ill: a systematic review and meta-analysis. *Crit Care* 2012; **16**: R66–R78.

43. Jiang Q. Natural forms of vitamin E: metabolism, antioxidant and anti-inflammatory activities and the role in disease prevention and therapy. *Free Rad Biol Med* 2014; **72**: 76–90.

44. Feranchak AP, Sokol RJ. Medical and nutritional management of cholestasis in infants and children. In: Suchy FJ, Sokol RJ, Balistreri WF, editors. Liver Disease in Children, 3rd edn. New York: Cambridge University Press, 2007, p. 213.

45. Baines M, Shenkin A. Lack of effectiveness of short-term intravenous micronutrient nutrition in restoring plasma antioxidant status after surgery. *Clin Nutr* 2002; **21**: 145–150.

46. Singer P, Berger MM, van den Berghe G, Biolo G, Calder P, Forbes A. ESPEN guidelines on PN: Intensive care. *Clin Nutr* 2009; **28**: 387–400.

47. Wanten G, Beunk J, Naber A, Swinkels D. Tocopherol isoforms in parenteral lipid emulsions and neutrophil activation. *Clin Nutr* 2002; **21**: 417–422.

48. Miller ER, Pastor-Barriuso R, Dalal D, Riemersma RA, Appel LJ, Guallar E. Meta-analysis: high dosage vitamin E supplementation may increase all-cause mortality. *Ann Intern Med* 2005; **142**: 37–46.

Chapter 3.6

Minerals in nutrition support

Avril Collinson[1] and Paula Murphy[2]
[1]Plymouth University, Plymouth, UK
[2]Derriford Hospital, Plymouth, UK

3.6.1 Introduction

Mineral (electrolytes and trace elements) deficiencies may occur during prolonged inadequate oral intake, malabsorption or severe illness due to increased requirements or losses. Mineral requirements have been established for healthy populations but how these requirements change during illness requires further study. This chapter critically reviews the dietary recommendations for key electrolytes and trace elements, and the impact of acute illness and undernutrition on requirements.

3.6.2 Electrolytes

Sodium

There is now consensus that reducing sodium intake reduces blood pressure and cardiovascular disease risk [1], but there is still debate as to the recommended level for optimum health. Country recommendations show the variation that exists (Table 3.6.1a).

Sodium is important for the regulation of fluid balance (see Chapter 3.1) but undernutrition and disease may alter sodium handling by the kidney, resulting in variations in requirements. Plasma sodium is determined by the ratio of solutes (primarily sodium and potassium salts) to total body water. Hyponatraemia can be seen in a wide range of conditions including trauma, cachexia, adrenal insufficiency, congestive cardiac failure, nephrotic syndrome, overuse of diuretics and fluid overload. Depending on the cause, hyponatraemia can be associated with normal, low or even high extracellular fluid content. Hypernatraemia can be seen in dehydration and conditions such as diabetes insipidus and Cushing's syndrome.

Sodium intake may need to be increased where there are gastrointestinal (GI) losses, such as excessive diarrhoea, vomiting, fistulae losses and in short bowel syndrome (SBS), as well as in the polyuric phase of chronic kidney disease (CKD). Stoma patients with losses >1200 mL/day may require an oral glucose-saline solution or intravenous (IV) sodium supplementation [2]. Sodium may need to be decreased in the oliguric/anuric phase of CKD, hypertension and cardiac failure, liver disease and oedematous patients.

Potassium

There is some variation in the recommended potassium requirements for healthy individuals (see Table 3.6.1a). Variation may be due to the limited evidence available that determines the precise level of potassium that will result in maximum health benefits. One systematic review found that an increased potassium intake via diet or supplementation (aiming for 3510–4690 mg/day) reduces blood pressure in individuals with hypertension [3].

Advanced Nutrition and Dietetics in Nutrition Support, First Edition. Edited by Mary Hickson and Sara Smith.
© 2018 John Wiley & Sons Ltd. Published 2018 by John Wiley & Sons Ltd.

Table 3.6.1a Daily oral or enteral requirements for electrolytes in healthy adults

	UK (RNI) 1991 [42] 19– >70 years	US (RDA) 1997–2011 [45] 19– >70 years	FAO/WHO 2004–2012 [46–48] 19– >70 years	SCF/EFSA 1993–2016 [49,50] >18 years	Australia (RDI) 2006 [51] 19– >50 years
Sodium	1600 mg	(19–50 years) 1500 mg (51–70 years) 1300 mg >70 years 1200 mg	<2000 mg* (WHO, 2012)	575–3500 mg Acceptable range (SCF, 1993)	460–920 mg (AI)
Potassium	3500 mg	4700 mg (AI)	No values >3510 mg* (WHO, 2012)	3500 mg (AI) (EFSA, 2016)	2800 mg (f) (AI) 3800 mg (m)
Calcium	(19–50 years) 700 mg (>50 years) 700 mg	(19–50 years) 1000 mg (>50 years) 1200 mg	(19–50 years) 1000 mg (>50 years) 1300 mg (f) (>65 years) 1300 mg (m)	>25 years 950 mg PRI (EFSA, 2015)	(19–50 years) 1000 mg (f) (19–70 years) 1000 mg (m) (>50 years) 1300 mg (f) (>70 years) 1300 mg (m)
Phosphorus	550 mg	700 mg	No values	550 mg (AI) (EFSA, 2015)	1000 mg
Magnesium	(19–50 years) 270 mg (f) 300 mg (m) (>50 years) 270 mg (f) 300 mg (m)	(19–30 years) 310 mg (f) 400 mg (m) (>30 years) 320 mg (f) 420 mg (m)	(19–65 years) 220 mg (f) 260 mg (m) (>65 years) 190 mg (f) 230 mg (m)	300 mg (f) 350 mg (m) (AI) (EFSA, 2015)	(19–30 years) 310 mg (f) 400 mg (m) (31– >70 years) 320 mg (f) 420 mg (m)

AI, adequate intake; f, female; m, male.

* Conditional recommendation – the guideline development group concluded that the desirable effects probably outweigh the undesirable effects.

Serum potassium is normally tightly regulated by the kidneys. Hyperkalaemia can occur due to an increased intake alongside renal impairment, a shift of potassium out of cells to the extracellular fluid or decreased excretion. Hyperkalaemia may also occur as a side effect of medications, such as potassium-sparing diuretics. If hyperkalaemia is severe (>7 mmol/L), it may cause cardiac arrhythmias and cardiac arrest. Evidence-based practice guidelines have been written for the dietetic management of hyperkalaemia in CKD patients [4,5]. Novel potassium-binding polymers are currently being tested to evaluate their long-term safety and efficacy in the management of hyperkalaemia [6].

Hypokalaemia can be caused by increased GI losses, via diarrhoea, vomiting, a shift of potassium into the intracellular compartment (e.g. insulin treatment for diabetic ketoacidosis), extrarenal potassium losses or certain medications (e.g. diuretics). If hypokalaemia is persistent, concurrent hypomagnesaemia should be sought as renal and GI potassium losses are higher in patients with magnesium depletion. Hypokalaemia can be corrected orally (e.g. Sando K) or intravenously.

Calcium

Calcium is the major component of hydroxyapatite, the predominant mineral in bone and teeth, and is essential to many fundamental processes in the body, such as muscle contraction and blood coagulation. Estimated calcium requirements for healthy individuals are shown in Table 3.6.1a. Variation is evident between countries due to different interpretations of human calcium balance data, since there are no reliable biochemical indicators to accurately assess calcium status. Plasma calcium is tightly regulated through complex physiological systems, such as parathyroid hormone (PTH), 1,25-dihydroxycholecalciferol (vitamin D) and calcitonin. Plasma concentrations may not accurately reflect total body calcium. Plasma calcium is bound to proteins, primarily albumin, so measurements are usually reported as 'adjusted calcium' if albumin is below the normal range.

Hypercalcaemia can be caused by a number of conditions, including malignancy, CKD and hyperparathyroidism. Treatment is aimed at addressing the cause of the hypercalcaemia. Hypocalcaemia may occur due to hypoparathyroidism or hypomagnesemia, which reduces the activity of PTH. CKD patients may experience hypocalcaemia due to a defect in the renal synthesis of active vitamin D, which is managed with active vitamin D analogues and calcium-containing phosphate binders [7]. Absorption of calcium may be impaired in individuals with fat malabsorption due to lack of vitamin D. Patients with malabsorption syndromes, for example, liver disease, coeliac disease, cystic fibrosis and those who have undergone bariatric surgery, are at risk of metabolic bone disease and have higher calcium requirements (8–12). There is little evidence on the efficacy of calcium supplementation and long-term clinical trials of both calcium and vitamin D supplements in these patients are warranted.

Some concerns have been raised with calcium supplementation and an increased risk of cardiovascular disease (CVD) [13,14], although these findings have not been supported by others [15,16]. An increased risk of developing type 2 diabetes has been reported in individuals at high cardiovascular risk with an increase in albumin-adjusted serum calcium concentrations [17]. Further research is needed to fully understand any potential risks, whilst clinical practice needs to balance the potential benefits for bone health with any adverse effects on cardiovascular risk.

Metabolic bone disease is a common complication in patients on home parenteral nutrition (HPN) although the specific impact of HPN on bone health is a matter of debate [18]. Bone mineral density assessment by dual-energy x-ray absorptiometry (DEXA) scanning is recommended on commencing HPN and 2 yearly thereafter [19].

Phosphorus

Phosphorus provides structure to bones and is required for biochemical processes, including energy production and pH regulation. Recommended daily requirements for phosphorus vary between 550 and 1000 mg/day (see Table 3.6.1a). Serum concentrations are regulated by PTH and vitamin D.

Hyperphosphataemia, which can occur in CKD, hypoparathyroidism and cell damage, may result in calcium phosphate deposition in soft tissues. Evidence-based practice guidelines have been written for the dietetic management of hyperphosphataemia in CKD patients [2,3]. Often dietary phosphorus restriction is not sufficient to manage hyperphosphataemia in these patients and phosphate binders are required.

Hypophospataemia can occur in hyperparathyroidism, refeeding syndrome, alcohol withdrawal and some genetic conditions (e.g. Fanconi's syndrome). Hypophosphatemia can be corrected orally (e.g. Phosphate Sandoz) or intravenously.

Magnesium

Magnesium is a cofactor for many enzyme systems. It is absorbed predominantly from the distal jejunum and ileum and excreted via the kidneys. Magnesium requirements can be seen in Table 3.6.1a. Some authors have questioned these recommendations and suggest a lower intake of 165 mg/day for healthy individuals regardless of age or gender [20].

Hypomagnesaemia can result from excessive losses (e.g. diarrhoea, vomiting, laxative abuse) and malabsorption syndromes (e.g. short bowel syndrome). A high incidence of magnesium deficiency (20–52%) has been found in critical illness and this is associated with a higher mortality rate [21]. Older people and those with type 2 diabetes are at higher risk of magnesium deficiency due to a decreased intake, reduced absorption and increased renal excretion [22]. A significant inverse association has been found between magnesium intake and diabetes risk [23]. Similarly, alcoholics are at an increased risk of hypomagnesaemia due to the diuretic action of alcohol coupled with a decreased intake [24]. Deficiency can lead to cardiac arrhythmias and disturb calcium homeostasis, leading to hypocalcaemia. This can be corrected with oral magnesium (e.g. MgO) or intravenously.

Hypermagnesaemia can be caused by conditions such as CKD and excessive ingestion of magnesium salts.

3.6.3 Trace elements

Zinc

Zinc is important for a healthy immune system, growth and wound healing. The daily oral requirement for zinc ranges from 3.0 to 16.3 mg/day (Table 3.6.1b). The range is wide as the World Health Organization (WHO) based zinc requirements in health on dietary zinc bioavailability and absorption efficiency.

Zinc requirements in disease states may be wide ranging due to the significant variation in GI or cutaneous losses in various clinical situations. Zinc deficiency is a major health problem in the developing world where zinc supplementation has been found to reduce the incidence and severity of diarrhoea in children [25]. Deficiency is known to cause a characteristic rash, poor wound healing and hair loss. Oral replacement will reverse the signs of deficiency within weeks. Zinc is an ingredient in many topical products to treat skin conditions but few studies support its use for accelerating would healing. A meta-analysis of 181 patients from six randomised controlled trials of oral zinc sulfate compared with a placebo for leg ulcers found no significant difference in time to ulcer resolution [26]. Despite its many essential roles in the body, few studies support supplementation in patients with normal zinc status.

Zinc toxicity is rare. Prolonged exposure to amounts greater than 40 mg/day (tolerable upper intake level) may suppress immunity, decrease HDL cholesterol concentrations and cause hypochromic microcytic anaemia and copper deficiency [27].

In stable patients receiving parenteral nutrition (PN), 2.5–6.5 mg is recommended (Table 3.6.2). Zinc content of available trace element additives in the UK and United States is outlined in Table 3.6.3. However, patients with high GI losses such as those with short bowel syndrome or high-output GI fistulae dependent on PN may require more.

Table 3.6.1b Daily oral or enteral requirements for trace elements in healthy adults

	UK (RNI) 1991 [42] 19–>70 years	US (RDA) 1997–2011 [45] 19–>70 years	FAO/WHO 2004–2012 [46–48] 19–>70 years	EFSA 2013–2015 [52] >18 years	Australia (RDI) 2006 [51] 19–>50 years
Zinc	7 mg (f) 9.5 mg (m)	8 mg (f) 11 mg (m)	3.0–9.8 mg (f) 4.2–14 mg (m)*	7.5–12.7 mg (f) 9.4–16.3 mg (m) (PRI) (EFSA, 2014)	8 mg (f) 14 mg (m)
Copper	1.2 mg	0.9 mg	N/A	1.3 mg (f) (AI) 1.6 mg (m) (EFSA, 2015)	1.2 mg (f) (AI) 1.7 mg (m)
Selenium	60 µg (f) 75 µg (m)	55 µg	19–65 years 26 µg (f) 34 µg (m) >65 years 26 µg (f) 34 µg (m)	70 µg (AI) (EFSA, 2014)	60 µg (f) 70 µg (m)
Manganese	No RNI SI above 1.4 mg	No RDA 1.8 mg (f) 2.3 mg (m) (AI)	N/A	3 mg (AI) (EFSA, 2013)	5 mg (f) (AI) 5.5 mg (m)
Chromium	No RNI SI >25 µg	No RDA (19–50 years) 25 µg (f) 35 µg (m) >50 years 20 µg (f) 30 µg (m) (AI)	N/A	No RDA	25 µg (f) (AI) 35 µg (m)
Molybdenum	No RNI SI 50–400 µg	45 µg	N/A	65 µg (AI) (EFSA, 2013)	45 µg
Iron	(19–50 years) 14.8 mg (f) 8.7 mg (m) (>50 years) 8.7 mg	(19–50 years) 18 mg (f) 8 mg (m) (>50 years) 8 mg	(19–50 years) 20–59 mg (f) 9–27 mg (m) (>50 years) 8–23 mg (f) 8–11 mg (m)*	16 mg (f premenopausal) 11 mg (f postmenopausal) 11 mg (m) (PRI) (EFSA, 2015)	(19–50 years) 18 mg (f) 8 mg (m) (>50 years) 8 mg (EFSA, 2015)
Iodine	140 µg	150 µg	110 µg (f) 130 µg (m)	150 µg (AI) (EFSA, 2014)	150 µg

AI, adequate intake; AR, average requirement; f, female; m, male; PRI, population reference intake; SI, safe intake.
* Range dependent on the Zn or Fe bioavailability of the diet.

Table 3.6.2 Recommended Adult Daily Parenteral Trace Element Requirements

	UK [52]	US [38]	Australia [39]
Zinc	3.2–6.5 mg	2.5–5 mg	3.2–6.5 mg
Copper	0.3–1.3 mg	0.3–0.5 mg	0.317–0.508 mg
Selenium	30–60 µg	20–60 µg	60–100 µg
Manganese	0.2–0.3 mg	0.06–0.1 mg	0.055 mg
Chromium	10–20 µg	10–15 µg	10–15 µg*
Molybdenum	19 µg	–†	19 µg§
Iron	1.2 mg	–†	1.1 mg*
Iodine	131 µg	–†	131 µg

* May not be necessary.
† Not routinely added in US.
§ Probably not necessary.

Table 3.6.3 Trace element content of selected IV trace element solutions

	UK (Additrace FK/10 mL)	UK (Nutryelt Baxter/10 mL)	US Multitrace 5 Concentrate – American Reagent/mL
Zinc	6.5 mg	10 mg	5 mg
Copper	1.3 mg	0.3 mg	1 mg
Selenium	32 µg	70 µg	60 µg
Manganese	0.27 mg	0.055 mg	0.5 mg
Chromium	10 µg	10 µg	10 µg
Molybdenum	19 µg	20 µg	–
Iron	1.1 mg	1.0 mg	–
Iodine	130 µg	130 µg	–

Iron

Daily requirements for iron vary widely depending on gender and age (see Table 3.6.1b). In iron deficiency, there is insufficient iron to maintain the normal physiological function of tissues, with prolonged deficiency leading to iron deficiency anaemia (IDA). Anaemia of chronic disease is due to inflammation and chronic immune activation. IDA is common in young children and women of child-bearing age and in many disease states. Haemoglobin concentrations can be used to assess the severity of IDA and response to oral iron supplementation can confirm IDA [28]. Transferrin saturation and serum ferritin values can help determine the presence of IDA. It is important to remember that iron status is influenced by the acute phase response, resulting in an increase in serum ferritin. Reasons for anaemia include malabsorption of iron (e.g. coeliac disease, Crohn's disease); chronic inflammation (e.g. obesity, cardiovascular disease); loss of blood (e.g. ulcerative colitis, ulcers, surgery); inadequate dietary intake (e.g. cancer cachexia); or high intake of absorption inhibitors.

The risk of anaemia is already high in obesity due to low-grade inflammation inducing hepcidin synthesis and subsequent decrease in iron absorption [29]; this is further exacerbated following malabsorptive procedures such as bariatric surgery [30]. A high incidence of anaemia is found in critical care patients, with 20–30% having moderate to severe anaemia [31]. IDA is also a common problem in CKD due to a reduction in erythropoietin production. Treatment includes erythropoiesis-stimulating agents with the addition of intravenous iron [32].

Treatment for IDA includes managing the underlying disease, so iron requirements are not suggested to be higher than normal recommendations although dietary counselling and/or supplementation may be required to increase concentrations. Concern has been expressed regarding excessive iron supplementation, as this can lead to GI side effects. A tolerable upper intake level has been set at 45 mg/day for adults >19 years [33]. In patients with genetic haemochromatosis, a condition which causes the body to absorb too much iron, avoidance of vitamin C and iron supplements is necessary [34].

Currently, there are no well-defined recommendations regarding the optimum level of iron in PN. Continued monitoring of iron status is recommended as both chronic iron overload and IDA can occur in patients on long-term PN.

Copper

Adult oral requirements for copper range from 0.9 mg/day to 1.7 mg/day (see Table 3.6.1b). There is substantial evidence that an optimal level of copper is required to maintain antioxidant defence and wound healing. Higher doses of copper are required in patients with excessive GI losses. Copper deficiency is rare but has been reported in adults following intestinal resection and bypass surgery. Other causes of deficiency include failure to supplement appropriately in patients on long-term PN andinappropriate zinc supplementation, as a high zinc intake will block the intestinal absorption of copper. Initial clinical signs are neutropenia and hypochromic microcytic anaemia that are unresponsive to iron supplementation.

Acute toxicity is rare but excess copper may cause harmful effects and has been reported in long-term PN patients in the presence of cholestasis. Approximately 80% of parenterally administered copper is excreted in bile, consequently it can accumulate in the liver in patients with impaired biliary excretion or cholestatic liver disease. Chronic toxicity is illustrated in Wilson's disease, a genetic disorder of copper

metabolism resulting in liver damage. Copper may be measured in plasma but results may be confounded by the acute phase response which increases caeruloplasmin synthesis. More than 90% of circulating copper is bound to caeruloplasmin. Changes in acute phase proteins are a direct response to infection, so care should be taken when assessing copper status while an inflammatory response is ongoing. Levels of C-reactive protein concentrations should be measured concurrently with copper concentrations to provide a context for interpreting the presence of acute phase response. Low plasma concentrations, on the other hand, can be considered a reliable measure of deficiency.

Guidelines for copper supplementation in PN initially produced by the American Medical Association (AMA) expert committee in 1979 [35] were revised in 2012 following the findings of balance studies where 0.3–0.5 mg/day was found to be the optimal copper dose [36] (see Table 3.6.2). A lower dose is recommended for patients with liver disease (e.g. 0.15 mg/day) and a higher amount (e.g. 0.4–0.5 mg/day) for patients with prolonged high GI fluid losses and burns patients. The commonly used trace element preparation in the UK (Additrace FK) contains 1.3 mg copper. This may be excessive for patients receiving long-term PN. The American Society for Parenteral and Enteral Nutrition (ASPEN) has made recommendations for changes to currently available US trace element products, including reduced daily dose of copper, based on excessive organ accumulation in patients who had received long-term PN [36].

Selenium

Selenium functions in the body as an antioxidant, in thyroid hormone metabolism, redox reactions, reproduction and immune function. Deficiency is rare but is seen in Keshan and Kashin–Beck's diseases involving the degeneration of organs and tissues. Recommended intakes of selenium have been calculated from the requirement for optimum plasma glutathione peroxidase activity, but it is unclear whether optimal health depends on maximisation of this enzyme. Possible benefits of higher intakes include protection against certain cancers, viral protection and immune function and CVD. Evidence for these benefits is inconclusive and consequently higher levels of intake have not been recommended when setting international recommended dietary intakes (RDIs). Selenium is toxic and intakes of 1500 μg/day or greater have been associated with abnormal signs.

Recommended oral intake ranges from 26 to 75 μg/day (see Table 3.6.1b). Selenium concentrations have been found to be lower in patients undergoing long-term haemodialysis, due in part to the removal of selenium from the blood. Restrictive diets and anorexia associated with uraemia and renal disease also contribute. Similarly, selenium has been found to be low in HIV due to inadequate intakes and excessive losses in diarrhoea and malabsorption. Patients with inflammatory bowel disease, GI fistulae or other intestinal disorders and patients following small bowel resection are likely to be depleted in selenium due to poor absorption but increased losses and low selenium intake may also contribute. Additional selenium is likely to be required in these cases. There is consensus that selenium should be routinely added to all PN formulas but there is ongoing debate about requirements. ASPEN increased the standard recommendation in adults to 60–100 μg/day in 2012 [36]. This is less than the currently available trace element additives (see Table 3.6.3) and is reflected in numerous reports of selenium deficiency in HPN patients.

Manganese

Manganese is associated with many enzymes and is an essential nutrient, yet no overt symptoms of manganese deficiency have been reported. In fact, toxicity is a greater concern than deficiency. RDAs have not been set by international organizations. Historically, it is recognised as a contaminant of PN solutions. The parenteral trace element additive widely used in the UK delivers 5 μmol (Additrace FK) yet normal manganese concentrations have been demonstrated to be maintained with supplementation of 1 μmol/day [37]. Because, like copper, a high proportion (90%) is excreted in bile, care should be taken when supplementing patients with cholestatic liver disease. Manganese deposits in the basal ganglia causing neurological toxicity have been shown on magnetic resonance imaging of home PN patients with elevated manganese concentrations [38].

Chromium

Dietary bioavailability of chromium is very low (0.4–2.5%). Absorption is in the small bowel but almost all chromium ingested is rapidly excreted in urine. Nonetheless, it is an essential trace metal, deficiency causing glucose intolerance. No recommended dietary intakes have been set worldwide, instead safe or adequate levels are outlined (see Table 3.6.1b). There have been no reports of chromium toxicity in adults [39]. Ingested trivalent chromium, the biologically active form, has a low level of toxicity due in part to its low level of absorption but when delivered by the parenteral route it may have a higher potential toxicity [40].

Chromium is not routinely monitored in patients due to the absence of reliable methods to assess status. Concentrations are reduced in acute illness which may contribute to the altered glucose metabolism characteristic of acute infection. Parenteral requirement ranges from 10 to 20 μg (see Table 3.6.2). If the absorption of oral chromium is 0.4–2.5%, then absorbed chromium from a standard adult oral diet is 0.1–0.9 μg/day, 10–100 times less than the recommended parenteral chromium. As chromium is excreted in the urine, patients with renal failure may be at risk of chromium toxicity and therefore may require restriction of parenteral chromium intake but there is no clear evidence to support this practice.

Trivalent chromium has been reported to be present as a significant contaminant in PN solutions, primarily from amino acid solutions and phosphate salts. Lipids may also contribute. PN solutions have been reported to contain contaminant chromium in amounts of 2.6–10.5 μg for a high-lipid formula, and 2.4–8.1 μg/day in a high-glucose formula [40]. The amount varies widely between manufacturers and between batches from the same manufacturer. Because of contaminant chromium, daily addition of chromium in PN might not be needed, but is still recommended until there is more evidence that contaminant amounts consistently meet requirements. Currently available trace element additives in the UK and US deliver 10 µg (see Table 3.6.3).

Additional studies are needed to determine how much chromium, if any, should be supplemented in PN and the effect of disease on chromium requirements.

Molybdenum

Molybdenum functions as a cofactor for a limited number of enzymes. RDA in the US is 45 µg/day (see Table 3.6.1b). No reference nutrient intake (RNI) has been set in the UK as mean dietary intakes far exceed the amount needed to avoid functional defects. Instead, a safe intake of between 50 and 400 µg/day has been suggested. Molybdenum has a low level of toxicity. One case of deficiency has been reported in a patient receiving PN (none in the diet) [41].

Molybdenum is thought to be a contaminant of PN solutions and is not added to trace element additive solutions in the US but continues to be included in the UK (see Table 3.6.3). The last published investigation into molybdenum contamination occurred over 30 years ago and the levels obtained cannot be generalised to the present time due to changes in packaging in the ensuing years [41]. In recent years, there has been a widespread change from glass to plastic containers and to needleless systems. Plastic is much less likely to contribute to trace element contamination than glass. Research is required to establish the impact of these changes in clinical practice. It is not routinely monitored due to the limitations of biochemical markers of molybdenum status. It is possible that supplementation may be necessary only for long-term PN patients as there are no significant data to warrant routine molybdenum supplementation in PN formulas.

Iodine

Iodine is an integral part of the thyroid hormones, thyroxine and tri-iodothyronine. Deficiency,

leading to thyroid enlargement and goitre development, is prevented in adults by daily oral intake of approximately 70 µg iodine (UK lower RNI). Oral requirements are outlined in Table 3.6.1b. The effects of disease on requirements is not known. Iodine is included in PN trace element additive solutions in the UK but it is not routinely supplemented in PN in the US, where parenteral requirements have not been established. Iodine deficiency would be expected to produce symptoms of hypothyroidism and has not been reported in adult PN patients. It is possible that PN contamination provides adequate levels to meet basal requirements.

3.6.4 Other trace elements

The human body also contains several other elements including silicon, boron, nickel, vanadium, arsenic and tin. Deficiency diseases for some of these have been described in animals but there is no firm evidence that any is essential for health in humans. RDAs have not been determined, due to a lack of sufficient data at the current time.

3.6.5 Mineral requirements for enteral and parenteral nutrition

Enteral nutrition

Micronutrients are routinely added to oral nutrition supplements and enteral formulas and trace metal intake can be easily established depending on daily formula volume. Enteral formulas are 'complete', that is, they meet or exceed the RNI in a range of volumes. However, this does not include the minerals sodium, potassium, chloride and in some cases magnesium also, due to the need to maintain acceptable osmolarity. This can affect some groups of patients (such as the elderly) in whom sodium and fluid homeostasis is depressed and low sodium intake could lead to depletion.

In many countries, micronutrient requirements are calculated using standard weights for different age groups in each gender [42]; consequently, enterally fed patients weighing significantly more may need their mineral intake adjusted accordingly to meet their needs. Mineral toxicity is unlikely as all formulas provide minerals below safe maximum intake levels. Monitoring micronutrient status in patients requiring long-term enteral nutrition is not routinely required, unless there are symptoms of deficiency or toxicity. These tests can be costly so sound clinical judgement is required.

Current practice is opinion based due to the lack of good-quality evidence in this area. Further research is needed to establish the micronutrient status of long-term enterally fed patients, to determine the bioavailability of trace metals in formulas and also the status of patients fed into the jejunum compared to the gastric route; there is some evidence that prolonged jejunal feeding may lead to iron and copper deficiency [43,44].

Parenteral nutrition

The intravenous administration of trace elements poses a risk of toxicity as the regulatory absorptive mechanism of the GI tract is bypassed and excretion may not be increased. The standard dosing ranges for electrolytes assume normal organ function without abnormal losses, so doses must be adjusted as clinically appropriate. The recommended adult daily parenteral trace element requirements and trace element content of selected intravenous solutions can be seen in Tables 3.6.2 and 3.6.3. Requirements for parenteral trace elements will vary among patients and further supplements may be appropriate in certain circumstances. For example, pancreatic fistula fluids have a high content of zinc, and biliary fistula fluid is rich in copper and manganese, resulting in increased losses and a need to provide additional supplementation. In other circumstances, there is a risk of toxicity, such as renal dysfunction, when selenium, molybdenum and chromium dose may need to be lowered to allow for reduced excretion. Supplementation with some metals, such as molybdenum and iodine, may be needed only for long-term PN and the impact of their use in trace element additives requires further study.

Mineral monitoring in acute illness

Serum electrolyte concentrations (Na, K, Ca, Mg, P) should be determined in acute illness and undernutrition and intake adjusted according to the results of regular laboratory analyses. However, plasma concentrations of many trace metals are influenced by the acute phase response and consequently concentrations fall or rise in trauma, infection and stress. Hence measurements taken in acutely ill patients should be interpreted with caution as they may not represent true deficiency, just redistribution which may be a beneficial adaptive response. When supplementation is considered necessary, serum concentrations should be checked to avoid toxicity, particularly in liver and renal insufficiency, intestinal fistulae, burns or patients receiving long-term PN.

References

1. Institute of Medicine. Sodium Intake in Populations: Assessment of Evidence. Washington: National Academies Press, 2013.
2. Nightingale JMD, Lennard-Jones JE, Walker ER, Farthing MJ. Oral salt supplements to compensate for jejunostomy losses: comparison of sodium chloride capsules, glucose electrolyte solution and glucose polymer electrolyte solution. *Gut* 1992; **33**:759–761.
3. Aburto, NJ, Hanson S, Gutierrez, H, et al. Effect of increased potassium intake on cardiovascular risk factors and disease: systematic review and meta-analyses. *BMJ* 2013; **346**: f1378.
4. EDTNA/ERCA. European guidelines for the nutritional care of adult renal patients. *Eur Dial Transplant Nurses Assoc/Eur Ren Care Assoc J* 2003; **29**: S1–S23.
5. Ash S, Campbell K, MacLaughlin H, et al. Evidence based practice guidelines for the nutritional management of chronic kidney disease. *Nutr Dietet* 2006; **63**(2): S33–S45.
6. Slomski A. Hyperkalemia controlled with 2 novel medications. *JAMA* 2015; **313**(4): 347.
7. National Kidney Foundation. KDOQI clinical practice guidelines for bone metabolism and disease in chronic kidney disease. *Am J Kidney Dis* 2003; **42**(Suppl 3): S1–S201.
8. Collier JD, Ninkovic M, Compston JE. Guidelines on the management of osteoporosis associated with chronic liver disease. *Gut* 2002; **50**(Suppl 1): i1–i9.
9. Ludvigsson JF, Bai JC, Biagi F, et al. Diagnosis and management of adult coeliac disease: guidelines from the British Society of Gastroenterology. *Gut* 2014; **63**(8): 1210–1228.

10. Fok J, Brown NE, Zuberbuhler P, Tabak J, Tom M. Low bone mineral density in cystic fibrosis patients. *Can J Diet Pract Res* 2002; **63**(4): 192–197.

11. Schulze KJ, O'Brien KO, Germain-Lee EL, Baer DJ, Leonard A, Rosenstein BJ. Efficiency of calcium absorption is not compromised in clinically stable prepubertal and pubertal girls with cystic fibrosis. *Am J Clin Nutr* 2003; **78**(1): 110–116.

12. Mechanick JI, Youdim A, Jones DB, et al. Clinical practice guidelines for the perioperative nutritional, metabolic, and nonsurgical support of the bariatric surgery patient – 2013 update cosponsored by American Association of Clinical Endocrinologists, The Obesity Society, and American Society for Metabolic & Bariatric Surgery. *Obesity* 2013; **21**(01): S1–S27.

13. Michaelsson K, Melhus H, Warensjo Lemming E, Wolk, A, Byberg L. Long term calcium intake and rates of all cause and cardiovascular mortality: community based prospective longitudinal cohort study. *BMJ* 2013; **346**: f228.

14. Xiao Q, Murphy RA, Houston DK, Harris TB, Chow WH, Park Y. Dietary and supplemental calcium intakes in relation to mortality from cardiovascular diseases in the NIH-AARP Diet and Health Study. *JAMA Intern Med* 2013; **173**(8): 639–646.

15. Nordin BEC, Lewis JR, Daly RM, et al. The calcium scare – what would Austin Bradford Hill have thought? *Osteoporos Int* 2011; **22**(12): 3073–3077.

16. Paik JM, Curhan GC, Sun Q, et al. Calcium supplement intake and risk of cardiovascular disease in women. *Osteoporos Int* 2014; **25**(8): 2047–2056.

17. Becerra-Tomas, N, Estruch R, Bull M, et al. Increased serum calcium levels and risk of type 2 diabetes in individuals at high cardiovascular risk. *Diabetes Care* 2014; **37**(11): 3084–3091.

18. Cohen-Solal M, Baudoin C, Joly F, et al. Osteoporosis in patients on long-term home parenteral nutrition: a longitudinal study. *J Bone Miner Res* 2003; **18**: 1989–1994.

19. National Institute for Clinical Excellence. Nutrition Support in Adults: Oral Nutrition Support, Enteral Tube Feeding and Parenteral Nutrition. NICE Clinical Guideline 32. London: NICE, 2006.

20. Hunt CD, Johnson LK. Magnesium requirements: new estimations for men and women by cross-sectional statistical analyses of metabolic magnesium balance data. *Am J Clin Nutr* 2006; **84**(4): 843–852.

21. Moskowitz A, Lee J, Donnino MW, Mark R, Celi LA, Danziger J. The association between admission magnesium concentrations and lactic acidosis in critical illness. *J Intens Care Med* 2016; **31**(3): 187–192.

22. Barbagallo M, Dominguez, LJ. Magnesium metabolism in type 2 diabetes mellitus, metabolic syndrome and insulin resistance. *Arch Biochem Biophys* 2007; **458**: 40–47.

23. Kim DJ, Xun P, Liu K, et al. Magnesium intake in relation to systemic inflammation, insulin resistance, and the incidence of diabetes. *Diabetes Care* 2010; **33**(12): 2604–2610.

24. Rivlin RS. Magnesium deficiency and alcohol intake: mechanisms, clinical significance and possible relation to cancer development (a review). *J Am Coll Nutr* 1994; **13**(5): 416–423.

25. Aggarwal R, Sentz J, Miller MA. Role of zinc administration in prevention of childhood diarrhoea and respiratory illnesses: a meta-analysis. *Pediatrics* 2007; **119**(6): 1120–1130.

26. Wilkinson EA, Hawke Cl. Does oral zinc aid the healing of chronic leg ulcers? A systematic literature review. *Arch Dermatol* 1998; **123**(12): 1556–1560.

27. Saper RB, Rash R. Zinc: an essential micronutrient. *Am Fam Physician* 2009; **79**(9): 768–772.

28. World Health Organization. Iron Deficiency Anaemia: Assessment, Prevention and Control: A Guide for Programme Managers. Geneva: World Health Organization, 2001.

29. Cepeda-Lopez AC, Aeberli I, Zimmermann MB. Does obesity increase risk for iron deficiency? A review of the literature and the potential mechanisms. *Int J Vitam Nutr Res* 2010; **80**: 263–270.

30. Weng TC, Chang CH, Dong YH, Chang YC, Chuang LM. Anaemia and related nutrient deficiencies after Roux-en-Y gastric bypass surgery: a systematic review and meta-analysis. *BMJ Open* 2015; **5**: e006964.

31. Walsh TS, Saleh ELD. Anaemia during critical illness. *Br J Anaesth* 2006; **97**(3): 278291.

32. National Kidney Foundation. KDOQI clinical practice guideline and clinical practice recommendations for anemia in chronic kidney disease: 2007 update of hemoglobin target. *Am J Kidney Dis* 2007; **50**: 471–530.

33. Institute of Medicine, Food and Nutrition Board. Dietary Reference Intakes for Vitamin A, Vitamin K, Arsenic, Boron, Chromium, Copper, Iodine, Iron, Manganese, Molybdenum, Nickel, Silicon, Vanadium and Zinc: A Report of the Panel on Micronutrients. Washington: National Academy Press, 2001.

34. Bacon B, Adams PC, Kowdley KV, Powell LW, Tavill AS. Iron diagnosis and management of hemochromatosis: practice guideline by the American Association for the Study of Liver Diseases. *Hepatology* 2011; **54**(1): 328–343.

35. [No authors listed] Guidelines for essential trace element preparations for parenteral use. *JAMA* 1979; **24**: 2051–2054.

36. Vanek VW, Borum P, Buchman A, et al. ASPEN position paper: recommendations for changes in commercially available parenteral multivitamin and multi trace element products. *Nutr Clin Pract* 2012; **27**(4): 440–491.

37. Takagi Y, Okada A, Sando K, Wasa M, Yoshida H, Hirabuki N. Evaluation of indices of in vivo manganese status and the optimal intravenous dose for adult patients undergoing home parenteral nutrition. *Am J Clin Nutr* 2002; **75**: 112–118.

38. Btaiche IF, Carver PL,Welsh KB. Dosing and monitoring of long term trace elements in long term home parenteral nutrition patients. *J Parenter Enteral Nutr* 2011; **35**: 736–747.

39. Osland EJ, Ali A, Isenring E, Ball P, Davis M, Gillanders L. Australasian Society for Parenteral and Enteral Nutrition guidelines for supplementation of trace elements during parenteral nutrition. *Asia Pacific J Clin Nutr* 2014; **23**(4): 545–554.

40. Moukarzel A. Chromium in parenteral nutrition: too little or too much? *Gastroenterology* 2009; **137**: S18–S28.

41. Abumrad NN, Schneider AJ, Steel D, Rogers LS. Amino acid intolerance during prolonged total parenteral nutrition reversed by molybdate therapy. *Am J Clin Nutr* 1981; **34**(11): 2551–2559.

42. Department of Health. Report 41: Dietary Reference Values for Food Energy and Nutrients for the United Kingdom. London: HMSO,1991.

43. Baxter YC, Goncalves Dias MC, Maculevicius J, et al. Iron deficiency anaemia in enteral nutrition, correlation with tube position. *Rev Hosp Clin Fac Med Sao Paulo* 1995; **50**(6): 330–333.

44. Nishwaki S, Iwashita M, Goto N, et al. Predominant copper deficiency during prolonged enteral nutrition through a jejunal tube compared to that through a gastrostomy tube. *Clin Nutr* 2011; **30**(5): 585–589.

45. Food and Nutritional Information Centre, National Agricultural Library. Dietary Reference Intakes. https://fnic.nal.usda.gov/dietary-guidance/dietary-reference-intakes (accessed 31 August 2017).

46. World Health Organization, Food and Agricultural Organization of the United Nations. Vitamin and Mineral Requirements in Human Nutrition, 2nd edn. Geneva: World Health Organization, 2004.

47. World Health Organization. Guideline: Potassium Intake for Adults and Children. Geneva: World Health Organization, 2012.

48. World Health Organization. Guideline: Sodium Intake for Adults and Children. Geneva: World Health Organization, 2012.

49. Scientific Committee on Food. Reports of the Scientific Committee on Food (31st series). Luxembourg: Commission of the European Community, 1993.

50. European Food Safety Authority. European Dietary Reference Values. www.efsa.europa.eu/sites/default/files/assets/DRV_Summary_tables_jan_17.pdf (accessed 15 September 2017).

51. National Health and Medical Research Council. Nutrient Reference Values for Australia and New Zealand including recommended dietary intakes. Canberra: NHMRC, 2006.

52. Shenkin A. Trace elements and vitamins in adult intravenous nutrition. In: Rombeau JL and Rolandeli RH, eds. Clinical Nutrition: Parenteral Nutrition. Philadelphia: W.B. Saunders, 2001, pp. 60–79.

SECTION 4

Nutritional interventions to prevent and treat undernutrition

Chapter 4.1

Population and community interventions to prevent and treat undernutrition

Lisa Wilson
Twickenham, Middlesex, UK

4.1.1 Introduction

However undernutrition is screened, diagnosed, treated or managed, it often begins and ends in the community. This is where people live their lives, make their food choices and eat their food. It is also often where nutritional status becomes compromised as a result of ill health, poor access to food, physical or mental health problems, low income, or long-term conditions which compromise health or a change in life circumstances affecting appetite, interest and diet.

Screening is a proven effective method of detecting patients who are at risk of undernutrition; the challenge for healthcare professionals is how to address what screening inevitably finds. In clinical settings, the picture is slightly clearer due to the relatively well-defined pathways of care indicating referral and management guidelines for inpatient undernutrition [1], but once a patient is discharged or if they are screened in the community, the evidence for the best way to manage undernutrition is lacking.

The challenge of managing undernutrition in the community is ensuring universal access to care and resources, particularly within groups or individuals who do not recognise that they may be at risk. In addition, general practitioners or family doctors lack training in nutrition so undernutrition can be missed or treated incorrectly [2]. Finally, a lack of public awareness can exacerbate the problem, especially in high-risk or vulnerable groups, such as housebound older people. This has meant that many interventions emerge via community groups, often as a part of local projects for which nutrition is not the main focus. This type of intervention relies on the drive and commitment of local individuals to succeed and can lead to an uneven distribution of support and information [3].

To tackle undernutrition in the community effectively, consideration must be given not only to the diagnosis, management and the role of health care professionals in clinical settings, but also the role of family, carers, social care and the wider aspects of a person's life which affect their nutritional intake [3]. Linked to this is the importance of taking into account food choice and preference when targeting interventions as, quite simply, if the food is not acceptable or appropriate to the person it will not be eaten [4]. The socioecological approach has been used to describe the myriad factors that influence an individual's nutritional intake, including individual factors, the social and physical environment and the broader environment of food supply. To effectively address undernutrition, this approach must be considered and multiple changes implemented across various areas [5].

While nutritional risk does not discriminate by age, gender or life circumstance, it disproportionately affects older people in the population [2].

Advanced Nutrition and Dietetics in Nutrition Support, First Edition. Edited by Mary Hickson and Sara Smith.
© 2018 John Wiley & Sons Ltd. Published 2018 by John Wiley & Sons Ltd.

For younger age groups, undernutrition is often a result of ill health or poverty, and failure to thrive in young children is a significant issue.

This chapter considers the population interventions that have proved successful in tackling undernutrition in the community. This includes any policy or project involving food or nutrition, which has been developed as a method of tackling the causes and consequences of undernutrition. The current policy with regard to undernutrition on a global, regional and national scale is briefly considered, providing context for two areas of focus: interventions to tackle food poverty and those to address undernutrition in vulnerable older people. These two groups are inextricably linked and food poverty among older people is of concern both in isolation and as part of the wider causes of undernutrition in this group.

4.1.2 Current policy on undernutrition

Policy on nutrition is a global, national and local issue, ranging from large-scale initiatives to small-scale local commitments to improve nutritional status in individuals. For many policymakers, motivation for policy intervention to tackle undernutrition comes from the association that poor nutrition has with morbidity and mortality. Therefore, nutrition interventions are often used to tackle these issues through diet and the encouragement of dietary change. This has been more apparent in the policy-level initiatives and backing given to the issue of obesity. Currently undernutrition lacks the public and political drive needed to become an area of major policy intervention, but some significant recent policy developments demonstrate an increased awareness of the importance of addressing undernutrition in the community.

International and European policy

In November 2014, the Food and Agricultural Organization (FAO) of the World Health Organization (WHO) published a declaration from the Second International Conference on Nutrition reaffirming the right of everyone to have access to safe, sufficient and nutritious food [6]. The declaration acknowledged the impact of undernutrition on the individual and society as well as the health and economic consequences.

On a European level, the European Innovation Partnership on Active and Healthy Ageing both includes and works with projects which are attempting to tackle undernutrition across all care settings [7]. The programme's overall aim, of increasing healthy life-years of European citizens by 2 years by 2020, recognises the beneficial impact that appropriate nutrition screening and intervention can have on health. These policies can provide a powerful tool for those working nationally and locally to create leverage and gain access to resources to tackle undernutrition in the community. For many countries in Europe, attaining political recognition of the issue of undernutrition is still some way off, and economic evidence is lacking.

National policy

The UK has done much to increase awareness of undernutrition and developing policy to tackle undernutrition across all care settings, although marked differences remain in the policy position of each of the four UK nations [8].

While there is still much to be done in the UK, pioneering work by the British Association of Parenteral and Enteral Nutrition (BAPEN) [9,10] and the Malnutrition Task Force [11] (Box 4.1.1) has led to increased awareness, political support and a commitment to change, as well as resources for interventions. In 2010, BAPEN responded to this local focus by producing a 'Toolkit for Commissioners', supporting the newly established health and well-being boards to ensure they meet quality standards in nutritional care when commissioning services [10]. While more clinical in focus, the tool can help develop policy locally on screening and monitoring in the community, and provides

---

Box 4.1.1   Undernutrition policy in the UK: the Malnutrition Task Force

The UK's Malnutrition Task Force is an independent group of experts across health, social care and local government united to address avoidable and preventable malnutrition in older people. The task force identified five best practice principles: raising awareness, working together, identifying malnutrition, personalising care support and treatment and monitoring and evaluating. In hospitals, care homes and in the community, it based pilot projects in five areas of the UK and published a series of guides and posters. The work of the task force highlights the need for local health and well-being boards, clinical commissioning groups and local authorities to work together to undertake joint strategic needs assessment to understand the scale of malnutrition, agree how it sits with competing local priorities and how addressing it can deliver a better nutritional care infrastructure that will provide wider benefits across the community.

---

support on the importance of multidisciplinary teams in tackling undernutrition.

In Canada and the US, there has been focus on measuring and monitoring food insecurity. In Canada specifically, PROOF (research to identify policy options to reduce food insecurity) has used food insecurity prevalence data to advocate around the impact of food insecurity and undernutrition on health and the need for public health policy [12]. In the US, investment has been focused on the Women, Infants and Children (WIC) programme to prevention food insecurity [13]. In Australia, funding strategies to alleviate food insecurity have been created, with a focus on the role local governments can play [14].

Regional and local policy

Increasingly, interventions are focused on a more local or individual level as financial responsibility is devolved from central to local government and health services. This means local areas are able to prioritise according to their demographic structure and patterns of health, putting resources where need is greatest and producing local policy and plans for action to tackle undernutrition [15,16]. While effective on a local level, this can lead to pockets of inspired and effective interventions sitting alongside areas where little or no action is taken as priorities lie elsewhere. In Australia, investment in local government has shown increased understanding of the issues of food insecurity and incorporation of inadequate access to nutritious food as a priority policy area [14].

4.1.3 Community interventions to tackle undernutrition

Community interventions generally take two forms: those which aim to support health or social care professionals to identify the causes of undernutrition and work from a more 'top-down' approach and those which work directly with vulnerable people to attempt to identify those malnourished or at risk of undernutrition.

Research has found that an education programme supported by a community dietetics service for patients 'at risk' of undernutrition increased nutritional knowledge and improved the reported management of undernourished patients in the community by healthcare professionals [17]. However, this type of evaluation does not demonstrate the impact of the increased knowledge on the nutritional status of those at risk. Similarly, projects that originate 'on the ground', responding to wider community needs, can struggle to demonstrate how their project has a measurable impact on individual nutritional status.

When considering interventions for undernutrition in the community, it is necessary to examine who may be the 'at-risk' groups – those who are more likely to experience undernutrition or its causes.

Older people have been found to be at significant risk of undernutrition [18]. It is estimated that 1 in 10 people over 65 in the UK are at risk and hospital admission studies have shown that 93% of undernutrition is in the community [18].

Much of the undernutrition occurring in the community can be linked to other experiences in a person's life. For older people, while some of this might be the result of underlying ill health or disease, other influences reported include depression or anxiety, social exclusion, problems with dental health, transport or mobility difficulties, poverty, the influence of medication on appetite or the body's ability to absorb nutrients, and access to food shops and other services [3,19].

While having a significant effect on health and well-being, undernutrition is preventable. The challenge is in raising awareness in the community and ensuring appropriate resources are allocated to prevention programmes and activities. Programmes of prevention have proved successful in addressing undernutrition among older people [3,20]. By developing tools to provide access to appropriate services, regular access to food and meals, and information for older people, their carers and families, projects are addressing some of the key risk factors for developing undernutrition [3,21]. Effective projects use food as a tool to develop relationships and prevent isolation as well as providing opportunities to link to other services, thereby addressing the causes of undernutrition. These might include preventing isolation, benefits advice, fuel poverty, legal issues and preventing abuse [21–23].

Cost–benefit analysis can be an effective tool in influencing policy and establishing community projects and interventions. Several types of intervention, including supplementation, lunch clubs and community meals, have been able to establish their economic benefit with regard to preventing undernutrition and its ensuing costs. Creating interventions in the community allows those living and working locally to contribute to the development of projects, outlining their needs and the factors preventing them from eating well.

A 2013 report for the UK Malnutrition Task Force [24] highlighted the cost savings and health benefits associated with community interventions. Increasingly, evaluation of such projects (which have been a low priority in the past) focuses on the benefits they can provide not only to the individual and community, but to the wider local or regional remit to address health inequalities, undernutrition and quality of life.

The challenge in measuring the effectiveness of food projects is that historically there has been a lack of evaluation or empirical evidence. However, this is changing as projects recognise the value of effective evaluation in addition to user feedback.

Lunch clubs

A lunch club is a venue where people can gather to eat lunch together in their community. It is usually based in a community centre, day centre or faith centre. It may be accompanied by activities, education or information sessions or simply be a place for people to meet and eat together. Some are accompanied by a small cost, subsidising local authority, voluntary sector or faith-based funding. A review of lunch clubs in Scotland found that they support older people living in their own homes to eat well, providing an opportunity to have a meal, at an affordable price, and meet with others in a social setting [22]. The clubs reviewed were run by a number of organisations including local authorities, which often provided transport, national organisations such as Royal Voluntary Service or Age UK or in some cases the private sector (e.g. pubs). They may take the form of a social club with a meal, a dedicated lunch club, some with activities added on, or community cafés, which may also provide training for café staff or developing skills for those aiming to get back into employment.

Small-scale observational studies have found that nutrient intake on a day attending a lunch club was higher than for other days of the week for micronutrients, but did not measure overall undernutrition [25]. Older people have reported that benefits include eating a wider range of foods and availability of affordable meals, stating that they would not bother to cook similar meals for themselves. In addition, they report that it is the only time they eat in the company of others, which improves their appetite [26]. Unfortunately, these studies are limited by small sample size and responses of those already attending the clubs, but the benefits the clubs provide are important to the older people who use these services, which can be forgotten when attempting to qualitatively measure this type of programme.

Shopping services

Shopping projects are an excellent means of addressing some of the biggest factors preventing older people eating well. Shopping services can take several forms and, like most projects, have evolved to meet the needs of the local area. Some provide transport to supermarkets to allow people to seek bargains and get their food carried home rather than struggle on the bus or manage with more expensive local shops [3,27]. These often also include a stop at a local café so users get a chance to socialise and chat to volunteers. Other successful projects use teleshopping or internet shopping, acting as a conduit for the older person who may not have internet access and brokering deals for delivery costs or payment systems with the retailer.

The most successful projects tend to involve multiple stakeholders and for shopping services, working with a local retailer or internet food provider can be a means to ensuring access for older people and sustainability for the project (Box 4.1.2). Partnering with a local retailer can ensure older people get the food they want, when they want it, from a local business that is invested in supporting their clients [27]. The next step for these projects is to determine the impact shopping services have on nutritional status and

---

Box 4.1.2 Case study: local shopping service, Age UK Oldham

Age UK Oldham developed a partnership with the local Co-operative supermarket, which provided an office, telephone and dedicated checkout in store. Older people not only got food delivered regularly, but the telephone ordering system contributed to a befriending service as well as establishing any need for further support with cooking or help at home. AGE UK staff visited the store on a client's behalf, with the 205 users in 2009 contributing £4000 a week to the takings of the store, meaning all stakeholders benefited from being involved [26].

---

currently only small-scale qualitative studies exist. This is in part because the focus of work in this area has been to take a holistic view of the quality of life and well-being of the individual, given that nutrition is interwoven through many other issues for older people (e.g. isolation, mental health and income).

Community meals

Community meals provide an invaluable service in providing food to vulnerable people in their own homes as well as social contact (also known at Meals on Wheels). The meal may be hot or frozen and reheated by the client or carer. Meals can be provided through a local authority based on eligibility criteria or through private contract. This type of service can be found in the USA, Canada, Japan, Australia and parts of Europe but models of delivery can vary [28], often relying on volunteers [29].

In the UK, evidence suggests that more people are receiving meals in their own home than are living in care homes, illustrating the importance of the service [30]. Other evaluations demonstrate the cost benefits of community meals; every £1 invested in community meals leads to a social return on investment of between £3.00–5.30 [24]. Meanwhile, research by a commercial community meal provider found that an annual additional subsidy of just over £5 million for community meals services would support 10% of the older population to remain in their own homes, saving £1.7 billion in health and social care, even if the projected cost of domiciliary care in 2020 was taken into account [31].

In other countries, 'community meals' are defined as meals shared outside the home, often by emergency food providers. These forms of community meal programmes struggle to meet increasing needs, relying on donations of food to prepare the meals. Data from Australia suggest that these services are only able to provide 66% of the food required to meet the needs of the hungry people requesting their service. Together with limited physical resources (including kitchen facilities, communal dining areas, etc.), this type of community meal is unlikely to be a sustainable solution to undernutrition [32].

4.1.4 Conclusions, challenges and the future

Community interventions are increasingly commissioned by clinical commissioning groups or local health and well-being boards. As such, they are subject to the same scrutiny as clinical resources and quite rightly have equal weighting with regard to referrals and support. This means that projects need to focus on structure, strategy, outcomes and evaluation as opposed to more reactive organic growth through which they have developed in the past. These changes follow an overall pattern of interventions developed for undernutrition considering not only the need for more food, but the circumstances under which the undernutrition occurred. By providing services and support appropriate to the individual rather than slotting them into a rigid 'programme', the underlying causes of undernutrition can be addressed and fully preventive measures, including screening, monitoring and support, implemented to break the cycle of undernutrition and prevent future ill health. It requires a new approach for all those involved in addressing undernutrition.

This requires an adjustment for clinicians who must acknowledge that community projects and community-based interventions have a role to play. It requires better training for general practitioners or family doctors on their role in diagnosing undernutrition in the community and consequently signposting or referring to a wider range of support services [33]. The role of informal carers (family and friends) needs to be better recognised and supported as they play a key part in maintaining the health and well-being of loved ones, as well as often being at risk of undernutrition themselves [34]. Lastly, it requires community projects to provide support and form partnerships to deliver solutions to those experiencing undernutrition in the community and understand their role in referring to doctors or dietitians where needed.

References

1. National Institute for Health and Clinical Excellence. Quality Standard for Nutrition Support in Adults. NICE Quality Standard 24. London: NICE, 2012.
2. Guest JF, Panca M, Baeyens JP, de Man F, Ljungqvist O, Pichard C, Wait S, Wilson L. Health economic impact of managing patients following a community-based diagnosis of malnutrition in the UK. *Clin Nutr* 2011; **30**(4): 422–429.
3. Wilson LC. Preventing Malnutrition in Older People: The Role of Community Food Projects. A report by the Caroline Walker Trust for Age Concern England, 2009.
4. Lau D. Role of food perceptions in food selection of the elderly. *J Nutr Elderly* 2008; **27**(3): 221–246.
5. Story M, Kaphingst KM, Robinson-O'Brien R, Glanz K. Creating healthy food and eating environments: policy and environmental approaches. *Ann Rev Public Health* 2008; **29**: 253–272.
6. Food and Agriculture Organization of the World Health Organization. Second International Conference on Nutrition. Rome: World Health Organization, 2014.
7. European Commission. European Innovation Partnership on Active and Healthy Ageing. http://ec.europa.eu/research/innovation-union/index_en.cfm?section=active-healthy-ageing (accessed 31 August 2017).
8. Caraher M, Crawley H, Lloyd S. Nutrition Policy Across the UK. London: Caroline Walker Trust, 2009.
9. Elia M, Stratton RJ. Calculating the cost of disease-related malnutrition in the UK in 2007 (public expenditure only). In: Combating Malnutrition: Recommendations for Action. Redditch: BAPEN, 2009.
10. Brotherton A, Stroud M, Simmonds N. Malnutrition Matters: Meeting Quality Standards in Nutrition Care. Redditch: BAPEN, 2010.
11. Malnutrition Task Force. www.malnutritiontaskforce.org.uk (accessed 31 August 2017).
12. PROOF. Food Insecurity Policy Research. http://proof.utoronto.ca (accessed 31 August 2017).
13. United States Department of Agriculture, Food and Nutrition Service. Women, Infants and Children. www.fns.usda.gov/wic/women-infants-and-children-wic (accessed 31 August 2017).
14. VicHealth. Food for All – Resources for Local Governments. www.vichealth.vic.gov.au/media-and-resources/publications/food-for-all-2005-10-program-evaluation-report (accessed 31 August 2017).
15. Wilson LC. A Nutrition Policy for Older People in Kensington and Chelsea. London: Royal Borough of Kensington and Chelsea and Kensington and Chelsea Primary Care Trust, 2009.
16. Dorset County Council and NHS Dorset. Nutritional Care Strategy for Adults: Action Plan. 2013. www.dorsetforyou.com/nutritional-care-strategy (accessed 31 August 2017).
17. Kennelly S, Kennedy N, Flanagan-Rughoobur G, Glennon-Slattery C, Sugrue S. An evaluation of a

community dietetics intervention on the management for healthcare professional. *J Hum Nutr Diet* 2010; **23**(6): 567–575.

18. Elia M, Russell C. Combatting Malnutrition: Recommendations for Action. Redditch: BAPEN, 2009.

19. European Nutrition for Health Alliance, British Association for Parental and Enteral Nutrition, International Longevity Centre-UK. Malnutrition Among Older People in the Community: Policy Recommendations for Change. London: European Nutrition for Health Alliance, 2006.

20. Jones J, Duffy M, Coull Y, Wilkinson H. Older People Living in the Community – Nutritional Needs, Barriers and Interventions: A Literature Review. Edinburgh: Scottish Government Social Research, 2009.

21. Age UK. Effectiveness of Day Services: Summary of Research Evidence. London: Age UK, 2011.

22. Community Food and Health Scotland. A Bite and A Blether: Case Studies from Scotland's Lunch Clubs. Glasgow: Community Food and Health Scotland, 2011.

23. Malnutrition Task Force. Malnutrition in Later Life: Prevention and Early Intervention. Best Practice Principles and Implementation Guide: A Local Community Approach. London: Malnutrition Task Force, 2013.

24. Wilson LC. A Review and Summary of the Impact of Malnutrition in Older People and the Reported Costs and Benefits of Interventions. London: Malnutrition Task Force, 2013.

25. Burke D, Jennings M, McClinchy J, Massey H, Westwood D, Dickinson A. Community luncheon clubs benefit the nutritional and social well-being of free-living older people. *J Hum Nutr Diet* 2011; **24**(3): 278.

26. Joseph Rowntree Foundation. How can Local Authorities with Less Money Support Better Outcomes for Older People? 2011. www.jrf.org.uk/sites/files/jrf/authorities-supporting-older-people-summary.pdf (accessed 31 August 2017).

27. Age Concern and Help the Aged. Prevention in Practice: Service Models, Methods and Impact. London: Age Concern and Help the Aged, 2009.

28. Winterton R, Warburton J, Oppenheimer M. The future for Meals on Wheels? Reviewing innovative approaches to meal provision for ageing populations. *Int J Soc Welf* 2013; **22**: 141–151.

29. O'Dwyer C, Timonen V. Doomed to extinction? The nature and future of volunteering for meals-on-wheels services. *Voluntas* 2009; **20**: 35–49.

30. Wilson LC. Personalisation and the Role of Community Meals: A Report from a Round Table Discussion on Personalisation and Community Meals Chaired by Baroness Greengross. London: International Longevity Centre, 2010.

31. Apetito. Meeting the Wider Funding Challenge: The Real Value of Community Meals on Wheels. Trowbridge: Malnutrition Task Force, 2013.

32. FairShare, SecondBite, VicRelief Foodbank. Community Food Programs in Victoria: A Report on the Food Needed and the Infrastructure Required. Victoria: VicHealth, 2011.

33. Audit Commission. Older People, Independence and Wellbeing: The Challenge for Public Services. London: Audit Commission and Better Government for Older People, 2004.

34. Carers UK. Malnutrition and Caring: The Hidden Cost for Families. London: Carers UK, 2012.

Institutional interventions to prevent and treat undernutrition

Adrienne Young

Department of Nutrition and Dietetics, Royal Brisbane and Women's Hospital, Brisbane, Australia

4.2.1 Introduction

Undernutrition is a common and costly problem in institutions where it has significant impact on health and service outcomes. Having nutrition support processes in place at a system level in institutions such as hospitals, residential aged care facilities, mental health facilities and prisons is critical to treat and prevent undernutrition.

This chapter will critically review system-level strategies aimed at creating a culture of nutrition support within institutions, improving food services and creating positive mealtime environments. It is important to note that recommendations in this chapter are largely derived from literature from the health services domain (hospitals and residential aged care facilities); however, some principles may translate to other institutions such as prisons and residential mental health and disability facilities.

4.2.2 Creating a culture of nutrition support within institutions

Creating an institutional culture where nutrition is valued by all stakeholders has been named as the first part of the solution for tackling the problem of undernutrition in institutions [1]. Key to creating this culture is taking a holistic and interdisciplinary approach to nutrition care, where responsibility and knowledge about nutrition no longer sit solely with the dietitian, but are on the agenda for all health professionals, managers and executives. Highlighting the fiscal impact of undernutrition, as well as the health implications for inpatients or residents, may help to inspire managers to address this critical issue by including nutrition within organisational plans, and by forming interdisciplinary governance committees to ensure that barriers are identified and action is taken, in order to meet nutrition service delivery targets and optimise inpatient or resident outcomes.

It is easy to say that 'nutrition is everyone's responsibility' but this can be difficult to operationalise with health professionals traditionally working within silos and often hesitant to step outside traditional role boundaries. Furthermore, when responsibility for nutritional care is spread across individuals or disciplines, accountability can be lost, and what was everyone's responsibility becomes 'nobody's job' [2]. It is important for there to be clear accountability and role delineation around who is responsible for each part of the nutrition care process, and for this to be clearly communicated and understood by all members of the healthcare team [1].

Another key principle of managing undernutrition in institutions is having clear processes for identifying inpatients or residents at risk of undernutrition in order to prioritise these people for nutrition assessment and intervention [1,3–5]. Embedding nutrition screening into

Advanced Nutrition and Dietetics in Nutrition Support, First Edition. Edited by Mary Hickson and Sara Smith.

routine clinical practice (e.g. integrating vali-dated screening tools into routine admission paperwork) has been highlighted as important, so that screening is not viewed as a burden or additional work for staff. Not only is screening important, but it is also necessary to have clear referral and action processes following nutrition screening, for example, having standardised electronic referral pathways and implementing basic nutrition support for an 'at-risk' consumer while awaiting a comprehensive dietitian assess-ment and nutrition care plan [1]. With decreas-ing lengths of stay in acute hospitals, it is important for clinicians to consider nutrition as the patient transitions from hospital back to the community. This is a vulnerable time for patients at risk of undernutrition, and improved discharge planning, follow-up and co-ordination of nutri-tion care need to be considered in order to prevent readmissions [6].

4.2.3 Improving food services

High-quality meals are an integral part of caring for those residing in institutions, especially where people rely on the institution for all or most of their nutrition. Unfortunately, the rele-vance and importance of food service are often undervalued and can be seen as a 'hotel service' where budgetary cuts can be introduced with minimal impact. Of course, there are differ-ences in food service systems between institu-tions based on inpatient or resident needs (for example, the nutritional needs of acute hospital inpatients differ from a prison population). Common to all institutions is the fact that most people look forward to mealtimes as meals mark the passage of time and are part of a famil-iar routine [7]. Despite this, food is often a cause for complaint, with the quality and deliv-ery of meals accentuating the patient's absence from home and home-style meals [8]. Given the serious health and fiscal implications of under-nutrition in institutions, it is important that high-quality food services meet the need of inpatients or residents, and are viewed as a cost-effective strategy for managing and preventing undernutrition.

There is limited published research to guide the design and delivery of food services outside the hospital and residential aged care settings, presenting significant opportunity for research in the prison, mental health and disability care settings to optimise nutritional intake of residents.

Food service systems and menu planning

There are several food production and delivery systems available to institutions (production: 'cook fresh', 'cook chill', 'cook freeze'; delivery: preplated, bulk delivery with plating at point of service). Studies suggest that consumer satisfaction, and in some cases dietary intake, is enhanced when inpatients or residents can make their meal choice close to the time of service (e.g. using same-day menus, room service or buffet-style service) [9]. While there are sub-stantial costs in setting up a point-of-service meal delivery system (e.g. costs associated with equipment, renovations and staff), long-term cost savings may be seen due to reduced waste and purchase of food [10].

The appropriate length of menu cycle is likely to be context specific, with longer cycles required in long-stay institutions such as residential care facilities and prisons. In fact, a longer menu cycle has been found to be associ-ated with reduced risk of undernutrition in resi-dential aged care facilities [11], as has a higher food budget [12]. When planning menus for acute hospitals, it is not enough to base the menu cycle length on average length of stay as hospital length of stay data are skewed. Acute hospital menus need to accommodate the needs of longer stay patients which have been found to occupy half of hospital beds and may represent those people most at risk of undernutrition [13].

One strategy to facilitate the implementation of high-quality and evidence-based food services is to develop standards or policies to outline the recommended food service systems and menus for the institution. Having standards or policies that are endorsed at a higher level (whether this is at the institutional, regional, or national level) creates a shared agreement to provide high-quality food services, and may assist with implementing and advocating for service improvements.

It is important for institutions to have systems in place to measure and monitor inpatient and resident satisfaction, and to use these data to design and deliver patient-centred food service systems. These data can be collected through interviews, focus groups and/or validated surveys. Examples of validated surveys include the Acute Hospital Foodservice Patient Satisfaction Questionnaire [14] and Resident Foodservice Satisfaction Questionnaire (for use in geriatric rehabilitation and aged care homes) [15]. Using qualitative methods to understand inpatient or resident experience may provide invaluable insight into how to improve service delivery and optimise nutritional intake [16].

Food fortification

Food fortification is an important strategy for treating and preventing undernutrition in hospitals and residential aged care facilities. Products commonly used to fortify foods include commercial nutrition supplements (e.g. protein powders) or food-based fortification (e.g. full-cream dairy, oils, cream, sauces). Thirteen studies (seven randomised controlled trials (RCT)) have evaluated the impact of fortified meals, snacks and/or drinks, with all studies showing increased dietary intakes and/or nutritional status [17–29]. Only three studies (two RCTs) have measured non-nutritional outcomes, with no difference seen in functional status or length of stay (despite improvements in dietary intake and/or weight) [19,20,23]. Functional improvements were observed in one RCT where food fortification was combined with a group exercise programme for aged care home residents [24], suggesting that multifaceted interventions may be important.

Particular care should be taken when planning menus for those requiring a restricted diet (for example, salt or fluid restriction for renal or heart failure, texture-modified diet for dysphagia). These restrictions can affect the palatability and variety of meals and may place these people at increased risk of undernutrition [30,31]. Food fortification and use of food moulds may improve dietary intakes of people requiring a texture-modified diet [31].

While food fortification is commonly used to improve the dietary intake of people admitted to or residing in institutions and is significantly cheaper than oral nutritional supplements (ONS) [26,32], success may be limited in practice without addressing other system-level barriers such as feeding assistance and supportive meal environment.

4.2.4 Creating positive mealtime environments

While many inpatients and residents look forward to mealtimes, descriptive studies reveal that mealtimes in hospitals and aged care homes can be unpleasant occasions and can be frequently interrupted by clinical activities such as doctors' rounds, nursing tasks and other health professionals' activities. Older people in hospitals and residential aged care facilities also may not receive the mealtime assistance they require, suggesting that strategies to create supportive mealtime environments, including dedicated feeding assistants, protected mealtimes, family-style dining and dining rooms, may be potential strategies to address undernutrition in institutions.

Dedicated feeding assistants

Four studies (two RCTs and two before-and-after studies) have evaluated the impact of feeding assistance by health assistants (dietetic assistants and healthcare assistants) or food service staff in the hospital setting. One RCT (using dietetic assistants to assist with meals and ONS) with low risk of bias showed significant improvement in clinical and nutritional outcomes [33] whereas another RCT (using healthcare assistants to plan and overcome mealtime barriers) with medium risk of bias showed no improvement in these outcomes [34]. Differences in implementation and/or evaluation may explain the heterogeneity of these results. Two before-and-after studies (one using nursing assistants to assist with meals and snacks, one using food service staff to assist and encourage snacks only) found improved dietary intake with feeding assistants compared with a historical control group [35,36]. A recent systematic review concluded that there is insufficient evidence on the impact of feeding assistance on the dietary intake of aged care home residents with dementia [37].

Volunteers have also been used to provide mealtime assistance to hospital patients. A systematic review evaluated the impact of a volunteer feeding assistance programme on the dietary intake and mealtime care provided to hospital inpatients [38]. While all studies reported high satisfaction with the volunteer programme and small improvements in energy and/or protein intake, most studied small samples and all had significant limitations in methodology. No studies have evaluated clinical outcomes of volunteer programmes.

While volunteer assistance programmes are highly acceptable to nurses, volunteers and institutions alike, studies report that recruiting and retaining a sufficient pool of volunteers to provide a meaningful service can be challenging [39]. It is also likely that the volunteer programme can only be implemented at the lunch meal [38]. The cost-effectiveness of volunteer feeding programmes has not been explored, which is crucial given the extensive training, assessment and supervision required to provide a safe volunteer feeding service [38]. Introducing dedicated feeding assistant roles does not guarantee an improvement in the level and quality of mealtime care. Large variation in the quality of care provided by paid feeding assistants has been observed in aged care homes [39], highlighting the importance of choosing highly motivated and dedicated assistants. Introducing a dedicated feeding assistant role also has the potential to further distance nurses from their role in providing nutritional care [40], inadvertently reducing the level of mealtime care as responsibility for this task shifts from nurses to the lone feeding assistant or volunteer. This was demonstrated in one study where patients reported receiving less attention by staff at mealtimes after the introduction of feeding assistants [41].

The 'red tray' system has been endorsed by the Royal College of Nursing (UK) as 'a simple way of alerting healthcare staff to the fact that a person requires help with eating' [42]. Despite widespread adoption throughout the NHS in the UK, and increasingly in Australia, there have been no studies evaluating the impact of red trays on mealtime practices or nutritional outcomes. One Australian study implemented red trays, amongst other strategies, and found improved weight outcomes for hospitalised patients [43]; however, the outcome of the use of red trays was not reported, making it difficult to determine the success of this strategy.

Protected mealtimes and mealtime environment

Florence Nightingale first wrote of the concept of protected mealtimes in 1859: 'Nothing shall be done on a ward whilst patients are having their meal'. Protected mealtimes is a strategy whereby staff activities are reprioritised to minimise non-urgent clinical activities and interruptions at mealtimes [44]. Protected mealtimes have been implemented in hospitals throughout the UK under recommendations from the National Patient Safety Agency and have been increasingly implemented in hospitals across Australia. Four before-and-after studies have evaluated the impact of protected mealtimes on dietary intake and mealtime care provided to hospital inpatients [35,45–47]. No studies have evaluated the impact of this strategy on functional or clinical outcomes of hospitalised patients. Outcomes are heterogeneous and appear to be linked to the efficacy of implementation and culture change. Three studies reported no/limited change in mealtime practices or dietary intake after the introduction of protected mealtimes [45–47]. The only study to suggest that protected mealtimes may improve dietary intake of hospital inpatients used an action research approach to implement change to mealtime practices and culture [35], in contrast to the other studies which primarily targeted knowledge deficits through posters and guideline dissemination.

Three studies have evaluated the effect of other meal environment interventions (family-style meals and ward dining rooms) on nutritional outcomes [48–50]. Enhancing the meal service in a residential aged care facility through family-style dining (where residents serve their own meals at the dining table), limiting unnecessary interruptions and designating staff to assist at mealtimes resulted in a significant increase in energy intake and maintenance of physical performance, weight and quality of life [49]. A similar study reported weight gain at 12 months, compared to stable weight in the control group [48]. These studies used a number of strategies to improve the mealtimes (including protected mealtimes and designating staff to assist at mealtimes) and it is possible that the multicomponent nature of these interventions enhanced their success. A systematic review concluded that interventions to improve mealtime ambience in aged care homes (through music, lighting, visual stimulation, increased meal choice and promoting conversation) may improve dementia-related behaviours such as aggression, agitation and confusion [51]. Most studies were small and reporting of study methods was poor; however, findings were similar across all studies, with most evidence for music interventions.

One study evaluated the introduction of a dining room in an acute hospital ward (with one dedicated staff member to assist and encourage intake) [50]. This study observed improved energy intake but no change in clinical outcomes, which may be explained by the underutilisation of the dining room by participants (accessed only an average of four times per participant). Sharing meals with caregivers resulted in significant weight gain for residents with dementia from two residential aged care facilities [52], as well as improved mealtime behaviours (resident–resident and staff–resident interactions, self-feeding) and staff satisfaction. A cross-sectional audit of 34 North American residential aged care facilities also found that residents were more likely to receive assistance and have their dietary

intake monitored if they ate in dining rooms, rather than individual rooms [53].

In summary, when implemented adequately, strategies to improve the mealtime environment (including dedicated feeding assistants, protected mealtimes and shared dining) present an opportunity to improve dietary intakes of people in hospitals and aged care homes. However, these strategies require complex changes to practice which can be difficult to achieve, perhaps explaining the disappointing results of studies thus far.

4.2.5 System-level nutrition processes: how to implement change into practice

It is easy to outline the evidence in favour of the aforementioned strategies and to ask health professionals and managers to simply implement them into practice. Audits and surveys of nutrition practices often show that there are gaps between what *should be* done and what *is* done, despite the best of intentions [54]. Institutions are complex systems and nutrition interventions often require changes to clinical routines or models of care which are particularly challenging to implement due to the complex interplay between professionals, social, environmental and political/economic contexts [55].

In the implementation science literature, there are a number of theoretical frameworks for implementing change into practice (e.g. Promoting Action on Research Implementation in Health Services [56], Theoretical Domains Framework [57]). Common themes from the implementation science literature highlight the following as critical factors for successful implementation.

- Acknowledging that change is a non-linear and time-intensive process.
- Need to understand the evidence and context (using research and local data from quantitative and qualitative sources).
- Critical importance of an experienced facilitator to enable change.
- Engaging the target group in designing and implementing the intervention.

- Champions and opinion leaders who can influence decision makers and peers to adopt change.
- Intervention strategies targeted at context-specific barriers, acknowledging that there is no one single universal strategy for successfully implementing change.

Staff education is frequently used as a behaviour change strategy to address the problem of undernutrition in institutions. The effectiveness of this strategy is likely to be limited unless the primary barrier is knowledge deficit. Therefore, clinicians should consider a range of other intervention strategies including, but not limited to, reminders at point of care, modelling and social strategies, environment restructuring, incentivisation and/or penalties, and audit and feedback [58]. Multifaceted interventions (food service improvements, nutrition screening, nutrition champions and/or ONS) have shown promise in treating and/or preventing undernutrition in the hospital setting [43,59], as have large-scale nutrition audits [60,61].

4.2.6 Summary

In summary, there is some evidence that institution-wide food service improvements (particularly food fortification) and mealtime interventions improve nutritional outcomes of inpatients or residents. The implementation approach is likely to be important, as mixed results in feeding assistant and protected mealtimes trials may be explained by differences in implementation success. Further high-quality research trials in all settings, but particularly in prisons and residential mental health and disability facilities, are required to strengthen the current available evidence.

References

1. Tappenden KA, Quatrara B, Parkhurst ML, Malone AM, Fanjiang G, Ziegler TR. Critical role of nutrition in improving quality of care: an interdisciplinary call to action to address adult hospital malnutrition. *J Parenter Enteral Nutr* 2013; **113**: 1219–1237.

2. Ross LJ, Mudge AM, Young AM, Banks M. Everyone's problem but nobody's job: staff perceptions and explanations for poor nutritional intake in older medical patients. *Nutr Diet* 2011; **68**: 41–46.

3. Leach B, Goodwin S. Preventing malnutrition in prison. *Nurs Stand* 2014; **28**: 50–56.

4. Arvanitakis M, Coppens P, Doughan L, van Gossum A. Nutrition in care homes and home care: recommendations – a summary based on the report approved by the Council of Europe. *Clin Nutr* 2009; **28**: 492–496.

5. Bryan F, Allan T, Russell L. The move from a long-stay learning disabilities hospital to community homes: a comparison of clients' nutritional status. *J Hum Nutr Diet* 2009; **13**: 265–270.

6. De van der Schueren M, Elia M, Gramlich L, et al. Clinical and economic outcomes of nutrition interventions across the continuum of care. *Ann NY Acad Sci* 2014; **1321**: 20–40.

7. Johns N, Edwards JS, Hartwell HJ. Hungry in hospital, well-fed in prison? A comparative analysis of food service systems. *Appetite* 2013; **68**: 45–50.

8. Johns N, Hartwell H, Morgan M. Improving the provision of meals in hospital. The patients' viewpoint. *Appetite* 2010; **54**: 181–185.

9. Mahoney S, Zulli A, Walton K. Patient satisfaction and energy intakes are enhanced by point of service meal provision. *Nutr Diet* 2009; **66**: 212–220.

10. Williams R, Virtue K, Adkins A. Room service improves patient food intake and satisfaction with hospital food. *J Pediatr Oncol Nurs* 1998; **15**: 183–189.

11. Carrier N, Ouellet D, West GE. Nursing home food services linked with risk of malnutrition. *Can J Diet Pract Res* 2007; **68**: 14–20.

12. Strathmann S, Lesser S, Bai-Habelski J, et al. Institutional factors associated with the nutritional status of residents from 10 German nursing homes (ErnSTES study). *J Nutr Health Aging* 2013; **17**: 271–276.

13. Vivanti AP, Banks MD. Length of stay patterns for patients of an acute care hospital: implications for nutrition and food services. *Austr Health Rev* 2007; **31**: 282–287.

14. Capra S, Wright O, Sardie M, Bauer J, Askew D. The Acute Hospital Foodservice Patient Satisfaction Questionnaire: the development of a valid and reliable tool to measure patient satisfaction with acute care hospital foodservices. *Foodservice Res Int* 2005; **16**: 1–14.

15. Wright OR, Capra S, Connelly LB. Foodservice satisfaction domains in geriatrics, rehabilitation and aged care. *J Nutr Health Aging* 2010; **14**: 775–780.

16. Mahadevan M, Hartwell HJ, Feldman CH, Ruzsilla JA, Raines ER. Assisted-living elderly and the mealtime experience. *J Hum Nutr Diet* 2014; **27**: 152–161.

17. Barton AD, Beigg CL, Macdonald IA, Allison SP. A recipe for improving food intakes in elderly hospitalized patients. *Clin Nutr* 2000; **19**: 451–454.

18. Gall MJ, Grimble GK, Reeve NJ, Thomas SJ. Effect of providing fortified meals and between-meal snacks on energy and protein intake of hospital patients. *Clin Nutr* 1998; **17**: 259–264.

19. Odlund Olin A, Osterberg P, Hadell K, Armyr I, Jerstrom S, Ljungqvist O. Energy-enriched hospital food to improve energy intake in elderly patients. *J Parenter Enteral Nutr* 1996; **20**: 93–97.

20. Munk T, Beck AM, Holst M, et al. Positive effect of protein-supplemented hospital food on protein intake in patients at nutritional risk: a randomised controlled trial. *J Hum Nutr Diet* 2014; **27**: 122–132.

21. Iuliano S, Woods J, Robbins J. Consuming two additional serves of dairy food a day significantly improves energy and nutrient intakes in ambulatory aged care residents: a feasibility study. *J Nutr Health Aging* 2013; **17**: 509–513.

22. Leslie WS, Woodward M, Lean ME, Theobald H, Watson L, Hankey CR. Improving the dietary intake of under nourished older people in residential care homes using an energy-enriching food approach: a cluster randomised controlled study. *J Hum Nutr Diet* 2013; **26**: 387–394.

23. Smoliner C, Norman K, Scheufele R, Hartig W, Pirlich M, Lochs H. Effects of food fortification on nutritional and functional status in frail elderly nursing home residents at risk of malnutrition. *Nutrition* 2008; **24**: 1139–1144.

24. Beck AM, Damkjær K, Beyer N. Multifaceted nutritional intervention among nursing-home residents has a positive influence on nutrition and function. *Nutrition* 2008; **24**: 1073–1080.

25. Lorefalt B, Wilhelmsson S. A multifaceted intervention model can give a lasting improvement of older peoples' nutritional status. *J Nutr Health Aging* 2012; **16**: 378–382.

26. Simmons SF, Zhuo X, Keeler E. Cost-effectiveness of nutrition interventions in nursing home residents: a pilot intervention. *J Nutr Health Aging* 2010; **14**: 367–372.

27. Castellanos VH, Marra MV, Johnson P. Enhancement of select foods at breakfast and lunch increases energy intakes of nursing home residents with low meal intakes. *JADA* 2009; **109**: 445–451.

28. Best RL, Appleton KM. Comparable increases in energy, protein and fat intakes following the addition of seasonings and sauces to an older person's meal. *Appetite* 2011; **56**: 179–182.

29. Stelten S, Dekker IM, Ronday EM, Thijs A, Boelsma E, Peppelenbos HW, de van der Schueren MAE. Protein-enriched 'regular products' and their effect on protein intake in acute hospitalized older adults; a randomized controlled trial. *Clin Nutr* 2015; **34**: 409–414.

30. Darmon P, Kaiser MJ, Bauer JM, Sieber CC, Pichard C. Restrictive diets in the elderly: never say never again? *Clin Nutr* 2010; **29**: 170–174.

31. Keller H, Chambers L, Niezgoda H, Duizer L. Issues associated with the use of modified texture foods. *J Nutr Health Aging* 2012; **16**: 195–200.

32. Allison SP. Hospital Food as Treatment. London: British Association for Parenteral and Enteral Nutrition, 1999.

33. Duncan DG, Beck SJ, Hood K, Johansen A. Using dietetic assistants to improve the outcome of hip fracture: a randomised controlled trial of nutritional support in an acute trauma ward. *Age Aging* 2006; **35**: 148–153.

34. Hickson M, Bulpitt, C, Nunes, M, et al. Does additional feeding support provided by health care assistants improve nutritional status and outcomes in acutely ill older in-patients? A randomised control trial. *Clin Nutr* 2004; **23**: 69–77.

35. Young AM, Mudge AM, Banks MD, Ross LJ, Daniels L. Encouraging, assisting and time to EAT: improved nutritional intake for older medical patients receiving Protected Mealtimes and/or additional nursing feeding assistance. *Clin Nutr* 2013; **32**: 543–549.

36. Lindman A, Rasmussen HB, Andersen NF. Food caregivers influence on nutritional intake among admitted haematological cancer patients – a prospective study. *Eur J Oncol Nurs* 2013; **17**: 827–834.

37. Liu W, Cheon J, Thomas SA. Interventions on mealtime difficulties in older adults with dementia: a systematic review. *Int J Nurs Stud* 2014; **51**(1): 14–27.

38. Green SM, Martin HJ, Roberts HC, Sayer AA. A systematic review of the use of volunteers to improve mealtime care of adult patients or residents in institutional settings. *J Clin Nurs* 2011; **20**: 1810–1823.

39. Remsburg RE. Pros and cons of using paid feeding assistants in nursing homes. *Geriatr Nurs* 2004; **25**: 176–177.

40. Pearson A, Fitzgerald M, Nay R. Mealtimes in nursing homes. The role of nursing staff. *J Gerontol Nurs* 2003; **29**: 40–47.

41. Lassen KO, Grinderslev E, Nyholm R. Effect of changed organisation of nutritional care of Danish medical inpatients. *BMC Health Serv Res* 2008; **8**: 168.

42. Royal College of Nursing. Supporting and Assisting People. www.rcn.org.uk/development/practice/cpd_online_learning/supporting_peoples_nutritional_needs/supporting_and_assisting_people.

43. Schultz TJ, Kitson AL, Soenen S, et al. Does a multidisciplinary nutritional intervention prevent nutritional decline in hospital patients? A stepped wedge randomised cluster trial. *e-SPEN J* 2014; **9**: e84–e90.

44. National Health Scheme. Protected Mealtimes Review – Findings and Recommendations Report. London: National Patient Safety Agency, 2007.

45. Hickson M, Connolly A, Whelan K. Impact of protected mealtimes on ward mealtime environment,

patient experience and nutrient intake in hospitalised patients. *J Hum Nutr Diet* 2011; **24**: 370–374.

46. Huxtable S, Palmer M. The efficacy of protected mealtimes in reducing mealtime interruptions and improving mealtime assistance in adult inpatients in an Australian hospital. *Eur J Clin Nutr* 2013; **67**: 904–910.

47. Chan J, Carpenter C. An evaluation of a pilot protected mealtime program in a Canadian hospital. *Can J Diet Pract Res* 2015; **76**: 1–5.

48. Mathey MF, Vanneste VG, de Graaf C, de Groot LC, van Staveren WA. Health effect of improved meal ambiance in a Dutch nursing home: a 1-year intervention study. *Prev Med* 2001; **32**: 416–423.

49. Nijs KA, de Graaf C, Kok FJ, van Staveren WA. Effect of family style mealtimes on quality of life, physical performance, and body weight of nursing home residents: cluster randomised controlled trial. *BMJ* 2006; **332**: 1180–1184.

50. Wright L, Hickson M, Frost G. Eating together is important: using a dining room in an acute elderly medical ward increases energy intake. *J Hum Nutr Diet* 2006; **19**: 23–26.

51. Whear R, Abbott R, Thompson-Coon J, et al. Effectiveness of mealtime interventions on behavior symptoms of people with dementia living in care homes: a systematic review. *J Am Med Dir Assoc* 2014; **15**: 185–193.

52. Charras K, Fremontier M. Sharing meals with institutionalized people with dementia: a natural experiment. *J Gerontol Soc Work* 2010; **53**: 436–448.

53. Simmons SF, Levy-Storms L. The effect of dining location on nutritional care quality in nursing homes. *J Nutr Health Aging* 2005; **9**: 434–439.

54. Duerksen DR, Keller HH, Vesnaver E, et al. Physicians' perceptions regarding the detection and management of malnutrition in Canadian hospitals: results of a Canadian Malnutrition Task Force survey. *J Parenter Enteral Nutr* 2015; **39**(4): 410–417.

55. Grol RPTM, Bosch MC, Hulscher MEJL, Eccles MP, Wensing M. Planning and studying improvement in patient care: the use of theoretical perspectives. *Milbank Q* 2007; **85**: 93–138.

56. Kitson AL, Rycroft-Malone J, Harvey G, McCormack B, Seers K, Titchen A. Evaluating the successful implementation of evidence into practice using the PARiHS framework: theoretical and practical challenges. *Implement Sci* 2008; **3**: 1.

57. Cane J, O'Connor D, Michie S. Validation of the theoretical domains framework for use in behaviour change and implementation research. *Implement Sci* 2012; **7**: 37.

58. Michie S, van Stralen MM, West R. The behaviour change wheel: a new method for characterising and designing behaviour change interventions. *Implement Sci* 2011; **6**: 42.

59. Bell JJ, Bauer JD, Capra S, Pulle RC. Multidisciplinary, multi-modal nutritional care in acute hip fracture inpatients – results of a pragmatic intervention. *Clin Nutr* 2014; **33**: 1101–1107.

60. Meijers JM, Candel MJ, Schols JM, van Bokhorst-de van der Schueren MA, Halfens RJ. Decreasing trends in malnutrition prevalence rates explained by regular audits and feedback. *J Nutr* 2009; **139**: 1381–1386.

61. Valentini L, Schindler K, Schlaffer R, et al. The first nutritionDay in nursing homes: participation may improve malnutrition awareness. *Clin Nutr* 2009; **28**: 109–116.

Chapter 4.3

Oral nutrition support to prevent and treat undernutrition

Christine Baldwin

Department of Nutritional Sciences, King's College London, London, UK

4.3.1 Introduction

The provision of oral nutrition support is often seen as one of the basic skills of the dietitian but in fact requires the ability to undertake assessments in complex environments and to make judgements about interventions based on evaluation of a number of factors. A distinction between different types of complexity was made by the Medical Research Council in its framework for the evaluation of complex interventions [1] and the distinctions are relevant to the consideration of provision of oral nutrition support interventions. An intervention might be considered complex because it is composed of 'a number of different components that may act both independently and inter-dependently' [1].

In addition, the system or setting within which the intervention takes place might also be complex and will affect the way that the intervention operates. People receiving oral nutrition support interventions will be in various settings from primary care-based settings to hospital and living in their own homes and the amounts of support available in each setting may vary considerably. Interventions vary from items of food and drink and proprietary oral nutritional supplements (ONS) through to alterations to aspects of the environment, such as enhancements to dining facilities or protected mealtimes designed to improve nutritional intake. Oral nutrition support, therefore, may be considered a complex intervention requiring considerable skill and judgement to implement appropriately.

4.3.2 Outcomes appropriate for the assessment of effectiveness of oral nutrition support

The association between poor nutritional status and adverse clinical outcomes is well established [2,3]. The rationale for the use of nutrition support is based on the premise that strategies to improve nutritional intake will result in improvements to nutritional status that translate into improvements in clinical and other healthcare-related outcomes. In order to scrutinise the evidence base for oral nutrition interventions, it is necessary to consider which outcomes might be most appropriate to assess their benefits. Traditionally, outcomes were defined in narrow terms and focused on areas of most interest to researchers, usually mortality and measures of morbidity in clinical settings and change in nutritional intake and impact on nutritional status in studies of nutrition support. Recent developments in the assessment of outcomes have broadened the definition to consider issues important to the patient such as quality of life, patient satisfaction and physical function as well as outcomes of interest to healthcare providers such as hospital admissions, length of stay

Advanced Nutrition and Dietetics in Nutrition Support, First Edition. Edited by Mary Hickson and Sara Smith.
© 2018 John Wiley & Sons Ltd. Published 2018 by John Wiley & Sons Ltd.

Table 4.3.1 Outcomes used in the assessment of oral nutrition interventions

Outcome	Parameters commonly measured
Nutritional intake	Energy and protein
	Micronutrients
Nutritional status	Weight
	Body composition
Clinical	Mortality
	Clinical function (generic and disease specific)
	Physical function
	Improvements in health
Patient related	Quality of life
	Satisfaction
	Patient experience
Healthcare utilisation and costs	Length of hospital stay
	Readmissions to hospital
	GP visits
	Cost-effectiveness

(LOS) and cost-effectiveness [4]. Outcomes used in the assessment of oral nutrition support interventions are shown in Table 4.3.1.

The use of nutritional markers as sole outcomes of studies has been criticised in that it relies on the assumption that they are intermediate or surrogate outcomes and any observed improvements will translate into improvements to clinical and healthcare outcomes [5]. An analysis of the outcomes of 99 randomised controlled trials (RCTs) of nutrition interventions found that although 75–100% of trials reported improvements to one or more nutritional outcomes, 50% or fewer trials reported improvements to clinical outcomes and in greater than 25% of trials, improvements in nutritional outcomes were associated with poorer clinical outcomes [5].

4.3.3 Oral nutrition support options

There are several strategies available to provide oral nutritional supplementation to nutritionally vulnerable individuals. The range of options and practical details associated with use in practice

have been reviewed [4]. The options and issues pertaining to their use in different settings are summarised in Table 4.3.2.

Choices about the type of oral nutrition support to offer to an individual may be governed by a number of factors. While dietitians are trained in detailed patient assessment and management, with estimates suggesting that there are up to 3 million nutritionally vulnerable patients in the UK, there are insufficient numbers of dietitians available to counsel every patient identified. Hence, initial management is often guided by management protocols linked to nutritional screening. National guidelines have frequently recommended a graded process starting with food-based interventions for individuals with lesser degrees of nutritional risk and introducing ONS, followed by referral to a dietitian for individuals with greater degrees of nutritional risk [4,6]. Many local policies have adopted or modified such approaches.

A review of 38 UK policies on the management of nutritionally vulnerable patients living in the community, identified by internet searching, revealed considerable variation in recommendations for both management and review, perhaps reflecting availability of local resources [7]. The recommended period for review of management varied, with 4 weeks being the most common but some recommending up to 12 weeks before review. Of particular note was the lack of reference to the goals to be achieved by the initiation of oral nutrition support, which could potentially make the patient review difficult and limits the ability to make judgements about the escalation of support offered [7].

A further driver of choice of nutrition support strategy has been the rising costs of ONS which, in some areas, has resulted in prescribing support initiatives aimed at ensuring the 'appropriateness' of ONS prescription and considering alternative strategies where possible. Proponents of this approach argue that the cost savings resulting from a reduction in prescribing can be used to fund specialist dietitians who can provide skilled assessment and management of patients across a range of healthcare settings [8,9]. The counter argument is that such an economically simple approach fails to consider

Table 4.3.2 Oral nutrition support options available, practical considerations for their use and the influence of patient setting

Oral nutrition support strategy	Options	Practical considerations	Influence of setting
Food based	Food fortification Increased intake (from increased portion sizes or frequency of eating) Additional snacks and nourishing drinks	**Positives** Food is familiar to patients, can be varied to suit individual tastes and to provide different textures and flavours Does not have any cost implications for healthcare services **Negatives** Requires dietitian time to educate the patient May not be suitable for patients unable to shop, cook and prepare food Associated with greater costs to the patient	All options are available to be used by individuals living in their own homes, in institutional settings and in hospital. Where individuals are living in their own homes, food-based options are provided as dietary counselling and require understanding of the instructions by the patient or their carers to be implemented. In institutional settings the use of food-based options requires high levels of staff awareness to implement as well as flexible catering systems
Oral nutritional supplements (ONS)	Balanced mixtures of macro- and micronutrients available as liquid feeds, puddings and powdered forms A range of different presentations and flavours, including fibre-containing, juice-like, yoghurt-like, etc. as well as formulations for specific clinical conditions, e.g. elemental supplements for patients with malabsorption Different products prescribable and available over the counter Modular supplements consisting of one or two nutrients only, e.g. fat-based or carbohydrate-based supplements	**Positives** Usually nutritionally complete Provided in easy-to use formulations, e.g. tetrapacks with straws Prescribable for many conditions, therefore low cost to patients Can be delivered to a patient's home **Negatives** Limited range of flavours leads to monotony and may reduce compliance The cost is borne by healthcare services	Similar to food-based options, ONS can be used in all healthcare settings as well as individuals living in their own homes. In free-living individuals, understanding of the prescription and instructions is required to enable optimal use. In institutional settings, ONS can be provided to patients without their explicit understanding but high levels of staff awareness are needed to implement as well as flexible catering systems
Supportive (aiming to increase nutritional intake)	Organisation initiatives (use of red trays, protected mealtimes, management protocols) Staff training Improvements to the environment (e.g. use of dining rooms and/or music) Modifications to food (e.g. flavour enhancements, fortification) Institution-wide strategies for the distribution of snacks and ONS (e.g. inclusion of ONS on prescription charts or provision of snacks with regular drinks rounds) Home-delivered meals	**Positives** Interventions can be integrated into the day-to-day running **Negatives** Often make additional demands on staff time Requires staff to understand the intervention and to change their behaviour	The majority of these initiatives are aimed at overcoming obstacles associated with the provision of oral nutrition support in institutional settings as well as supporting improved nutritional intake and do not lend themselves to use in free-living individuals. Exceptions to this are training which can be provided to carers and free-living individuals and the use of home-delivered meals. An emerging intervention is the use of electronic media (e.g. telemedicine) to facilitate compliance with nutritional prescriptions

the overall implications for healthcare, and the impact on outcomes such as hospital admissions, readmissions and length of stay is unknown [9]. In order to make informed choices about choice of oral nutritional support strategy, it is necessary to critically evaluate the evidence base for individual modalities.

4.3.4 Evidence for food-based options

Dietary counselling provided to individuals

Dietary advice or dietary counselling can be used to deliver food-based oral nutrition support interventions to individuals. A systematic review published in 2011 identified 12 RCTs of dietary advice compared with usual care conducted in 1053 patients from a range of different clinical backgrounds [10]. There were small but significant improvements in both energy intake and weight in groups receiving dietary advice compared with those receiving usual care (mean difference (MD) 258 kcal, 95% confidence interval (CI) 0.7–516, P=0.05 and MD 1.5 kg, 95% CI 0.3–2.6, P=0.01 respectively), although the heterogeneity was high in each of these analyses, suggesting that the studies might not be similar enough to justify combining. A series of subgroup analyses were undertaken to attempt to identify any subgroups who benefited from the intervention but that might have been obscured by combining all studies together, but no effects were seen in analyses according to clinical background, age, proportion of patients defined as malnourished or at nutritional risk, study quality and length of intervention [11]. No effects were seen on mortality hospital admissions and nutritional status, with the exception of mid-arm muscle circumference where data from two small studies suggested significant benefits (MD 0.5 cm, 95% CI –0.09 to 1.09, P=0.09) associated with receiving dietary advice compared with routine care.

The number of studies identified for these analyses was small, representing only 1053 participants, and the quality of studies was low, so it is not possible to be certain whether the effects

seen represent the real potential of this type of intervention. More studies are needed to confirm and expand on these findings [12].

The majority of included studies provided little detail on the intervention given beyond describing it as 'individualised'. One study used provision of additional snacks to individuals with cancer living in their own homes as the method of nutrition support [13] and another study used dietary advice to patients with chronic obstructive pulmonary disease (COPD) to recommend a range of methods of support, including inclusion of snacks between meals, addition of desserts to meals, change from low-fat to higher fat products, taking breakfast and energy-dense meal choices when away from home as well as the provision of milk powder to be used in fortification of food [14].

In the study by Dixon, compliance with the intervention, in patients with cancer, was assessed by research nurses on monthly visits to the patient's home [13]. By the ninth visit, the mean number of snacks taken was 13.5 (SD 3.1) per subject and subjects were noted to be mostly leaving puddings and baked goods. Supplementary snacks were fully consumed only 8% of the time and 82% of products had been partially consumed. In the study by Weekes et al., compliance was assessed over a 6-month period using 5-day food diaries and there was high compliance overall, with 87% of patients with COPD making some changes to their diet [15]. One hundred percent compliance was reported with advice to take additional snacks and in choosing energy-dense meals when away from home. The lowest levels of compliance were reported for advice to change from low-fat to higher fat alternatives. Compliance with advice on food fortification, assessed by 5-day dietary diaries, was high, with 79% of those being advised complying but the foods that patients chose to fortify varied considerably, with the majority adding milk powder to hot and cold drinks and breakfast products.

It is important to be mindful that the assessments of compliance reported above occurred in the context of trials and may not reflect compliance outside this controlled environment. More research is needed to provide understanding of patient compliance and satisfaction with different forms of nutrition support as well as the importance of regular review of prescriptions for nutrition interventions.

There are no systematic reviews examining costs or cost-effectiveness of dietary interventions. A small study of 59 patients with COPD compared the costs attributed to hospital admissions, LOS and hospitalisation in patients randomised to receive individualised dietary counselling and food fortification or usual care. Costs were lower in patients receiving the dietary intervention and patients experienced significantly greater weight gain and improvements in respiratory quality of life [16].

This group of 12 RCTs of dietary advice provides some evidence for the overall benefits to intake and nutritional status of this form of nutrition support but the evidence for functional, clinical and patient-centred benefits is lacking. In addition, there is insufficient detail about the different methods of food-based intervention to provide an evidence base for practice in this area.

4.3.5 Oral nutrition supplements

Oral nutrition supplements have been widely used to improve nutritional intake in patients from a range of clinical backgrounds and healthcare settings. The evidence for their benefit derives from more than 230 individual RCTs, as well as studies using non-randomised designs, and has been extensively summarised in systematic reviews and meta-analyses. A recent overview identified 31 systematic reviews of ONS-based interventions in undernourished and nutritionally vulnerable patients [17]. Eleven of 31 reviews were of studies in patients from all clinical backgrounds combined and 20 were in specific clinical conditions, including patients with dementia, hip fracture, liver disease, COPD, cancer, stroke, diabetes, kidney disease and perioperative patients. Outcomes were reported in meta-analyses (22 reviews) or in narrative only, and included nutritional, functional, clinical and healthcare-related outcomes. The results of findings from the meta-analyses and numerical summaries presented in the systematic reviews are summarised in Table 4.3.3.

Overall, six of 31 reviews reported on energy intake with four meta-analyses in patients from mixed clinical backgrounds (n=3), patients with COPD (n=1), stroke patients (n=1) and those with cancer (n=1). All found significantly greater energy intake ranging from mean between group differences of 234 to 430 kcal per day in those receiving ONS compared with those receiving usual care. Two reviews reported results in narrative with 66–68% of RCTs demonstrating significantly greater intake associated with receiving ONS [17,18]. Eleven of 31 reviews in groups from all clinical backgrounds combined (n=7) and in patients with COPD, dementia and liver cirrhosis included meta-analyses of data on weight change. All but two reviews, one in mixed groups of patients and one small review in patients with liver cirrhosis [18,19], demonstrated significantly greater weight gain, ranging from a MD of 0.72 to 3.5 kg in those receiving ONS compared with usual care. The wide range probably reflects differences in the length of intervention, follow-up and the clinical background of patients.

A small number of reviews reported on physical (n=5) and clinical function (n=7). Physical function was assessed by handgrip or quadriceps strength in groups of patients from mixed clinical backgrounds and in patients with COPD. The results were mixed and the analyses included small numbers of patients, with significant benefits ranging from a MD of 1.76 kg in a clinically mixed group of patients to a standardised mean difference of 0.57 kg in people with COPD (see Table 4.3.3). Significant reductions in total complications in groups that received ONS were seen in six of 10 analyses across a range of patient groups. The studies that reported no effect of ONS on total complications were in two reviews of patients with hip fracture and one small review of women undergoing surgery for ovarian cancer. Infectious complications were reported in four reviews (six analyses) and were reduced in patients with liver disease and perioperative patients.

Table 4.3.3 Summary of findings on nutritional, functional and healthcare outcomes for ONS from individual systematic reviews and meta-analyses

	Nutritional outcomes		Physical function	Clinical function		Mortality (reported in 17 studies, 25 analyses)	Outcomes of healthcare	
	Energy intake (reported in 6 reviews)	**Weight** (reported in 12 reviews, 13 analyses)	**Muscle strength** (reported in 5 reviews)	**Total complications** (reported in 8 reviews, 10 analyses)	**Infectious complications** (reported in 4 reviews, 6 analyses)		**LOS** (reported in 8 studies, 14 analyses)	**Hospital readmissions** (reported in 3 studies, 3 analyses)
All clinical backgrounds combined	**Significant improvement** 1 review (2 meta-analyses) 2 reviews (narrative summary, 66–68% of RCTs demonstrated improvement)	**Significant improvement** 8 of 9 reviews	**Significant improvement** 1 of 3 reviews	**Significant improvement** 6 of 7 analyses	**Significant improvement** 0 reviews	**Significant improvement** 7 of 16 analyses	**Significant improvement** 2 of 11 analyses (perioperative patients and mixed patients receiving high protein ONS)	**Significant improvement** 2 of 3 analyses
Specific clinical conditions	**Significant improvement** 3 reviews (COPD, stroke and cancer)	**Significant improvement** 3 of 4 analyses	**Significant improvement** 1 of 2 reviews	**Significant improvement** 0 of 3 analyses (hip fracture, liver disease and surgical)	**Significant improvement** 3 of 6 analyses (perioperative and liver disease n=2))	**Significant improvement** 0 of 9 analyses	**Significant improvement** 0 of 3 reviews and analyses	**No data**

COPD, chronic obstructive pulmonary disease; LOS, length of stay; ONS, oral nutritional supplement.

Outcomes related to healthcare included mortality, length of hospital stay and hospital readmissions and were reported in several reviews. There were significant reductions in mortality in only seven of 25 meta-analyses in patients from mixed clinical backgrounds and none of the eight analyses in individual patient groups. There was limited evidence of a benefit to LOS, with only two of 14 analyses reporting a significant reduction ranging from 2 to 3.8 days in perioperative patients and in groups receiving high-protein ONS. Few reviews conducted meta-analyses of hospital readmissions, with two of three analyses finding significantly fewer admissions in patients who received ONS.

Despite the large number of RCTs and systematic reviews to examine the benefits of ONS in the management of nutritionally vulnerable patients, the overall conclusions about benefit to outcomes remains patchy. There is consistent evidence of benefits to energy intake and body weight across a range of patient groups as well as evidence of reductions in total complications and infectious complications in some groups. The nutritional benefits reported frequently failed to translate into improvements in mortality (only seven of 24 analyses reporting benefit) and to LOS and few reviews have examined hospital readmissions with inconsistent findings. The small size of included studies and lack of power to estimate outcomes related to healthcare might in part explain the poor results in relation to this outcome.

Systematic reviews are seen as the highest level of evidence but examination of the quality of the identified reviews using the AMSTAR tool [20] revealed several with methodological weaknesses. Only nine of 31 reviews were judged to be of high quality, eight of which were published in the Cochrane Library. The remaining reviews had many aspects that might have led to publication bias resulting from biased study inclusion, and failure to identify all the relevant studies. In addition, although not a quality criterion specifically, scrutiny of the studies included in the reviews suggests wide variation in inclusion criteria, with some reviews including studies of food-based interventions

combined with ONS but attributing the benefits to ONS. Conclusions about use of ONS in nutritionally vulnerable patients must therefore be made with caution.

Evidence from the highest quality reviews suggested ONS were associated with reductions in mortality and improvements in weight in older people. Perioperative patients had fewer complications and reduced length of hospital stay and patients with liver disease experienced fewer infectious complications. ONS in stroke patients were associated with increased energy intake and reduced risk of pressure ulcers. It is of note that no adverse outcomes were identified.

One of the key issues raised in relation to use of ONS relates to compliance, with patients reporting taste fatigue, feelings of fullness and other gastrointestinal symptoms. A systematic review of 46 studies (4328 participants) estimated the pooled mean percent compliance as 78% with a range from 37% to 100%. Compliance was reported to be higher in studies in the community (81%) than in hospital (67%) [21]. The methods used to assess compliance varied across studies and included counts of ONS, patient report, use of food diaries and direct observations of consumption, highlighting the lack of gold standard and potential errors in assessment. As with food-based interventions, the information on compliance was all collected from patients included in trials. It is not known if the benefits observed in these situations can be translated to patients outside this setting. If patients fail to take ONS as prescribed then the benefits will be limited and careful attention and monitoring have been advised to maximise use [4].

Two recent systematic reviews have examined the costs and cost-effectiveness of ONS in both hospital and community settings. The authors cautiously concluded that ONS in both settings were associated with cost advantages and may be cost-effective because of their beneficial effects on clinical and healthcare outcomes [22,23]. These conclusions were based on small numbers of studies, few of which were prospective studies or had cost as a primary outcome. The groups of patients included in the studies were heterogeneous with patients from different clinical backgrounds, with varying nutritional status and the interventions included ONS given with and without dietary counselling, making it difficult to attribute all the effects to ONS alone. The included studies used different methodological designs, were of variable quality and in many the cost analyses were undertaken retrospectively. The authors acknowledge the considerable limitations of their analyses and suggest that more studies are needed, particularly examining the cost-effectiveness of ONS across the boundaries of care rather than in one setting in isolation. Given the types of policies currently driving the use of ONS and food-based interventions, studies that directly compare outcomes, particularly functional and patient-centred outcomes, as well as cost-effectiveness of these interventions are urgently needed.

4.3.6 Food-based interventions combined with oral nutrition supplements

An online survey of the practices of 207 dietitians in the UK on the provision of oral nutrition support interventions suggested that dietitians were significantly more likely to use food-based interventions combined with ONS rather than either intervention alone (62% versus 34% food-based alone and 4% ONS alone, P<0.001) (Gibbs et al., unpublished). The evidence for dietary advice given with ONS has been examined in a Cochrane systematic review [10]. Fourteen RCTs (1070 participants) from a variety of clinical backgrounds were identified although few studies reported the outcomes of interest. Significant improvements to energy intake and weight were observed (MD 213 kcal, 95% CI -0.9 to 426, P=0.05 and MD 2.2 kg, 95% CI 1.2–3.3, P<0.0001 respectively), although heterogeneity in the analyses was moderate to high. No difference in mortality was observed between groups. There were too few data on other outcomes to allow meaningful conclusions to be drawn.

4.3.7 Supportive strategies aiming to improve oral nutrition intake

The majority of research into the use of supportive nutrition interventions has been carried out in institutional settings. Seven recent systematic reviews have been undertaken in this area [24–30], examining the use of supportive interventions from a range of perspectives. Three reviews included studies from residential and long-term care settings only [27,29,30], one review was of studies in acute care [28] and two included studies from a range of settings [24,31]. Two reviews included only patients with dementia [29,30]. The level of evidence included varied, with four reviews including both randomised and non-randomised studies [26–28,30], the reviews by Whear et al. [29] and Kimber et al. [24] included only non-randomised studies and the review by Baldwin et al. [25] included only RCTs.

Overall, despite the number of studies and systematic reviews undertaken, there remains limited evidence to justify the use of supportive interventions. There is considerable variation in the extent to which review authors have been able to summarise and estimate the magnitude and direction of effect on outcomes. Five of the seven reviews do not undertake a meta-analysis [24,26,28–30], with the review by Vucea et al. [26] being a scoping review only. The review by Abbott et al. [27] of mealtime interventions in residential care identified 37 studies and undertook some analysis of data, concluding that there was some evidence of an effect of supportive interventions on nutritional intake but inconsistent evidence of whether this translated to benefits to weight. The review by Lui et al. included a narrative summary but also used a grading of strength of evidence (based on methodological bias within studies, amount of evidence and number of participants included in studies), which suggested moderate evidence of an effect of ONS on energy intake, weight and body mass index and of staff training on eating time and feeding difficulties [30]. The review by Baldwin et al. (25) explored the effects of similar interventions grouped together as well as an analysis of all interventions combined for data on mortality and weight. There was low-quality evidence of improved weight and survival in groups receiving supportive interventions compared with routine care but insufficient evidence on other outcomes to reach a conclusion [31].

The systematic reviews discussed above largely focused on the use of supportive interventions in institutional settings. Two studies were of training for carers of people with dementia living at home [32,33] and three studies of the provision of home-delivered meals were identified in the reviews by Gibbs et al. and Kimber et al. [24]. Small improvements to energy intake (ranging from a mean difference of 12 kcal/day after 6 months in one study and a mean change of 121 kcal per day after 8 weeks in the second study) [34,35] and weight (mean change 1.86, SD 5.3 in the intervention group and -1.04, SD 5.2 in the control group) [36] in groups receiving home-delivered meals and improvements to weight and body composition in people with dementia [33], but no differences were reported between groups in mortality and Activities of Daily Living. More studies are required to fully understand the benefits of these interventions in nutritionally vulnerable people living in their own homes.

4.3.8 Summary

The efficacy of oral nutrition support interventions has been examined for each strategy individually and some similarities and differences in outcomes identified. All interventions (food-based, ONS and supportive strategies) have been demonstrated to be effective at increasing nutritional intake and some aspects of nutritional status but there were differences between nutrition support strategies in terms of their effects on other outcomes, with some evidence of benefit to complications, clinical and healthcare outcomes in reviews of ONS that were not apparent in the reviews of food-based interventions or supportive interventions. Some of the differences most probably relate to differences in the size of the evidence base, with more than 230 RCTs of ONS compared with fewer than

30 studies of food-based interventions and around 40 RCTs of supportive interventions. Despite the stronger evidence for benefits of ONS to clinical and healthcare outcomes, there remains discordance between reviews and it is difficult to explain the variation.

No adverse events were reported for any mode of intervention. In practice, decisions about nutrition support are largely made after nutritional assessment, which takes into consideration the complex nature of the patient's usual habits, preferences and wishes as well as the complicated nature of the patient's environment. Greater attention is needed to characterise the benefits of oral nutrition support to aid these complex decisions. There is also a need for greater focus on functional and patient-centred outcomes.

References

1. Shiell A, Hawe P, Gold L. Complex interventions or complex systems? Implications for health economic evaluation. *BMJ* 2008; **336**(7656): 1281–1283.
2. Corish CA, Kennedy NP. Protein-energy undernutrition in hospital in-patients. *Br J Nutr* 2000; **83**(6): 575–591.
3. Norman K, Pichard C, Lochs H, Pirlich M. Prognostic impact of disease-related malnutrition. *Clin Nutr* 2008; **27**(1): 5–15.
4. Gandy J. Manual of Dietetic Practice. Hoboken: John Wiley & Sons, 2014.
5. Koretz RL. Death, morbidity and economics are the only end points for trials. *Proc Nutr Soc* 2005; **64**(3): 277–284.
6. Holdoway A, Brotherton A, Mason P, McGregor I, Pryke R. Managing malnutrition in the community. *Br J Gen Pract* 2013; **63**(610): 233–234.
7. Holdoway A. Strategies to identify and manage malnutrition in the community: a difference of opinion. A review of locally-developed oral nutrition support guidance across the UK. *CN Focus* 2012; **4**(1): 13–15.
8. Creighton S. Managing adult malnutrition in the community. The role for appropriate prescribing. *CN Focus* 2013; **5**(2): 43–45.
9. Stratton RJ, Elia M. Encouraging appropriate, evidence-based use of oral nutritional supplements. *Proc Nutr Soc* 2010; **69**(4): 477–487.
10. Baldwin C, Weekes CE. Dietary advice with or without oral nutritional supplements for disease-related malnutrition in adults. *Cochrane Database Syst Rev* 2011; **9**: CD002008.

11. Baldwin C, Weekes CE. Dietary counselling with or without oral nutritional supplements in the management of malnourished patients: a systematic review and meta-analysis of randomised controlled trials. *J Hum Nutr Diet* 2012; **25**(5): 411–426.

12. Baldwin C, Weekes CE, Campbell KL. Measuring the effectiveness of dietetic interventions in nutritional support. *J Hum Nutr Diet* 2008; **21**(4): 303–305.

13. Dixon J. Effect of nursing interventions on nutritional and performance status in cancer patients. *Nurs Res* 1984; **33**(6): 330–335.

14. Weekes CE, Emery PW, Elia M. Dietary counselling and food fortification in stable COPD: a randomised trial. *Thorax* 2009; **64**(4): 326–331.

15. Weekes CE, Pateras C, Maxted H, Elia M, Emery PW. Compliance with dietary counselling in outpatients with chronic obstructive pulmonary disease. *Clin Nutr* 2008; **3**(Suppl): 115–116.

16. Weekes CE, Emery PW, Elia M. Dietary counselling and food fortification in malnourished outpatients with chronic obstructive pulmonary disease; a post hoc cost analysis. Presented at ESPEN Conference, 2006.

17. Baldwin C, Weekes CE. What is the quality of the evidence supporting the role of oral nutritional supplements (ONS) in the management of malnutrition? *Clin Nutr* 2016; **35**(Suppl 1): OR07.

18. Ney M, Vandermeer B, van Zanten SJ, Ma MM, Gramlich L, Tandon P. Meta-analysis: oral or enteral nutritional supplementation in cirrhosis. *Aliment Pharmacol Ther* 2013; **37**(7): 672–679.

19. Stratton RJ, Elia M. A critical, systematic analysis of the use of oral nutritional supplements in the community. *Clin Nutr* 1999; **18**: 29–84.

20. Shea BJ, Grimshaw JM, Wells GA, Boers M, Andersson N, Hamel C, Porter AC, Tugwell P, Moher D, Bouter LM. Development of AMSTAR: a measurement tool to assess the methodological quality of systematic reviews. *BMC Med Res Methodol* 2007; **7**(1): 10.

21. Hubbard GP, Elia M, Holdoway A, Stratton RJ. A systematic review of compliance to oral nutritional supplements. *Clin Nutr* 2012; **31**(3): 293–312.

22. Elia M, Normand C, Laviano A, Norman K. A systematic review of the cost and cost effectiveness of using standard oral nutritional supplements in community and care home settings. *Clin Nutr* 2016; **35**(1): 125–137.

23. Elia M, Normand C, Norman K, Laviano A. A systematic review of the cost and cost effectiveness of using standard oral nutritional supplements in the hospital setting. *Clin Nutr* 2016; **35**(2): 370–380.

24. Kimber K, Gibbs M, Weekes CE, Baldwin C. Supportive interventions for enhancing dietary intake in malnourished or nutritionally at risk adults: a systematic review of nonrandomised studies. *J Hum Nutr Diet* 2015; **28**(6): 517–545.

25. Baldwin C, Kimber KL, M G, Weekes CE. Supportive interventions for enhancing intake in malnourished or nutritionally at-risk adults. *Cochrane Database Syst Rev* 2016; **12**: CD009840.

26. Vucea V, Keller HH, Ducak K. Interventions for improving mealtime experiences in long-term care. *J Nutr Gerontol Geriatr* 2014; **33**(4): 249–324.

27. Abbott RA, Whear R, Thompson-Coon J, Ukoumunne OC, Rogers M, Bethel A, Hemsley A, Stein K. Effectiveness of mealtime interventions on nutritional outcomes for the elderly living in residential care: a systematic review and meta-analysis. *Ageing Res Rev* 2013; **12**(4): 967–981.

28. Cheung G, Pizzola L, Keller H. Dietary, food service, and mealtime interventions to promote food intake in acute care adult patients. *J Nutr Gerontol Geriatr* 2013; **32**(3): 175–212.

29. Whear R, Abbott R, Thompson-Coon J, Bethel A, Rogers M, Hemsley A, Stahl-Timmins W, Stein K. Effectiveness of mealtime interventions on behavior symptoms of people with dementia living in care homes: a systematic review. *J Am Med Dir Assoc* 2014; **15**(3): 185–193.

30. Liu W, Cheon J, Thomas SA. Interventions on mealtime difficulties in older adults with dementia: a systematic review. *Int J Nurs Stud* 2014; **51**(1): 14–27.

31. Gibbs M, Baldwin C, Weekes CE, Kimber KL. Supportive interventions for enhancing dietary intake in malnourished or nutritionally at-risk adults. *Cochrane Database Syst Rev* 2016; **12**: CD009840.

32. Salvà A, Andrieu S, Fernandez E, Schiffrin EJ, Moulin J, Decarli B, Rojano-i-Luque X, Guigoz Y, Vellas B, NutriAlz Group. Health and nutrition promotion program for patients with dementia (NutriAlz): cluster randomized trial. *J Nutr Health Aging* 2011; **15**(10): 822–830.

33. Pivi GA, da Silva RV, Juliano Y, Novo NF, Okamoto IH, Brant CQ, Bertolucci PH. A prospective study of nutrition education and oral nutritional supplementation in patients with Alzheimer's disease. *Nutr J* 2011; **10**: 98.

34. Frongillo EA, Isaacman TD, Horan CM, Wethington E, Pillemer K. Adequacy of and satisfaction with delivery and use of home-delivered meals. *J Nutr Elder* 2010; **29**(2): 211–226.

35. Roy MA, Payette H. Meals-on-wheels improves energy and nutrient intake in a frail free-living elderly population. *J Nutr Health Aging* 2006; **10**(6): 554–560.

36. Kretser AJ, Voss T, Kerr WW, Cavadini C, Friedmann J. Effects of two models of nutritional intervention on homebound older adults at nutritional risk. *J Am Diet Assoc* 2003; **103**(3): 329–336.

Chapter 4.4

Enteral nutrition to prevent and treat undernutrition

Matthieu Joerger and Stéphane M. Schneider
Archet University Hospital, Nice, France

4.4.1 Introduction

Enteral nutrition (EN) is a nutritional therapy that delivers nutrition into the gastrointestinal (GI) tract, either through a nasal or oral tube, or through a GI stoma [1]. It provides many physiological, metabolic, safety and cost advantages over other methods of feeding. Enteral nutrition is used for patients who are unable to ingest sufficient food and/or oral nutritional supplements (ONS) orally with a functional accessible GI tract, or for whom oral intake is contraindicated (unconscious patients, unsafe swallow) [2]. The route and type of appliance used will depend on the individual circumstances of the patient. Most commonly, formulas that are nutritionally complete are administered via nasogastric or nasojejunal tubes (short term) or gastrostomy or jejunostomy tubes (long term) [3]. Specialised formulas also exist for patients with malabsorption, renal, intestinal or hepatic diseases, diabetes and in perioperative or intensive care units (ICU). A dietitian, nutritionist or nutrition support team can advise on the appropriate route of enteral nutrition and choice of formula and devise a suitable feeding regimen [3].

4.4.2 Enteral nutrition formulas

The main EN formulas available on the market can be distinguished by their degree of polymerization and their total energy content.

Polymeric formulas contain whole proteins, semi-elemental formulas contain small peptides and elemental formulas contain amino acids (Table 4.4.1) [4].

The choice of formula varies depending on the patient [4,5]. This must be tailored to the patient's specific needs, taking into account their disease, nutritional status, nutrient and water requirements, whether or not their GI tract is fully functional, the assumed duration of the nutrition, cost and specific features of the different forms available, the aggressiveness of the treatment regimen and/or the disease and the administration site for EN.

With patients outside the ICU and not at risk of refeeding syndrome, total intake should provide 25–35 kcal/kg/day, including 0.8–1.5 g protein/kg/day, and 30–35 mL fluid/kg, also accounting for additional losses from drains and fistulas [3]. However, the preferred approaches to calculating energy, protein and fluid requirements vary depending upon a variety of factors and are addressed within the chapters on requirements (Section 3) and specific clinical conditions (Section 5).

Fibre-rich formula

Dietary fibre is an important part of a healthy diet and it is commonly added to EN formulas [6], with potential benefits in GI tract function, gut health, immunity, blood glucose and serum lipid control. Fibres from a variety of sources, either alone or as part of a mixture, are added to

Advanced Nutrition and Dietetics in Nutrition Support, First Edition. Edited by Mary Hickson and Sara Smith.
© 2018 John Wiley & Sons Ltd. Published 2018 by John Wiley & Sons Ltd.

Table 4.4.1 Enteral nutrition formulations

	Description/ indications	Energy (kcal/mL)	Protein (% energy)	Fat (% energy)	Carbohydrate (% energy)	Osmolality (mOsm/kg)
Standard formula	No special requirements	1.0–1.2	15%	30%	55%	300–500
High-protein standard formula	Increased protein requirement	1.0–1.2	20%	30%	50%	300–500
High-energy formula (1.5 kcal/mL)	High energy requirements or fluid restriction	1.5	20%	30%	50%	500–650
High-energy formula (2 kcal/mL)	High energy requirements or fluid restriction	2.0	15%	40%	45%	450–800
Semi-elemental formula	Minimal fibre and other residue, protein as peptides	1.0	20%	10%	70%	320–520
Elemental formula	Minimal fibre and other residue, protein as free amino acids	1.0	15–20%	3–15% (varies widely between products)	70–85%	500–730

EN formulas. Fibres from different sources offer differing characteristics such as solubility, fermentability and viscosity [6,7].

The approach to EN has been changed by the possibility of incorporating different fibres into enteral formulas without aggravating the risk of tube obstruction. While in the early days of clinical nutrition, products used to contain fibre from a single source, present-day thinking is that blended fibres from multiple sources more closely resemble a regular diet and may provide a greater range of benefits for the patient (Table 4.4.2). Supplementation with single fibre sources, both soluble and insoluble, has been shown to cause GI side effects such as bloating, flatulence and abdominal pain. By combining multiple fibres in lower doses, it may be possible to achieve the desired benefits without exceeding the tolerance level for any one fibre. Furthermore, it emerged from a meta-analysis covering 51 studies on fibre-supplemented enteral formulas that fibre significantly reduced the incidence of diarrhoea in acute cases, especially in populations with a high baseline incidence of this condition [8]. However, the effect was significant only in patients not on the intensive care unit (ICU). The principal factor in these results was the presence of partially hydrolysed guar gum [9]. A meta-analysis and systematic review further indicated that fibre significantly reduced bowel frequency when baseline frequency was high and increased it when it was low, so that the presence of fibre is shown to have an important moderating effect [8].

Future studies will need to compare various mixed-fibre blends in order to determine the optimum fibre combinations and doses to produce the desired end-results in a range of patient populations.

Diabetes-specific formula

There is an increasing prevalence of diabetes across the globe, along with frequent insulin resistance, in patients under metabolic stress.

Table 4.4.2 Summary of current recommendations for use of fibre in enteral nutrition

1. Source	Recommendations
Fibre Consensus Panel	To prevent EN-induced diarrhoea in postsurgical and in critical ill patients, supplementing EN with partially hydrolysed guar gum is effective. (Recommendation A)
	Fermentable and viscous fibres (e.g. oat β-glucan) are effective for glycaemic control, but the available studies make it difficult to ascertain to what extent fibre supplementation contributes to the beneficial effects of the diabetes formulas. (No recommendation)
	Short-term studies showed that soy polysaccharides or soy polysaccharides combined with oat fibre increased daily stool weight and frequency. There is only one pilot study showing a beneficial effect of adding soy polysaccharides to control bowel habits in patients on long-term enteral nutrition. (Recommendation C)
European Society for Clinical Nutrition and Metabolism	A fibre intake of 15–30 g/day is advisable for patients receiving EN.
	In non-ICU patients or those requiring long-term EN, a mixture of bulking and fermentable fibre is the best approach.
	Dietary fibre can contribute to normalisation of GI tract function in elderly patients. In acute illness, fermentable fibre is effective in reducing diarrhoea in patients after surgery and in critically ill patients (guar gum and pectin are superior to soy polysaccharides).
Society for Critical Care Medicine and American Society for Parenteral and Enteral Nutrition	If there is evidence of diarrhoea, soluble fibre-containing or small peptide formulations may be utilised. (Grade E)
	Soluble fibre may be beneficial for the fully resuscitated, haemodynamically stable critically ill patient receiving EN who develops diarrhoea. Insoluble fibre should be avoided in all critically ill patients. Both soluble and insoluble fibre should be avoided in patients at high risk for bowel ischaemia or severe dysmotility. (Grade C)

EN, enteral nutrition; ICU, intensive care unit.
The guidelines referred to in this table use various grading systems to show the strength of the evidence supporting any given recommendation. For the precise meaning of grades used in any specific guideline, please refer to that document directly. Broadly speaking, grade A is strong evidence and grade C is weaker etc. The exact meaning of each classification should therefore be taken with reference to the original publication.
Source: Adapted from Klosterbuer et al. [7].

Standard formulas may compromise glycaemic control in these patients, due to rapid gastric emptying and rapid nutrient assimilation. For this reason, diabetes-specific formulas designed principally to achieve glycaemic control have been developed [6].

'Classic' diabetes-specific formulas contain fructose and starch as the main source of carbohydrates. Newer formulas have replaced part of the carbohydrates with monounsaturated fatty acids, up to 35% of total energy, and may also have additional dietary fibre [6]. These nutrients may facilitate glycaemic management by delaying gastric emptying (fat and fibre), delaying intestinal absorption of carbohydrate (fibre), and producing lower glycaemic responses (fructose). A high proportion of monounsaturated fatty acids may also have beneficial effects on lipid profiles.

A systematic review and meta-analysis examining the impact of oral or enteral diabetes-specific formulas showed a lower postprandial rise in blood glucose and peak blood glucose concentrations in patients with diabetes when diabetes-specific formulas were used [10]. There is no consistent effect on clinical outcomes, however, and their availability and use vary considerably across the world.

Immune-enhancing formula

Numerous clinical trials and meta-analyses have suggested benefits of immunonutrition. The immunonutrients (or pharmaconutrients) backed by some evidence include glutamine, arginine, nucleotides, ω-3 polyunsaturated fatty acids, some micronutrients and probiotics [11]. Immunonutrition comprises varying concentrations of all these ingredients but the ideal dosages are not well defined. There is neither a single indication for immunonutrition nor a universal immune-enhancing formula.

Immune-enhancing formula in pre-operative and peri-operative surgery

The European Society for Clinical Nutrition and Metabolism (ESPEN) has proposed enteral immunonutrition (arginine, ω-3 fatty acids and nucleotides) for undernourished patients preoperatively for major GI surgery, and perioperatively for oncology surgical patients. In both these situations, grade A level evidence demonstrates that immunonutrition reduces postoperative morbidity and length of stay [12].

A recent systematic review showed that perioperative administration of enteral arginine, ω-3 fatty acids, and nucleotides significanty reduced infection rate and length of stay in patients with upper and lower GI cancer surgery, albeit with no effect on mortality [13]. The most pronounced benefits of immunonutrition were found in subgroups of high-risk and undernourished patients. French clinical guidelines on perioperative nutrition recommend the use of the same postoperative pharmaconutrition in undernourished patients [14].

Immune-enhancing formula in critical illness

In contrast with the perioperative period, interest in immunonutrition in the ICU has steadily decreased over the years [15], due to the lack of benefit and in some cases harm resulting from its use. For example, arginine, a nitric oxide precursor, is now contraindicated in septic shock patients. On the other hand, emerging evidence has suggested that glutamine supplementation should be considered in patients with a critical illness associated with a catabolic response [16]. However, other evidence contradicts this opinion, such as the REDOX trial [17], which studied the effect of high-dose supplemental glutamine (intravenous and enteral) and antioxidants in critically ill ventilated patients with multiorgan failure, and showed an increased 28-day mortality in glutamine-supplemented patients. A systematic review including 3013 patients (ICU, burn and trauma patients) showed that immuno-modulating formulas reduced the number of secondary infections (odds ratio (OR) 0.63, 95% confidence interval (CI) 0.47–0.86) but had no effect on mortality or length of stay [18]. All three parameters were significantly lower only in ICU patients receiving fish oil; mortality (OR 0.42, 95% CI 0.26–0.68), secondary infections (OR 0.45, 95% CI 0.25–0.79) and length of stay (weighed mean difference -6.28 days, 95% CI -9.92 to -2.64 days). This suggests that, with the exception of immuno-modulating formulas containing a high concentration of fish oil, other immuno-modulating formulas have limited clinical benefits in critically ill ICU, burn or trauma patients.

Canadian clinical practice guidelines recommend the use of a standard, polymeric enteral formula to be initiated within 24–48 hours after admission to ICU [19]. Arginine-containing enteral products are not recommended, but products containing fish oil, borage oil and antioxidants should be considered for patients with acute respiratory distress syndrome, and glutamine-enriched formulas for patients with severe burns and trauma.

American guidelines for the provision and assessment of nutrition support therapy in the critically ill adult patient warrant the use of immune-enhancing formulas in well-defined populations (major elective surgery, trauma, burns, head and neck cancer, and critically ill patients on mechanical ventilation), caution being necessary in patients with severe sepsis (for surgical ICU patients grade A evidence; for medical ICU patients grade B evidence) [11]. Where ICU patients do not meet the criteria for immune-modulating formulations, they should receive standard enteral formulations (grade B evidence).

Liquidised food

The practice of using liquidised food for EN, or the administration through a patient's feeding tube of food that has been puréed using a blender, has recently gained popularity despite the availability of commercially prepared, nutritionally complete formulas [20]. The advice given in the UK is that commercially prepared nutritionally complete formulations be administered as recommended by the tube manufacturer, following a full process of dietetic assessment and review. Providing all patients with liquidised meals would be regarded as a retrograde step and is not advocated by the British Dietetic Association. This mode of nutrition is not seen as a routine alternative to commercially available formulas; interest in liquidised food largely stems from parents or is explored as a possibility for children intolerant to EN.

This mode of nutrition may be used in children with gastrostomy tubes who suffer retching, gagging or vomiting with their current enteral formula but who are growing satisfactorily. It is not an appropriate technique for infants under 6 months, jejunally fed patients, immunocompromised patients or those intolerant to bolus feeding with a strict volume limit. In addition, potential patients must be medically stable, gaining weight satisfactorily and with a well-healed gastrostomy site (Box 4.4.1).

There are clearly complex issues in responding to patients' or carers' requests for liquidised feeding, including assessing patient suitability, the risk to the patient, the medical and dietetic support required and the associated professional and ethical issues of providing this support. Even when the patient's family has requested a move to liquidised food, carers (including family members) must be thoroughly trained in its use before any decision is made to change the formula.

The British Dietetic Association has developed a practice toolkit for patients or carers

---

Box 4.4.1   Important elements to consider when assessing patient suitability for liquidised food as a form of enteral nutrition

Organisational considerations
- Patient, parent or carer requests liquidised food as enteral nutrition
- Family has adequate financial and material resources (e.g. blender, refrigeration, access to ingredients including clean water supply and multivitamins)
- Family displays time, motivation, interest and understanding of commitment required
- Registered dietitian is available for oversight, including recipe development and patient monitoring

Clinical considerations
- Patient is at least 6 months old
- Patient is medically stable with appropriate weight gain
- Patient is not immunocompromised or undergoing immunosuppressive therapy

Nutritional considerations
- Patient does not have multiple food allergies
- Patient does not require continuous feeding
- Tube is a gastrostomy tube (not jejeunostomy)
- Gastrostomy site is well healed
- Tube is at least 14 French in diameter
- Patient does not have severe volume limitation (e.g. delayed gastric emptying, fluid restriction)
- Energy requirements can be met using the liquidised diet

Source: Adapted from Heyland et al. [19].

requesting liquidised food via gastrostomy tube. This includes details on patient selection, risk assessment, preparing, storing and delivery of liquidised food and patient assessment and monitoring [21].

Complications can include tube blockage (prevented by using a specialised blender, a tube size 14 French or higher and flushing the tube), poor volume tolerance and bacterial contamination [22]. The latter can be prevented by, among other things, using uncontaminated water and thorough cooking and correct refrigeration of ingredients, as well as proper flushing between food boluses. Any liquidised food not used within 24 hours of being made must be discarded.

4.4.3 Disease-specific formula

The future of EN depends in part on the development of specific products for a disorder or a given clinical situation. These disease-specific formulas have been developed for several conditions. Well-designed clinical trials may or may not be available (mostly not). Moreover, many of the trials have been done with 'cocktails' of active nutritional ingredients, making it difficult to identify the effective intervention. Pharmaceutical effects are claimed for many specialty enteral formulas (e.g. reduced infections, reduced time on the ventilator) but they also charge pharmaceutical prices (8–10 times more expensive than standard formulas). Moreover, enteral formulas are classed as medical foods, not drugs, and are regulated differently. It is up to the clinician to evaluate the evidence that supports the claims regarding these disease-specific formulas.

Crohn's disease

Artificial nutrition is one of the treatments for Crohn's disease but is less used in adults than in children, and is mostly preferred in situations of undernutrition and corticosteroid resistance.

Of 15 relevant trials comparing different EN formulations for the treatment of active Crohn's disease, 11 compared one (or more) elemental formula with a non-elemental one, three compared enteral diets of similar protein composition but different fat composition, and one compared non-elemental diets differing only in glutamine enrichment [23]. The result of a meta-analysis of 10 trials covering 334 patients was that the efficacy of elemental versus non-elemental formulas showed no difference (OR 1.10, 95% CI 0.69–1.75). Subgroup analyses revealed no statistically significant differences between elemental, semi-elemental and polymeric formulas.

Guidelines from ESPEN state that in the treatment of active Crohn's disease, free amino acid, peptide-based and whole-protein formulas have no significantly different effects on disease activity, and free amino acid or peptide-based formulas are not generally recommended [5]. Moreover, modified enteral formulas (fat modified, ω-3, fatty acids, glutamine, TGF-β enriched) are not recommended because no clear benefits have been shown (grade A). In adults, EN should be employed as the sole therapy in the acute phase mainly when treatment with corticosteroids is not feasible, and combined therapy (EN plus drugs) should be employed in undernourished patients as well as in those with inflammatory stenosis of the GI tract EN is regarded as the first-line therapy for children with Crohn's disease.

Liver disease

'Liver-specific' formulas contain reduced aromatic amino acids and increased branched chain amino acids (BCAA), therefore reducing the risk of hepatic encephalopathy while carrying a lower splanchnic extraction. However, they are more expensive and often lower in protein than standard formulas.

For alcoholic steatohepatitis, whole-protein formulas are generally recommended (grade C) and high-energy formulas are advised in patients with ascites (grade C) [24]. Use of BCAA-enriched formulas is recommended for patients with hepatic encephalopathy arising during EN (grade A). For liver cirrhosis, whole-protein formulas are generally recommended (grade C) [24].

Short-bowel syndrome

Although this is a typical indication for parenteral nutrition (PN), continuous additional EN in limited amounts can be used, depending on enteral fluid loss, to improve intestinal adaptation (grade C) [5]. No specific substrate composition is required, but peptide-based formulas (elemental and semi-elemental) are frequently used. Recommendations concerning the quantity and type of fat are controversial. Patients with an intact jejunum may benefit from a modified fat regimen, replacing some long-chain triglycerides with 20–60 g medium-chain triglycerides per day. For patients with a jejunostomy, the relative proportions of carbohydrate and fat are not significant. A regimen to accelerate intestinal adaptation with recombinant growth hormone, glutamine and special formula [25] (low fat, high carbohydrates) is not generally recommended because of inconclusive results (grade C) [5].

Renal failure

Patients with renal failure are an extremely heterogeneous population, and consequently their nutritional requirements may differ widely. Nutritional status is one of the main factors determining outcomes.

In acute renal failure, monitoring micronutrient status is crucially important because excessive supplementation may result in toxicity. Standard formulas are suitable for the majority of patients (grade C) and were originally developed in an effort to delay the need for dialysis as long as possible [26]. Typically, they are energy-dense (2.0 kcal/mL) products with relatively low protein concentrations and modified electrolytes and are generally too low in protein for dialysed and acutely ill patients [27].

In conservatively treated chronic renal failure, energy intake of 35 kcal/kg/day is associated with better nitrogen balance and is recommended in stable chronic renal failure for patients in the ideal body weight range ± 10% (grade A). Moreover, essential amino acids and ketoanalogues, in association with very low-protein formulas, are recommended to preserve renal function (grade B) [26].

Chronic obstructive pulmonary disease

Enteral nutrition in combination with exercise and anabolic pharmacotherapy has the potential to improve nutritional status and function. In stable chronic obstructive pulmonary disease, there is no additional advantage of disease-specific low-carbohydrate, high-fat ONS compared to standard high-protein or high-energy ONS [28].

4.4.4 Administering enteral nutrition

Starter regimen

Traditionally, patients were initially started on low-volume and diluted feeding regimens and gradually built up to a full-volume, full-strength diet. This was thought to reduce the incidence of bloating and abdominal pain. However, often the only result of such 'build-up' diets was to provide inadequate nitrogen and energy. Typically, EN is now introduced at gradually increasing rates on the first day of feeding, with the aim of achieving full (or nearly full) requirements at the end of the first day. EN is usually begun at a low rate (about 50–75 mL/h) and increased in stages to about 100–150 mL/h after tolerance is demonstrated. Bolus feeding may cause more problems with bloating and diarrhoea [29].

The only indication of a starter diet is in patients at risk of refeeding syndrome. Excessively fast refeeding may cause profound metabolic disturbances (hypophosphataemia, hypomagnesaemia, hypokalaemia, hyperglycaemia, hypovitaminosis B1), with a resulting failure of various organs in variable degrees of severity. Prescription of nutrition support for these patients should not exceed a maximum limit of 10 kcal/kg/day, levels being increased gradually to meet or exceed full needs by 4–7 days [3].

Choice of route

The ASPEN enteral nutrition practice recommendations state that EN systems can be classified into two categories: one is a short-term nutrition system lasting for less than 4 weeks in the acute phase of disease, whereas the second is a long-term EN system lasting over 4 weeks at the chronic stage (gastrostomy and jejunostomy) [2]. The position of the distal end will depend on the risk of aspiration.

Short-term feeding (up to 4 weeks)

A nasogastric tube remains the reference route of administration for EN when this is planned for a period of under a month (Figure 4.4.1). This technique involves the insertion of a fine-bore feeding tube (French gauge 5–9) via the nose into the stomach. Bolus or pump feeding can be used with a nasogastric tube [3]. The major risk is of bronchial aspiration [1]. In order to prevent this, the distal tip of the tube should be confirmed as correctly positioned in the prepyloric region of the gastric antrum. Confirmation of this position can be either via an x-ray or pH paper indicating pH less than 5.5.

Intrajejunal administration of EN considerably reduces the risk of aspiration in patients who are at very high aspiration risk [1,3]. Because of this, it should be reserved for patients who are at high risk of bronchial aspiration. A nasojejunal route for EN on the ICU is not required except where there is gastric feeding intolerance, according to ASPEN (grade B) and ESPEN (grade C) guidelines [2].

Long-term feeding (longer than 4 weeks)

Percutaneous endoscopic gastrostomy (PEG) has become the reference route for EN lasting for more than 4 weeks (see Figure 4.4.1). PEG is used earlier than 4 weeks in specific situations: when upper aerodigestive tract cancers requiring radiochemotherapy are diagnosed, at the onset of weight loss in a patient with amyotrophic lateral sclerosis and after 2–4 weeks following a cerebrovascular accident in a patient with persistent dysphagia.

Patients unable to swallow safely (e.g. dysphagia following stroke) or to consume sufficient energy and nutrients orally should have an initial 2–4-week trial of nasogastric EN [2,3]. Surgical jejunostomy should be preferred for long-term postpyloric EN as this reduces the risk of bronchial aspiration and the incidence of aspiration pneumonia [30].

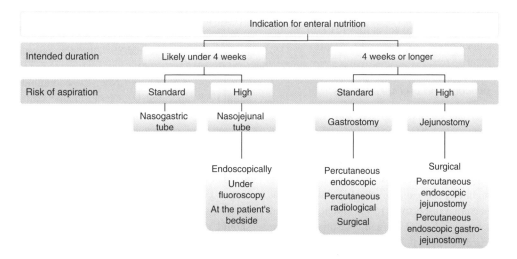

Figure 4.4.1 Gastrointestinal access for enteral nutrition. Source: Adapted from Anker et al. [28] with permission from Elsevier

Choice of delivery mode

The delivery mode can be chosen according to the needs of the patient [29]. A relatively large amount of formula can be delivered several times per day (intermittent or bolus feeding) or smaller amounts continuously during the day (continuous feeding). A patient may also start with continuous feeding and gradually move to intermittent feeding [2,31].

Intermittent or bolus feeding

This involves the delivery of 100–300 mL over a period of 10–30 minutes and can be given 4–6 times a day depending on the patient's individual feeding regime. Administration can be with a syringe but using only the barrel as a funnel to allow the formula to infuse using gravity. The plunger from the syringe should not be used to push formula through. Bolus feeding can also be administrated with bolus feed gravity sets. If there are any signs of intolerance, then another feeding method should be sought. Flushing feeding tubes with 30 mL of water before and after intermittent feedings is recommended by ASPEN adult guidelines [2]. Intermittent feedings are more often used in stable patients. This promotes greater independence and is suitable for ambulatory use, consistent with physical activity. It is therefore a good indication for patients who have preserved their ability to move about and who are at lower risk of aspiration pneumonia.

Continuous and cyclical infusions

Pumps can be set to deliver formula at rates between 5 and 500 mL/h, within 10% accuracy, for adults and this can be constant over 24 hours or with a break of a few hours. When continuous feeding is administered only during the daytime or nightime, it is called cyclical feeding (diurnal or nocturnal respectively) [32]. Cyclical EN can restore physiological alternating fasting-nutrition. The recommended flow rate is 200–250 mL/h during the day and 100–120 mL/h at night.

Continuous feeding should be considered in the initial phase of refeeding in patients with severe protein energy undernutrition (at risk of refeeding syndrome), GI disorders or jejunal administration. Continuous feeding should also be used in patients at high risk of aspiration pneumonia and when slow rates of enteral formula are required, such as in the neonatal population or in a patient unable to tolerate large volumes of formula [2]. It has been established that some GI complications (e.g. diarrhoea) are less common if nutrients are administered slowly and continuously, rather than as a bolus. Flushing feeding tubes with 30 mL of water every 4 hours during continuous infusion is recommended by ASPEN adult guidelines [2].

Enteral nutrition in the community

Home EN is used principally for providing nutrition to patients with a functional intestinal tract but a degree of oropharyngeal or oesophageal failure [31]. An ESPEN survey of home EN in Europe has shown that 49% of all patients started on home EN in 1998 had underlying neurological problems (usually cerebrovascular accidents) and 27% had head and neck cancer; 85% of these patients were suffering from dysphagia [33]. EN is also sometimes used to treat patients with anorexia and those with energy demands exceeding their ability to take nutrition orally. Most patients receiving home EN have long-term feeding tubes sited; in the European study, 58% of patients were fed through a PEG tube and 29% through nasoenteral tubes.

Patients who receive EN in the community should be supported by a co-ordinated multidisciplinary team (dietitians, district, care home or homecare company nurses, general practitioners) [3]. A close liaison between the multidisciplinary team, patients and caregivers is mandatory in respect of diagnoses, prescriptions, practical arrangements and potential problems. Such patients and their carers should receive an individualised care plan setting out the overall objectives, as well as a monitoring plan, training and information on the management of tubes, delivery systems and regimen, describing all procedures for setting up feeding, using infusion pumps, and all likely risks and ways of troubleshooting common problems [34]. They should also be given an instruction manual containing both routine and emergency telephone numbers so that they are able to contact a healthcare professional who understands the needs and potential problems of people on home EN, plus arrangements for delivery of equipment, supplies and formula, with appropriate contact details for any home-care company involved [3].

4.4.5 Outcomes of patients treated with enteral nutrition

Clinical outcomes

Undernutrition is linked to poor clinical outcomes. Systematic reviews and meta-analyses have high-lighted the advantages of EN in patients suffering from, or at risk of, undernutrition (Table 4.4.3)

[35]. Meta-analysis of trials with various patient groups suggests that mortality rates (OR 0.48, 95% CI 0.30–0.78) and complication rates (OR 0.50, 95% CI 0.35–0.70) are significantly lower with EN than with patients receiving routine care [36,37]. They have also indicated fewer complications with EN in those undergoing GI surgery compared with routine care or PN.

Nutrition, costs and economic benefits

Most literature on undernutrition has concentrated on the clinical or health consequences. Little attention has been given to the economic implications [38]. This may be because it is hard to set a monetary value on the physical and psychological manifestations of undernutrition. It can increase healthcare costs by delaying recovery and rehabilitation and increase the risk of medical complications. Action on nutrition

Table 4.4.3 Improvements in outcome with enteral nutrition in benign and malignant disease

Patient group	Significant benefits to clinical and functional outcome with EN from randomised controlled trials
Burns	Fewer wound infections
Chronic obstructive pulmonary disease	Improved maximal expiratory pressure and sustained inspiratory pressure (endurance)
Critically ill/trauma	Lower number of infective complications
	Attenuation of increases in intestinal permeability
	Improved immune function
Gastrointestinal surgery	Earlier return of gastrointestinal function
	Lower rate of reoperations
	Lower mortality
	Attenuation of increases in gut permeability
	Improved wound healing rate
	Lower rate of postoperative complications, including infective complications
	Shorter length of stay
	Less use of parenteral nutrition
Liver disease	Improved liver function
	Lower mortality rate
	Lower complication rate, including viral complications
Malignancy	Improved physical and emotional functioning and dyspnoea symptoms
Orthopaedics	Shorter rehabilitation time
	Shorter length of stay in very thin patients

Source: Adapted from Stratton et al. [35].

has the potential to provide cost-effective preventive care and treatment. However, while limited data exist on the economic and other effects of such action, the cost of disease-related undernutrition in the United Kingdom is established at a figure well over £7.3 billion per year [38].

In a US cost-effectiveness study [39], the authors set out to describe the clinical and economic implications that might result from greater use of EN in critically ill adults. The results demonstrate that the administration of immune-modulating substrates preoperatively or perioperatively or upon admission to hospital could be an important cost reduction strategy. The far lower rate of postoperative or postadmission complications translates into significant cost savings and improved cost-effectiveness compared with the alternative (standard enteral formulas). The net cost savings for the medical patient (after taking the increased costs of administering an immune-modulating formula into account) amount to US$2066. The result of the same calculations for surgical and trauma patients yielded US$688 and US$308 net cost savings per patient respectively. This study shows that specialised nutritional formulations are a cost-effective way for hospitals to improve clinical outcomes while cutting resource consumption and total cost.

The authors of a clinical and economic evaluation of EN set out to estimate the costs and effectiveness of greater use of EN compared with PN and other therapies for the treatment of critically ill adult patients in the US [40]. Including data on costs per adverse event and costs per inpatient day, they calculated the potential resultant savings for each patient switched from PN to EN therapy. Compared to PN, EN savings from reduced adverse event risks average nearly US$1500 per patient; savings from reduced hospital length of stay amount to nearly US$2500 per patient. Moving 10% of parenterally treated adult patients in the US to EN would save US$35 million annually owing to fewer adverse events, and another US$57 million through shorter hospital stays. Evidence of the benefits, both clinical and economic, achieved through EN bears out the ASPEN guidelines advocating its use wherever possible in critically ill hospital patients [40].

Notes

The guidelines referred to throughout this chapter use various grading systems to show the strength of the evidence supporting any given recommendation. For the precise meaning of the grades used in any specific guideline, please refer to that document directly. Broadly speaking, grade A is strong evidence and grade C is weaker. The exact meaning of each classification should therefore be taken with reference to the original publication.

References

1. Lloyd DA, Powell-Tuck J. Artificial nutrition: principles and practice of enteral feeding. *Clin Colon Rectal Surg* 2004; **17**(2): 107–118.
2. Bankhead R, Boullata J, Brantley S, et al. Enteral nutrition practice recommendations. *J Parenter Enteral Nutr* 2009; **33**(2): 122–167.
3. National Institute for Health and Clinical Excellence. Nutrition Support for Adults: Oral Nutrition Support, Enteral Tube Feeding and Parenteral Nutrition. NICE Clinical Guideline 32. www.nice.org.uk/guidance/CG32 (accessed 2 September 2017).
4. Sharma K, Joshi I. Formulation of standard (Nutriagent std) and high protein (Nutriagent protein plus) ready to reconstitute enteral formula feeds. *Int J Sci Tech Res* 2014; **3**(5): 28–35.
5. Lochs H, Dejong C, Hammarqvist F, et al. ESPEN guidelines on enteral nutrition: gastroenterology. *Clin Nutr* 2006; **25**(2): 260–274.
6. Lochs H, Allison SP, Meier R, et al. Introductory to the ESPEN guidelines on enteral nutrition: terminology, definitions and general topics. *Clin Nutr* 2006; **25**(2): 180–186.
7. Klosterbuer A, Roughead ZF, Slavin J. Benefits of dietary fiber in clinical nutrition. *Nutr Clin Pract* 2011; **26**(5): 625–635.
8. Elia M, Engfer MB, Green CJ, Silk DB. Systematic review and meta-analysis: the clinical and physiological effects of fibre-containing enteral formulae. *Aliment Pharmacol Ther* 2008; **27**(2): 120–145.
9. Whelan K, Schneider SM. Mechanisms, prevention, and management of diarrhea in enteral nutrition. *Curr Opin Gastroenterol* 2011; **27**(2): 152–159.

10. Elia M, Ceriello A, Laube H, Sinclair AJ, Engfer M, Stratton RJ. Enteral nutritional support and use of diabetes-specific formulas for patients with diabetes: a systematic review and meta-analysis. *Diabetes Care* 2005; **28**(9): 2267–2279.

11. Martindale RG, McClave SA, Vanek VW, et al. Guidelines for the provision and assessment of nutrition support therapy in the adult critically ill patient: Society of Critical Care Medicine and American Society for Parenteral and Enteral Nutrition: executive summary. *Crit Care Med* 2009; **37**(5): 1757–1761.

12. Weimann A, Braga M, Harsanyi L, et al. ESPEN guidelines on enteral nutrition: surgery including organ transplantation. *Clin Nutr* 2006; **25**(2): 224–244.

13. Braga M, Wischmeyer PE, Drover J, Heyland DK. Clinical evidence for pharmaconutrition in major elective surgery. *J Parenter Enteral Nutr* 2013; **37**(5 Suppl): 66S–72S.

14. Chambrier C, Sztark F, Societe Francophone de nutrition clinique et metabolism, Societe francaise d'anesthesie et reanimation. French clinical guidelines on perioperative nutrition. Update of the 1994 consensus conference on perioperative artificial nutrition for elective surgery in adults. *J Visc Surg* 2012; **149**(5): e325–336.

15. Kreymann KG, Berger MM, Deutz NE, et al. ESPEN guidelines on enteral nutrition: intensive care. *Clin Nutr* 2006; **25**(2): 210–223.

16. McClave SA, Martindale RG, Vanek VW, et al. Guidelines for the provision and assessment of nutrition support therapy in the adult critically ill patient: Society of Critical Care Medicine (SCCM) and American Society for Parenteral and Enteral Nutrition (A.S.P.E.N.). *J Parenter Enteral Nutr* 2009; **33**(3): 277–316.

17. Heyland D, Muscedere J, Wischmeyer PE, et al. A randomized trial of glutamine and antioxidants in critically ill patients. *N Engl J Med* 2013; **368**(16): 1489–1497.

18. Marik PE, Zaloga GP. Immunonutrition in critically ill patients: a systematic review and analysis of the literature. *Intens Care Med* 2008; **34**(11): 1980–1990.

19. Heyland DK, Dhaliwal R, Drover JW, Gramlich L, Dodek P. Canadian clinical practice guidelines for nutrition support in mechanically ventilated, critically ill adult patients. *J Parenter Enteral Nutr* 2003; **27**(5): 355–373.

20. Johnson TW, Spurlock A, Pierce L. Survey study assessing attitudes and experiences of pediatric registered dietitians regarding blended food by gastrostomy tube feeding. *Nutr Clin Pract* 2015; **30**(3): 402–405.

21. British Dietetic Association. Practice Toolkit: Liquidised Food via Gastrostomy Tube. www.bda. uk.com/professional/practice/clinical_practice_ guidance/bda_clinical_policy_state (accessed 2 September 2017).

22. Pentiuk S, O'Flaherty T, Santoro K, Willging P, Kaul A. Pureed by gastrostomy tube diet improves gagging and retching in children with fundoplication. *J Parenter Enteral Nutr* 2011; **35**(3): 375–379.

23. Zachos M, Tondeur M, Griffiths AM. Enteral nutritional therapy for induction of remission in Crohn's disease. *Cochrane Database Syst Rev* 2007; **1**: CD000542.

24. Plauth M, Cabre E, Riggio O, et al. ESPEN guidelines on enteral nutrition: liver disease. *Clin Nutr* 2006; **25**(2): 285–294.

25. Kumpf VJ. Pharmacologic management of diarrhea in patients with short bowel syndrome. *J Parenter Enteral Nutr* 2014; **38**(1 Suppl): 38S–44S.

26. Cano N, Fiaccadori E, Tesinsky P, et al. ESPEN guidelines on enteral nutrition: adult renal failure. *Clin Nutr* 2006; **25**(2): 295–310.

27. Stratton RJ, Bircher G, Fouque D, et al. Multinutrient oral supplements and tube feeding in maintenance dialysis: a systematic review and meta-analysis. *Am J Kidney Dis* 2005; **46**(3): 387–405.

28. Anker SD, John M, Pedersen PU, et al. ESPEN guidelines on enteral nutrition: cardiology and pulmonology. *Clin Nutr* 2006; **25**(2): 311–318.

29. Stroud M, Duncan H, Nightingale J. Guidelines for enteral feeding in adult hospital patients. *Gut* 2003; **52**(Suppl 7): vii1–vii12.

30. Schneider SM, Barnoud D, Bouteloup C, et al. Enteral access techniques in adults. *Nutr Clin Metab* 2009; **23**(3): 168–169.

31. Cawsey SI, Soo J, Gramlich LM. Home enteral nutrition: outcomes relative to indication. *Nutr Clin Pract* 2010; **25**(3): 296–300.

32. Hébuterne X, Broussard JF, Rampal P. Acute renutrition by cyclic enteral nutrition in elderly and younger patients. *JAMA* 1995; **273**(8): 638–643.

33. Hébuterne X, Bozzetti F, Moreno Villares JM, et al. Home enteral nutrition in adults: a European multicentre survey. *Clin Nutr* 2003; **22**(3): 261–266.

34. CREST. A Model for Managing Enteral Tube Feeding. Belfast: CREST, 2004. www.irspen.ie/ wp-content/uploads/2014/10/CREST_A_model_ for_managing_enteral_tube_feeding.pdf (accessed 2 September 2017).

35. Stratton RJ, Green CJ, Elia M. Evidence base for enteral tube feeding. In: Stratton RJ, Green CJ, Elia M, editors. Disease-Related Malnutrition: An Evidence-Based Approach to Treatment. Wallingford: CABI, 2003, pp. 237–275.

36. Braunschweig CL, Levy P, Sheean PM, Wang X. Enteral compared with parenteral nutrition: a meta-analysis. *Am J Clin Nutr* 2001; **74**(4): 534–542.
37. Thomson A. The enteral vs parenteral nutrition debate revisited. *J Parenter Enteral Nutr* 2008; **32**(4): 474–481.
38. Elia M. Nutrition and health economics. *Nutrition* 2006; **22**(5): 576–578.
39. Strickland A, Brogan A, Krauss J, Martindale R, Cresci G. Is the use of specialized nutritional formulations a cost-effective strategy? A national database evaluation. *J Parenter Enteral Nutr* 2005; **29**(1 Suppl): S81–91.
40. Cangelosi MJ, Auerbach HR, Cohen JT. A clinical and economic evaluation of enteral nutrition. *Curr Med Res Opin* 2011; **27**(2): 413–422.

Chapter 4.5

Parenteral nutrition to prevent and treat undernutrition

Ronit Das¹ and Timothy Bowling²
¹Royal Derby Hospital, Derby, UK
²Nottingham University Hospitals NHS Trust, Nottingham, UK

4.5.1 Indications for parenteral nutrition

Artificial nutrition support is appropriate in any situation in which a patient's nutritional needs become greater than their receptive or absorptive ability. Enteral nutrition is usually the preferred route [1]. Enteral nutrition has fewer side effects, it is more physiological, avoids systemic mineral deposition and is not immunosuppressive. There is additional evidence that enteral nutrition promotes gut mucosal integrity and may prevent bacterial translocation [2]. Enteral nutrition is also cheaper in terms of formulation and access.

When the gastrointestinal tract is not available or accessible, nutrition can be provided by the parenteral route (parenteral nutrition or PN). Although more invasive, if managed appropriately, it is safe [3]. Common indications for PN are set out in Box 4.5.1 [4].

4.5.2 Routes of parenteral nutrition

Central venous access for PN delivery is now the clinical standard. Previous use of peripheral venous access for short-term nutritional delivery resulted in unacceptable rates of local complications, including site infection and thrombophlebitis. Central access in the form of peripherally inserted central catheters (PICC), subclavian or internal jugular lines has now become standard. Long-term PN utilising PICC and tunnelled subclavian lines is most common [4,5].

The central venous catheter needs to be placed in a sterile and aseptic manner. Following the initial appropriate placement, a strict 'clean' technique must be adhered to during accessing and maintenance.

A PN catheter should not be used for any purpose other than PN delivery. The exception to this is the critical care patient requiring venous access for various reasons (e.g. nutrition, antibiotics, inotropic support) with multilumen lines. In such situations, one lumen should be used exclusively for PN. Dressing changes should be at least every 48 hours. Patients and carers should be educated to recognise the initial stages of infection or complications. In addition to this, patients should have ready access to PN-specific medical services if nutrition support is being delivered in the community [5].

4.5.3 Formulation of parenteral nutrition

There are multiple ready-made 'standard' PN formulations of varying nutrient content. The challenge over the last two decades has been whether novel substrates should be added to 'standard' PN formulations to improve clinical outcomes and cost-effectiveness. There have been many studies looking especially at lipids

Advanced Nutrition and Dietetics in Nutrition Support, First Edition. Edited by Mary Hickson and Sara Smith.
© 2018 John Wiley & Sons Ltd. Published 2018 by John Wiley & Sons Ltd.

Box 4.5.1   Indications for parenteral nutrition

Short term feeding (<28 days)
Non-functioning GI tract, e.g. prolonged ileus, intra-abdominal malignancy
Proximal gut fistula
Preoperatively only if severely undernourished (e.g. BMI <17 kg/m^2) and oral/enteral feeding not possible
Postoperatively only when oral or enteral feeding is contraindicated
Where requirements cannot be fully met orally/enterally, e.g. multiorgan failure, major trauma, burns
Postchemotherapy mucositis

Long-term feeding (>28 days)
Following extensive bowel resection, e.g. Crohn's disease, gut infarction
Extensive Crohn's with malabsorption
High-output fistula
Radiation enteritis
Motility disorders, e.g. pseudo-obstruction, visceral myopathy or neuropathy

Source: Reproduced from Jones [4] with permission of BAPEN.

---

and protein sources, but most have been small and with heterogeneous patient groups, mainly in the context of critical care and surgery, making results difficult to interpret. This has necessitated a number of meta-analyses to synthesise the plethora of information, in an attempt to clarify a confusing area of clinical practice. The jury, however, remains very much out as to whether these activities are proving effective [6,7].

Lipids

Intravenous fat emulsions typically provide 20–40% of the daily energy requirement in PN. Lipids are essential energy-dense molecules (9 kcal/g). Lipid emulsions, as part of PN, are effective in maintaining body weight [8], even in high catabolic states such as malignancy, sepsis and pancreatitis-related systemic inflammatory response syndrome (SIRS). While essential in preventing fatty acid deficiency and meeting energy targets, initial use of lipid emulsions produced variable results. Lipid emulsions derived from soybean oil and cottonseed oil were associated with a number of adverse immunological effects, such as reduced migration and phagocytosis of granulocytes, resulting in increased rates of infections and sepsis [9,10]. Early reports of cottonseed oil emulsion-induced haemolytic anaemia led to withdrawal from use [11].

Numerous investigations into the commonly used soybean oil-derived lipid emulsions have failed to precisely characterise the immunomodulatory mechanism [12]. High content of polyunsaturated fatty acids (PUFA) in these derivations have been identified as possibly causative [12]. While saturated fatty acids serve primarily as an energy source, PUFAs are integral as structural lipids, as in lipid membranes. Long-chain PUFAs synthesised from essential fatty acids (linoleic acid and α-linolenic acid) affect numerous membrane properties and cellular transport. In particular, the n-6 PUFA arachidonic acid is a precursor to proinflammatory mediators such as leukotrienes, prostaglandins and thromboxanes, intravenous delivery of which may adversely affect the immune response [13].

These concerns have led to the development of lipid emulsions in which the bioactive n-6 PUFA is replaced by less bioactive fatty acids. Emulsions derived from coconut, olive and in particular fish oil, which is high in anti-inflammatory n-3 PUFAs, seem to produce fewer immunological issues [13]. However, in terms of clinical efficacy, a recent meta-analysis of ω-3 fatty acids in critical care did not demonstrate any benefit on length of stay in critical care or mortality [14] (Table 4.5.1).

Emulsion delivery in PN also may play a role in worsening oxidative stress. Reactive oxygen species (ROS) can be produced by neutrophils and macrophages as part of the immune response. This effect is normally balanced by the activity of antioxidant enzymes and molecules,

Table 4.5.1 Key studies raising concerns over use of parenteral nutrition (PN) lipids in hospitalised patients

Study	Design	Results	Conclusion
A prospective, randomised, double-blind, multicentre trial to assess the safety and effectiveness of a lipid emulsion (PN) enriched with n-3 fatty acids from fish oil Wichmann 2007 [15]	Patients (n=256) undergoing abdominal surgery were randomised to PN or high n-3 FA PN. Length of ICU stay, hospital stay and complication rates reviewed	Lipoplus group n=127, Intralipid group n=129 – PN initiated immediately following surgery and ended on day 6 post-op Significantly shorter hospital stay in Lipoplus group, 17.2 versus 21.9 days	Increased delivery of n-3 fatty acids is safe, and produces shorter hospital stay in postabdominal surgery patients
A prospective, randomised trial of intravenous fat emulsion administration in trauma victims requiring total parenteral nutrition. Battistella 1997 [16]	Polytrauma patients (n=60) receiving PN were randomised to receive fat emulsion PN or non-fat emulsion PN	Length of hospital stay (days): Lipid: 39 ± 24 No lipid: 27 ± 16 Intensive care unit stay (days): Lipid: 29 ± 22 No lipid = 18 ± 12 Mechanical ventilation days: Lipid: 27 ± 21 No lipid: 15 ± 12 Total ICU infections: Lipid: 72 in 30 patients No lipid: 39 in 27 patients	PN with fat emulsions early in PN had: Increased susceptibility to infection Prolonged pulmonary failure Longer hospital and ICU stays
A prospective, randomised trial of patients undergoing abdominal surgery – receiving standard PN versus PN and additional n-3 FA source Weiss 2007 [17]	Abdominal surgery patients randomised to receive Lipoven or Lipoven and additional Omegaven (rich in N-3 FAs, constituted from fish oil only)	Mean ICU stay: 4.1 days (Lipoven + Omegaven) vs 9.1 days (Lipoven only) Mean hospital stay: 17.8 days (Lipoven + Omegaven) vs 23.5 days (Lipoven only) Five serious instances of infection in each group. Additional measurement of IL-6 as inflammatory marker	Apparent immunomodulatory effect of n-3 fatty acid from fish source Downregulation of inflammatory response and smaller immune suppression effect in n-3 FA group Shorter ICU and hospital stay in additional n-3 FA group
A prospective randomised trial of patients undergoing laparotomy to receive PN containing MCT/LCT emulsion or LCT emulsion only Grau 2003 [18]	Prospective, randomised, double-blind trial of patients undergoing both planned and emergency laparotomy. Randomisation of 72 patients to perioperative PN containing MCT/LCT emulsion or LCT LE only	Intra-abdominal abscess formation: MCT/LCT group 2 of 26 vs 10 of 31 in LCT group Intrahospital mortality: MCT/LCT group 4 of 26 vs 11 of 31 in LCT group Stratified analysis, patients without cancer treated with MCT/LCT presented significantly fewer intra-abdominal abscesses (2/14) than those with LCT (5/8) and a significantly lower mortality	PN composed of MCT/LCT emulsions protected against the development of intra-abdominal abscesses in comparison to LCT-only PN. This effect was more notable in patients without cancer

FA, fatty acid; ICU, intensive care unit; IL, interleukin; LCT, long-chain triglyceride; LE, lipid emulsion; MCT, medium-chain triglyceride.

preventing collateral cellular damage [19]. A key effect of ROS activity is lipid peroxidation [20], in which ROS react with unsaturated lipids, producing apoptosis-inducing lipid peroxides. Polyunsaturated fatty acids may provide reactive potentials for ROS in critical illness states, resulting in an increased risk of oxidative damage [21]. The generation of increased oxidative stress in critical illness may play a role in multiorgan dysfunction and sepsis. In order to avoid these sequelae, antioxidant infusions, most commonly vitamin E (α-tocopherol), can be added to lipid emulsions during critical illness.

The evidence base for the use of variable-length fatty acids is evolving. There are virtually no data outside critical care, and even within critical care, there remains a lack of consensus [22] regarding best practice for lipid constituents. Further trials are required to evaluate the appropriate roles of variable-source lipid emulsions.

Proteins

Protein is usually delivered at a rate of 1.5 g/kg/day, but in the presence of catabolism an increased requirement is common. Critical care, post trauma or surgery, burns or ongoing dialysis all increase the risk of negative nitrogen balance and therefore may require a protein delivery of up to 2–2.5 g/kg/day [23]. Alternatively, in those awaiting renal replacement therapy, a net increase in nitrogen balance may necessitate decreasing PN protein delivery to less than 1 g/kg/day [24].

Parenteral nutrition solutions contain mixed amino acid preparations, which deliver all nine essential amino acids, with a varying composition of non-essential amino acids. There exist limited data from randomised, double-blind, appropriately sized clinical trials to define optimal doses of amino acids in PN. It is, however, clear that the lack of a complete complement of amino acids results in loss of lean body mass [25].

Glutamine is unique in having a largely supportive evidence base. It is required by immune cells both as a primary fuel and as a nitrogen donor for nucleotide precursor synthesis. *In vivo* studies have demonstrated that optimum monocyte, lymphocyte and neutrophil function

is dependent on glutamine stores [26]. A meta-analysis of 550 publications found a decreased hospital stay in those receiving increased glutamine PN [27]. The greatest benefit was seen in the surgical patient subgroup, in which septic complications were reduced.

A prospective, double-blind, controlled, randomised multicentre trial conducted across 16 intensive care units in France compared glutamine supplementation in 114 patients [28]. Those in the glutamine intervention group suffered fewer episodes of infection, though no change in 6-month survival. Against glutamine, supplementation in the recent SIGNET trial demonstrated that glutamine or selenium supplementation in critical care patients did not improve clinical outcomes or length of stay in the intensive care unit [29]. A subsequent meta-analysis still supported glutamine use in surgical and critical care, but the perceived benefits were weakened by the SIGNET trial findings [30].

Parenteral delivery of arginine results in the release of growth hormone, insulin-like growth factor and gut catecholamines. It additionally leads to the upregulation of nitric oxide pathways and has a direct effect on vascular volume and local vasodilation. It is probable that arginine is immunomodulatory, though trial evidence has not definitively shown benefit or harm with its use. There is limited evidence that in severe sepsis, arginine supplementation results in worsening haemodynamic instability, cytotoxicity and organ dysfunction [31]. A randomised, multicentre, controlled trial across 33 Italian units found an increased mortality in the intervention group receiving higher arginine nutrition [32]. Twenty-one of the 39 patients suffering severe shock in the study received an 'immunonutrition' intervention. The hypothesis of improved immune outcomes with arginine supplementation has not been adequately demonstrated.

Parenteral nutrition delivery of essential amino acids is safe in the context of routine nutrition support. However, despite the wealth of data looking at the benefits of supplementing single or multiple amino acids, the literature remains confusing and findings inconclusive. The most persuasive evidence related to glutamine until the SIGNET trial was reported [26–32]. Therefore, the clinical and cost-effectiveness case has still not been made with regard to amino acid or 'immunomodulatory' diets in routine clinical practice.

4.5.4 Monitoring

An individualised care plan should co-ordinate the multiple teams involved with PN provision and identify specific PN goals [33]. Patients and carers should be trained to recognise and respond to their nutritional delivery system and potential PN complications [33]. Monitoring venesection should be performed by appropriately trained staff as inappropriate venesection technique can lead to complications (infection) and spurious results. Those on longer term community-based PN should be looked after by specialist teams with appropriate expertise [33].

Biochemical monitoring should initially be daily. With stabilisation, the frequency of monitoring can be decreased to weekly and then monthly (Table 4.5.2). Standard recommendations or guidelines for the routine use of anthropometric measurements do not exist and therefore this is largely performed based on local expertise-driven practice.

4.5.5 Complications of parenteral nutrition

Immediate complications

The immediate risks of PN relate to the central venous catheter insertion (i.e. nerve injury, arterial injury, pneumothorax, haemopericardium). There have been limited reports of hypersensitivity to the fat emulsion component of PN. Reactions may range from pruritus to anaphylaxis, but even mild reactions are relatively uncommon [35].

Short-term complications (<30 days)

Line complications

An artificial device within the central circulation risks thrombosis, line sepsis and embolic phenomena. Between 5% and 10% patients suffer from line infection of varying severity [36]. A minority of patients suffer thromboembolic complications. There is no established link between nutrition type and the rate of line-specific infections. PICC lines have been reported to have increased rates of thrombophlebitis in comparison to subclavian lines, but there have not been reports of increased line infection with either [37].

Table 4.5.2 Monitoring of parenteral nutrition (PN)

Timing	Measurements
Pre-PN and first 24 hours of initiation	Serum: potassium, phosphate, magnesium, calcium, TSH, triglycerides, blood sugar, liver function tests, serum creatinine Patient: hypersensitivity reaction, weight, fluid status Investigations: ECG, urine dipstick
Short term (24 hours to 14 days)	Serum: potassium, phosphate, magnesium, calcium, TSH, triglycerides, blood sugar, liver function tests, serum creatinine (blood tests every 1–2 days) Patient: weight, vascular access site, dermatological manifestations, fluid status
Long term (>14 days)	Serum: potassium, phosphate, magnesium, calcium, TSH, triglycerides, blood sugar, liver function tests, serum creatinine, parathyroid hormone (blood tests every 1–4 weeks depending on patient stability) Patient: weight, vascular access site, dermatological manifestations, fluid status Investigations: bone densitometry, vitamins A, D, E, selenium, copper, zinc, manganese (3–6 monthly)

ECG, electrocardiogram; TSH, thyroid stimulating hormone.
Source: Koletzko et al. [34] with permission of German Medical Sciences.

Refeeding syndrome

Upon initiation of PN, there exists a risk of refeeding syndrome, especially in those with recent weight loss >10%, little or no intake for over 5 days and recurring electrolyte abnormalities. In undernutrition or starvation, there is a preferential utilisation of fat and protein stores as energy sources. This non-carbohydrate metabolism results in the utilisation and depletion of electrolytes. While serum phosphate concentrations are typically normal in starved patients, intracellular stores are in fact low. The reintroduction of carbohydrates results in an insulin tide and stimulates the cellular uptake of phosphate, potentially resulting in profound hypophosphataemia. While there may exist a parallel hypokalaemia or hypomagnesaemia, phosphate deficit seems to be the key refeeding syndrome feature. The clinical signs of onset can be vague and vigilance in electrolyte monitoring is required [33]. A more detailed review of the pathophysiological mechanisms of refeeding syndrome is provided in Chapter 2.4.

Hyperglycaemia

Hyperglycaemia in those receiving PN has been associated with an increased risk of cardiac complications, infection, systemic sepsis, renal dysfunction and death [38] Its presence is an independent predictor of poorer outcome and demonstrably increases in-hospital mortality[38]. When exposed to physiological stressors such as trauma, major surgery or critical illness, patients may develop insulin resistance as a result of an increased glucocorticoid state [39]. Physiological stress when combined with intravenous carbohydrate delivery may result in hyperglycaemia. Any PN solution delivering dextrose over a rate of 4–5 mg/kg/min significantly increases this incidence [40].

Randomised controlled trial (RCT) evidence suggests that lower energy PN formulations in which dextrose or carbohydrate load has been minimised result in less extreme hyperglycaemic periods and consequent lower insulin requirements [41]. A prospective RCT involving 1548 patients in an intensive care setting found that intensive insulin therapy for hyperglycaemia control reduced in-hospital mortality by 34%, bloodstream infections by 46% and acute renal failure requiring renal support by 41%. While only a minority of those recruited to this study received extended PN, its conclusions have been taken to support the normoglycaemia ideal [42]. Patients receiving PN should have close monitoring of blood sugars upon initiation of PN, and regular interval checks once established on PN. The method of hyperglycaemia control should balance formulation carbohydrate load, insulin use in the acute phase and dynamic long-term monitoring.

Long-term complications (>30 days)

Cholestasis/liver injury

The continuation of PN in the longer term is associated with deranged liver function tests (LFT) in 15–85% of patients [43]. The pathogenesis of this remains unclear and may relate to a number of factors, including ratio and concentrations of fat and carbohydrates, the absence of enteric nutrients during PN, potential unrecognised hepatotoxins within PN solutions and possible elements of immune variability given vascular delivery of nutrients [44]. Deranged LFTs can reflect cholestasis and steatosis, which occasionally proceed to cirrhosis. There are no markers or factors in the identification of patients at higher risk of liver injury and cholestasis. Jaundice, LFT derangement and cholestasis may resolve completely following PN cessation. Improvement in liver function can occur if the lipid source is changed from soybean and olive oil to fish oil [45]. Overall, the incidence of PN-associated liver disease has been decreasing in the adult population and this may reflect the recognition that fat concentrations >1 g/kg are a significant risk factor and the use of more liver-friendly fat formulations in recent years.

Metabolic bone disease

Those receiving long-term PN are at risk of metabolic bone disease, which is characterised by patchy osteomalacia and low bone turnover

Table 4.5.3 Monitoring of patients with suspected parenteral nutrition (PN)-related bone disease

Parameter	Rationale
Calcium, magnesium, phosphate	Weekly, followed by monthly (post month 2)
PTH	Malabsorption/hypoparathyroidism
25-hydroxyvitamin D	Malabsorption
TSH	Suspected hyperparathyroidism
Urine: N telliopeptide collagen 24-hour excretion of calcium and magnesium	Proof of metabolic bone disease, followed by regular monitoring every 6–12 months
X-ray/DEXA	As confirmation of bone disease – indicated by suspicion/PN > months

DEXA, dual-energy x-ray absorptiometry; PTH, parathyroid hormone; TSH, thyroid stimulating hormone.

(Table 4.5.3). Initially thought to be a consequence of aluminium toxicity, the syndrome is now thought to relate to suboptimal nutritional support, physical inactivity and drugs [46]. An adequate delivery of calcium, phosphate and vitamin D should be ensured. The use of steroids over the short term should be monitored, with consideration of bone mineral density scanning. In suspected loss of density, bisphosphonates have been shown to improve markers [47].

Vitamin and mineral deficiencies

Vitamin and mineral deficiencies (or excesses) can occur in anyone on longer term PN. The clinical manifestations are many and varied and beyond the scope of this chapter. However, appropriate monitoring (see earlier) should avoid these problems.

4.5.6 Conclusion

Parenteral nutrition is a safe and effective therapy. To minimise the risks and complications, its use should be confined to healthcare professionals and teams with appropriate expertise, and in such hands it is usually life-saving and can be life-prolonging. Demand for in-hospital and community PN rises every year, mainly on the basis of increasing surgical intervention for sick patients. Healthcare systems need to be able to adapt to changing demography and increasing demand.

References

1. McClave S, Martindale R, Vanek V, et al. Guidelines for the provision and assessment of nutrition support therapy in the adult critically ill patient. *J Parenter Enteral Nutr* 2009; **33**(3): 277–316.
2. Nakasaki H, Mitome T, Tajima T, Ohnishi N, Fujii K. Gut bacterial translocation during total parenteral nutrition in experimental rats and its countermeasure. *Am J Surg* 1998; **175**(1): 38–43.
3. Messing B, Crenn P, Beau P, Boutron-Ruault MC, Rambaud JC, Matuchansky C. Long-term survival and parenteral nutrition dependence in adult patients with the short bowel syndrome. *Gastroenterology* 1999; **117**(5): 1043–1050.
4. Jones B. Home Parenteral Nutrition in the United Kingdon – A Position Paper. British Association for Parenteral & Enteral Nutrition. www.bapen.org.uk/pdfs/hpn.pdf (accessed 2 September 2017).
5. Pittiruti M, Hamilton H, Biffi R, MacFie J, Pertkiewicz M. ESPEN guidelines on parenteral nutrition: central venous catheters (access, care, diagnosis and therapy of complications). *Clin Nutr* 2009; **28**(4): 365–377.
6. Kochevar M, Guenter P, Holcombe B. ASPEN statement on parenteral nutrition standardization. *J Parenter Enteral Nutr* 2007; **31**(5): 441–448.
7. Singer P, Berger M, van den Berghe G, Bioli G, Calder P, Forbes A, Griffiths R, Kreymanh G, Leverve X, Pichard C. ESPEN guidelines on parenteral nutrition: intensive care. *Clin Nutr* 2009; **28**(4): 387–400.
8. Meguid M, Schimmel E, Johnson WC, Meguid V, Lowell BC, Bourinski J, Nasbeth DC. Reduced metabolic complications in TPN: pilot study using fat to replace one third of glucose calories. *J Parenter Enteral Nutr* 1982; **6**(4): 304–307.
9. Jarstrand C, Berghem L, Lahnborg G. Human granulocyte and reticuloendothelial system function during intralipid infusion. *J Parenter Enteral Nutr* 1978; **2**(5): 663–670.

10. Nordenstrom J, Jarstrand C, Wiernik A. Decreased chemotactic and random migration of leukocytes during intralipid infusion. *Am J Clin Nutr* 1979; **32**(12): 2416–2422.

11. Alexander C, Zieve L. Fat infusions – toxic effects and alterations in fasting serum lipids following prolonged use. *Arch Intern Med* 1961; **107**(4): 514–528.

12. Wanten GJ, Calder PC. Immune modulation by parenteral lipid emulsions. *Am J Clin Nutr* 2007; **85**(5): 1171–1184.

13. Adolph M, Heller AR, Koch T, Koletzko B, Kreymann KG, Krohn K. Lipid emulsions – guidelines on parenteral nutrition. *Ger Med Sci* 2009; **7**(22): Doc22.

14. Palmer A, Ho C, Ajibola O, Avenall A. The role of w-3 fatty acid supplemented parenteral nutrition in critical illness in adults: a systematic review and meta-analysis. *Crit Care Med* 2013; **41**(1): 307–316.

15. Wichmann MW, Thul P, Czarnetzki HD, Morlion BJ, Kemen M, Jauch KW. Evaluation of clinical safety and beneficial effects of a fish oil containing lipid emulsion (Lipoplus, MLF541): data from a prospective, randomized, multicenter trial. *Crit Care Med* 2007; **35**(3): 700–706.

16. Battistella FD, Widergren JT, Anderson JT, Siepler JK, Weber JC, MacColl K. A prospective, randomized trial of intravenous fat emulsion administration in trauma victims requiring total parenteral nutrition. *J Trauma* 1997; **43**(1): 52–58.

17. Weiss G, Meyer F, Matthies B, Pross M, Koenig W, Lippert H. Immunomodulation by perioperative administration of n-3 fatty acids. *Br J Nutr* 2002; **87**(Suppl 1): S89–94.

18. Grau T, Ruiz de Adana JC, Zubillaga S, Fuerte S, Giron C. Randomized study of two different fat emulsions in total parenteral nutrition of malnourished surgical patients; effect of infectious morbidity and mortality. *Nutr Hosp* 2003; **18**(3): 159–166.

19. Mishra M. Oxidative stress and role of antioxidant supplementation in critical illness. *Clin Lab* 2007; **53**(3-4): 199–209.

20. Goodyear-Bruch C, Pierce JD. Oxidative stress in critically ill patients. *Am J Crit Care* 2002; **11**(6): 543–551.

21. Hardy G, Allwood MC. Oxidation of intravenous lipid emulsions. *Nutrition* 1997; **13**(3): 230–233.

22. Edmunds C, Brody R, Parrott J, Stankorb S, Heyland D. The effects of different IV fat emulsions on clinical outcomes in critically ill patients. *Crit Care Med* 2014; **42**(5): 1168–1177.

23. Parrish CR, Madsen H, Frankel E. The hitchhiker's guide to parenteral nutrition management for adult patients. *Practical Gastroenterol* 2006; **40**: 40–68.

24. Druml W. Nutritional management of acute renal failure. *Am J Kidney Dis* 2001; **37**(1 Suppl 2): S89–S94.

25. Singer P, Berger MM, van den Berghe G, et al. ESPEN guidelines on parenteral nutrition: intensive care. *Clin Nutr* 2009; **28**(4): 387–400.

26. Andrews FJ, Grffiths RD. Glutamine: essential for immune nutrition in the critically ill. *Br J Nutr* 2002; **87**(Suppl 1): S3–S8.

27. Novak F, Heyland DK, Avenell A, Drover JW, Su X. Glutamine supplementation in serious illness: a systematic review of the evidence. *Crit Care Med* 2002; **30**(9): 2022–2029.

28. Dechelote P, Hasselmann M, Cynober L, et al. L-alanyl-L-glutamine dipeptide-supplemented total parenteral nutrition reduces infectious complications and glucose intolerance in critically ill patients: the French controlled, randomized, double-blind, multicenter study. *Crit Care Med* 2006; **34**(3): 598–604.

29. Andrews PJD, Avenell A, Noble DW, Campbell MK, Croal BL, Simpson WG, Vale LD, Battison CG, Jenkinson DJ, Cook JA. The SIGNET Trials Group – randomized trial of glutamine and/or selenium supplemented parenteral nutrition for critically ill patients. *BMJ* 2011; **342**: d1542.

30. Bollhalder L, Pfeil A, Tomonaga Y, Schwenkglenks M. A systematic literature review and meta-analysis of randomized clinical trials of parenteral glutamine supplementation. *Clin Nutr* 2013; **32**(2): 213–223.

31. Suchner U, Heyland DK, Peter K. Immune-modulatory actions of arginine in the critically ill. *Br J Nutr* 2002; **87**(Suppl 1): S121–S132.

32. Bertolini G, Iapichino G, Radrizzani D, et al. Early enteral immunonutrition in patients with severe sepsis: results of an interim analysis of a randomized multicentre clinical trial. *Intens Care Med* 2003; **29**(5): 834–840.

33. National Institute for Health and Care Excellence. Nutritional Support in adults: Oral Nutrition Support, Enteral Tube Feeding and Parenteral Nutrition – Costing Report 2006. www.nice.org.uk/guidance/cg32/resources/costing-report-pdf-194884669 (accessed 2 September 2017).

34. Koletzko B, Jauch KW, Verwied-Jorky S, Krohn K, Mittal R. Working group for developing the guidelines for parenteral nutrition of the German Association for Nutritional Medicine. *Geriatr Med Sci* 2009; **7**: Doc27.

35. Nagata MJ. Hypersensitivity reactions associated with parenteral nutrition: case report and review of the literature. *Ann Pharmacother* 1993; **27**(2): 174–177.

36. Ryan J, Abel RM, Abbott WM, et al. Catheter complications in total parenteral nutrition – a prospective study of 200 consecutive patients. *N Engl J Med* 1974; **290**(14): 757–761.

37. Cowl CT, Weinstock JV, Al-Jurf A, Ephgrave K, Murray JA, Dillon K. Complications and cost associated with parenteral nutrition delivered to hospitalized patients through either subclavian or peripherally inserted central catheters. *Clin Nutr* 2000; **19**(4): 237–243.

38. Cheung N, Napier B, Zaccaria C, Fletcher JP. Hyperglycemia is associated with adverse outcomes in patients receiving total parenteral nutrition. *Diabetes Care* 2005; **28**(10): 2367–2371.

39. Ferris H, Kahn C. New mechanisms of glucocorticoid-induced insulin resistance: make no bones about it. *J Clin Invest* 2012; **122**(11): 3854–3857.

40. Rosmarin DK, Wardlaw GM, Mirtallo J. Hyperglycemia associated with high, continuous infusion rates of total parenteral nutrition dextrose. *Nutr Clin Pract* 1996; **11**(4): 151–156.

41. Ahrens C, Barletta JF, Kanji S, Tyburski JG, Wilson RF, Janisse JJ, Devlin JW. Effect of low-calorie parenteral nutrition on the incidence and severity of hyperglycemia in surgical patients: a randomized controlled trial. *Crit Care Med* 2005; **33**(11): 2507–2512.

42. Van den Berghe G, Wouters P, Weekers F, et al. Intensive insulin therapy in critically ill patients. *N Engl J Med* 2001; **345**(19): 1359–1367.

43. Cavicchi M, Beau P, Crenn P, Degott C, Messing B. Prevalence of liver disease and contributing factors in patients receiving home parenteral nutrition for permanent intestinal failure. *Ann Intern Med* 2000; **132**(7): 525–532.

44. Forchielli M, Walker WA. Nutritional factors contributing to the development of cholestatsis during total parenteral nutrition. *Adv Pediatr* 2003; **50**: 245–267.

45. Venecourt-Jackson E, Hill SJ, Walmsley RS. Successful treatment of parenteral nutrition associated liver disease in an adult by use of a fish oil based lipid source. *Nutrition* 2013; **29**(1): 356–358.

46. Cohen-Solal M, Baudoin C, Joly F, Vahedi K, d'Aoust L, de Vernejoul MC, Messing B. Osteoporosis in patients on long-term home parenteral nutrition: a longitudinal study. *J Bone Miner Res* 2003; **18**(11): 1989–1994.

47. Nishikawa RA. Intravenous pamidronate improves bone mineral density in home parenteral nutrition patients. *Clin Nutr* 2003; **22**(1): S88.

Undernutrition and nutrition support in clinical specialties

Chapter 5.1

Nutrition support in paediatrics

Rosan Meyer[1] and Luise Marino[2]

[1]Imperial College London, London, UK
[2]University Hospital Southampton Foundation Trust, Southampton, UK

5.1.1 Introduction

Childhood is a dynamic, ever-changing period when children undergo an orderly and predictable sequence of neurodevelopmental and physical growth. This sequence is influenced continuously by a variety of factors (nutritional and environmental), making each infant's developmental path unique [1]. Nutritional requirements vary depending on age, growth velocity, activity and the different stages of development of the brain and organs [2]. This fact sets paediatric nutrition support apart from that of adults as the management of any paediatric disorder has as its background the objective of achieving optimal growth and development, in addition to managing nutritional requirements imposed by the underlying diagnosis. Supplemental to this is that childhood is also the time for the development of an emotional and social association with food that may have far-reaching implications for growth, development but also psychological well-being [3,4]. These factors should be taken into account when planning nutrition support and are summarised in Table 5.1.1.

Although there are unique evidence-based nutritional requirements for many types of paediatric diagnoses, the unifying side effect of many disorders is undernutrition which has an impact on morbidity and mortality [5,6].

5.1.2 Definition of undernutrition in paediatrics

Many terms are used interchangeably for undernutrition, including malnutrition, faltering growth and failure to thrive, but they do not necessarily describe the same level of undernutrition (Box 5.1.1) [9]. Faltering growth is most commonly defined as a deceleration of weight in children <2 years of age of more than 2 centiles over a period of time and describes the process of crossing growth centiles [9]. Conversely, malnutrition is defined by the World Health Organization (WHO) as a measurement ≤2 z-scores height for age or weight for height, and is the equivalent of the 2nd centile or less in the UK-WHO growth chart [10].

Authors have in the past used growth faltering as a definition for developed countries and malnutrition for developing countries, which implies that children in developed countries are monitored more frequently and picked up earlier, which is clearly not the case. Therefore, any child, irrespective of the environment, should have their growth reviewed on a regular basis [9].

In this chapter, undernutrition is used as the over-arching term for both faltering growth and malnutrition as defined by the WHO. However, it should be noted that wherever appropriate to

Advanced Nutrition and Dietetics in Nutrition Support, First Edition. Edited by Mary Hickson and Sara Smith.
© 2018 John Wiley & Sons Ltd. Published 2018 by John Wiley & Sons Ltd.

Table 5.1.1 Factors and their implications unique to the nutritional management of paediatrics [1,7,8]

Factor	Implication
Continuing growth	Increased energy and protein requirements
	Increased micronutrient requirements, in particular calcium, iron, vitamin D and zinc
Varying growth velocity	Energy and protein requirements require constant adjustments
Development of oral motor skills	Texture of food requires adjustment in addition to the equipment depending on developmental stage
Development of feeding behaviour	Requires feeding routine and behavioural management

---

Box 5.1.1 Different criteria used to describe undernutrition [9,11]

Inadequate growth or weight gain for >1 month in a child of <2 years of age

Weight crossing more than 2 centiles >1 month in child <2 years of age (1 centile on the UK-WHO growth chart = 0.68 SD)

Weight loss or no weight gain for >3 months in a child >2 years of age

Changes in weight for age downward of more than 1 SD in 3 months for children <1 year of age on growth charts

Change in weight for height downward of more than 1 SD in 3 months for children ≥1 year of age on growth charts

Decrease in height velocity 0.5–1 SD/year at <4 years of age and 0.25 SD/year at >4 years of age

Decrease in height velocity >2 cm from preceding year during early/mid puberty

SD, standard deviation = 1 z-score.

---

the supportive literature, faltering growth or malnutrition is used as defined by the appropriate criteria.

5.1.3 Prevalence of undernutrition in paediatrics

The worldwide prevalence of children being underweight (low weight for age) is 16%, but stunting (low height for age) is much higher at 26% [12]. In the UK, the prevalence of faltering growth amongst healthy infants at the 6–8-weeks check has been reported as being 6.1% [13] and it is thought that between 5% and 9% of the general infant and toddler population develop growth faltering at some point during infancy [13,14]. The prevalence of stunting in the general UK population is reported as 5.6% [15]. While these data are difficult to compare to other countries, due to varying definitions being used, Grimberg et al. [14] observed that 9% of children in urban USA paediatric primary care practices

had growth faltering (defined as height <5th percentile or z-score dropping by ≥1.5 SD before age 18 months or ≥1 SD thereafter). In Europe, prevalence data exist mainly in the context of undernutrition during hospital admission.

Acute and chronic undernutrition is much more prevalent in the hospitalised population and amongst those children with chronic disease. The prevalence of undernutrition in hospitalised children in middle-income countries, such as South Africa and Turkey, ranges from 34% to 40% [16,17], compared to 14–24% amongst hospitalised children in European countries (including the UK) [18,19]. A large multicentre European study found that 7% of paediatric hospital admissions had a body mass index (BMI) ≤ −2 z-score with a higher prevalence of undernutrition in infants (10.8%) [20]. In a tertiary specialist paediatric hospital, Pichler et al. reported that 27% of children admitted were classified as being undernourished [14% moderate: z-score < −2 to −3, and 13% severe: z-score ≤ −3] with a further decline in growth parameters during hospitalisation increasing the prevalence to 32% at discharge (11% moderate, 21% severe) [21]. It is important to note that the latter study was based on weight for age only.

The prevalence of undernutrition within a hospital setting has remained unchanged for 20 years [22]. It is therefore important that healthcare professionals recognise undernutrition early in order to provide timely nutrition support and thereby preventing ongoing faltering growth.

5.1.4 Common causes of undernutrition in paediatrics

Causes of undernutrition are often classified as illness (previously organic) and non-illness (previously non-organic) related. Illness-related undernutrition is associated with medical disease whereas non-illness-related undernutrition is linked to environmental and socioeconomic factors, including poor food security, maternal deprivation and depression, and a dysfunctional mother–child relationship [23–26]. In the past, it was thought that of children who were undernourished, 90–95% had non-illness-related growth faltering and 5–10% was illness related. However, it is now recognised that there is significant overlap between illness-related and non-illness -related undernutrition. Ramsay et al. found that 57% of infants had inefficient sucking at 2 months of age, which lead to compensatory feeding in 45% and this in turn was linked to poor growth [25]. These infants were classified with non-illness-related growth faltering but had subtle neurodevelopmental disorders and pathophysiology (i.e. delayed sucking ability), but were otherwise medically well. An example of this is where a child has experienced gastro-oesophageal reflux as an infant leading to textural hypersensitivity (exhibited by gagging on lumpier textures), with associated maternal anxiety, further affecting nutrient intake and resulting in growth faltering [27,28]. In addition, where food availability and quality are the primary cause of undernutrition, childhood infections result in further nutrient loss and altered metabolism, which also

demonstrates the overlap between illness-related and non-illness-related undernutrition [26].

Illness-related undernutrition in paediatrics

The causes for undernutrition in children with chronic disease are multifactorial and linked to increased macronutrient and micronutrient requirements, altered metabolism, increased nutrient losses through stool and urine, reduced dietary intake and disordered feeding [27–30]. In a hospital setting, the most vulnerable children are those <2 years of age with multiple medical problems and with an inpatient stay of >1 month [21] (Figure 5.1.1).

Non-illness-related undernutrition in paediatrics

The most common cause for non-illness-related undernutrition is poor food availability and food quality in developing countries and a disrupted mother–child relationship in developed countries, which may occur for various reasons, including neglect [12,31]. In addition, toddlers are notoriously fussy eaters which can occur in up to 50% of all toddlers and young children [32,33]. Being picky can narrow the variety of foods consumed by young children [33], increasing their risk of being underweight and wasted, especially in children <3 years of age [34]. The Millennium study in the UK found that 16.7% and 19.8% of 8- and 12-month-old infants respectively had severe avoidant feeding behaviour that affected weight gain [35]. The same research group also found that mothers with high depression scores were more than twice as likely to have weight faltering infants up to 4 months [36].

5.1.5 Pathophysiology of undernutrition in paediatrics

Although there may be concomitant factors related to underlying illness/infection and environment, the net effects of diets deficient in macronutrients and micronutrient for both illness/non-illness-related undernutrition remain the same.

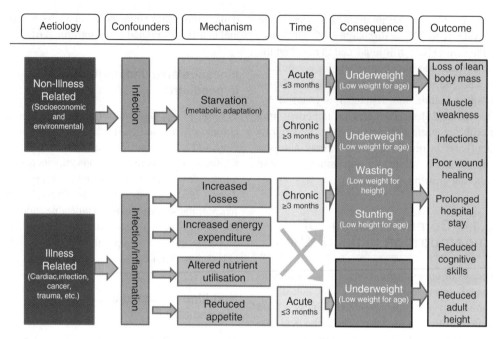

Figure 5.1.1 Progression of undernutrition with associated short-term and long-term consequences. Source: Adapted from Mehta et al. [24].

Table 5.1.2 Hormones and growth factors that affect nutritional status

Hormone	Affected by nutrient restriction	Effect on growth
Insulin	Reduced	Stimulates growth
Growth hormone	Increased	Stimulates growth
IGF-1	Reduced	Stimulates growth
IGF binding protein 1	Increased	Inhibits growth
Leptin	Reduced	Stimulates growth
Glucocorticoids	Increased	Inhibit growth
Thyroid hormones	Reduced	Stimulate growth
Vitamin D, zinc, iron, vitamin A, B-vitamins	Reduced	Required for optimal growth
Sex hormones	Reduced	Stimulate growth

IGF, insulin-like growth factor.
Source: Adapted from Gat-Yablonski and Phillip [26].

A negative energy balance will lead to reduced plasma concentrations of insulin, insulin-like growth factor-1 (IGF-1), thyroid hormone, leptin and sex hormones and increased concentrations of glucocorticoids and IGF binding protein-1 and -7. In addition to this, other factors, including cytokines in illness-related undernutrition and vitamin D (amongst other micronutrients), have an impact on IGF (Table 5.1.2).

However, in addition to the hormonal effects and micronutrient deficiencies, there are a number of interrelated energy regulatory systems in cells which may also be involved in the pathophysiology of undernutrition. These include microRNAs (which function in RNA silencing and posttranscriptional regulation of gene expression), transcription factors (e.g. hypoxia-inducible factor 1α), energy-protein sensing enzyme implicated in growth (e.g. mammalian target of rapamycin), histone modification influencing gene regulation and autophagy [26]. By way of example, autophagy has also been identified as affecting growth. Authopagy is a catabolic process that results in the autophagosome-dependent lysosomal degradation of bulk cytoplasmic content, abnormal protein aggregates and excess of damaged cells. Nutrient insufficiency may increase the autophagic response, in particular in the epiphyseal growth plates (affecting longitudinal growth). Generally, when the restriction is short, this process may be reversible but when it is prolonged, cell numbers may be reduced and growth stunted [26].

5.1.6 Consequences of undernutrition in paediatrics

There are both short- and long-term consequences of undernutrition. In the hospital setting, acute undernutrition has been linked to poor wound healing, increased infection, muscle weakness and subsequently an increased length of hospital stay (see Figure 5.1.1) [20,24,37–40]. The latter has in particular been shown in a recent multicentre European study, which recruited 2567 patients (median age: 4.7 years; interquartile range 1.4–11.1 years) from 14 centres in 12 countries. The findings of this study indicated that the children with a BMI ≤ -2 had a significant increase in length of hospital stay of 1.3 days [20].

Health-related quality of life (HRQL) is also affected by undernutrition, with the data from Hecht et al. indicating that 15.1% of children with poor weight gain had a worse score for HRQL [20]. There are also data on the impact of nutritional status on HRQL in chronic diseases like cancer and cystic fibrosis. Brinksma et al. found the undernourished children with cancer had worse physical and social functioning [41]. On the other hand, Bodnar et al. found that children with a low BMI (≤ -2 z-score) with cystic fibrosis had significantly lower scores in the eating, body image and treatment burden domains [42].

The long-term consequences of undernutrition are in particular related to height growth (see Figure 5.1.1). Being short in stature as a result of faltering growth is more harmful for health in the long term compared to being acutely underweight [16], which seems to have little impact on cognitive development compared to severe and prolonged undernutrition [43]. Being stunted as a result of growth faltering is associated with poorer neurodevelopmental outcomes, in particular reduced cognition [44]. In addition, stunting has also been linked to delayed walking, motor skill and language development [43–45]. Lastly, stunting has also been linked to shorter adult height and increased all-cause mortality [15].

5.1.7 Identifying undernutrition in paediatrics

Nutritional screening in paediatrics

Anthropometry and growth charts have traditionally been used to assess growth and to screen for chronic undernutrition. Although this is an essential part of paediatric nutritional care, it will not identify children with subtle growth faltering or those at risk of deterioration as a result of an acute medical condition [46]. Due to the work pressures in hospital, plotting growth data can be time-consuming and, most importantly, requires training for both plotting and interpretation.

It has been proposed that nutritional screening tools may be more appropriate to identify nutritional risk and could be utilised by nursing staff to screen for undernutrition that is then subsequently diagnosed by a dietitian following a detailed nutritional assessment [47]. Several paediatric nutritional screening tools exist, including the STAMP tool [48], the STRONGkids tool [49] and the Yorkhill screening tool [47], among others [50,51]. Currently, there is no consensus on the ideal method for the screening and assessment of nutritional risk in children admitted to hospital and there is insufficient evidence to recommend one nutritional screening tool over another based on their predictive accuracy [50]. It is, however, recommended that all

Box 5.1.2 Approaches to determining whether a child has acute or chronic undernutrition

Does the child have acute undernutrition?
Normal length/height but low weight for height or low weight for age. This normally represents an acute event of short duration, e.g. following a short episode of illness.

Does the child have chronic undernutrition?
Short length for age but normal weight for height/length even though underweight for age, e.g. chronic illness such as end-stage renal failure.

Does the child have acute-on-chronic undernutrition?
Short length/height for age but low weight for height/length and underweight for age, e.g. chronic illness such as end-stage renal failure with a recent lower respiratory tract infection.

members of the healthcare team should collaborate to ensure that screening for nutrition risk/undernutrition becomes an integral part of routine paediatric care [51]. It is important to note that screening does *not* replace the assessment of nutritional status, which is described in further detail below.

Nutritional assessment in paediatrics

To identify a child with undernutrition, it is important to review their growth record, considering the trend of growth. A growth curve that is flattening represents early growth faltering with a slowing in weight gain velocity; a growth curve where lines are being crossed, for example where there is weight loss or no weight gain, suggests an undernourished child. Children with growth curves that are either flattening or show downward crossing of centiles would be considered to have undernutrition, with action required in both [52]. It is also important to establish if a child has acute or chronic undernutrition, as this will affect the nutritional management. There are a number of different ways to establish this (Box 5.1.2).

5.1.8 Frequency of monitoring, catch-up growth and follow-up in paediatrics

All children with faltering growth should be followed up monthly with defined dietary and catch-up goals for nutritional rehabilitation [53].

When catch-up growth of 1–2 centiles or weight for height of >100% or 1 SD for the reference standards have been achieved, nutritional supplementation should be reviewed [54]. Following catch-up, it is important to continue monitoring patients at age-appropriate intervals [55].

Although it is important to aim for catch-up growth early, ideally prior to 2 years of age, Prentice et al. highlighted in their study that substantial height catch-up occurs between 24 months and mid-childhood and again between mid-childhood and adulthood [56]. Catch-up is therefore possible at any stage of childhood and healthcare professionals should aim for optimal dietary management to enable this. The same group also highlighted the time of growth of different body systems which also need to be taken into account (Figure 5.1.2).

5.1.9 Nutrient requirements during undernutrition in paediatrics

Energy and protein requirements in paediatrics

When promoting catch-up growth, WHO/FAO/UNU guidelines focus on the accrual of lean body mass with an optimal balance between lean body mass and fat mass (73% lean, 27% fat mass) [5,57,58]. Optimal catch-up growth is dependent not only on sufficient energy delivery, but also on adequate protein (Table 5.1.3).

An ideal protein energy (P:E) ratio for catch-up growth resulting in lean body mass accretion,

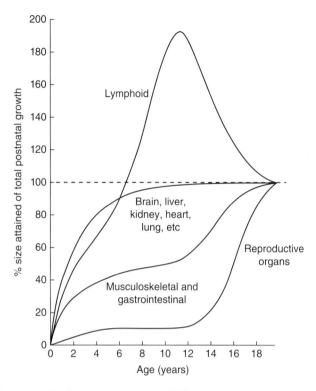

Figure 5.1.2 Timing of growth of body systems during childhood. Source: Prentice et al. [56] reproduced with permission from the American Society for Nutrition.

Table 5.1.3 Theoretical energy and protein intake for 5, 10 and 20 g/kg/day catch-up growth

Required catch-up growth	Protein requirements (g/kg/day)	Energy requirements (kcal/kg/day)	Protein energy ratio (%)*
5 g/kg/day	1.82	105	6.9
10 g/kg/day	2.82	126	8.9
20 g/kg/day	4.82	167	11.5

* The % energy from protein (i.e. 1.82 g of protein, 105 kcal = 6.9% energy from protein).
Source: reproduced from Joint WHO/FAO/UNU Expert Consultation [5], with permission from the World Health Organization.

rather than deposition of adipose tissue, has been shown to be 8.9–12% [5,6]. Enriching nutritional supplements with modular additions of fat and carbohydrate alone often results in a P:E ratio of 4.5–6% which does not favour optimal catch-up growth in growth faltering infants [57,58].

With respect to nutrition rehabilitation (the process of improving nutrient intake and feeding practice), it is important to set growth goals,

such as achieving a weight for height or height for age of greater than < −1–0 z-score. In younger children <5 years of age with moderate growth faltering (e.g. z-score ≤ −1 or downward crossing of ≥2 centiles for weight or height), it is usual to expect a weight gain of 10 g/kg/day. In children whose weight gain is 5–10 g/kg/day, it is important to review whether intake targets are being met and/or whether there is ongoing infection/inflammation. Poor weight gain is <5 g/kg/day and in these children a review of biochemistry (particularly growth factors) and intake should be considered. In older children >5 years of age, weight gain may be slower but 5–10 g/kg/day should still be achievable [24].

Vitamin and mineral requirements

In addition to protein and energy, children with undernutrition also require vitamin and mineral supplementation. Multiple micronutrient supplementation (including vitamin A, D, zinc, iron) has been shown to be effective in promoting catch-up growth in children under the age of 5 years and supplementation should be considered routine in growth faltering children [57,59].

Iron deficiency anaemia (IDA) affects up to 17% of children under 5 years of age in the UK, mostly from ethnic minorities and socioeconomically deprived groups [60]. Evidence suggests that even mild anaemia can have a long-term detrimental influence on mental and psychomotor development although there are many confounders which could influence the prevalence of IDA, including poverty, maternal education and prematurity [61,62].

In developing countries, zinc supplementation of 10 mg/day in infants <6 months of age and 20 mg/day in infants >6 months of age and children has been shown to significantly reduce morbidity in children with diarrhoeal disease and pneumonia [62,63]. Zinc supplementation has also been shown to be effective in promoting linear growth [59,62,63].

5.1.10 Feeding advice as part of the management of undernutrition in paediatrics

Feeding is a skill acquired during the first 2 years of life which involves the progressive acquisition of motor skills, maturation of sensory systems and psychosocial aspects, including communication. Feeding skills develop through practice and keen observance along with developmentally appropriate complementary feeding choices within a responsive feeding environment. However, this sensitive period can be disrupted as a result of altered feeding patterns aiming to promote catch-up growth [31,35,64]. This can lead to regression of feeding skills, acceptance of new foods and/or textures, altered motivation and feeding practices leading to parental frustration and anxiety which is mirrored back to the infant/child. Therefore, it is important that when nutrition support for growth faltering is initiated, the potential impact is explained to the parents and is recognised as a potential trigger for feeding difficulties [31]. Additionally, if nasogastric or gastrostomy feeding is required, it is necessary to provide parents with feeding advice on how to maintain oral motor skills and avoid sensory hypersensitivity arising from the placement of a nasogastric tube or absence of oral stimulation [65].

5.1.11 Nutrition intervention for infants and children with faltering growth

Nutrition intervention for infants and children with faltering growth focuses on the use of oral nutrition support and enteral nutrition. Parenteral nutrition would not be routinely used unless there was a disease-specific requirement.

Oral nutrition support in paediatrics

Enriched home foods can initially be tried in children where undernutrition is not too severe (i.e. downward crossing of 1 centile), but if this approach fails then the use of oral nutritional supplements should be tried [66]. Energy-dense ready-to-feed infant formulas that deliver energy and protein at an appropriate P:E ratio have been shown to significantly improve growth and nitrogen status [67]. Although not ideal, it may be necessary to manipulate standard formulas for some diagnoses where ready-to-use (RTU) infant formulas are not available, with modular additions. However, it is important to pay attention to the P:E ratio, the osmolality and renal solute load when suggesting this as a mode of treatment. In many cases, the manipulation of feeds may lead to symptom exacerbation and

Table 5.1.4 Comparison of energy and protein provided in standard infant formula (SIF) compared to protein energy-enriched (PEE) infant formula

Volume mL/kg	SIF protein g/kg	SIF energy kcal/kg	PEE protein g/kg	PEE energy kcal/kg
100 mL	1.3	67	2.6	100
110 mL	1.4	73	2.9	110
120 mL	1.5	80	3.1	120
130 mL	1.7	87	3.3	130
140 mL	1.8	93	3.6	140
150 mL	1.9	100	3.9	150

suboptimal catch-up growth, and so where possible this practice should be avoided [68–70]. The older child may also require nutritionally complete oral nutritional supplements, if initial nutritional treatment with enriched home foods has failed (Table 5.1.4).

Enteral nutrition in paediatrics

If growth remains suboptimal, the placement of a nasogastric tube (NGT) may be required for short-term nutrition support. However, if a NGT is required for >4 weeks, the placement of a gastrostomy tube may need to be considered [66]. Enteral nutrition should be commenced with appropriate food for special medical purposes in the form of RTU nutritionally complete formulas [66,71]. The nutrition care plan should be discussed with the carers, including advice on oral food intake, feeding management and maintaining oral motor skills [33,72].

There has been a recent escalation in parental requests for liquidised food as a replacement for nutritionally complete RTU sterile formulas (see section 4.4.2). However, in order to promote optimal growth and continued development, nutrition support in children with complex medical needs should at least meet nutrition requirements for macronutrients and micronutrients [66,73]. Until now, RTU formulas have been the accepted form of providing nutrition support as they are well studied and have been shown to support continued growth and meet nutrient requirements [66,74,75]. There is a perception that liquidised diets are more 'natural' [76,77] and at face value, this appears to be a nutritious

offering, particularly with the use of fresh vegetables and fruit. Recipes for liquidised feeds assume that the quality and quantity of macronutrients and micronutrients in the foods used are optimal, but it is known that where the foods are sourced from, the cooking methods and storage (i.e. light exposure) affect their nutrient content. Therefore, the theoretical calculations of ingredients often do not reflect the actual content [77].

Sullivan et al. found the nutrition content of blended diets from nutritionally suitable recipes created and analysed using dietary analysis software were in practice very different from the theoretical content [78]. Fluctuations in the nutrition composition of 16–50% have been described in liquidised feeds using the same recipe. The authors concluded that liquidised feeds have an inconsistent level of macronutrients and micronutrients and were unlikely to deliver optimum nutrients based on recipes developed [8–10].

To date, there has only been one study considering the growth of children on liquidised feeds. Pentiuk et al. found that over time, children gained an average of 6.2 g/day (median 5 g/day; range –8 to 28.9 g/day) [79]. Further analysis on these data indicated that 48% of the cohort had a significant decline in their weight-for-age z-scores during the study period which suggests the liquidised feeds were not sufficient to support adequate growth. Healthcare professionals therefore need to be aware that current research highlights some significant concerns related to the use of liquidised feeds and families requesting such a diet should have an appropriate risk assessment.

References

1. Johnson CP, Blasco PA. Infant growth and development. *Pediatr Rev* 1997; **18**(7): 224–242.

2. Paulino AC, Constine LS, Rubin P, Williams JP. Normal tissue development, homeostasis, senescence, and the sensitivity to radiation injury across the age spectrum. *Semin Radiat Oncol* 2010; **20**(1): 12–20.

3. Varni JW, Bendo CB, Shulman RJ, et al. Interpretability of the PedsQL gastrointestinal symptoms scales and gastrointestinal worry scales in pediatric patients with functional and organic gastrointestinal diseases. *J Pediatr Psychol* 2015; **40**(6): 591–601.

4. Cooper PJ, Whelan E, Woolgar M, Morrell J, Murray L. Association between childhood feeding problems and maternal eating disorder: role of the family environment. *Br J Psychiatry* 2004; **184**: 210–215.

5. Joint WHO/FAO/UNU Expert Consultation. Protein and Amino Acid Requirements in Human Nutrition. Geneva: World Health Organization, 2007.

6. World Health Organization, UNICEF. WHO Child Growth Standards and The Identification of Severe Acute Malnutrition in Infants and Children. Geneva: World Health Organization, 2009.

7. Prentice A, Schoenmakers I, Laskey MA, DeBono S, Ginty F, Goldberg GR. Symposium on 'nutrition and health in children and adolescents' session 1: nutrition in growth and development. *Proc Nutr Soc* 2006; **65**(4): 348–360.

8. Carruth BR, Skinner JD. Feeding behaviors and other motor development in healthy children (2–24 months). *J Am Coll Nutr* 2002; **21**(2): 88–96.

9. Olsen EM, Peterson J, Skovgaard JM, Weile B, Jorgensen T, Wright CM. Failure to thrive: the prevalence and concurrance of anthropometric criteria in a general infant population. *Arch Dis Child* 2007; **92**: 109–114.

10. World Health Organization. Global Database on Child Growth and Malnutrition: Child Growth Indicators and Their Interpretation. www.who.int/nutgrowhdb/about/introudction/en/index2.html (accessed 3 September 2017).

11. World Health Organization. Child Growth Standards: Training Course and Other Tools. www.who.int/childgrowth/training/en/ (accessed 3 September 2017).

12. Oruamabo RS. Child malnutrition and the millennium development goals: much haste but less speed? *Arch Dis Child* 2015; **100**(Suppl 1): S19–S22.

13. McDougall P, Drewitt RF, Hungin APS, Wright CM. The detection of early weight faltering at the 6–8 week check and its association with family factors, feeding and behairoural development. *Arch Dis Child* 2009; **94**: 549–552.

14. Grimberg A, Ramos M, Grundmeier R, et al. Sex-based prevalence of growth faltering in an urban pediatric population. *J Pediatr* 2009; **154**: 567–572.

15. Ong KK, Hardy R, Shah I, Kuh D. Childhood stunting and mortality between 36 and 64 years: the British 1946 Birth Cohort Study. *J Clin Endocrinol Metab* 2013; **98**(5): 2070–2077.

16. Victora CG, de Onis M, Hallal PC, Blossner M, Shrimpton R. Worldwide timing of growth faltering: revisiting implications for interventions. *Pediatrics* 2010; **125**(3): e473–e480.

17. Marino LV, Goddard E, Workman L. Determining the prevalence of malnutrition in hospitalized paediatric patients. *S Afr Med J* 2006; **96**(9 Pt2): 993–995.

18. Joosten KF, Hulst JM. Prevalence of malnutrition in pediatric hospital patients. *Curr Opin Pediatr* 2008; **20**(5): 590–596.

19. Pawellek I, Dokoupil K, Koletzko B. Prevalence of malnutrition in paediatric hospital patients. *Clin Nutr* 2008; **27**(1): 72–76.

20. Hecht C, Weber M, Grote V, et al. Disease associated malnutrition correlates with length of hospital stay in children. *Clin Nutr* 2015; **34**(1): 53–59.

21. Pichler J, Hill SM, Shaw V, Lucas A. Prevalence of undernutrition during hospitalisation in a children's hospital: what happens during admission? *Eur J Clin Nutr* 2014; **68**(6): 730–735.

22. Sullivan PB. Malnutrition in hospitalised children. *Arch Dis Child* 2010; **95**(7): 489–490.

23. Ramsay M, Gisel EG, McCusker J, Bellavance F, Platt R. Infant sucking ability, non-organic failure to thrive, maternal characteristics, and feeding practices: a prospective cohort study. *Dev Med Child Neurol* 2002; **44**(6): 405–414.

24. Mehta NM, Corkins MR, Lyman B, et al. Defining pediatric malnutrition: a paradigm shift toward etiology-related definitions. *J Parenter Enteral Nutr* 2013; **37**(4): 460–481.

25. Ramsay M, Gisel EG, Boutry M. Non-organic failure to thrive: growth failure secondary to feeding-skills disorder. *Dev Med Child Neurol* 1993; **35**(4): 285–297.

26. Gat-Yablonski G, Phillip M. Nutritionally-induced catch-up growth. *Nutrients* 2015; **7**(1): 517–551.

27. Haas AM. Feeding disorders in food allergic children. *Curr Allergy Asthma Rep* 2010; **10**(4): 258–264.

28. Rommel N, de Meyer A, Feenstra L, Veereman-Wauters G. The complexity of feeding problems in 700 infants and young children presenting to a tertiary care institution. *J Pediatr Gastroenterol Nutr* 2003; **37**: 75–84.

29. Cartwright MM. The metabolic response to stress: a case of complex nutrition support management. *Crit Care Nurs Clin North Am* 2004; **16**(4): 467–487.

30. Hogan SE. Energy requirements of children with cerebral palsy. *Can J Diet Pract Res* 2004; **65**(3): 124–130.

31. Levy Y, Levy A, Zangen T, et al. Diagnostic clues for identification of nonorganic vs organic causes of food refusal and poor feeding. *J Pediatr Gastroenterol Nutr* 2009; **48**(3): 355–362.

32. Jacobi C, Agras WS, Bryson S, Hammer LD. Behavioral validation, precursors, and concomitants of picky eating in childhood. *J Am Acad Child Adolesc Psychiatry* 2003; **42**(1): 76–84.

33. Harding C, Faiman A, Wright J. Evaluation of an intensive desensitisation, oral tolerance therapy and hunger provocation program for children who have had prolonged periods of tube feeds. *Int J Evid Based Health* 2010; **8**(4): 268–276.

34. Ekstein S, Laniado D, Glick B. Does picky eating affect weight-for-length measurements in young children? *Clin Pediatr* 2010; **49**(3): 217–220.

35. Wright CM, Parkinson KN, Drewett RF. How does maternal and child feeding behavior relate to weight gain and failure to thrive? Data from a prospective birth cohort. *Pediatrics* 2006; **117**(4): 1262–1269.

36. Wright CM, Parkinson KN, Drewett RF. The influence of maternal socioeconomic and emotional factors on infant weight gain and weight faltering (failure to thrive): data from a prospective birth cohort. *Arch Dis Child* 2006; **91**(4): 312–317.

37. Mehta NM, Bechard LJ, Cahill N, et al. Nutritional practices and their relationship to clinical outcomes in critically ill children – an international multicenter cohort study*. *Crit Care Med* 2012; **40**(7): 2204–2211.

38. Goiburu ME, Goiburu MM, Bianco H, et al. The impact of malnutrition on morbidity, mortality and length of hospital stay in trauma patients. *Nutr Hosp* 2006; **21**(5): 604–610.

39. De Souza MF, Leite HP, Koch Nogueira PC. Malnutrition as an independent predictor of clinical outcome in critically ill children. *Nutrition* 2012; **28**(3): 267–270.

40. Pichler J, Horn V, Macdonald S, Hill S. Sepsis and its etiology among hospitalized children less than 1 year of age with intestinal failure on parenteral nutrition. *Transplant Proc* 2010; **42**(1): 24–25.

41. Brinksma A, Sanderman R, Roodbol PF, et al. Malnutrition is associated with worse health-related quality of life in children with cancer. *Support Care Cancer* 2015; **23**(10): 3043–3052.

42. Bodnar R, Kadar L, Holics K, et al. Factors influencing quality of life and disease severity in Hungarian children and young adults with cystic fibrosis. *Ital J Pediatr* 2014; **40**: 50.

43. Rudolf MCJ, Logan S. What is the long term outcome for children who fail to thrive? *Arch Dis Child* 2005; **90**: 925–931.

44. Sudfeld CR, Charles MD, Danaei G, et al. Linear growth and child development in low- and middle-income countries: a meta-analysis. *Pediatrics* 2015; **135**(5): e1266–e1275.

45. Dewey KG, Begum K. Long-term consequences of stunting in early life. *Matern Child Nutr* 2011; **7**(Suppl 3): 5–18.

46. Gerasimidis K, Macleod I, Maclean A, et al. Performance of the novel Paediatric Yorkhill Malnutrition Score (PYMS) in hospital practice. *Clin Nutr* 2011; **30**(4): 430–435.

47. Gerasimidis K, Macleod I, Finlayson L, et al. Introduction of Paediatric Yorkhill Malnutrition Score – challenges and impact on nursing practice. *J Clin Nurs* 2012; **21**(23–24): 3583–3586.

48. McCarthy H, Dixon M, Crabtree I, Eaton-Evans MJ, McNulty H. The development and evaluation of the Screening Tool for the Assessment of Malnutrition in Paediatrics (STAMP(c)) for use by healthcare staff. *J Hum Nutr Diet* 2012; **25**(4): 311–318.

49. Hulst JM, Zwart H, Hop WC, Joosten KF. Dutch national survey to test the STRONGkids nutritional risk screening tool in hospitalized children. *Clin Nutr* 2010; **29**(1): 106–111.

50. Huysentruyt K, Devreker T, Dejonckheere J, De Schepper J, Vandenplas Y, Cools F. The accuracy of nutritional screening tools in assessing the risk of under-nutrition in hospitalized children: a systematic review of literature and meta-analysis. *J Pediatr Gastroenterol Nutr* 2015; **61**(2): 159–166.

51. Becker PJ, Nieman CL, Corkins MR, et al. Consensus statement of the Academy of Nutrition and Dietetics/American Society for Parenteral and Enteral Nutrition: indicators recommended for the identification and documentation of pediatric malnutrition (undernutrition). *J Acad Nutr Diet* 2014; **114**(12): 1988–2000.

52. World Health Organization. Guidelines for an Integrated Approach to the Nutritional Care of HIV-Infected Children (6 Months–14 Years). Preliminary Version for Country Introduction. Chart Booklet. Geneva: WHO, 2009.

53. UNICEF. IMCI integrated management of childhood illness. Geneva: WHO, 2005.

54. Amthor RE, Cole SM, Manary MJ. The use of home-based therapy with ready-to-use therapeutic food to treat malnutrition in a rural area during a food crisis. *J Am Diet Assoc* 2009; **109**(3): 464–467.

55. Himes JH. Minimal time intervals for serial measurements of growth with recumbent length of stature of individual children. *Acta Paediatr* 1999; **88**: 120–125.

56. Prentice AM, Ward KA, Goldberg GR, et al. Critical windows for nutritional interventions against stunting. *Am J Clin Nutr* 2013; **97**(5): 911–918.

57. Golden MH. Proposed recommended nutrient densities for moderately malnourished children. *Food Nutr Bull* 2009; **30**(3 Suppl): S267–S342.

58. Pencharz PB. Protein and energy requirements for 'optimal' catch-up growth. *Eur J Clin Nutr* 2010; **64**(Suppl 1): S5–S7.

59. Ramakrishnan U, Nguyen P, Martorell R. Effects of micronutrients on growth of children under 5 y of age: meta-analyses of single and multiple nutrient interventions. *Am J Clin Nutr* 2009; **89**(1): 191–203.

60. Aggett PJ, Agostoni C, Axelsson I, et al. Iron metabolism and requirements in early childhood: do we know enough? A commentary by the ESPGHAN Committee on Nutrition. *J Pediatr Gastroenterol Nutr* 2002; **34**(4): 337–345.

61. Freeman VE, Mulder J, van't Hof MA, Hoey HM, Gibney MJ. A longitudinal study of iron status in children at 12, 24 and 36 months. *Public Health Nutr* 1998; **1**(2): 93–100.

62. Bhaskaram P. Micronutrient malnutrition, infection, and immunity: an overview. *Nutr Rev* 2002; **60**(5 Pt 2): S40–S45.

63. Doherty CP, Crofton PM, Sarkar MA, et al. Malnutrition, zinc supplementation and catch-up growth: changes in insulin-like growth factor I, its binding proteins, bone formation and collagen turnover. *Clin Endocrinol* 2002; **57**(3): 391–399.

64. Levine A, Bachar L, Tsangen Z, et al. Screening criteria for diagnosis of infantile feeding disorders as a cause of poor feeding or food refusal. *J Pediatr Gastroenterol Nutr* 2011; **52**(5): 563–568.

65. Zangen T, Ciarla C, Zangen S, et al. Gastrointestinal motility and sensory abnormalities may contribute to food refusal in medically fragile toddlers. *J Pediatr Gastroenterol Nutr* 2003; **37**(3): 287–293.

66. Braegger C, Decsi T, Dias JA, et al. Practical approach to paediatric enteral nutrition: a comment by the ESPGHAN committee on nutrition. *J Pediatr Gastroenterol Nutr* 2010; **51**(1): 110–122.

67. Clarke SE, Evans S, MacDonald A, Davies P, Booth IW. Randomized comparison of a nutrient-dense formula with an energy-supplemented formula for infants with faltering growth. *J Hum Nutr Diet* 2007; **20**: 329–339.

68. Pereira-da-Silva L, Pitta-Gros DM, Virella D, Serelha M. Osmolality of elemental and semi-elemental formulas supplemented with nonprotein energy supplements. *J Hum Nutr Diet* 2008; **21**(6): 584–590.

69. Meyer R, Venter C, Fox AT, Shah N. Practical dietary management of protein energy malnutrition in young children with cow's milk protein allergy. *Pediatr Allergy Immunol* 2012; **23**(4): 307–314.

70. Ziegler EE, Fomon SJ. Potential renal solute load of infant formulas. *J Nutr* 1989; **119**(Suppl 12): 1785–1788.

71. King C, Davis T. Nutritional treatment of infants and children with faltering growth. *Eur J Clin Nutr* 2010; **64**(Suppl 1): S11–S13.

72. Dello SL, Principato F, Sinibaldi D, et al. Feeding dysfunction in infants with severe chronic renal failure after long-term nasogastric tube feeding. *Pediatr Nephrol* 1997; **11**(1): 84–86.

73. Bott L, Husson MO, Guimber D, et al. Contamination of gastrostomy feeding systems in children in a home-based enteral nutrition program. *J Pediatr Gastroenterol Nutr* 2001; **33**(3): 266–270.

74. Jalali M, Sabzghabaee AM, Badri SS, Soltani HA, Maracy MR. Bacterial contamination of hospital-prepared enteral tube feeding formulas in Isfahan, Iran. *J Res Med Sci* 2009; **14**(3): 149–156.

75. Baniardalan M, Sabzghabaee AM, Jalali M, Badri S. Bacterial safety of commercial and handmade enteral feeds in an Iranian teaching hospital. *Int J Prev Med* 2014; **5**(5): 604–610.

76. O'Flaherty T, Santoro K, Pentuik S. Calculating and preparing a pureed-by-gastrostomy-tube (PBGT) diet by paediatric patients with retching and gagging postfundoplication. *Infant Child Adoles Nutr* 2011; **3**(6): 361–364.

77. Santos VF, Morais TB. Nutritional quality and osmolality of home-made enteral diets, and follow-up of growth of severely disabled children receiving home enteral nutrition therapy. *J Trop Pediatr* 2010; **56**(2): 127–128.

78. Sullivan MM, Sorreda-Esguerra P, Santos EE, et al. Bacterial contamination of blenderized whole food and commercial enteral tube feedings in the Philippines. *J Hosp Infect* 2001; **49**(4): 268–273.

79. Pentiuk S, O'Flaherty T, Santoro K, Willging P, Kaul A. Pureed by gastrostomy tube diet improves gagging and retching in children with fundoplication. *J Parenter Enteral Nutr* 2011; **35**(3): 375–379.

Chapter 5.2

Nutrition support in anorexia nervosa

Maria Gabriella Gentile[1] and Lisa Chiara Fellin[2]

[1]Department of Clinical Nutrition, A.O. Niguarda, Arese, Italy
[2]University of East London, London, UK

5.2.1 Introduction

Sociocultural, biological and psychological factors can all contribute to the aetiology of eating disorders. In economically developed countries, the excessive value placed on thinness can encourage extreme dieting and weight control practices [1]. The conflict between the stigmatisation of fatness, myth of thinness and easy access to highly palatable foods can lead to strict dieting and bingeing and in some cases to eating disorders [1]. In addition, negative comparisons between the 'self' and the 'ideal' body shape can affect self-esteem, comparisons and power struggles within and outside the family. Family processes can play a role in the maintenance of eating disorders, but also in seeking help and recovery, given the egosyntonic nature of this disorder [1–3].

Eating disorders are mental health disorders defined by abnormal eating habits that negatively affect a person's physical or mental health. They include bulimia nervosa, anorexia nervosa (AN), binge eating disorders and other specified feeding or eating disorders [4–6]. The *Diagnostic and Statistical Manual of Mental Health Disorders* (DSM) provides diagnostic criteria to assist in the diagnosis and care of individuals with eating disorders [4]. Table 5.2.1 provides a comparison of the classification of bulimia nervosa and anorexia nervosa.

5.2.2 Anorexia nervosa

Anorexia nervosa (AN) is a potentially life-threatening eating disorder characterised by self-starvation, excessive weight loss and negative body image. Epidemiological trends in AN are difficult to ascertain because detection by self-reporting may not be reliable in a disorder characterised by secrecy and denial. Trends can also be affected by changes in diagnostic criteria over time. The worldwide prevalence of AN in women is estimated at 0.3–1%, with a yearly incidence of 8 cases/100 000 population [4]. The National Institute for Health and Care Excellence reports a prevalence of 1 in 250 females and 1 in 2000 males in the UK [5]. How much of the prevalence in females can be attributed to biological rather than social factors remains uncertain. While most common in females, approximately 10–15% of all individuals with anorexia are male. AN can affect individuals of all ethnicities and all ages, but the onset of AN most commonly occurs during adolescence [4–6].

Anorexia nervosa presents the highest mortality rates of all psychiatric disorders (up to 5–6%) [7] and is the third most common chronic disease among female adolescents [8]. An individual diagnosis of AN is made based on the detailed DSM criteria, as outlined in Box 5.2.1 [4].

Advanced Nutrition and Dietetics in Nutrition Support, First Edition. Edited by Mary Hickson and Sara Smith.
© 2018 John Wiley & Sons Ltd. Published 2018 by John Wiley & Sons Ltd.

Table 5.2.1 DSM classification of bulimia nervosa and anorexia nervosa

Disorder	Remarks

Anorexia nervosa	• Persistent restriction of energy intake leading to significantly low body weight (in context of what is minimally expected for age, sex, developmental trajectory and physical health)
	• Either an intense fear of gaining weight or of becoming fat, or persistent behaviour that interferes with weight gain (even though already of significantly low weight)
	• Disturbance in the way one's body weight or shape is experienced, undue influence of body shape and weight on self-evaluation, or persistent lack of recognition of the seriousness of the current low body weight
	• Subtypes:
	  ○ Restricting type
	  ○ Binge-eating/purging type

Bulimia nervosa	• Recurrent episodes of binge eating. An episode of binge eating is characterised by both of the following:
	  ○ Eating, in a discrete period of time (e.g. within any 2-hour period), an amount of food that is definitely larger than most people would eat during a similar period of time and under similar circumstances
	  ○ A sense of lack of control over eating during the episode (e.g. a feeling that one cannot stop eating or control what or how much one is eating)
	• Recurrent inappropriate compensatory behaviour in order to prevent weight gain, such as self-induced vomiting, misuse of laxatives, diuretics or other medications, fasting, or excessive exercise
	• The binge eating and inappropriate compensatory behaviours both occur, on average, at least once a week for 3 months
	• Self-evaluation is unduly influenced by body shape and weight.
	• The disturbance does not occur exclusively during episodes of anorexia nervosa

Source: *Diagnostic and Statistical Manual of Mental Health Disorders* [4] with permission of the American Psychiatric Association.

Consequences of undernutrition in anorexia nervosa

Undernutrition, disordered eating and weight behaviours can explain most of the biological findings in AN as well as much of the emotional and cognitive disorders and psychological distress. Severe undernutrition causes measurable adverse effects on body composition, functions and clinical outcomes. In patients with AN, the primary risk factors for developing medical complications due to undernutrition are the degree and speed of weight loss and the chronicity of the illness [9,10]. Weight loss greater than approximately 15–20% of ideal body weight often leads to gastroparesis, that is, delayed emptying of the stomach. The main symptoms are bloating, upper quadrant pain and early satiety which can be severe [11]. It has also been observed that weight loss with a body mass index (BMI) less than 12 kg/m^2 can produce mild elevation (2–3 times normal) of transaminases [12].

Sex hormones are affected in both males and females with AN, with low concentrations of hypothalamic gonadotrophin-releasing hormone, pituitary hormone, luteinising hormone, follicle-stimulating hormone, oestrogen and testosterone being reported. Usually these symptoms appear very early, even in mild undernutrition. These abnormalities affect potency, fertility and bone density, and cause amenorrhoea [10].

Additionally, bone marrow can be adversely affected by AN. Specifically, anaemia and leucopenia occur in approximately one-third of AN patients and thrombocytopenia occurs in 10%.

Box 5.2.1 Diagnostic criteria for anorexia nervosa

A Restriction of energy intake relative to requirements, leading to a significantly low body weight in the context of age, sex, developmental trajectory and physical health. *Significantly low weight* is defined as a weight that is less than minimally normal or, for children and adolescents, less than that minimally expected.
B Intense fear of gaining weight or of becoming fat, or persistent behaviour that interferes with weight gain, even though at a significantly low weight.
C Disturbance in the way in which one's body weight or shape is experienced, undue influence of body weight or shape on self-evaluation, or persistent lack of recognition of the seriousness of the current low body weight.

Specify type of eating disorder
Restricting type: During the last 3 months, the individual has not engaged in recurrent episodes of binge eating or purging behaviour (i.e. self-induced vomiting or the misuse of laxatives, diuretics or enemas). This subtype describes presentations in which weight loss is accomplished primarily through dieting, fasting and/or excessive exercise.
  Binge-eating/purging type: During the last 3 months, the individual has engaged in recurrent episodes of binge eating or purging behaviour (i.e. self-induced vomiting or the misuse of laxatives, diuretics or enemas).

Specify remission status
In partial remission: After full criteria for anorexia nervosa were previously met. Criterion A (low body weight) has not been met for a sustained period, but either Criterion B (intense fear of gaining weight or becoming fat or behaviour that interferes with weight gain) or Criterion C (disturbances in self-perception of weight and shape) is still met.
  In full remission: After full criteria for anorexia nervosa were previously met, none of the criteria have been met for a sustained period of time.

Specify current severity
The minimum level of severity is based, for adults, on current BMI (see below) or, for children and adolescents, on BMI percentile. The ranges below are derived from WHO categories for thinness in adults; for children and adolescents, corresponding BMI percentiles should be used. The level of severity may be increased to reflect clinical symptoms, the degree of functional disability and the need for supervision.

Mild: BMI >17 kg/m^2
Moderate: BMI 16–16.99 kg/m^2
Severe: BMI 15–15.99 kg/m^2
Extreme: BMI <15 kg/m^2

Source: *Diagnostic and Statistical Manual of Mental Health Disorders* [4] with permission of the American Psychiatric Association.

As disease severity worsens and BMI falls, the frequency of these abnormalities is greater, with upwards of 75% of patients demonstrating cytopenias [10].

Thyroid abnormalities have also been reported in individuals with AN, with low concentrations of total thyroxine and tri-iodothyronine (T$_3$) being observed, with concentrations of T$_3$ usually decreasing in proportion to the degree of weight loss [10]. However, it should be noted that the thyroid stimulating hormone is usually within normal ranges. Furthermore, a number of cardiac abnormalities associated with AN have been described in the literature, including pericardial and valvular pathology, changes in left ventricular mass and function, conduction abnormalities, bradycardia, hypotension and dysregulation in peripheral vascular; usually they are proportional to the degree of weight loss [10].

The brain is especially vulnerable to undernutrition, which causes shrinking and many behavioural and psychosocial effects such as rigidity, emotional dysregulation and abnormal social behaviour [13]. Some studies have demonstrated that AN is associated with variable, but usually significant, brain atrophy [14]. On magnetic resonance imaging, severe cases of AN may present with enlarged ventricles and decreased cortical substance. However, research has shown that regional grey and global grey and white matter volumes were similar for women long-term recovered from AN and age-matched healthy controls [14,15].

Patients with AN very commonly have impaired bone structure and reduced bone strength. Osteoporosis or osteopenia has been reported in 85% of women with a diagnosis of AN [16]. Weight restoration may correct many of these reversible symptoms, but bone and brain alterations may be irreversible [4–6].

5.2.3 Nutritional assessment in anorexia nervosa

Assessment of adults with AN should be person centred, involve family and significant others unless there are clear contraindications, take a multidisciplinary approach and tailor management based on stage of illness severity and symptom profile [2,4–6,17,18]. An initial comprehensive evaluation should include a thorough anthropometric, biochemical, clinical, dietary and environmental assessment in order to inform nutrition intervention strategies and monitor their impact. A summary of the relevant parameters commonly considered in practice is provided below.

Anthropometry

It is common to undertake routine measurement of weight, height, calculation of BMI, weight change, weight history and body composition (e.g. lean body mass), in addition to exploring reasons for the inability to restore weight, fears about weight gain and body image disturbance.

Biochemistry

It is recommended that serum tests to detect hypokalaemia, hypoglycaemia, hypophosphataemia, hypomagnesaemia, metabolic alkalosis or acidosis are undertaken, in addition to liver function tests and relevant blood tests to investigate undernutrition-induced bone marrow suppression such as neutropenia, and low lymphocytes [4–6,17–19].

Clinical

A detailed clinical history, full physical examination, pulse rate, blood pressure (seated and standing), electrocardiogram, temperature and checks on amenorrhoea or irregular menses are recommended, in addition to a bone mineral density scan, if the person has been underweight for 6 months or longer with or without amenorrhoea [20,21].

Psychiatric comorbidities should also be assessed, including anxiety, depression, substance misuse, suicidality and personality disorders. However, it is important to be aware that depression, obsessional thinking, anxiety and other psychiatric symptoms could represent the reversible effects of undernutrition on the brain [13].

Dietary and environmental

Nutritional history should include levels of dietary restriction, fluid intake, excessive exercise, purging, bingeing, use of medications to lose or maintain low weight (laxative, diuretics), disordered eating behaviours, such as eating apart from others, prolonged mealtimes and division of food into very small pieces. Social circumstances should also be considered, as should the presence of additional stressors interfering with the patient's ability to eat, such as intercurrent illnesses, inadequate social supports, severe disabling symptoms of bulimia that have not responded to outpatient treatment and severe family problems such as depression, alcoholism and eating disorders.

A summary of the relevant markers used as a risk assessment for the identification of major complications in AN patients is provided in Table 5.2.2; these findings should be used to determine if immediate hospital admission is required. Hospitalisation is indicated for those at high risk of life-threatening medical complications, extremely low weights and other uncontrolled symptoms [2,4–6,17,18].

Table 5.2.2 Nutritional and clinical markers for risk assessment in AN patients

	Very high risk	High risk
Anthropometry	BMI <13 kg/m² Recent weight loss of ≥1 kg/week	BMI 13–15 kg/m² Recent weight loss of <0.5 kg or less /week
Biochemical abnormalities	Hypophosphataemia Hypokalaemia Hypo- or hypernatraemia Raised transaminases Hypoglycaemia	Hypophosphataemia Hypokalaemia Hypo- or hypernatraemia
Hydration status	Severe dehydration from fluid refusal or overhydration from excessive fluid intake	Moderate dehydration or overhydration
Cardiovascular system	Heart rate (awake) <40 bpm Low blood pressure: Systolic (mmHg) <80 Diastolic (mmHg) <50 Marked orthostatic changes in systolic blood pressure Raised QTc (>450 ms) Non-specific T-wave changes Low core temperature <35.5 °C tympanic	Heart rate (awake) 40–50 bpm Low blood pressure: Systolic (mmHg) <90 Diastolic (mmHg) <60
Activity and exercise	High levels of uncontrolled exercise in the context of severe undernutrition	Moderate levels of uncontrolled exercise in the context of undernutrition

BMI, body mass index; bpm = beats per minute.

5.2.4 Nutritional, psychological and pharmacological intervention in anorexia nervosa

Evidence for effective AN treatment is still poor; guidelines and position papers agree on defining the best treatment as a multidisciplinary approach involving a team of medical and mental health staff, dietitians and nurses trained in the treatment of eating disorders. Treatment simultaneously involves appropriate nutritional, psychological and pharmacological interventions (Box 5.2.2) [4–6,18]. As much as possible, family members and other professionals should also be involved because symptom minimisation, poor insight and lack of understanding of the seriousness of symptoms are common in AN patients. In addition, due to the nature of the condition, long-term follow-up will be required [2,5,6,18].

All international guidelines recommend treatment as an outpatient or day patient, with hospital admission required for those at risk of medical and/or psychological compromise. Guidelines [2,4–6,17] consistently agree that when possible, AN patients should be engaged and treated before they reach severe emaciation to improve outcomes [5]. This requires both early identification and intervention. Effective monitoring and engagement of patients at severely low weight, or with falling weight, should be a priority and patients should be hospitalised before becoming medically unstable. The patient's general medical status will assist in determining whether psychiatric or medical hospitalisation is indicated.

Discharge from hospital should only occur when the person is medically stabilised and when nutrition intervention has reversed any cognitive effects of starvation, so that the patient can benefit from outpatient or day patient

---

Box 5.2.2 Summary of the nutritional, psychological and pharmacological management of anorexia nervosa

Nutritional rehabilitation

Establishment of expected rates of controlled weight gain to reach healthy weight

    Personalised nutritional programmes

    Vitamin supplementation (especially thiamine and group B vitamins)

    Mineral supplementation (especially phosphorus)

    Very frequent monitoring of serum phosphate, potassium, magnesium

    Reduce or restrict physical activity and always carefully supervise and monitor

    Monitoring of body weight and the reactions associated with weight gain (e.g. anxiety)

Management of behaviours

Food avoidance and concealment

    Exercising

    Falsifying weight

    Excessive water drinking

    Hiding drugs

Psychosocial interventions

Cognitive behavioural therapy

    Individual psychotherapy

    Group psychotherapy

    Psychoeducation programme for patients and parents

    Family therapy

Pharmacological interventions

Psychotropic medications when patients show significant comorbid psychopathology such as obsessive-compulsive disabling symptoms, depression or anxiety

    Vitamin and mineral supplementation, e.g. vitamin D, phosphorus, potassium, magnesium, calcium, zinc, motility agents (as fibre)

---

psychotherapy (often several weeks of nutrition are required to achieve this). Prior to discharge, individuals should have had trials of leave to demonstrate that they can eat outside hospital, and they need a direct link with appropriate outpatient monitoring, support and treatment.

Outpatient home treatment is the most common method of intervention if the patient's symptoms are less severe or improving. Each individual will undergo a unique course of treatment, with personal factors taken into account such as current weight, level of motivation and condition of health. This usually means that specialist dietary plans must be made in order to correct the imbalances and not cause additional problems.

The general goals for intervention in AN are as follows [1,2,4,5,18].

(1) Treat physical complications and correct nutritional deficiencies.

(2) Restore patients to a healthy body weight for physiological function (i.e. return of ovulatory menses in female patients, normal hormone concentrations in male patients).

(3) Help patients reassess and change core dysfunctional AN-related cognitions and feelings and provide psychoeducation regarding healthy nutrition and eating patterns.

(4) Treat psychological issues and possible associated psychiatric conditions.

(5) Provide family counselling and therapy.

Whilst nutrition intervention and weight restoration are basic goals in the treatment of patients with AN and will result in improvements in the majority of clinical and psychological derangements, clear guidelines are still lacking. US [2] and NICE guidelines [5] similarly suggest an expected average weight gain in AN inpatients and outpatients of 0.5–1 kg/week in the inpatient setting and 0.5 kg/week in the outpatient setting (requiring approximately 3500–7000 additional kcals a week to achieve), but the guidelines do not consider the optimal quantity and quality of nutrients that are most critical to achieve treatment goals. It should also be recognised that there will be significant individual variability and weight gain may be slower, but the aim should be for progressive weight restoration.

For many years, recommendations for the commencement of regimens for AN inpatients have been cautious. UK and Australian guidelines have recommended nutritional regimens starting with as little as 200–600 kcal/day, that is, an initial refeeding rate of between 10 and 20 kcal/kg/day [2,5]. In contrast, in the United States the usual recommendations are to commence nutritional regimens around 1200 kcal/day, progressing slowly to full requirements by adding 200 kcal every other day [2,17]. Both UK and US treatment guidelines for AN recommend average inpatient weight gain rates between 0.5 and 1.4 kg/week to avoid refeeding syndrome.

Refeeding syndrome in AN

Refeeding syndrome is characterised by rapid mineral, electrolyte and fluid shifts that can result in severe medical sequelae, including cardiac arrhythmias, cardiac arrest, muscle weakness, haemolytic anaemia, delirium, seizures, coma and even death [18,22–24]. The majority of current guidelines aim to avoid refeeding syndrome mainly by restricting the intake of energy. Refeeding of severely undernourished patients poses two very complex and conflicting tasks: to avoid refeeding syndrome caused by a too fast correction of undernutrition and avoid underfeeding caused by an overly cautious nutritional rehabilitation.

Energy intake should ideally be prescribed based on indirect calorimetric measurements, particularly in severely undernourished bedrest patients. Where indirect calorimetry is not possible for the measurement of basal metabolic rate, clinical evaluation investigating any medical complications and the current level of medical risk should be used. Some studies have demonstrated a reduction of approximately 20%

of estimated basal metabolic rate in AN undernourished patients, based on the Harris–Benedict formula [22,23].

The risk of refeeding syndrome with associated hypophosphataemia is largely correlated to the degree of undernutrition and how this is managed, that is, the amount of energy, vitamins and macro/micronutrients supplied [25]. Supplementation of additional phosphate when basal serum values are normal may also be required to prevent hypophosphataemia. Phosphate requirements can vary extensively and in severe AN (BMI below 15 kg/m^2) strict daily monitoring of serum concentrations is required [22].

Initial refeeding may be associated with mild transient fluid retention, but patients who abruptly stop laxatives or diuretic may develop marked fluid retention caused by secondary hyperaldosteronism and in such cases, a competitive aldosterone antagonist diuretic may be required (21). Patients may also experience abdominal bloating or delayed gastric emptying or constipation. The latter can be ameliorated with stool softeners and/or fibre intake.

A systematic review of 27 studies (96% were observational/prospective or retrospective and performed in hospital) of refeeding in AN observed that more recently published studies (12 studies since 2010) utilised approaches starting with higher energy prescriptions than currently recommended (e.g. 1400 kcal/day), without an increase in risk [26]. Based on this and other findings of the review, the following recommendations were proposed [26].

- In mildly and moderately undernourished patients, lower energy refeeding is overly conservative.
- Both meal-based approaches or combined nasogastric and meals can be used to administer higher energy intakes.
- Higher energy prescriptions have not been associated with increased risk for the refeeding syndrome under close medical monitoring with electrolyte correction.
- In severely undernourished inpatients, there is insufficient evidence to change the current standard of care.

- Parenteral nutrition is not recommended; only one study used it.
- Nutrient compositions within recommended current dietary guidelines are appropriate.

Food interventions

Nutrition intervention in AN should be regarded as a process developing through different levels, including improving intakes from ordinary food, use of oral nutritional supplements or use of artificial nutrition support, and that these are not mutually exclusive. Patients should primarily be encouraged, but not forced, to eat the planned amount of food. Dietary inquiries through either daily diet diaries (outpatients) or food record charts (inpatients) should be used to monitor intakes. Patients should be supported to choose their own meals and be given a personalised structured meal plan that ensures nutritional adequacy and inclusion of all major food groups. There should be a particular emphasis on foods rich in phosphorus and protein, such as semi-hard or hard cheese, to assist in the prevention of hypophosphataemia [5,6,17,18].

Oral nutrition supplements

In AN, supplementing the diet with oral nutritional supplements may be useful to achieve the prescribed energy goal and can be a very effective strategy to achieve weight gain. Methods of nutritional provision include supervised meals and high-energy, high-protein oral liquid supplements [6,18,27–29]. When patients are prescribed oral or enteral nutritional supplements, consideration should be given to the use of high-energy supplements (e.g. 2 kcal/mL) to reduce gastric discomfort. Moreover, supplements should be rich in phosphate (e.g. milk) to help avoid refeeding syndrome. Total daily fluid intakes can easily exceed safe levels, and the recommendation is a maximum total of 30–35 mL/kg/24h of fluid from all sources, as refeeding oedema is well recognised [18].

Food intake should be adequately monitored by dietitians and nurses to avoid likely concealment. Secrecy and concealment of disordered eating are common. Patients may fake eating, hide food, avoid eating with others, drink water or use hidden objects to modify weight and secretly binge and purge and take excessive exercise [6,18,21].

Enteral nutrition

Criteria for the use of artificial nutrition support are not clearly established in AN, and there is a lack of consensus about optimal patient population, dosing timing and duration of treatment. However, in life-threatening conditions, artificial nutrition support should be considered. The following criteria have been proposed to identify eligible patients [30].

- Severe undernutrition (BMI $\leq$13 kg/m^2) and willing intake less than 100% of energy needs or with body weight not increasing.
- Unwilling to take dietary treatment or refusing any oral intake (accepting only artificial nutrition).
- Has a BMI between 13 and 15 kg/m^2 with measured resting metabolic rate lower than 70% of estimated basal metabolic rate according to the Harris–Benedict formula. If it is not possible to measure metabolic rate, use clinical evaluation, investigating any medical complications and the current level of medical risk.

Enteral nutrition is preferred if there is a functional accessible gastrointestinal tract. On very rare occasions where enteral nutrition is unfeasible, parenteral nutrition may be indicated [2,5,6,26]. Use of the nasogastric route demonstrates a lower risk of complications and is more cost-effective; the most comfortable nasogastric tubes are small (6–9 French units), made from silicon and polyurethane [28,30]. To significantly reduce fluid overload and gastric discomfort, a commercially high energy (1.7–2.2 kcal/mL), polymeric lactose-free, high-nitrogen fluid formula is recommended [23,29,30]. To minimise the risk of complications, enteral nutrition should be closely monitored and regulated via an electronically operated pump.

Compulsory treatment

As previously highlighted, severe acute or chronic undernutrition can lead to structural and functional changes in the central nervous system and as a consequence, at extremely low weights AN patients may be unable to make their own decisions. Therefore, in severe cases of AN where the patient refuses life-saving treatment, compulsory treatment should be considered. The frequency of compulsory treatment in AN has been reported from six studies from the UK, Australia, Japan, Germany and the USA and ranges from 13% to 44% [31].

However, whilst compulsory treatment may provide the opportunity to prevent fatal complications, the potential adverse effects on the therapeutic alliance should be considered [6]. The short-term weight gain response of compulsorily treated AN patients has been shown to be comparable to those admitted voluntarily and many of those who are treated on an involuntary (compulsory) basis later agree that treatment was necessary and remain therapeutically engaged [6]. However, research also suggests that patients can change their minds in retrospect about compulsory treatment and that they are often subject to compulsory treatment and coercion even without formal compulsory treatment orders, particularly if parents are consenting [32]. Furthermore, studies have demonstrated that patients receiving compulsory treatment compared with voluntary treatment have a higher severity of symptoms, higher comorbidity, more preadmissions, longer duration of illness and greater incidence of self-harm [31,33]. It is therefore evident that future research should focus on the most effective AN treatment, and on the longer term effects of compulsory treatment.

As a consequence of the above, compulsory treatment in AN inpatients has caused considerable controversy for ethical and legal aspects and legislation varies across different countries. Legislation in both New Zealand and Australia allows for compulsory assessment or treatment based on a person with AN having impaired decision-making capacity, and being unable or unwilling to consent to interventions required to preserve life [6]. The Mental Health Act 1983 for England and Wales, the Mental Health (Care and Treatment) (Scotland) Act 2008 and the Mental Health (Northern Ireland) Order 1986 allow for compulsory treatment of patients with eating disorders.

The specific assessment criteria informing compulsory admission and treatment are:

- the presence of a mental disorder (e.g. AN)
- inpatient treatment is appropriate (e.g. for refeeding), necessary and available
- such treatment is necessary for the health or safety of the patient.

For compulsory treatment, the Mental Health Act 1983 (amendments 2007) also requires a recommendation from a psychiatrist, a second recommendation from another doctor (generally the general practitioner or another psychiatrist) and an application from an approved mental health practitioner (formerly an approved social worker) [5]. In the US, to be subject to compulsory treatment (civil commitment), a person with a substantial mental health disorder must pose a risk of harm to herself or others because of the disorder [34]. That risk can be evidenced via an action, attempt or threat to do direct physical harm, or it might inhere in the potential for developing grave disability through neglect of one's basic needs, such as failing to eat adequately. If the evidence shows that an eating-disordered behaviour has placed the patient at imminent risk of permanent injury or death, it is possible to consider satisfied the legal criteria that justify court-ordered psychiatric hospitalisation [34].

References

1. Treasure J, Claudino AM, Zucker N. Eating disorders. *Lancet* 2010; **375**: 583–593.
2. American Psychiatric Association. Treatment of patients with eating disorders (3ʳᵈ ed). *Am J Psychiat* 2006; **163**(Suppl 7): 4–54.
3. Ugazio V, Negri A, Fellin L. Freedom, goodness, power and belonging: the semantics of phobic, obsessive-compulsive, eating, and mood disorders. *J Constr Psychol* 2015; **28**(4): 1–23.

4. Diagnostic and Statistical Manual of Mental Disorders (DSM-5®), 5th edn. Virginia: American Psychiatric Association, 2013.

5. National Institute for Health and Care Excellence. Eating Disorders – Core Interventions in the Treatment and Management of Anorexia Nervosa and Related Disorders. www.nice.org.uk (accessed 3 September 2017).

6. Hay P, Chinn D, Forbes D, et al. Royal Australian and New Zealand College of Psychiatrists clinical practice guidelines for the treatment of eating disorders. *Aust N Z J Psychiatry* 2014; **48**; 997–1009.

7. Sullivan PF. Mortality in anorexia nervosa. *Am J Psychiatry* 1995; **152**(7); 1073–1074.

8. Fisher M, Golden NH, Katzman DK, et al. Eating disorders in adolescents: a background paper. *J Adolesc Health* 1995; **16**: 420–437.

9. Miller KK, Steven K, Grinspoon SK, et al. Medical findings in outpatients with anorexia nervosa. *Arch Intern Med* 2005; **165**(5): 561–566.

10. Mehler PS, Brown C. Anorexia nervosa – medical complications. *J Eat Disord* 2015; **3**: 11.

11. Kamal N, Chami T, Andersen A, Rosell FA, Schuster MM, Whitehead WE. Delayed gastrointestinal transit times in anorexia nervosa and bulimia nervosa. *Gastroenterology* 1991; **101**(5): 1320–1324.

12. Hanachi M, Melchior JC, Crenn P. Hypertransaminasemia in severely malnourished adult anorexia nervosa patients: risk factors and evolution under enteral nutrition. *Clin Nutr* 2013; **32**(3): 391–395.

13. Keys A, Brozek J, Henschel A. The Biology of Human Starvation. Minneapolis: University of Minnesota Press, 1950.

14. Ehrlich S, Burghardt R, Weiss D, Salbach-Andrae H. Glial and neuronal damage markers in patients with anorexia nervosa. *J Neural Transm* 2008; **115**(6): 921–927.

15. Lázaro L, Andrés S, Calvo A, Cullell C, Moreno E. Normal gray and white matter volume after weight restoration in adolescents with anorexia nervosa. *Int J Eat Disord* 2013; **6**(8): 841–848.

16. Fazeli PK, Klibanski A. Bone metabolism in anorexia nervosa. *Curr Osteoporos Rep* 2014; **12**(1): 82–89.

17. American Dietetic Association. Position statement: nutritional intervention in the treatment of anorexia nervosa, bulimia nervosa, and other eating disorders. *J Am Diet Assoc* 2006; **106**(12): 2073–2082.

18. Marpisan Group. Marpisan: Management of Really Sick Patients with Anorexia Nervosa. College Report CR162. London: Royal College of Physicians, 2010.

19. Nishida T, Sakakibara H. Association between underweight and low lymphocyte count as an indicator of malnutrition in Japanese women. *J Womens Health* 2010; **19**(7): 1377–1383.

20. Mehler PS, Wilnkelman AB, Andersen DM, et al. Nutritional rehabilitation: practical guidelines for refeeding the anorectic patient. *J Nutr Metab* 2010; **1**: e10.

21. Gentile MG. Pseudo Bartter syndrome from surreptitious purging behaviour in anorexia nervosa. *J Nutr Disord Ther* 2012; **2**: 107.

22. Gentile MG, Manna GM. Refeeding hypophosphatemia in malnutrition patients: prevention and treatment. *Clin Nutr* 2011; **31**: 429.

23. Gentile MG, Pastorelli P, Ciceri R, et al. Specialized refeeding treatment for anorexia nervosa patients suffering from extreme undernutrition. *Clin Nutr* 2010; **29**: 627–632.

24. O'Connor G, Nicholls D, Hudson L, Singhal A. Refeeding low weight hospitalized adolescents with anorexia nervosa: a multicenter randomized controlled trial. *Nutr Clin Pract* 2016; **31**(5): 681–689.

25. O'Connor G, Nicholls D. Refeeding hypophosphatemia in adolescents with anorexia nervosa: a systematic review. *Nutr Clin Pract* 2013; **28**(3): 358–364.

26. Garber AK, Sawyer SM, Golden NH, et al. A systematic review of approaches to refeeding in patients with anorexia nervosa. *Int J Eat Disord* 2016; **49**(3): 293–310.

27. Philipson TJ, Snider JT, Lakdawalla DN, et al. Impact of oral nutritional supplementation on hospital outcomes. *Am J Manag Care* 2013; **19**: 121–128.

28. Kells M, Kelly-Weeder S. Nasogastric tube feeding for individuals with anorexia nervosa: an integrative review. *J Am Psychiatr Nurses Assoc* 2016; **22**(6): 449–468.

29. Gentile MG, Manna GM, Ciceri R, et al. Efficacy of inpatient treatment in severely malnourished anorexia nervosa patients. *Eat Weight Disord* 2008; **13**: 191–197.

30. Gentile MG. Nutritional management of anorexia in critical care. In: Nutrition in Critical Care. Cambridge: Cambridge University Press, 2014.

31. Thom RP, Mossman D. Imposing treatment on patients with eating disorders: what are the legal risks? *Curr Psychiatry* 2016; **15**(3): 54, 56–59.

32. Clausen L, Jones A. A systematic review of the frequency, duration, type and effect of involuntary treatment for people with anorexia nervosa, and an analysis of patient characteristics. *J Eat Disord* 2014; **2**: 29.

33. Elzakkers IFFM, Danner UN, Hans W, Hoek HW. Compulsory treatment in anorexia nervosa: a review. *Int J Eat Disord* 2014; **47**: 845–852.

34. Tan J, Hope T, Stewart A, Fitzpatrick R. Control and compulsory treatment in anorexia nervosa: the views of patients and parents. *Int J Law Psychiatry* 2003; **26**: 627–645.

Chapter 5.3

Nutrition support in older adults

Kathryn Rochette
Sunnybrook Health Sciences Centre, Toronto, Canada

5.3.1 Introduction

Worldwide, in 2010, there were an estimated 524 million older adults (people over the age of 65) and it is estimated that this number will triple by the year 2050 [1]. In a report compiled by Age UK, approximately 17% of the population in the UK will be over the age of 65 in 2015, with almost 5% of the population over the age of 80 and approximately 20% will live to become centenarians [2]. The UK Office for National Statistics estimates that for those who reach the age of 65 years, men can expect to live to 83.6 years and women 86.1 years [2]. Similar longevity trends have been reported in developed countries, with Canada reporting an average life expectancy of 85.7 years for those aged 65 years in 2009 [3] and Australia reporting a life expectancy of 87.1 years for women and 84.4 years for men aged 65 years [4].

5.3.2 Prevalence of undernutrition

Current estimates suggest that 32% of older adults admitted to UK hospitals are undernourished at the time of their admission [5]. A 2005 study of 22 007 Spanish older adults found that 4.3% of those screened utilising the Mini Nutritional Assessment (MNA) tool were undernourished and a further 25.4% were at risk of undernutrition [6]. Additional studies focused on long-term care units in Europe have found the prevalence of undernutrition older adults to be between 36% and 85% [7]. It is therefore anticipated that in future the prevalence of undernutrition could increase due to the increasing number of older adults.

5.3.3 Causes of undernutrition in older adults

There are many causes of undernutrition in older adults. Between the ages of 40 and 70 years, the average person can expect their energy intake to decrease by approximately 25% as a result of a phenomenon known as the anorexia of ageing [8]. Physiological changes, including changes to taste and smell, xerostomia, loss of dentition, reduced mobility due to conditions such as arthritis and decreased eyesight, can affect food intake by making food less appealing to consume and more difficult to obtain and prepare [7–9]. Other factors such as polypharmacy, cognitive decline, social isolation and alcohol consumption may lead to undernutrition in older adults whilst physical inactivity and depression may lead to either over- or undernutrition [8,9].

Physiological causes of undernutrition in older adults

In the UK, it is estimated that cataracts develop in approximately 42% of those over the age of 75 [2]. This can affect a person's ability to both obtain and prepare food. Poor dentition or the absence of natural teeth, estimated at 23% of older adults in the UK [2], will also affect the

Advanced Nutrition and Dietetics in Nutrition Support, First Edition. Edited by Mary Hickson and Sara Smith.
© 2018 John Wiley & Sons Ltd. Published 2018 by John Wiley & Sons Ltd.

types of foods consumed, including a reduction in the consumption of fresh fruits and vegetables and meat [10]. Olfactory changes associated with ageing can lead to a decreased interest in food and impairment of the cephalic phase of digestion, through decreases in salivation, pancreatic, gastric and intestinal secretions and delayed digestion [8]. Age-related changes to the gastrointestinal (GI) tract. including decreased gastric secretion of HCl, intrinsic factor and pepsin, can lead to decreased absorption of B12, folate and iron. Bacterial overgrowth and decreased lactase production also affect nutrient absorption [8]. Xerostomia decreases taste sensation and increases the risk for dental caries and gum disease, making chewing and swallowing more difficult [8].

Dysphagia often develops in older adults as a result of either ageing or another disease process, such as Parkinson's, Alzheimer's, stroke or other neurological disorders such as multiple sclerosis. It was estimated in 2010 that up to 40% of older adults in the United States had some form of dysphagia and that 55% of older adults with dysphagia are at risk of undernutrition [11]. Dysphagia can lead to undernutrition as people self limit the types of foods and liquids they consume and can develop a fear of eating after a significant aspiration and the lack of visual appeal of texture-modified foods.

Cognitive impairment in older adults

In 2014, approximately one in 14 older adults in the UK had a diagnosis of dementia, with Alzheimer's being the most prevalent [12]. Approximately 44% of individuals with dementia are undernourished versus 25% of age-matched healthy dementia-free individuals and an associated increase in mortality has been observed [13]. Several associated behaviours lead to either weight loss or weight gain. People may forget they have eaten and constantly seek and consume food, leading to weight gain. In contrast, dietary intake can decrease as food becomes less recognisable and behaviours such as prolonged chewing and spitting can lead to substantial weight loss [13]. Other repetitive behaviours such as pacing can lead to an increase

in energy requirements [14]. Physiological changes such as dysphagia and dyspraxia also occur in late-stage dementia that negatively impact on intake.

Social factors leading to undernutrition in older adults

Social factors can also lead to undernutrition in older adults. The UK Office for National Statistics (2011) demonstrate that 24% of older men and 13% of older report consuming alcohol five or more days per week. This is higher than the average of 16% and 9% respectively for all age groups [2] and may be related to depression and grief. Depression is noted to affect 40% of older adults residing in care homes [2]. Men with depression are more likely to be undernourished than women [9]. Alcohol takes the place of other more nutrient-dense foods in older adults who already have diminished appetites. Social isolation is also linked with depression and decreased food intake.

Polypharmacy in older adults

Polypharmacy (taking six or more medications) negatively affects intake as a result of drug–nutrient interactions and side effects such as delayed gastric emptying, nausea, altered metabolism and absorption of nutrients, and diarrhoea [15]. The provision of medication at mealtimes may also decrease intake of food as a result of the volume of liquid required to take medications.

5.3.4 Consequences of undernutrition

There are many consequences of undernutrition, including higher risk of pressure ulcers, sarcopenia, sarcopenic obesity, increased morbidity and mortality rates and increased healthcare costs.

Pressure ulcers

Pressure ulcers are often linked to prolonged bedrest, wheelchair dependence and hospitalisation. Patients who are undernourished stay in hospital approximately 50% longer than well-nourished patients, putting them at greater risk of developing pressure ulcers [16]. A study involving 31 381 patients in German and Dutch hospitals and nursing homes demonstrated a prevalence of pressure ulcers of 9.1–43% in nursing homes and 18–41.4% in hospitals [17]. Proteolysis occurs with the generation of proinflammatory cytokines that are released during periods of infection. Increased time in bed may be a result of decreased muscle strength and physical activity linked with this proteolysis or sarcopenia [18]. Regardless of the cause, the risk of developing pressure ulcers increases.

Sarcopenia

There are many definitions of what constitutes sarcopenia. Common to each is an age-related loss of muscle strength related to decreased muscle mass, including a decrease in muscle quality and decreases in both contractility and fibre size [19]. Decreased muscle strength is a strong predictor of frailty, morbidity and mortality. A study in the US utilising data from the NHANES III and the National Medical Care Utilisation and Expenditures Survey determined that approximately 45% of the older adults were sarcopenic, with approximately 50% of these experiencing physical disability. The study also determined that sarcopenia added $860 (males) and $933 (females) in healthcare costs for each person with sarcopenia, accounting for approximately 1.5% of total healthcare expenditure in the year 2000 [20].

Sarcopenic obesity

Sarcopenic obesity (SO), like sarcopenia, does not have a concrete definition. Essentially, it is muscle wasting in the context of increased adipose tissue, but the extent of muscle wasting required to increase the risk of morbidity and mortality is not clear, nor is the cut-off point for adiposity [21,22]. Excess adipose tissue increases the risk of multiple comorbidities such as insulin resistance, diabetes, cardiovascular disease, hypertension and stroke. The causes of SO are multifactorial, including diet, physical activity level, insulin resistance, vascular and proinflammatory cytokines [22].

In one meta-analysis, depending on the definition used, SO occurred in 10–50% of people over the age of 80 years and 3.4–12.4% of those aged 60 and over [19,23]. SO has been associated with increased mortality, in particular in patients with end-stage renal disease. It is also linked to increased morbidity in cardiovascular disease where disease rates are 23% higher than in those with sarcopenia or obesity [22,24]. It can also be used as a predictor in hospitalised older adults of nosocomial infection risk [24]. Decreases in functional status are also reported among community-dwelling older adults with SO, including decreased ability to complete activities of daily living, decreased aerobic capacity, balance and walking ability [25]. This reduced independent function can affect quality of life [22].

Quality of life

Quality of life is affected both physically and mentally by undernutrition as a result of weakness and physical disability caused by loss of muscle mass and lower haemoglobin concentrations increased rates of infection, decreased recovery from illness, wound healing and longer lengths of stay in hospital [9,16]. The multiple comorbidities associated with undernutrition such as chronic obstructive pulmonary disease and cardiac cachexia also affect quality of life by limiting an individual's ability to consume adequate amounts of food and participate in activities of daily living [23].

5.3.5 Assessment and diagnosis of undernutrition in older adults

Anthropometry

The use of weight alone as an anthropometric measure in older adults is problematic. Older adults may have significant muscle wasting that is masked by excess adipose tissue (see Sarcopenic obesity, abov) or oedema and weight may therefore not adequately reflect body composition [22]. The use of additional anthropometric measures such as mid-upper arm circumference and skinfold thickness can provide a better indication of body composition [26]. Measurement of standing height is not always appropriate due to potential difficulties in obtaining height for reasons such as presence of kyphosis [27].

Use of body mass index in older adults

In a study of 5888 community-dwelling American adults aged 65 or older [28], it was found that having a BMI of 18.5 kg/m² was associated with worse health outcomes than those who had a BMI of 18.5–24.9 kg/m². In addition, it was observed that a BMI of 25–29.9 kg/m² was not often associated with worse outcomes than those of a 'normal' BMI at age 65 and could be associated with significantly better outcomes [28]. Another American study involving nearly 13 000 people over the age of 65, in a 7-year follow-up, found that those with a BMI of 25–29.9 kg/m² appeared to have the longest disability-free life expectancy and the lowest hazard ratio for mortality when compared to those with BMI categories greater than 35 kg/m² and less than 25 kg/m² in the study [29]. Those with a BMI of higher than 30 kg/m² and less than 18.5 kg/m² were significantly more likely to experience disability. When BMI was examined as a single value and not in categories, as they are often referenced, it was found that a BMI of 24 kg/m² was linked to the best health outcomes for those 65 or older. The results also showed that individuals aged 75 or greater with a BMI of 27–29 kg/m² had the lowest mortality rates. This is a striking contrast to what has been reported for adults aged 55 or younger where the lowest mortality rates are found in those with a BMI of 18.5–20 kg/m² [29].

Older adults with BMI >25 kg/m²

Based upon results from the National Diet and Nutrition Survey (2008–2009 and 2009–2010), it is estimated that approximately one-third of women over 65 years of age are obese, while another 7% are morbidly obese (BMI >40 kg/m²). Approximately one-third are overweight (BMI >25 kg/m² and <30 kg/m²) and one-third are of a normal BMI (18.5–24.9 kg/m²) while only approximately 1% are under a normal BMI of 18.5 kg/m² as defined by the World Health Organization (WHO) and National Institute for Health and Care Excellence (NICE) [30]. In men, 16% were found to be of normal BMI, 54% were found to be overweight and 31% were found to be obese.

While higher rates of morbidity and mortality are observed in younger people at the extremes of the BMI scale (morbidly obese and severely underweight), older adults do not appear to have significantly increased morbidity or mortality risks associated with being in the overweight category of a BMI of 25–29.9 kg/m² [28,29]. It is theorised that higher BMIs are associated with better outcomes for several reasons. First, in the setting of metabolic stressors such as the flu or surgery, there are more reserves to draw from during recovery as it may take longer for an older adult to recover from illness and energy intakes typically decline during this time [29]. Second, moderate subcutaneous fat stores associated with BMIs in the mid to high 20s can also provide a cushioning barrier between bony prominences such as the spine and a bed during periods of bedrest, decreasing the risk of bedsores developing [18,31]. Third, there is some evidence that BMIs in the overweight category may be protective against some types of fractures following falls [32]. It should be kept in mind, however, that obesity continues to lead to poorer outcomes in terms of reduced mobility, increased joint pain and increased surgical recovery time [28,29].

Older adults with BMI <18.5 kg/m²

While it may not seem that undernutrition is a significant issue in older adults, with reports of just 2% of women and 1% of men with a BMI less than 18.5 kg/m², there is current debate within the literature as to whether or not this cut-off is too low. When an undernutrition definition of 'BMI under 20 kg/m², loss of appetite and or unexplained weight loss' was applied to the

UK population, it was found that 1.2 million community-dwelling people over 65 met the definition of undernutrition while another 100 000 living in institutional care also met the definition [33,34].

Biochemistry

There are several biochemical markers of specific concern for the nutritional well-being of older adults. Cobalamin (vitamin B12) concentrations should be monitored in older adults as the body's ability to absorb cobalamin decreases with age [35]. Compounding this decreased absorption, meat is the primary source of cobalamin and meat intake may decline in the older adult population as a result of becoming edentulous or due to its relatively higher cost [35]. Low concentrations of cobalamin may lead to pernicious anaemia and have also been implicated in the development of vascular dementia [35]. Similarly, serum iron and transferrin concentrations should be monitored for the development of iron deficiency anaemia, particularly in older adults taking antacid medications or with limited meat intake and in the setting of chronic inflammation or chronic kidney disease for the anaemia of chronic disease [35]. Serum vitamin D concentration should be monitored as deficiency is common among institutionalised older adults [35].

Clinical

Clinical assessment of the older adult is done in the same manner as for the general adult population. Observation of hair, skin, nails, extremities and mucous membranes will yield the same results as for the general adult population. It should be kept in mind that skin cell turnover declines with age and as such there may be slight variations in appearance of skin and hair that do not directly correlate with a nutrient deficiency [26]. Use of a validated screening tool such as the Subjective Global Assessment (SGA), which incorporates specific consideration of gastrointestinal symptoms such as nausea, vomiting, diarrhoea and anorexia, changes in functional capacity and a physical examination of subcutaneous fat stores and muscle wasting, oedema

and ascites, can assist in determining the extent of undernutrition in older populations [35].

Dietary

Dietary assessment of older persons can be difficult. Many dietary assessment tools such as the 24-hour food recall and the food frequency questionnaire rely on an individual's memory. It can be challenging to obtain accurate information from a population that is more likely to have cognitive impairment [26]. Dietary assessment of those in hospital or living in institutions is best done through direct observation or utilising methods such as calorie counts where the amount of food consumed is recorded by a healthcare provider directly following a meal [26].

Environmental

Decreased eyesight, mobility and impaired senses such as taste and smell can make meal preparation and consumption more difficult and less appealing [26]. Medications used for depression and Parkinson's may also cause taste alterations that lead to decreased intake of food [26]. Social isolation and dining areas that are not pleasurable (i.e. when patients are placed in the corridor near the nursing station for mealtime observation) can also lead to decreased food intake [6]. Interventions targeted at correcting these environmental challenges are discussed below.

5.3.6 Nutritional interventions

Targeted nutrition interventions can decrease the incidence of morbidity and mortality in the undernourished older adult population. The goal of these interventions is not curative in nature; however, they may slow disease progression and improve quality of life. Goals associated with nutrition interventions include slowing weight and muscle loss, providing adequate protein for the prevention and recovery from pressure ulcers, and correcting specific nutrient deficiencies [14].

Nutrition interventions need to take into account individual goals of care and may include alterations to the type and timing of meals, the use of oral nutrition supplements or the use of enteral or parenteral nutrition. Depending upon the disease state of the individual, modifications to energy, macronutrients or micronutrients may be required. Table 5.3.1 provides a summary of the key micronutrients to consider.

ESPEN guidelines indicate that the majority of sick older adults require approximately 30 kcal/kg/day and 1 g protein/kg/day [14]. These modifications should first be made through altering food items, providing assistance at mealtimes or altering the meal pattern to small frequent meals [14]. If social isolation is thought to contribute to decreased intake, the creation of a pleasant and communal dining environment and encouragement from caregivers may be an appropriate intervention [8]. If modifications to food items and dining environments are not sufficient, oral nutrition supplements such as enteral formulas should be considered.

Oral nutrition supplements

Oral nutrition supplements (ONS) have a beneficial effect on undernourished older adults. They can improve energy and protein intake and increase weight, but their use may not significantly improve mortality rates in some disease states (i.e. end-stage dementia) [14]. Several ESPEN recommendations supported by grade A evidence have been made for oral nutrition supplements in older adults [14]. First, ONS should be used in patients who are undernourished or at risk of undernutrition to increase energy, protein or micronutrient intake. Second, it is recommended that ONS should be used to improve nutritional status in frail older adults as well as to reduce complications in older adults after hip fractures and orthopaedic surgery. Lastly, there is evidence that ONS with high protein content can reduce the risk of developing pressure ulcers in older adults [14].

The most significant benefits from ONS are seen in those who are undernourished and either in hospital or long-term care. A Cochrane review including 62 trials (n = 10 187 randomised patients) found protein energy supplementation provided a weight change benefit of 2.2% (95%

confidence interval (CI) 1.8–2.5) in 42 trials and a significant improvement in mortality results only when participants (n = 2461) were defined as undernourished (relative risk (RR) 0.79, 95% CI 0.64–0.97) [36]. Undernourished patients who receive ONS may benefit from a reduction in complications (i.e. pressure ulcers); however, it does not lead to shorter hospital stays or improved functional status [7,37]. When possible, it is recommended that when administering medications to older adults at risk of undernutrition, they be given with a energy-dense oral nutrition supplement instead of water [15] as part of a med pass programme. Timing of ONS needs to be considered (i.e. between meals or as part of a med pass programme) so as not to interfere with the oral intake of food items [7,14].

Enteral nutrition

The use of enteral nutrition for older adults should be carefully considered. Multiple considerations regarding the patient's own goals of care and their underlying disease state should be taken into account [14]. In addition, assessment prior to initiating tube feeding should determine if the person's quality of life can be improved by enteral nutrition, what effects long-term enteral nutrition may have on their living situation and whether the intervention is congruent with the patient's expressed end-of-life wishes [14]. Should enteral nutrition be initiated, ESPEN guidelines recommend percutaneous endoscopic gastrostomy tubes over nasogastric tubes as the preferred delivery route for long-term nutrition support (>4 weeks) in older adults [14].

Pressure ulcers

Both hydration and nutrition are important in maintaining the integrity of skin and tissue as well as supporting repair after injury [18]. Weight loss and undernutrition are associated with the development and prolonged healing of pressure ulcers [18]. Adequate energy intakes are required for protein sparing so as to maximise collagen synthesis [18]. Recent recommendations suggest the use of the Mifflin St Jeor equation for healthy obese individuals or 30 kcal/kg (125.4 kj/kg) for

Table 5.3.1 Summary of key micronutrient requirements in older adults

Nutrient	Importance in older adult population	Recommended intakes
Calcium	Calcium intake is inadequate in approximately 56% of women and 62% of men over the age of 70 according to NHANES data. The amount of calcium required increases with age as intestinal absorption of calcium and vitamin D decreases and urinary excretion increases	Adequate intake (AI) I is 1200 mg/day for men and women over 51 years of age Recommended nutrient intake (RNI) 700 mg/day for older adults (65 and above)
Cobalamin (B12)	Deficiency occurs in the older adult population as intestinal absorption decreases with age as well as atrophic gastritis and ileal disease	Recommended daily amount (RDA) is 2.4 µg/day for men and women over 51 years of age RNI 1.5 µg/day for older adults (65 and above) Intramuscular injections of B12 are often required to correct this deficiency
Folate	Estimated that up to 25% of women over the age of 65 years in Europe are deficient in folate. Lower serum folate and cobalamin concentrations are linked to increased homocysteine concentration. These elevated homocysteine concentrations have been implicated as a risk factor for osteoporosis and functional decline	RDA is 400 µg/day for men and women over 51 years of age RNI 200 µg/day for older adults
Iron	Approximately 20% of older adults have atrophic gastritis, which decreases the body's ability to absorb iron	The recommended treatment for iron deficiency is 325 mg of iron sulfate three times per day until iron concentration stabilise RNI 8.7 mg/day for older adults
Thiamin (B1)	Supplementation is often required in the context of alcohol abuse and prolonged poor nutrient intake and thiamin is therefore a nutrient of concern for many older adults	RDA is 1.2 mg/day for men and 1.1 mg/day for women over 51 years of age RNI 0.7–0.8 mg older women: 0.9 mg older men
Vitamin D	Older adults residing in institutions are at risk of developing vitamin D deficiencies due to their lack of exposure to sunlight. Vitamin D deficiency has been linked to reduced mobility, increased risk of falls and fracture as well as increased levels of depression. Vitamin D3 has been linked to a decreased mortality rate though vitamin D2 does not significantly reduce mortality	AI for men and women is 15 µg/day 51–70 years of age and 20 µg/day over 70 years of age RNI 10 µg/day for older adults
Zinc	Adults over the age of 70 years commonly have inadequate intakes of zinc. Zinc deficiency is of particular concern in older adults as it is required for normal immune function, decreased risk of skin breakdown and improved wound healing	RDA is 11 mg/day for men and 8 mg/day for women over 51 years of age. Low-dose supplementation of 40–50 mg/day is recommended to avoid copper deficiency RNI 9.5 µg/day for older men, 7.0 µg/day for older women

Source: Montgomery et al. [35], Detsky et al. [40].

a non-obese individual when calculating the energy needs for a patient with pressure ulcers [18]. Protein requirements of 1.25–1.5 g/kg have been suggested for those with pressure ulcers in the context of undernutrition (18). Some evidence of improved healing has been shown with arginine supplementation of 6–9 g daily and glutamine supplements when combined with an oral nutrition supplement for stage 3 and 4 pressure ulcers [18]. Ascorbic acid, while necessary for collagen synthesis, has not been found to improve pressure ulcer healing. Zinc is required for protein, DNA and RNA synthesis. Zinc deficiencies can develop in patients with decreased nutritional intake and increased wound exudate. If a zinc deficiency is suspected, 40 mg/day of elemental zinc should be provided until the deficiency is corrected to assist with wound healing. Prolonged supplementation with zinc may lead to copper deficiencies, which in turn decrease wound healing [18]. Additional hydration should be provided to those with fevers and high exudate losses as a result of their wound [18].

Dementia

The European Society for Parenteral and Enteral Nutrition published guidelines on nutrition and dementia in 2015 [38]. Of the 26 recommendations made, only three were given a high grade of evidence and three others had a moderate grade of evidence. Recommendations with a high grade were:

- not to provide w-3 fatty acid supplements to persons with dementia for the correction of cognitive impairment
- to encourage the use of ONS for patients with early to moderate dementia to improve nutritional status for those with insufficient oral intake as a result of apraxia of eating, increased activity levels, forgetting to eat, etc.
- not to initiate enteral nutrition in patients with severe or end-stage dementia [14,38].

Recommendations with a moderate grade of evidence were:

- provide meals in a pleasant home-like atmosphere

- not to provide ONS to prevent further cognitive decline
- not to use vitamin E supplements for the prevention of cognitive decline (38).

Protein and amino acid supplementation

Protein and amino acid supplementation has been reviewed extensively within the older adult population. Dietary protein is important in older and frail adults to mitigate the loss of muscle tissue that results from decreased intake, ageing and reduced activity levels which can contribute to the development of sarcopenia but there is insufficient evidence to make specific recommendations on supplementation [21]. Protein supplementation on its own has shown a slight reduction in pressure ulcer occurrence while in hospital and a reduced risk of complications following hip fractures but no other significant improvements in terms of morbidity and mortality [36].

With regard to amino acid supplementation, leucine, a branch chain amino acid, has been postulated to be beneficial in improving muscle synthesis in older adults but unequivocal evidence of its benefit is lacking [39].

Physical activity

According to national statistics published in 2009, approximately 25% of older adults in England meet the minimum recommendations for physical activity required to achieve health benefits [2]. In 2013, an ESPEN expert group published guidelines on physical activity and protein requirements to preserve muscle mass, thus helping to prevent the complications associated with sarcopenia, sarcopenic obesity and undernutrition [39]. The key recommendations included a protein intake of 1.0–1.2 g/Kg/day of protein for healthy older adults in conjunction with daily aerobic activity and progressive resistance training (usually 2–3 sets of 8–12 repetitions of the exercise) 2–3 times per week for 12 weeks to preserve lean muscle mass [39].

References

1. National Institute on Aging. Global Health and Aging. https://www.nia.nih.gov/sites/default/files/2017-06/global_health_aging.pdf (accessed 3 September).

2. Age UK. Later Life in the United Kingdom. www.ageuk.org.uk/Documents/EN-GB/Factsheets/Later_Life_UK_factsheet.pdf?dtrk=true (accessed 3 September 2017).

3. Statistics Canada. Life Expectancy, at Birth and At Age 65, by Sex and by Province and Territory. www.statcan.gc.ca/tables-tableaux/sum-som/l01/cst01/health72a-eng.htm (accessed 3 September 2017).

4. Australian Institute of Health and Wellfare. Life Expectancy. www.aihw.gov.au/deaths/life-expectancy/ (accessed 3 September 2017).

5. Russell CA, Elia M. Nutrition Screening Surveys in Hospitals in England, 2007–2011. Redditch: British Association for Parenteral and Enteral Nutrition (BAPEN), 2014.

6. Cuervo M, García A, Ansorena D, Sanchez-Villegas A, Martínez-González MA, Astiasaran I, Martinez JA. Nutritional assessment interpretation on 22 007 Spanish community-dwelling elders through the Mini Nutritional Assessment test. *Public Health Nutr* 2009; **12**(01): 82–90.

7. Abbott R, Whear R, Thompson-Coon J, et al. Effectiveness of mealtime interventions on nutritional outcomes for the elderly living in residential care: a systematic review and meta-analysis. *Ageing Res Rev* 2013; **12**(4): 967–981.

8. Nieuwenhuizen W, Weenen H, Rigby P, Hetherington M. Older adults and patients in need of nutritional support: review of current treatment options and factors influencing nutritional intake. *Clin Nutr* 2010; **29**(2): 160–169.

9. Johansson Y, Bachrach-Lindström M, Carstensen J, Ek A. Malnutrition in a home-living older population: prevalence, incidence and risk factors. A prospective study. *J Clin Nurs* 2009; **18**(9): 1354–1364.

10. Savoca MR, Arcury TA, Leng X, Chen H, Bell RA, Anderson AM, Kohrman T, Frazier RJ, Gilbert GH, Quandt SA. Severe tooth loss in older adults as a key indicator of compromised dietary quality. *Public Health Nutr* 2010; **13**(4): 466–474.

11. Rofes L, Arreola V, Almirall J, et al. Diagnosis and management of oropharyngeal dysphagia and its nutritional and respiratory complications in the elderly. *Gastroenterol Res Pract* 2011; **2011**: 1–13.

12. Alzheimer's Society demographics and statistics, 2013. www.alzheimers.org.uk (accessed 3 September 2017).

13. Allen V, Methven L, Gosney M. Use of nutritional complete supplements in older adults with dementia: systematic review and meta-analysis of clinical outcomes. *Clin Nutr* 2013; **32**(6): 950–957.

14. Volkert D, Berner YN, Berry E, Cederholm T, Bertrand PC, Milne A, Palmblad J, Sobotka L, Stanga Z, Lenzen-Grossimlinghaus R, Krys U. ESPEN guidelines on enteral nutrition: geriatrics. *Clin Nutr* 2006; **25**(2): 330–360.

15. Heuberger R, Caudell K. Polypharmacy and nutritional status in older adults. *Drugs Aging* 2011; **28**(4): 315–323.

16. Edington J, Boorman J, Durrant ER, et al. Prevalence of malnutrition on admission to four hospitals in England. *Clin Nutr* 2000; **19**(3): 191–195.

17. Tannen A, Dassen T, Halfens R. Differences in prevalence of pressure ulcers between the Netherlands and Germany – associations between risk, prevention and occurrence of pressure ulcers in hospitals and nursing homes. *J Clin Nurs* 2008; **17**(9): 1237–1244.

18. Posthauer ME, Banks M, Dorner B, Schols JM. The role of nutrition for pressure ulcer management: National Pressure Ulcer Advisory Panel, European Pressure Ulcer Advisory Panel, and Pan Pacific Pressure Injury Alliance white paper. *Adv Skin Wound Care* 2015; **28**(4): 175–188.

19. Stenholm S, Harris T, Rantanen T, Visser M, Kritchevsky S, Ferrucci L. Sarcopenic obesity: definition, etiology and consequences. *Curr Opin Clin Nutr Metab Care* 2008; **11**(6): 693–700.

20. Janssen I, Shepard D, Katzmarzyk P, Roubenoff R. The healthcare costs of sarcopenia in the United States. *J Am Geriatr Soc* 2004; **52**(1): 80–85.

21. Beasley J, Shikany J, Thomson C. The role of dietary protein intake in the prevention of sarcopenia of aging. *Nutr Clin Pract* 2013; **28**(6): 684–690.

22. Prado C, Wells J, Smith S, Stephan B, Siervo M. Sarcopenic obesity: a critical appraisal of the current evidence. *Clin Nutr* 2012; **31**(5): 583–601.

23. Saka B, Kaya O, Ozturk G, Erten N, Karan M. Malnutrition in the elderly and its relationship with other geriatric syndromes. *Clin Nutr* 2010; **29**(6): 745–748.

24. Prado C, Lieffers J, McCargar L, et al. Prevalence and clinical implications of sarcopenic obesity in patients with solid tumours of the respiratory and gastrointestinal tracts: a population-based study. *Lancet Oncol* 2008; **9**(7): 629–635.

25. Zamboni M, Mazzali G, Fantin F, Rossi A, di Francesco V. Sarcopenic obesity: a new category of obesity in the elderly. *Nutr Metab Cardiovasc Dis* 2008; **18**(5): 388–395.

26. Ahmed T, Haboubi N. Assessment and management of nutrition in older people and its importance to health. *Clin Interv Aging* 2010; **5**(1): 207–216.

27. Stratton R, King C, Stroud M, Jackson A, Elia M. 'Malnutrition Universal Screening Tool' predicts mortality and length of hospital stay in acutely ill elderly. *Br J Nutr* 2006; **95**(2): 325.

28. Diehr P, O'Meara E, Fitzpatrick A, Newman A, Kuller L, Burke G. Weight, mortality, years of healthy life, and active life expectancy in older adults. *J Am Geriatr Soc* 2008; **56**(1): 76–83.

29. Al Snih S, Ottenbacher KJ, Markides KS, Kuo YF, Eschbach K, Goodwin JS. The effect of obesity on disability vs mortality in older Americans. *Arch Intern Med* 2007; **167**(8): 774.

30. Bates B, Lennox A, Bates C, Swan G. National Diet and Nutrition Survey. Headline Results from Years 1 and 2 (Combined) of the Rolling Programme (2008/2009–2009/2010). www.gov.uk/government/uploads/system/uploads/attachment_data/file/216484/dh_128550.pdf (accessed 3 September 2017).

31. Van Gilder C, MacFarlane G, Meyer S, Lachenbruch C. Body mass index, weight, and pressure ulcer prevalence. *J Nurs Care Qual* 2009; **24**(2): 127–135.

32. Premaor M, Compston J, Fina Avilés F, et al. The association between fracture site and obesity in men: a population-based cohort study. *J Bone Miner Res* 2013; **28**(8): 1771–1777.

33. National Institute for Health and Care Excellence. Obesity Prevention. NICE Clinical Guideline No. 43. www.nice.org.uk/guidance/cg43 (accessed 3 September 2017).

34. Elia M, Russell C. Combating Malnutrition: Recommendations for Action. www.bapen.org.uk/pdfs/reports/advisory_group_report.pdf (accessed 3 September 2017).

35. Montgomery S, Streit S, Beebe M, Maxwell P. Micronutrient needs of the elderly. *Nutr Clin Pract* 2014; **29**(4): 435–444.

36. Milne AC, Potter J, Vivanti A, Avenell A. Protein and energy supplementation in elderly people at risk from malnutrition. Cochrane Database Syst Rev 2005; **2**: CD003288.

37. Milne AC, Avenell A, Potter J. Meta-analysis: protein and energy supplementation in older people. *Ann Intern Med* 2006; **144**(1): 37.

38. Volkert D, Chourdakis M, Faxen-Irving G, Frühwald T, Landi F, Suominen MH, Vandewoude M, Wirth R, Schneider SM. ESPEN guidelines on nutrition in dementia. *Clin Nutr* 2015; **34**(6): 1052–1073.

39. Deutz NE, Bauer JM, Barazzoni R, Biolo G, Boirie Y, Bosy-Westphal A, Cederholm T, Cruz-Jentoft A, Krznariç Z, Nair KS, Singer P. Protein intake and exercise for optimal muscle function with aging: recommendations from the ESPEN Expert Group. *Clin Nutr* 2014; **33**(6): 929–936.

40. Detsky AS, McLaughlin JR, Baker JP, et al. What is subjective global assessment of nutritional status? *J Parenter Enteral Nutr* 1987; **11**(1): 8–13.

41. Public Health England. Government Dietary Recommendations: Government Recommendations for Food Energy and Nutrients for Males and Females Aged 1–18 Years and 19+ Years. www.gov.uk/government/uploads/system/uploads/attachment_data/file/618167/government_dietary_recommendations.pdf (accessed 3 September 2017).

Chapter 5.4

Nutrition support in neurological disorders

Filomena Gomes

Cereneo AG and Kantonsspital Aarau, Vitznau, Switzerland

5.4.1 Introduction

Worldwide, neurological disorders present a major public health challenge and constitute 12% of the total deaths, including 9.9% due to stroke, 0.73% due to dementia, 0.18% due to Parkinson's disease and 0.03% due to multiple sclerosis [1].

Several neurological conditions can significantly affect nutritional status. Depending on the area of the nervous system affected and the extent of the damage, individuals may present difficulties in purchasing, preparing, chewing, swallowing and delivering food to the mouth. These impairments, in conjunction with confusion, decreased alertness and depression, leave these patients at risk of undernutrition, which can further deteriorate their condition.

Given that stroke is the most prevalent neurological disorder and that the causes of undernutrition and recommendations for nutritional support are similar among the different neurological conditions (e.g. multiple sclerosis (MS) and motor neuron diseases (MND)), this chapter will focus primarily on the management of stroke. Other neurological conditions such as dementia and spinal cord injury are covered elsewhere (see Chapters 5.3, 5.5).

Stroke

Stroke is defined as an acute onset of focal (at times global) neurological deficit of presumed vascular origin that lasts more than 24 hours. The site and extent of the damage caused by the interruption of blood supply to the brain cells determine whether the stroke is fatal or causes permanent or temporary disabilities, including motor and sensory impairment, impaired cognitive function, dysphagia and dysarthria (slurred speech), among others.

Ischaemic strokes are due to blood vessel occlusion and account for approximately 85% of all strokes, while haemorrhagic strokes are less frequent (15%) and lead to bleeding in the brain from a ruptured blood vessel, which may be weakened (e.g. by an aneurysm), abnormally formed or subject to trauma [2]. Ischaemic strokes are usually divided into large artery atherosclerosis, cardioembolism (arterial occlusion due to an embolus arising from the heart) and small vessel occlusion (lacunar infarcts, with lesions smaller than 1.5 cm), the remainder being due to a miscellany of much rarer (or undetermined) causes [3].

Stroke affects 15 million people worldwide every year, is a major cause of death (more than 6 million per year) and physical disability, and has a significant impact on patients, carers and health services, making it a costly disease [4]. Risk factors for stroke are reported to be different between ischaemic and haemorrhagic strokes [5] (e.g. dyslipidaemia is only associated with an increased risk of ischaemic strokes [6]), between first and recurrent strokes[7], between very old (≥80 years old) and younger (<80 years) stroke

Advanced Nutrition and Dietetics in Nutrition Support, First Edition. Edited by Mary Hickson and Sara Smith.

patients [8], and between different ethnic groups [9]. Nutrition-related risk factors include hypertension, diabetes, dyslipidaemia, hyperhomocysteinaemia and a poor diet, for example low consumption of fish, fruit and vegetables; low intake of antioxidants, n-3 polyunsaturated fatty acids, potassium, calcium, vitamin D, folic acid, vitamins B6 and B12; high intake of salt, alcohol, total and saturated fat [10–12].

Multiple sclerosis

Multiple sclerosis is defined as a chronic autoimmune, inflammatory neurological disease of the central nervous system, where the myelin and axons are attacked and destroyed to varying degrees, interfering with the transmission of nerve signals. Signs and symptoms vary widely, depending on the amount of damage and which nerves are affected. MS and other demyelinating diseases most commonly result in vision loss, muscle weakness, muscle stiffness and spasms, fatigue, loss of co-ordination and dizziness, sensory disturbances, bladder and bowel dysfunction, speech and swallowing problems.

The course of MS is highly varied and unpredictable, but in the most common form (affecting 85% of patients) periods of relapse or exacerbation of symptoms are followed by periods of remission; in a smaller proportion of patients (10%), symptoms continue to worsen gradually from the beginning [1,13]. Ms is reported to affect approximately 2.5 million people worldwide, is more prevalent in women and in people of northern European descent and is mostly diagnosed between the ages of 20 and 45, but its precise cause is unknown. There is no cure for multiple sclerosis; treatment typically focuses on shortening the duration and decreasing the frequency of acute exacerbations, and providing symptomatic relief [1,13].

Amyotrophic lateral sclerosis

Motor neuron diseases are a group of progressive neurological disorders that selectively destroy motor neurons. Amyotrophic lateral sclerosis (ALS) is the most common form of MND in adults, affecting both upper and lower motor neurons. With an annual incidence of 2 in 100 000 people, ALS is considered to be a rare but severe neurological disorder, with no cure and an average survival time of 3 years, although a small proportion of patients survive more than 10 years [14,15]. Familial causes comprise approximately 5% of ALS cases and the cause of the remaining sporadic cases is unknown; it is more common in men and commonly manifests between the ages of 55 and 65 years. The progressive muscle weakness begins in the legs and hands and, as motor nerves deteriorate, most voluntary muscles are paralysed and there is difficulty in breathing, speaking and swallowing, but the senses of sight, smell, touch, hearing and taste remain intact [15].

5.4.2 Undernutrition: prevalence, causes and consequences

The prevalence of undernutrition has been reported to be between 6% and 62% following stroke [16] and this variation is probably due to differences in criteria and the timing of assessment, as well as differences in patient characteristics.

Undernutrition at the point of admission is associated with increased mortality and morbidity. In a cohort of 3012 stroke patients, enrolled in the Feed Or Ordinary Diet (FOOD) trial (a multicentre randomised trial evaluating various feeding policies), those classified as undernourished on admission to hospital had a 2.32 increased risk of death at 6 months when compared with those with a normal nutritional status, and also had statistically significant higher rates of pneumonia, other infections, pressure sores and gastrointestinal haemorrhages [17]. Further deterioration of nutritional status occurs in a proportion of patients post stroke, not only during hospital stay (it has been demonstrated that the proportion of undernourished patients increases significantly during hospital stay, from 9% to 65% [18]) but also after discharge, as demonstrated in a study with 305 stroke survivors, in which one-quarter of the patients suffered weight loss (>3 kg) at 4 and 12 months post stroke [19].

There is a wide range of factors that can affect food choices, preparation and consumption post stroke, that have a negative impact on nutritional status, including disease-related factors (such as disease- or drug-induced anorexia, postural instability, visual and communication deficits, lip closure and chewing difficulties due to facial weakness, gastrointestinal symptoms and dysphagia) and psychological and social factors (such as depression, social isolation, financial issues and lack of access to social care services) [20].

In MS, the typical symptoms that affect nutrient intake and can lead to undernutrition include reduced mobility, tremor, poor sight, dysphagia, cognitive difficulties, depression, the side effects of drugs and their interaction with nutrients (which can, in turn, cause fatigue and worsening of disease symptoms) [21].

In patients with ALS, factors such as depression, anxiety, difficulty communicating needs, fatigue, sialorrhoea (excessive salivation), shortness of breath at meals, chewing and swallowing problems can all contribute to deterioration in nutritional status. As the disease progresses, decreases in body fat, lean body mass and nitrogen balance, and an increase in resting energy expenditure (an estimated additional 10% [22]) have been observed. Consequently, undernutrition exacerbates muscle weakness, impairs respiratory and immune system function and can negatively impact on prognosis [14,23].

5.4.3 Screening and assessment of nutrition status in neurological disorders

Screening for risk of undernutrition is recommended at the time of hospital admission, with regular reassessment thereafter [24,25]. The predictive validity of the Malnutrition Universal Screening Tool (MUST) has been evaluated in a prospective UK study of 543 stroke patients (mean age 75 years, 87% ischaemic stroke, 29% high risk of undernutrition) [25]. Results demonstrated that MUST accurately identified those who were more likely to have negative outcomes. The greater the risk of undernutrition assessed on admission to hospital, the greater the risk of mortality, length of hospital stay and hospitalisation costs at 6 months post-stroke, as demonstrated in Table 5.4.1 [26].

Patients with stroke who are identified as being at high risk of undernutrition should then be referred to a nutrition specialist (e.g. dietitian) for a thorough nutrition assessment, to identify nutritional problems and to deliver a tailored nutrition intervention (plan). There is currently no 'gold standard' for the assessment of nutritional status, and variety of methods may be used [16], which usually includes a combination of several markers [20,21,23].

Anthropometry

Body mass index (BMI) reflects chronic malnutrition, justifying the importance of obtaining

Table 5.4.1 Mortality, length of hospital stay and hospitalisation costs in patients following stroke, according to risk of undernutrition as determined by the Malnutrition Universal Screening Tool (MUST)

Risk of undernutrition (MUST)	Mortality (hazard ratio (95% confidence interval)) *Univariate Cox proportional hazards model*	Cumulative length of hospital stay (median number of days) *Kruskal–Wallis test P < 0.001*	Hospitalisation costs (median, in £) *Kruskal–Wallis test P < 0.001)*
Low	Reference	14	4920
Medium	4.9 (2.3–10.5)	19	6490
High	9.3 (5.6–15.30	48	8720

Source: Adapted from Gomes et al. [26] with permission from Elsevier.

accurate records of weight and height (or alternative measures) on a regular basis, during hospitalisation and after discharge [20]. Equally important is the assessment of recent unintentional weight loss (greater than 10% over 3–6 months, or more than 5% in 1–3 months) as, regardless of BMI, this parameter is an independent predictor of poor outcome in many diseases. In the stroke population, it has been shown that unintentional weight loss prior to stroke affects one in every five patients and is associated with statistically significant higher rates of mortality, length of hospital stay and costs at 6 months post stroke [27]. In a retrospective study of 63 ALS patients, weight loss of more than 10% at the time of diagnosis was associated with a shorter survival (17 ± 6 months versus 35 ± 26 months) [14]. Although relevant, measures of skeletal muscle mass, fat mass and function may be influenced by factors secondary to the neurological condition (e.g. muscle atrophy due to immobility) [16].

Biochemistry

The use of some biochemical markers such as serum albumin and transferrin to assess nutritional status is discouraged as they can be affected independently by other factors associated with stroke; instead, they should be considered as markers of acute illness and metabolic stress [16]. However, laboratory data are required to assess nutritional and hydration status, to monitor the adequacy of the nutrition interventions and to correct any existent metabolic imbalances. Some vitamin deficiencies, such as B6, B9 and B12, are particularly relevant for stroke patients, not only because they are more common in the elderly population (and 75% of strokes occur in older adults), but also because they are inversely related to hyperhomocysteinaemia, which in turn leads to endothelial dysfunction, atherogenesis and vascular damage [11]. In fact, a recent meta-analysis has identified a positive correlation between hyperhomocysteinaemia and cervical artery dissection, a recognised cause of ischaemic strokes [28].

Clinical

A careful clinical examination provides useful information to identify potential nutritional deficiencies (e.g. oedema, skin rash, thinning of the hair [21]). Existing comorbidities (e.g. diabetes) or other factors such as swallowing difficulties and constipation, affecting a significant proportion of stroke, MS and ALS patients, should be taken into consideration for the development of an individualised nutrition care plan [20].

Dietary and environmental

A dietary assessment is needed to define adequacy of macro- and micronutrient intakes, and to identify deficiencies which can lead to further deterioration in neurological conditions. The method of assessment will depend on the nutrient or food of concern (e.g. fluids, protein, vitamin D or essential fatty acids, such as docosahexaenoic acid, the predominant structural fatty acid in the central nervous system), the care setting (e.g. hospital, nursing home or home) and the patient's ability to provide accurate information [20]. The development of an individualised care plan to maximise nutritional and fluid intakes should also take into consideration the level of swallowing function, level of alertness, any associated communication difficulties, changes in care settings and possible dependence on others for preparing food and for feeding.

5.4.4 Nutrition intervention

Patients with intact swallowing function

The effect of oral nutritional supplements (ONS) on undernourished stroke patients was evaluated in a Cochrane review [29]. ONS were associated with significantly reduced pressure sores (odds ratio (OR) 0.56, 95% confidence interval (CI) 0.32–0.96), increased energy intake (mean difference 430 kcal/day; 95% CI 142–719) and protein intake (mean difference 17.28 g/day; 95% CI 1.99–33), and had no effect on mortality or functional dependency, but it should be noted that the authors included a study that provided antioxidants and ω-3 fatty acids, and many of the included studies did not use a validated method to assess undernutrition or included well-nourished individuals. While a few of the included studies suggest beneficial effects of ONS or other forms of oral nutrition support in undernourished patients, there is no evidence to support their routine use in adequately nourished patients [30].

Patients with impaired swallowing function

Dysphagia affects up to 50% patients in the acute phase after stroke, and this reduction in the co-ordination of pharyngeal muscles increases the risk of undernutrition dehydration, chest infection, pneumonia and death. Half of these patients recover within 2 weeks; some die and others require long-term enteral nutrition [29].

Depending on the severity of the dysphagia and the level of alertness, modified-texture diets (MDT) and thickened fluids can be offered. The aim of changing the food consistency to mechanically soft or puréed meals and thickening fluids is to reduce the need for oral manipulation and to enable the safe transition of food and fluids to the oesophagus. However, these diets tend to be less nutritionally dense, offer fewer food choices and are less appealing than normal diets, which explain why patients on MTD fail to meet their nutrition and hydration requirements [31,32]. Thus, other nutrition support strategies, such as food fortification or use of supplemental enteral formula and fluids, may be useful although their efficacy has not been studied.

In the last decade, different countries have proposed different descriptors of types and textures of foods to be used for the management of dysphagia. As a consequence, the comparison of study findings can be problematic. Recently, an International Dysphagia Diet Standardisation Initiative (IDDSI) has developed new global standardised terminology and definitions to describe texture-modified foods and thickened liquids. The initiative primarily aims to improve patient safety, but the use of a common language also supports researchers working in this field.

In 2016, the multidisciplinary IDDSI Committee published a dysphagia diet framework, consisting of a continuum of eight levels, where drinks are measured from levels 0 to 4, while foods are measured from levels 3 to 7, and levels are identified by numbers, text labels and colour codes. A summary of the framework is presented in Table 5.4.2 [33].

Table 5.4.2 Summary of the International Dysphagia Diet Standardisation Initiative framework

	IDDSI label			
Level	Foods	Drinks	IDDSI colour	Example of key characteristics
7	Regular	-	Black	Normal everyday foods with various textures
6	Soft and bite sized	-	Blue	Can be eaten with fork, spoon or chopsticks
5	Minced and moist	-	Orange	Can be eaten with fork or spoon
4	Puréed	Extremely thick	Green	Usually eaten with a spoon/cannot be sucked through a straw
3	Liquidised	Moderately thick	Yellow	Can be drunk from a cup/can be eaten with a spoon
2	-	Mildly thick	Pink	Flows off a spoon
1	-	Slightly thick	Grey	Thicker than water
0	-	Thin	White	Flows like water

Source: Adapted from International Dysphagia Diet Standardisation Committee [33].

Enteral nutrition

When oral intake is not safe or sufficient to meet requirements, patients should be considered for enteral nutrition with a nasogastric tube (NGT). Some stroke guidelines recommend that this should be done within 24 hours of admission [24], while others suggest it should be implemented within 72 hours [34].

In one of the three studies included in the large multicentre FOOD trial, dysphagic patients were randomised to receive early enteral nutrition (<1 week) versus avoid any enteral nutrition for at least 1 week. While no significant difference was observed, it could be argued that the group receiving early enteral nutrition showed a trend towards a reduced mortality by 5.8% (P=0.09) [30]. There may be a potential benefit of early initiation of enteral nutrition in dysphagic patients (particularly in those with premorbid undernutrition) but it should be noted that this trial is limited by the fact that those with a clear indication for early enteral nutrition were not recruited (only those whose attending physician was unsure about the adequate nutrition therapy were included) [34]. Where a NGT needs frequent replacement, nasal bridles may be a useful alternative and have been demonstrated to increase the volume of enteral formula and fluid delivered and to correct eletrolyte disturbances [35]. When long-term enteral nutrition is required (>4 weeks), gastrostomy feeding should be considered, as this is associated with high formula delivery and a trend for a lower mortality, although more research is needed [29].

Recommendations specific to ALS and MS

In ALS, proactive nutrition management and education are suggested as the standard of care [15]. The aim of nutrition support is to prevent undernutrition and dehydration and to enhance quality of life. The appropriate diet consistency is determined throughout the progression of the disease and, similar to stroke, in patients with impaired oral intake a percutaneous endoscopic gastrostomy (PEG) is recommended to stabilise weight and prolong survival [15,36]. Forced vital capacity is a parameter defined as the volume of air that can be exhaled after maximum inhalation, and is used as part of monitoring disease progression [15]. Given that morbidity and mortality rates during PEG placement increase as the forced vital capacity falls, some authors suggest PEG placement while that parameter is above 50% of predicted [15,36], but further studies are required to determine the optimal time for PEG placement and its impact on quality of life [37].

In MS, several nutrients such as polyunsaturated fatty acids and vitamin D have been investigated but further research is needed to reach definitive conclusions about their role in disease progression [21,38].

Common food–drug interactions

Particular attention needs to be paid to some common food–drug interactions in neurological diseases, besides the general principles of drug administration via enteral feeding [39]. Vitamin K and n-3 fatty acids are important nutrients in the diet of the stroke patient but they have the potential to interact with the frequently used anticoagulant and antiplatelet medication. Similarly, statins are often prescribed to this patient population, so grapefruit and its juice may need to be avoided, depending on the type of statin being taken. For patients with ALS, riluzole (a drug used for the inhibition of presynaptic release of glutamate, to prolong survival in 2–3 months) must be taken 1 hour before a meal or 2 hours after due to reduced absorption [39].

Other considerations

Obesity (based on either BMI or on measures of abdominal obesity) has been identified as a risk factor for a first stroke and planned weight loss has been proven to reduce high blood pressure, a major risk factor for stroke. In this context, some guidelines for secondary prevention of stroke recommend that overweight and obese patients should be advised to lose weight [24]. Weight management (towards a 'normal' BMI) is also commonly addressed while providing nutrition support and advice for secondary prevention.

However, there is a growing body of evidence demonstrating that overweight (BMI 25–30 kg/m²) and/or obese (BMI >30 kg/m²) stroke patients have a better survival, when compared to those at 'normal' weight, and this has been demonstrated in ischaemic and haemorrhagic strokes, in first and recurrent strokes, and in different ethnicities [40,41]. The level of reduction in mortality risk observed in over a dozen studies varies according to the methodology used (e.g. there are differences in the defined BMI cut-offs, group of reference, follow-up period, confounders used in the multivariable analyses) and the study population (ischaemic versus haemorrhagic stroke, first versus recurrent stroke, different countries).

Furthermore, other studies have shown that obesity is paradoxically associated with better functional recovery and a lower risk of recurrent strokes. For instance, in a study of 1521 patients with an acute (first or recurrent) stroke or a transient ischaemic attack, Doehner et al. found the risk of death or high dependency was 0.60 (95% CI 0.39–0.91) and the risk of death or recurrent stroke was 0.56 (95% CI 0.37–0.86) in the group of obese patients, when compared with the normal weight group [42].

It should be noted that, as yet, no specific biological mechanism has been identified to explain this 'obesity paradox'. In addition, to date, all studies have been observational (many of them retrospective and subanalysis of clinical trials) and no randomised controlled trial has been conducted to assess the effect of weight loss on outcomes of obese stroke patients. Hence, this is an area that requires more research. However, in light of this emerging evidence, the American guidelines on secondary prevention have introduced a new (level C) recommendation which states that '(…) the usefulness of weight loss among patients with a recent TIA or ischemic stroke and obesity is uncertain' [43]. Independently of these uncertainties, there is evidence that the quality of the diet has an important role in the secondary prevention of strokes, which needs to be taken into consideration by dietitians when providing dietary counselling for stroke patients [10].

References

1. World Health Organization. Neurological Disorders: Public Health Challenges. www.who.int/mental_health/neurology/neurological_disorders_report_web.pdf (accessed 3 September 2017).
2. Wolfe C, Rudd T. The Burden of Stroke. White Paper http://safestroke.eu/wp-content/uploads/2016/07/FINAL_Burden_of_Stroke.pdf (accessed 3 September 2017).
3. Adams HP, Bendixen BH, Kappelle LJ, et al. Classification of subtype of acute ischemic stroke. Definitions for use in a multicenter clinical trial. TOAST. Trial of Org 10172 in Acute Stroke Treatment. *Stroke* 1993; **24**(1): 35–41.
4. World Health Organization. WHO STEPS Stroke Manual: The WHO STEPwise Approach to Stroke Surveillance. www.who.int/chp/steps/Manual.pdf (accessed 3 September 2017).
5. O'Donnell MJ, Xavier D, Liu L, et al. Risk factors for ischaemic and intracerebral haemorrhagic stroke in 22 countries (the INTERSTROKE study): a case-control study. *Lancet* 2010; **376**(9735): 112–123.
6. Tirschwell DL, Smith NL, Heckbert SR, Lemaitre RN, Longstreth WT Jr, Psaty BM. Association of cholesterol with stroke risk varies in stroke subtypes and patient subgroups. *Neurology* 2004; **63**(10): 1868–1875.
7. Carroll K, Eliahoo J, Majeed M, Murad S. Stroke incidence and risk factors in a population-based prospective cohort study. *Health Stat Q* 2001; **12**: 18–26.
8. Cristensen L, Krieger D, Cristensen H. Risk factors for stroke are different in the very old. *Int J Stroke* 2010; **40**.
9. Hajat C, Tilling K, Stewart JA, Lemic-Stojcevic N, Wolfe CDA. Ethnic differences in risk factors for ischemic stroke – a European case-control study. *Stroke* 2004; **35**(7): 1562–1567.
10. Hookway C, Gomes F, Weekes CE. Royal College of Physicians Intercollegiate Stroke Working Party evidence-based guidelines for the secondary prevention of stroke through nutritional or dietary modification. *J Hum Nutr Diet* 2015; **28**(2): 107–125.
11. Gariballa S. Nutrition and Stroke: Prevention and Treatment. Hoboken: Blackwell Publishing, 2004.
12. Lakkur S, Judd SE. Diet and stroke: recent evidence supporting a Mediterranean-style diet and food in the primary prevention of stroke. *Stroke* 2015; **46**: 2007–2011.
13. Goldenberg MM. Multiple sclerosis review. *P&T* 2012; **37**(3): 175–184.
14. Limousin N, Blasco H, Corcia P, et al. Malnutrition at the time of diagnosis is associated with a shorter disease duration in ALS. *J Neurol Sci* 2010; **297**(1–2): 36–39.
15. Greenwood DI. Nutrition management of amyotrophic lateral sclerosis. *Nutr Clin Pract* 2013; **28**(3): 392–399.
16. Foley N, Teasell R, Richardson M, Serrato J, Finestone H. Nutritional Interventions Following Stroke. Evidence-Based Review of Stroke

Rehabilitation. www.ebrsr.com/evidence-review/16-nutritional-interventions-following-stroke (accessed 3 September 2017).

17. FOOD Trial Collaboration. Poor nutritional status on admission predicts poor outcomes after stroke: observational data from the FOOD trial. *Stroke* 2003; **34**(6): 1450–1456.

18. Mosselman MJ, Kruitwagen CLJJ, Schuurmans MJ, Hafsteinsdottir TB. Malnutrition and risk of malnutrition in patients with stroke: prevalence during hospital stay. *J Neurosci Nurs* 2013; **45**(4): 194–204.

19. Joonsson AC, Lindgren I, Norrving B, Lindgren A. Weight loss after stroke: a population-based study from the Lund Stroke Register. *Stroke* 2008; **39**(3): 918–923.

20. Smithard D, Weekes CE. Swallowing and nutritional complications. In: Bhalla A, Birns J, editors. Management of Post-Stroke Complications. Switzerland: Springer International Publishing, 2015.

21. Habek M, Hojsak I, Brinar VV. Nutrition in multiple sclerosis. *Clin Neurol Neurosurg* 2010; **112**(7): 616–620.

22. Braun MM, Osecheck M, Joyce NC. Nutrition assessment and management in amyotrophic lateral sclerosis. *Phys Med Rehabil Clin North Am* 2012; **23**(4): 751–771.

23. Salvioni C, Stanich P, Almeida C, Oliveira A. Nutritional care in motor neurone disease/ amyotrophic lateral sclerosis. *Arq Neuropsiquiatr* 2014; **72**: 157–163.

24. Royal College of Physicians. Stroke Guidelines. www.rcplondon.ac.uk/sites/default/files/national-clinical-guidelines-for-stroke-fourth-edition.pdf (accessed 3 September 2017).

25. Scottish Intercollegiate Guidelines Network. Management of Patients with Stroke: Identification and Management of Dysphagia. www.sign.ac.uk/assets/sign119.pdf (accessed 3 September 2017).

26. Gomes F, Emery PW, Weekes CE. Risk of malnutrition is an independent predictor of mortality, length of hospital stay, and hospitalization costs in stroke patients. *J Stroke Cerebrovasc Dis* 2016; **25**(4): 799–806.

27. Gomes F, Emery PW, Weekes CE. Weight loss prior to stroke is associated with increased mortality and length of hospital stay at 6 months post-stroke. *Int J Stroke* 2013; **8**(Suppl 3): 39.

28. Luo H, Liu B, Hu J, Wang X, Zhan S, Kong W. Hyperhomocysteinemia and methylenetetrahydrofolate reductase polymorphism in cervical artery dissection: a meta-analysis. *Cerebrovasc Dis* 2014; **37**(5): 313–322.

29. Geeganage C, Beavan J, Ellender S, Bath PM. Interventions for dysphagia and nutritional support in acute and subacute stroke. *Cochrane Database Syst Rev* 2012; **10**: CD000323.

30. Dennis M, Lewis S, Cranswick G, Forbes J. FOOD: a multicentre randomized trial evaluating feeding policies in patients admitted to hospital with a recent stroke. *Health Technol Assess* 2006; **10**(2): 1–91.

31. Foley N, Finestone H, Woodbury MG, Teasell R, Greene-Finestone L. Energy and protein intakes of acute stroke patients. *J Nutr Health Aging* 2006; **10**(3): 171–175.

32. Whelan K. Inadequate fluid intakes in dysphagic acute stroke. *Clin Nutr* 2001; **20**(5): 423–428.

33. International Dysphagia Diet Standardization Committee. What is the IDDSI Framework? http://iddsi.org/framework/ (accessed 3 September 2017).

34. Wirth R, Smoliner C, Jäger M, Warnecke T, Leischker AH, Dziewas R. Guideline clinical nutrition in patients with stroke. *Exp Transl Stroke Med* 2013; **5**(1): 14.

35. Gomes F, Hookway C, Weekes CE. Royal College of Physicians Intercollegiate Stroke Working Party evidence-based guidelines for the nutritional support of patients who have had a stroke. *J Hum Nutr Diet* 2014; **27**(2): 107–121.

36. Miller RG, Jackson CE, Kasarskis EJ, et al. Practice parameter update: the care of the patient with amyotrophic lateral sclerosis: drug, nutritional, and respiratory therapies (an evidence-based review): report of the Quality Standards Subcommittee of the American Academy of Neurology. *Neurology* 2009; **73**(15): 1218–1226.

37. Katzberg HD, Benatar M. Enteral tube feeding for amyotrophic lateral sclerosis/motor neuron disease. *Cochrane Database Syst Rev* 2011; **1**: CD004030.

38. Farinotti M, Vacchi L, Simi S, Di Pietrantonj C, Brait L, Filippini G. Dietary interventions for multiple sclerosis. *Cochrane Database Syst Rev* 2012; **12**: CD004192.

39. White R, Bradnam V. Handbook of Drug Administration via Enteral Feeding Tubes. London: Pharmaceutical Press, 2007, p. 569.

40. Kim BJ, Lee SH, Jung KH, et al. Dynamics of obesity paradox after stroke, related to time from onset, age, and causes of death. *Neurology* 2012; **79**(9): 856–863.

41. Vemmos K, Ntaios G, Spengos K, et al. Association between obesity and mortality after acute first-ever stroke the obesity-stroke paradox. *Stroke* 2011; **42**(1): 30–36.

42. Doehner W, Schenkel J, Anker SD, Springer J, Audebert HJ. Overweight and obesity are associated with improved survival, functional outcome, and stroke recurrence after acute stroke or transient ischaemic attack: observations from the TEMPiS trial. *Eur Heart J* 2012; **34**(4): 268–277.

43. Kernan WN, Ovbiagele B, Black HR, et al. Guidelines for the prevention of stroke in patients with stroke and transient ischemic attack: a guideline for healthcare professionals from the American Heart Association/American Stroke Association. *Stroke* 2014; **45**(7): 2160–2236.

Chapter 5.5

Nutrition support in spinal cord injury

Samford Wong

National Spinal Injuries Centre, Aylesbury, UK

5.5.1 Introduction

The annual incidence of spinal cord injury (SCI) throughout the world is 15–40 cases per million [1]. It is estimated that there are around 10 000 new cases in the US and around 500–700 new cases each year in the UK. The American Spinal Injury Association Impairment Scale (AIS) focuses on 10 key muscles and 10 key sensory points to be tested during neurological assessment [2]. Figures 5.5.1 and 5.5.2 illustrate the neurological evaluation according to the International Standard of Neurological Classification of Spinal Cord Injuries [2].

Spinal cord injury can affect both motor and sensory dermatomes.

- Tetraplegia (quadriplegia): this results from damage to cervical cord segments causing impairment or loss of function in all four limbs.
- Paraplegia: function of the lower limbs is impaired or lost as a result of damage to the thoracic, lumbar or, to a lesser extent, sacral cord segments. In both paraplegia and tetraplegia there is impairment of autonomic function, including bladder and bowel control.
- Complete (AIS: A) and incomplete lesions (AIS: B–D): in a complete lesion, all neurological function is lost below the level of the lesion. In an incomplete lesion, there is partial preservation of neurological function and any combination of motor (muscle), sensory (feeling) or autonomic function may be spared. (Nerves of the autonomic system control those body functions which are not under conscious control.) Brown–Séquard syndrome or central cord syndrome describes different patterns of incomplete lesion usually occurring as a result of neck injuries.
- Muscle wasting: post-injury muscle wasting results in a reduction of lean body mass and, in the longer term, immobility encourages an increase in total body fat.
- Autonomic dysreflexia (AD): people with SCI above T6 level can experience AD, a group of abnormal signs and symptoms triggered by a noxious stimulus below the level of lesion that causes an increase in autonomic activity. It is characterised by a sudden, severe headache secondary to an uncontrolled elevation of blood pressure, flushing and profuse sweating. If untreated, the hypertension may progress to fatal complications, such as cerebral haemorrhage or acute myocardial infarction. The most common nutrition-related stimuli are an overdistended bladder, bowel impaction, urinary tract infection and pressure ulcers.

5.5.2 Causes and mechanisms of undernutrition after spinal cord injury

Metabolic response

After SCI, the pathology, in the acute phase, encompasses an array of pathophysiological processes, including initiation of a robust inflammatory reaction and immune response. This is

Advanced Nutrition and Dietetics in Nutrition Support, First Edition. Edited by Mary Hickson and Sara Smith.
© 2018 John Wiley & Sons Ltd. Published 2018 by John Wiley & Sons Ltd.

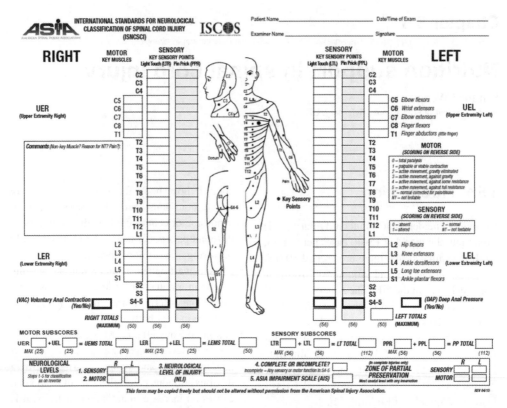

Figure 5.5.1 International standards for neurological classification of spinal cord injury. Reproduced with permission of the American Spinal Injury Association

characterised in part by the synthesis of cytokines and a co-ordinated infiltration of the injured cord by peripheral monocytes. Furthermore, patients may already be suffering from undernutrition [3]. Negative energy balance will result in depletion of glycogen stores and rapid increase in the utilisation of body fat and protein for energy provision. Patients frequently develop hypercatabolism [4] and a delayed supply of nutrition will result in the depletion of whole-body energy stores, loss of lean muscle mass and, ultimately, loss of gastrointestinal mucosal integrity and compromise of the immune system [5].

It has been shown that this negative nitrogen balance is common in the period after SCI although it may not be present until the second or third week post injury [6]. The inflammatory stress response also contributes to the catabolic process after injury. Inflammatory cytokines and stress hormones cause a shift in substrate utilisation and increase the basal metabolic rate. Protein stores could become depleted if no nutrition intervention is initiated, resulting in undernutrition [7].

Swallowing dysfunction

Patients with SCI may also suffer from swallowing dysfunction that hinders their ability to tolerate oral food, which may occur as a result of lying flat. Studies have reported that 16% of patients have dysphagia after SCI [8]. Ventilator support and tracheotomy may also present physical barriers to eating and drinking. Kirshblum et al. suggested that the presence of a tracheostomy appears to be a risk factor in causing dysphagia [9]. If dysphagia remains undetected

Muscle Function Grading

0 = total paralysis
1 = palpable or visible contraction
2 = active movement, full range of motion (ROM) with gravity eliminated
3 = active movement, full ROM against gravity
4 = active movement, full ROM against gravity and moderate resistance in a muscle specific position
5 = (normal) active movement, full ROM against gravity and full resistance in a functional muscle position expected from an otherwise unimpaired person
5* = (normal) active movement, full ROM against gravity and sufficient resistance to be considered normal if identified inhibiting factors (i.e. pain, disuse) were not present
NT = not testable (i.e. due to immobilization, severe pain such that the patient cannot be graded, amputation of limb, or contracture of > 50% of the normal ROM)

Sensory Grading

0 = Absent
1 = Altered, either decreased/impaired sensation or hypersensitivity
2 = Normal
NT = Not testable

When to Test Non-Key Muscles:

In a patient with an apparent AIS B classification, non-key muscle functions more than 3 levels below the motor level on each side should be tested to most accurately classify the injury (differentiate between AIS B and C).

Movement	Root level
Shoulder: Flexion, extension, abduction, adduction, internal and external rotation **Elbow:** Supination	C5
Elbow: Pronation **Wrist:** Flexion	C6
Finger: Flexion at proximal joint, extension. **Thumb:** Flexion, extension and abduction in plane of thumb	C7
Finger: Flexion at MCP joint **Thumb:** Opposition, adduction and abduction perpendicular to palm	C8
Finger: Abduction of the index finger	T1
Hip: Adduction	L2
Hip: External rotation	L3
Hip: Extension, abduction, internal rotation **Knee:** Flexion **Ankle:** Inversion and eversion **Toe:** MP and IP extension	L4
Hallux and Toe: DIP and PIP flexion and abduction	L5
Hallux: Adduction	S1

ASIA Impairment Scale (AIS)

A = Complete. No sensory or motor function is preserved in the sacral segments S4-5.

B = Sensory Incomplete. Sensory but not motor function is preserved below the neurological level and includes the sacral segments S4-5 (light touch or pin prick at S4-5 or deep anal pressure) AND no motor function is preserved more than three levels below the motor level on either side of the body.

C = Motor Incomplete. Motor function is preserved at the most caudal sacral segments for voluntary anal contraction (VAC) OR the patient meets the criteria for sensory incomplete status (sensory function preserved at the most caudal sacral segments (S4-S5) by LT, PP or DAP), and has some sparing of motor function more than three levels below the ipsilateral motor level on either side of the body.
(This includes key or non-key muscle functions to determine motor incomplete status.) For AIS C – less than half of key muscle functions below the single NLI have a muscle grade ≥ 3.

D = Motor Incomplete. Motor incomplete status as defined above, with at least half (half or more) of key muscle functions below the single NLI having a muscle grade ≥ 3.

E = Normal. If sensation and motor function as tested with the ISNCSCI are graded as normal in all segments, and the patient had prior deficits, then the AIS grade is E. Someone without an initial SCI does not receive an AIS grade.

Using ND: To document the sensory, motor and NLI levels, the ASIA Impairment Scale grade, and/or the zone of partial preservation (ZPP) when they are unable to be determined based on the examination results.

Steps in Classification

The following order is recommended for determining the classification of individuals with SCI.

1. Determine sensory levels for right and left sides.
The sensory level is the most caudal, intact dermatome for both pin prick and light touch sensation.

2. Determine motor levels for right and left sides.
Defined by the lowest key muscle function that has a grade of at least 3 (on supine testing), providing the key muscle functions represented by segments above that level are judged to be intact (graded as a 5).
Note: in regions where there is no myotome to test, the motor level is presumed to be the same as the sensory level, if testable motor function above that level is also normal.

3. Determine the neurological level of injury (NLI)
This refers to the most caudal segment of the cord with intact sensation and antigravity (3 or more) muscle function strength, provided that there is normal (intact) sensory and motor function rostrally respectively.
The NLI is the most cephalad of the sensory and motor levels determined in steps 1 and 2.

4. Determine whether the injury is Complete or Incomplete.
(i.e. absence or presence of sacral sparing)
If voluntary anal contraction = No AND all S4-5 sensory scores = 0 AND deep anal pressure = No, then injury is Complete.
Otherwise, injury is Incomplete.

5. Determine ASIA Impairment Scale (AIS) Grade:

Is injury Complete? If YES, AIS=A and can record ZPP (lowest dermatome or myotome on each side with some preservation)

NO ↓

Is injury Motor Complete? If YES, AIS=B
(No=voluntary anal contraction OR motor function more than three levels below the motor level on a given side, if the patient has sensory incomplete classification)

NO ↓

Are at least half (half or more) of the key muscles below the neurological level of injury graded 3 or better?

NO → AIS=C   YES → AIS=D

If sensation and motor function is normal in all segments, AIS=E
Note: AIS E is used in follow up testing when an individual with a documented SCI has recovered normal function. If at initial testing no deficits are found, the individual is neurologically intact; the ASIA Impairment Scale does not apply.

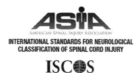

ASIA
AMERICAN SPINAL INJURY ASSOCIATION
INTERNATIONAL STANDARDS FOR NEUROLOGICAL CLASSIFICATION OF SPINAL CORD INJURY

ISCOS
INTERNATIONAL SPINAL CORD SOCIETY

Figure 5.5.2 International standards for neurological classification of spinal cord injury. Reproduced with permission of the American Spinal Injury Association

and untreated, aspiration pneumonia could result. It is recommended that a swallow assessment is performed prior to oral feeding in all cases of cervical SCI. In cases of severe dysphagia, an alternative route of nutrition may be required.

5.5.3 Nutrition-related complications in spinal cord injury

Complications in the acute phase

Gastrointestinal complications

Gastrointestinal factors such as dysphagia, ileus, gastrointestinal bleeding, diarrhoea or constipation, early satiety and abdominal injuries may adversely affect a patient's nutritional status. In addition, a compromised GI tract due to spinal shock could lead to gastric content aspiration and abdominal distension which could comprise dietary intake and ventilation [10].

Gut paralysis (ileus) and distension may cause an inadequate evacuation that can lead to nausea and vomiting, high gastric residual, anorexia, poor lung expansion and inadequate venous return [11]. For this reason, it is mandatory to check the patient's bowel movement daily.

Hyponatraemia

Spinal cord injury carries a 20–35% risk of hyponatraemia which is more common with complete injuries [12,13]. One of the secondary complications of hyponatraemia is visual disturbance. The pathophysiology is related to partially blocked sodium conservation (sympathetic denervation of the kidney or impaired blood flow), enhanced water conservation (in the competition between hypovolaemia and hyponatraemia, hypovolaemia wins and exerts its volume-building effects), and increased fluid intake [14]. It has been shown that in AIS A and B, the higher the level of injury, the greater the correlation between reduced sodium conservation, hypotension, polydipsia and hyponatraemia [14].

Anaemia

Anaemia is common immediately post SCI, even without substantial blood loss, and may contribute to respiratory dysfunction and occurrence of pressure ulcers [15]. A study of 28 C3–C7-injured subjects found that 82% had decreased red blood cell mass. Although decreased red cell mass was common, no subjects had below normal blood volumes and the process of erythropoiesis did not seem to be altered [15]. This led the authors to hypothesise that quadriplegics may need less oxygen (and therefore oxygen-carrying capacity) to maintain function [15]. Of note, iron or folic acid supplements may not correct anaemia, but normal haemoglobin concentration may be attained only after a chronic disease, such as pressure ulcer, urinary tract infection, folic acid deficiency due to psychosocial maladjustment, is eliminated [16]. Low-quality evidence supports the use of an erythrocyte transfusion strategy to optimise haemoglobin, especially if surgery for pressure ulcer closure is planned [17].

Protein loss

Serum albumin is found to be lower in patients with SCI. A study evaluating the nutritional status of 51 patients at 2, 4 and 8 weeks post injury found nutrient deficiencies that occurred with varying frequencies, including low albumin [18]. Most depressed parameters improved with time but albumin remained consistently low. Barco et al. noticed that despite the negative nitrogen balance, prealbumin increased as protein and energy intake increased over the duration of the 4-week postinjury study (based on 2 g/kg admission body weight) [19]. Hypoalbuminaemia was reported as an independent predictor for long hospital stay [19].

Patients with recurrent hypoalbuminaemia should be considered for detailed nutritional assessment.

Bladder and urinary infections

Due to the need for long-term bladder catheterisation, patients are particularly vulnerable to infections of the urinary tract or kidneys. Cranberry juice is taken by some people with SCI in the belief that it might help in preventing bladder infections [20]. The small number of studies on this topic reported inconclusive findings, although there is some evidence that cranberry juice may reduce urinary tract infections but it may also contribute to weight gain. A Cochrane review of studies in otherwise healthy adults indicated that, while there is some evidence of beneficial effects from regular cranberry consumption in women, there were no statistically significant differences when the results of a much larger study were included. The optimum dosage or method of administration (e.g. juice or tablets) remains unknown and further, better designed trials are needed [21].

Complications in the chronic phase

Obesity

Obesity is a common secondary complication of SCI in the longer term and is associated with adverse metabolic consequences. Total energy expenditure is compromised due to a reduced basal metabolic rate (BMR) secondary to muscle atrophy and a reduction in physical activity level. Studies suggested that up to 65.8% of patients with SCI are overweight (BMI >25 kg/m^2), and up to 30% are obese (BMI >30 kg/m^2) [22]. In addition, it has been proposed that the BMI cut-off definitions for overweight and obesity should be changed to 22 kg/m^2 as overweight and >25 kg/m^2 as obese, in view of the body composition changes occurring with SCI [23].

Not all clinical rehabilitation centres will have access to an indirect calorimeter to measure BMR [24], but predictive equations should be used with caution as they tend to overestimate measured requirements by 5–32%, most markedly in tetraplegia [25]. Measured BMR has been found to be 14–27% lower in people with SCI than in able-bodied controls [24], which explains the problem with the use of predictive equations. Two possible mechanisms to explain reduced BMR have been proposed: a change in body composition resulting in reduced fat-free mass and an altered sympathetic nervous system activity. The higher level SCI lesions are associated with markedly decreased sympathetic activity.

Pressure ulcers

Patients with SCI are susceptible to pressure ulcers [5,26]. After SCI, an individual's ability to feel pain in a pressure area is impaired due to sensation loss, and they are also unable to shift weight naturally due to mobility loss [26]. A pressure ulcer generally arises as a result of sustained pressure on the soft tissue layers over bony prominences. While tissues can withstand large pressures for brief periods, continuous pressures above the arterial capillary pressure can impair the flow of nutrients and oxygen to the tissues. In addition, continuous pressure greater than the venous capillary closing pressure over a long period of time can impede the return of blood flow and lead to accumulation of toxic metabolites, lymphatic stasis and tissue damage [27]. Reactive capillary dilation, increased vascular permeability, oedema, blistering and thrombosis that follow culminate in a downward spiral of tissue necrosis and ulceration [27].

There is minimal research investigating the relationship between nutritional status and prevention and/or healing of pressure ulcers. One observational study comparing healing rate of pressure ulcers in patients with SCI found that receipt of 9 g of arginine resulted in a significantly shorter mean healing time when compared with historical controls [28]. A recent guideline published in America made an attempt to quantify amounts of nutrients needed to prevent pressure ulcers or optimise the healing process once a pressure ulcer occurs [29] (see Table 5.5.1).

Osteoporosis

It has been clearly demonstrated that bone density decreases in the first few weeks after SCI and continues to worsen for 3–8 years [30]. Vitamin D deficiency, disuse or poor circulation could all contribute to the development of this low bone density and increased porosity. A cross-sectional study of 89 men with complete SCI found that bone loss was greatest in the epiphyses and was reduced by 50% in the femur

Table 5.5.1 Energy, protein, fluid and micronutrient needs for patients with SCI and pressure ulcer

Needs	SCI with pressure ulcers
Energy	Pressure ulcer stage II: BMR × 1.2
	Pressure ulcer stage III–IV: BMR × 1.5
Protein	Pressure ulcer stage II: 1.2–1.5 g/kg BW/day
	Pressure ulcer stage III–IV:1.5–2.0 g/kg BW/day
Fluid	No pressure ulcer: max 30–40 mL/kg BW/day; min 1.0 mL/kg BW/day
	Additional fluid: 10–15 mL/kcal/day for those using air-fluidised beds set high temperature (>31–34 °C)
Micronutrients	Daily vitamin and mineral supplement as RDA
	Vitamin A 10 000–50 000 IU per day
	Pressure ulcer stage I–II: vitamin C 100–200 mg/day
	Pressure ulcer stage III–IV: vitamin C 1000–2000 mg/day
	Zinc – 50 mg elemental zinc, twice a day; higher dose should be limited to 2–3 weeks
	Iron to correct iron deficiency anaemia

BMR, basal metabolic rate estimated by the Harris–Benedict formula; BW, body weight; IU, international unit; RDA, recommended daily allowance; SCI, spinal cord injury.

and 60% in the tibia [31]. Vitamin D deficiency is common after SCI due to limited sunlight exposure in the chronic phase, and vitamin D supplements should be considered.

Renal calculi

Individuals with SCI have a greater risk for urolithiasis, primarily as a result of recurrent bladder infections, increased retention of calcium by the bladder and kidneys or poor hydration. Longer duration of SCI, the completeness of lesion and resulting immobility all increase the risk [32]. To help prevent bladder infections, the recommended fluid intake is at least 2.5 litres of water-based fluids per day. Dietary restriction of calcium is not indicated [32].

Neurogenic bowel dysfunction

Neurogenic bowel dysfunction (NBD) is one of the many impairments that result from SCI and is often quoted as being one of the most distressing problems individuals have to face [33]. Following SCI, there is a spinal shock in the initial stages and during this period reflex-mediated defaecation is less active [34]. In the later stages, studies have reported delayed gastric emptying, prolonged colon transit time [35] and low colonic compliance [36]. There are two patterns of NBD.

- Upper motor neuron or reflexive bowel syndrome which generally occurs in cervical and thoracic injury. Upper motor neuron syndrome results in constipation with faecal retention behind a spastic anal sphincter.
- Lower motor neuron or areflexive bowel syndrome which generally occurs in lumbar or sacral injury where the conus or nerve roots are damaged. Lower motor neuron bowel syndrome produces constipation with a high risk of frequent incontinence through a lax external sphincter mechanism.

The two types of NBD require different bowel management programmes; adjustments in dietary intake (particularly dietary fibre) may be required to produce an ideal stool consistency. Chemical stimulants are commonly used in patients with upper motor neuron syndrome

where a softer stool is required, and a high fibre intake with adequate fluids may therefore be helpful. Manual evacuation is commonly used with lower motor neuron where a harder and drier stool is required; therefore a lower fibre intake can be helpful.

Spinal cord injury results in delayed gut transit times in both the acute and chronic stages. The factor associated with colorectal dysfunction is complete SCI. If enteral nutrition is required, it is best to start with a non-fibre formula and gradually introduce fibre within toleration. Additional fluids may be necessary due to the slower colonic transit time which results in increased reabsorption of fluid. In practice, at least 2.5 litres or more is usually recommended. The British SCI centres have updated guidelines on bowel management following SCI and provide recommendations on fluid requirement and fibre intake [37]. Further research is needed to determine the optimal dietary fibre intake for individuals with SCI.

5.5.4 Assessment and diagnosis of undernutrition in spinal cord injury

Nutritional screening in patients with spinal cord injuries

Nutritional screening is an important step in detecting and ultimately preventing undernutrition. A disease-specific nutrition screening tool, the Spinal Nutrition Screening Tool (SNST) (Figure 5.5.3), based on eight parameters (BMI, age, level of SCI, presence of comorbidities, skin condition, diet, appetite and ability to eat), has been developed and validated for use on patients with SCI [38]. Healthcare professionals are recommended to screen patients before transfer to and during their stay in a SCI centre.

Assessing the degree of weight loss since injury

Postinjury weight loss is a common consequence of SCI. The early stages of SCI are immediately marked by reduced energy expenditure, and extensive nitrogen losses that may last from weeks to several months. Most patients will be able to recall their preinjury weight, but measuring current weight can be difficult. Appropriate weighing scales may be unavailable (bed or hoist scales), unemptied catheter or stoma bags lead to inaccurate weights, and dependence on a ventilator can mean weighing is not feasible.

Other anthropometric measurements

Standing height, required to calculated BMI, is often impossible to measure accurately due to immobility, but self-reported height or measurements of other body segments can be used as an alternative, such as ulna length, knee height, arm

Complete all boxes on admission and action as indicated by score.

Estimated/reported preinjury weight (kg)	Estimated/reported height (m)	Preinjury BMI (use BMI chart to calculate)

Score each risk factor, using highest score if more than one is relevant.
Total up column scores to obtain risk score and record below.

Current BMI or Weight Loss Since Injury	Age (yrs)	Level of SCI	Other Medical Conditions	Skin Conditions	Diet	Intake	Ability to Eat
0 BMI (18.5 – 22) or "Minimal" Wt Loss (under 5%)*	1 18-30	1 S1-S5	0 None	0 Intact	0 Normal diet and fluids or established NG/PEG feed	0 Eating all meals or tolerating full enteral feed	0 Not applicable as on NG/PEG feed
1 BMI (22.5 – 25) or "Some" Wt Loss (5-10%)*	2 31-60	2 L1-L5	1 Chronic conditions eg. Pain/ substance abuse	1 Grade 1 ulcer	1 Introductory NG/PEG feed	1 Under half meal or NG/PEG feed tolerated	0 Able to eat independently
3 BMI over 25 or BMI under 18.5 or "Moderate" Wt Loss (11-15%)*	3 Over 60	3 T1-T12	2 Acute trauma eg. head injury/ fractures	2 Grade 2 ulcer	2 Modified texture diet	2 Minimal diet, or reduced NG/PEG feed	2 Requires some help
4 BMI over 40 Or BMI under 16 or "Marked" Wt Loss (over 15%)*	4 Under 18	5 C1-C8	3 Within 1 week of surgery/ ongoing infection	3 Grade 3 ulcer	3 Nil by mouth for more than 5 days	3* Vomiting and diarrhoea or not tolerating NG/PEG feed	3 Needs to be fed
			4 Ventilated (non-invasive)	5 Grade 4 ulcer			
*calculate current BMI and % weight loss using spinal adapted BMI and % weight loss charts			5 Fully ventilated with tracheostomy			* Investigate cause and treat	

Date	Column Score	Column Score	Column Score	Column Score	Column Score	Column Score	Column Score	Column Score	RISK SCORE

Transfer total score overleaf and choose appropriate action plan according to identified risk category.
Complete table below to update nutritional risk scores and document weight changes.

Figure 5.5.3 Spinal Nutrition Screening Tool

Date	Risk Score	Risk Level (L/M/H)	Latest Weight (dated)	Current BMI or % Loss	Variance and Comments	Referred to Dietitian	Review Date	Nurse's Signature

Implement action plan according to risk, document actions in nursing management plan.

Score	Risk	Action Plan	
10 and under	**Low Rehab**	Suggest healthy coded menu choices to avoid inappropriate weight gain	**Repeat score each month**
	Low Acute	Suggest 'small appetite' menu choices If eating less than half meals complete 3-day food chart and offer 2 Build–Up Soups/Shakes* a day **Intake needs monitoring, after Day 3 escalate to Dietitian or discontinue**	**Repeat score each week**
11–15	**Moderate Rehab and Acute**	Encourage appropriate menu choices as above If eating less than half of meals complete 3-day food chart and offer 2 Build-Up Soups/Shakes* a day **Intake needs monitoring, after day 3 escalate to dietitian or discontinue**	**Repeat score each week**
Above 15	**High Rehab and Acute**	Encourage appropriate menu choices as above If eating less than half of meals offer 2 supplement drinks a day, e.g. Fortisip/Fortijuice* as prescribed by doctor or dietitian Complete 3-day food chart for nutritional assessment **Needs action, refer to Dietitian**	**Repeat score each week**

Figure 5.5.3　(Continued)

or demi-span. Caution should be used with these measurements as they have been shown to have poor agreement with standing height. In addition, arm anthropometric measurement, such as mid-upper arm circumference, triceps skinfold and mid-arm muscle circumference, could be used as surrogate for BMI.

5.5.5　Nutrition intervention

Assessment of the need for nutrition support is necessary in all trauma patients, and early enteral nutrition support has been associated with improved outcomes.

Timing of first feeding after spinal cord injury

Intestinal paralysis is prominent during the acute phase of SCI. Regurgitation and vomiting may occur and result in aspiration pneumonia. The Consortium of Spinal Cord Medicine recommended consideration of enteral nutrition within 24–48 hours after admission if the patient could not meet their nutritional need orally [39]. The enteral route should be considered before parenteral nutrition due to the increased risk of infectious complications and lower incidence of hyperglycaemia [40]. A pilot study by Dvorak et al. on the timing of the first feeding post injury showed no difference in the incidence of infection, nutritional status, feeding complications, number of ventilator hours or length of stay between patients receiving early (<72 hours after injury) versus late (>120 hours after injury) enteral nutrition [41]. Nevertheless, artificial nutrition support should be commenced as soon as possible and after assessment by a trauma centre dietitian. There is no evidence that early enteral feeding cannot be safely administered in the early stage of SCI [42].

Energy and protein requirements

After SCI, patients have reduced metabolic activity and actual energy needs are at least 10% below predicted needs [1]. In the absence of indirect calorimeter measurements, adjusting the standard equations may provide an adequate estimate for the initial phase. The American Dietetic Association [43] recommends that energy needs should be estimated with the Harris–Benedict formula, using admission body weight, an injury factor of 1.2 to 1.4 and an activity factor of 1 [44]. Alternatively, if a patient with SCI is in the rehabilitation phase, the energy need can be estimated by using the following factors [25]: 22.7 kcal per kg of body weight per day for tetraplegics and 27.9 kcal per kg per day for paraplegics.

Protein requirements of 2.0 g per kg of body weight per day are recommended for patients during the acute phase [43]. This is reduced to 0.8–1.0 g per kg body weight per day during rehabilitation and long-term phases, for maintenance of protein status in the absence of pressure ulcers or infection [28,43].

5.5.6 Summary

To improve the health of individuals with SCI, clinicians should be aware of the impact of undernutrition body functions, physical capability, consequences and complications such as pressure ulcers, obesity, osteoporosis and metabolic syndrome. Patients with SCI should be nutritionally screened on admission, during rehabilitation and long-term phases to detect undernutrition and micronutrient deficiency. There is a need for more research in this area in order to provide nutritional recommendations for SCI patients.

As with non-SCI traumas, it is preferential to use the enteral over the parenteral route if the GI tract is functional, in order to help maintain integrity and function as well as reduce risk of infections. Where indicated, dietary supplementation through food fortification, extra snacks and prescribed oral nutritional supplements may be of benefit in both the acute and chronic phases of SCI.

References

1. Sekhon LH, Fehlings MG. Epidemiology, demographics, and pathophysiology of acute spinal cord injury. *Spine* 2001; **26**(Suppl 24): S2–S12.
2. American Spinal Injury Association. International Standards for Neurological Classification of Spinal Cord Injury. http://asia-spinalinjury.org/wp-content/uploads/2016/02/International_Stds_Diagram_Worksheet.pdf (accessed 3 September 2017).
3. Hausmann ON. Post-traumatic inflammation following spinal cord injury. *Spinal Cord* 2003; **41**: 369–378.
4. Kaufman HH, Rowlands BJ, Stein DK, Kopaniky DR, Gildenberg PL. General metabolism in patients with acute paraplegia and quadriplegia. *Neurosurgery* 1985; **16**(3): 309–313.
5. Cruse JM, Lewis RE, Roe DL, Dilioglou S, Blaine MC, Wallace WF, Chen RD. Facilitation of immune function, healing of pressure ulcers, and nutritional status in spinal cord injury patients. *Exp Mol Pathol* 2000; **68**: 38–54.
6. Hadley MN. Nutrition support after spinal cord injury. *Neurosurgery* 2002; **50**: S81–S84.
7. Bissit PA. Nutrition in acute spinal cord injury. *Crit Care Nurs Clin North Am* 1990; **2**: 375–384.
8. Seid RO, Nusser-Muller-Busch R, Kurzweil M, Niedeggen A. Dysphagia in acute tetraplegics: a retrospective study. *Spinal Cord* 2010; **48**: 197–201.
9. Kirshblum S, Johnston MV, Brown J, O'Connor KC, Jarosz P. Predictors of dysphagia after spinal cord injury. *Arch Phys Med Rehabil* 1999; **80**: 1101–1105.
10. Merli G, Crabbe S, Doyle L, et al. Mechanical plus pharmacological prophylaxis for deep vein thrombosis in acute spinal cord injury. *Paraplegia* 1992; **30**: 558–562.
11. Fealey RD, Szurszewski JH, Merritt JL, et al. Effect of traumatic spinal cord transection on human upper gastrointestinal motility and gastric emptying. *Gastroenterology* 1984; **87**: 69–75.

12. Biyani A, Inman CG, el Masry WS. Hyponatremia after acute spinal injury. *Injury* 1993; **24**(10): 671–673.

13. Karlsson AK, Krassioukov AV. Hyponatremia-induced transient visual disturbances in acute spinal cord injury. *Spinal Cord* 2004; **42**: 204–207.

14. Frisbie JH. Salt wasting, hypotension, polydipsia, and hyponatremia and the level of spinal cord injury. *Spinal Cord* 2007; **45**: 563–568.

15. Huang CT, DeVivo MJ, Stover SL. Anemia in acute phase of spinal cord injury. *Arch Phys Med Rehabil* 1990; **71**: 3–7.

16. Perkash A, Brown M. Anemia in patients with traumatic spinal cord injury. *J Am Parapleg Soc* 1989; **50**: 353–358.

17. Cullis JO. Diagnosis and management of anaemia of chronic disease: current status. *Br J Haematol* 2011; **154**: 289–300.

18. Barco KT, Smith RA, Peerless JR, Plaisier BR, Chima CS. Energy expenditure assessment and validation after acute spinal cord injury. *Nutr Clin Pract* 2002; **17**: 309–313.

19. Wong S, Derry F, Jamous A, Hirani SP, Grimble G, Forbes A. Do nutritional risk associate with adverse clinical outcomes in spinal cord injured patients admitted to a spinal centre? *Eur J Clin Nutr* 2013; **68**: 125–130.

20. Hess MJ, Hess PE, Sullivan MR, Nee M, Yalla SV. Evaluation of cranberry tablets for the prevention of urinary tract infections in spinal cord injured patients with neurogenic bladder. *Spinal Cord* 2008; **46**: 622–626.

21. Jepson RG, Williams G, Craig JC. Cranberries for preventing urinary tract infections. *Cochrane Database Syst Rev* 2012; **10**: CD001321.

22. Gupta N, White KT, Sandford PR. Body mass index in spinal cord injury – a retrospective study. *Spinal Cord* 2006; **44**: 92–94.

23. Laughton GE, Buchholz AC, Martin Ginis KA, Goy RE. Lowering body mass index cutoffs better identifies obese persons with spinal cord injury. *Spinal Cord* 2009; **47**: 757–762.

24. Buchholz AC, Pencharz PB. Energy expenditure in chronic spinal cord injury. *Curr Opin Clin Nutr Metab Care* 2004; **7**: 635–639.

25. Cox SA, Weiss SM, Posuniak EA, Worthington P, Prioleau M, Heffley G. Energy expenditure after spinal cord injury: an evaluation of stable rehabilitating patients. *J Trauma* 1985; **25**: 419–423.

26. Krause JS, Broderick L. Patterns of recurrent pressure ulcers after spinal cord injury: identification and protective factors 5 or more years after onset. *Arch Phys Med Rehabil* 2004; **85**: 1257–1264.

27. Mak AF, Zhang M, Tam EW. Biomechanics of pressure ulcer in body tissues interacting with external forces during locomotion. *Ann Rev Biomed Eng* 2010; **12**: 29–53.

28. Brewer S, Deneves K, Pearce L, et al. Effect of an arginine containing nutritional supplement on pressure ulcer healing time in community spinal patients. *J Wound Care* 2010; **19**: 311–316.

29. Consortium for Spinal Cord Medicine. Pressure Ulcer Prevention and Treatment Following Injury: A Clinical Practice Guideline for Health-Care Providers, 2nd edn. Washington: Paralyzed Veterans of America, 2014.

30. Wilmet E, Ismail AA, Heliporn A, Welraeds D, Bergman P. Longitudinal study of the bone mineral content and of soft tissue composition after spinal cord section. *Paraplegia* 1993; **33**: 674–677.

31. Freehafer AA. Limb fractures in patients with spinal cord injury. *Arch Phys Med Rehabil* 1995; **76**: 823–827.

32. Bartel P, Krebs J, Wollner J, Gocking K, Pannek J. Bladder stones in patients with spinal cord injury: a long-term study. *Spinal Cord* 2014; **52**: 295–297.

33. Lynch AC, Wong C, Anthony A, Dobbs BR, Frizelle FA. Bowel dysfunction following spinal cord injury: a description of bowel function in a spinal cord injured population and comparison with age and gender matched control. *Spinal Cord* 2000; **38**(12): 717–723.

34. Atkinson PP, Atkinson JLD. Spinal shock – a review. *Mayo Clin Proc* 1996; **71**: 384–389.

35. Nino-Murcia M, Stone JM. Colonic transit in spinal cord-injured patients. *Invest Radiol* 1990; **25**: 109–112.

36. Glick MR, Meshkinpour H, HaldemanS, Hoehler F, Downey N, Bradley WE. Colonic dysfunction in patients with thoracic spinal cord injury. *Gastroenterology* 1984; **86**: 87–94.

37. Multidisciplinary Association of Spinal Cord Injured Professionals. Guidelines for Management of Neurogenic Bowel Dysfunction in Individuals with Central Neurological Conditions. www.rnoh.nhs.uk/sites/default/files/sia-mascip-bowelguidenew2012.pdf (accessed 3 September 2017).

38. Wong S, Derry F, Jamous A, Hirani SP, Grimble G, Forbes A. Validation of the Spinal Nutrition Screening Tool (SNST) in patients with spinal cord injuries (SCI) result from a multicentre study. *Eur J Clin Nutr* 2012; **66**: 382–387.

39. Consortium for Spinal Cord Medicine. Early Acute Management in Adults with Spinal Cord Injury: A Clinical Practice Guideline for Health-Care Providers. Washington: Paralyzed Veterans of America, 2008.

40. Gramlich L, K Kichian, Prinilla J. Does enteral nutrition compared to parenteral nutrition result in better outcomes in critically ill adult patients? A systematic review of literature. *Nutrition* 2004; **20**: 843–848.

41. Dvorak MF, Noonan VK, Bélanger L, et al. Early versus late enteral feeding in patients with acute

cervical spinal cord injury: a pilot study. *Spine* 2004; **29**(9): E175–180.

42. Rowan CJ, Gillanders LK, Paice RL, Judson JA. Is early enteral feeding safe in patients who have suffered spinal cord injury? *Injury* 2004; **35**(3): 238–242.

43. American Dietetic Association. Spinal Cord Injury (SCI) Guideline. www.andeal.org/topic.cfm?cat=3485 (accessed 3 September 2017).

44. Rodriguez DJ, Benzel EC, Clevenger FW. The metabolic response to spinal cord injury. *Spinal Cord* 1997; **35**: 599–604.

Chapter 5.6

Nutrition support in pulmonary and cardiac disease

Peter F. Collins

School of Exercise and Nutrition Sciences, Queensland University of Technology, Brisbane, Australia

5.6.1 Undernutrition in cardiopulmonary disease

Chronic obstructive pulmonary disease

Chronic obstructive pulmonary disease (COPD) is a lung disease characterised by persistent airflow limitation that is usually progressive and associated with an enhanced chronic inflammatory response [1]. Across the European region, an estimated 66 million people live with the disease and it is predicted to rise to the third leading cause of mortality globally by 2020. In the UK, COPD is a major cause of morbidity and mortality with around 30 000 deaths per year and an estimated 3.7 million individuals with the disease [2]. The symptoms of COPD include shortness of breath (dyspnoea), chronic cough and chronic sputum production, and these are known to negatively impact on an individual's ability to meet their nutritional requirements. In addition, the disease is characterised by stable periods punctuated by episodes of acute worsening of these symptoms or exacerbations. These exacerbations are often inflammatory in nature and further compromise nutritional intake.

The relationship between weight loss and COPD has been reported for over 100 years. Interestingly, attempts to describe the different COPD phenotypes observed in relation to the different nutritional states led to the classic descriptions of the emphysematous (pink puffer) and bronchitic (blue bloater) COPD types. The emphysematous patient is characteristically thin, with visible muscle wasting, breathless with marked hyperinflation of the chest. The bronchitic patient is often overweight in appearance, which can hide clinically relevant fat-free mass depletion; they may not be particularly breathless at rest but have severe central cyanosis (bluish-purple discoloration of the skin due to oxygen desaturation). With most patients presenting a mixed picture of the two forms of airflow limitation, clinicians in the 1960s started to refer to them under the umbrella term of COPD. This could explain why research into the nutritional management of the two distinct nutritional phenotypes of COPD has been lacking [3].

Clinically relevant unintentional weight loss (5% in 3 months or 10% in 6 months) is found in 25–40% of COPD patients [4]. However, the prevalence varies between the inpatient and outpatient setting with up to 45% of outpatients and 60% of inpatients reported to be at risk [5]. Nutritional intake in COPD patients has been found to be severely impaired prior to hospitalisation, remaining low during the first few days of admission and only returning to the habitual level on discharge [6].

Chronic heart failure

Chronic heart failure (CHF) is also a leading cause of morbidity and mortality, affecting an estimated 26 million people worldwide [7].

Advanced Nutrition and Dietetics in Nutrition Support, First Edition. Edited by Mary Hickson and Sara Smith.

CHF is a complex clinical syndrome resulting in structural abnormalities of the heart and/or cardiac dysfunction, impairing the ability of the heart to pump blood around the body. CHF is characterised by similar symptoms to COPD, such as dyspnoea and fatigue, having a similar impact on an individual's nutritional status. Complex interactions exist between the pulmonary and cardiovascular systems due to the codependent functionality of the heart and lungs, in order to first oxygenate the blood (pulmonary) and then pump it around the body (cardiology). It is therefore not surprising that a disease of either organ is likely to affect the other. CHF can lead to pulmonary oedema; this accumulation of fluid can impair the diffusive capacity of the lungs, leading to respiratory failure. Conversely, COPD can cause right-sided heart failure (cor pulmonale) secondary to increased demands placed on the right heart as it works against increased pulmonary arterial blood pressure.

Due to the complexity of CHF, its association with disease-related undernutrition has not been explored in such great detail as other clinical conditions. However, its association with wasting (cardiac cachexia) has long been known, Hippocrates around 400 BC first described cardiac cachexia in Greek citizens suffering from a condition in which 'the flesh is consumed and becomes water…the shoulders, clavicles, chest, and thighs melt away' [8]. Cardiac cachexia is defined as unintentional weight loss of more than 6% in 6 months (excluding presence of oedema) and its prevalence is estimated at 12–15% [4]. The presence of a cachectic state in CHF has been found to be a strong independent risk factor for mortality [9].

5.6.2 Mechanisms for weight loss and muscle wasting

While diseases of the cardiac and respiratory systems can cause undernutrition, undernutrition can also negatively affect both the heart and lungs. Undernutrition causes loss of body tissue and whilst cardiac tissue is relatively spared during periods of starvation, nutritional depletion does lead to loss of lung tissue and reduction in

size and function of the muscles associated with breathing, such as the diaphragm. It is often difficult to establish the exact causality when it comes to undernutrition in these chronic wasting diseases, as it may develop over time due to the progressive nature of the diseases impacting on nutritional intake. Conversely, the presence of undernutrition may accelerate disease progression; for example, undernutrition leading to the wasting of respiratory muscles may impair the ability to expectorate, predisposing to increased frequency of infective exacerbations and further declines in nutritional status.

Whilst the aetiology of undernutrition in cardiopulmonary diseases is complex, its development in COPD and CHF shares several key similarities (Figure 5.6.1). Diseases involving the cardiopulmonary system often lead to undernutrition through a variety of mechanisms, centring on the impact symptoms have on an individual's ability to consume enough food to meet their nutritional requirements (dyspnoea, dryness of mouth, early satiety and abdominal discomfort, and fatigue). These symptoms can occur due to the disease itself, such as in COPD where hyperinflated lungs result in a flattening of the diaphragm and increased intrathoracic pressure, which can impact on gastric volume and feeling of satiety.

In addition, altered neuroendocrine and immunological processes have a significant effect on the balance between catabolism and anabolism, with elevated systemic inflammation contributing to anorexia and reduced functional capacity. It is this elevated inflammation that has been observed to increase energy expenditure at rest in both COPD and CHF patients. The energy demands of breathing are only about 2% of basal metabolic rate (BMR) in normal subjects, and the contribution of cardiac tissue to BMR is considerably higher [10]. However, in patients with respiratory disease, BMR may be elevated by 15–20%. Despite patients with COPD and CHF having elevated resting energy expenditures, total energy requirements may not be elevated and have been found to be reduced [11] with reduced physical activity more than accounting for any basal energy increase due to the disease. In patients with CHF and cachexia, total

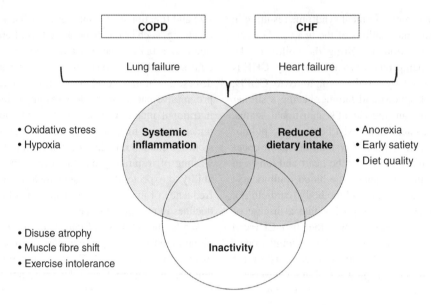

Figure 5.6.1 Disease-related undernutrition.

energy expenditure (TEE) has been found to be reduced by 10–20% compared to non-cachectic patients [12].

Therefore, whilst the aetiology of undernutrition in cardiopulmonary diseases is complex, it would appear that it is related predominantly to a reduction in dietary intake and ability to utilise nutrition appropriately rather than an inability to achieve elevated requirements. This has important implications for the methods, timing, composition and amount of nutrition support to provide to patients and is likely to be dependent on their stage of lung or heart disease and whether they are stable or acutely unwell.

5.6.3 Consequences of undernutrition

Along with increased mortality, undernutrition in COPD also presents both an economic and an operational burden to healthcare systems. Undernutrition has been found to be independently associated with a significant increase in hospitalisation rate, duration of hospital stay and subsequent healthcare costs [13]. With an increasing focus on reducing durations of hospital stay, only the sickest patients remain

hospitalised. Therefore, in order for nutrition support to be effective, malnourished patients need to be promptly identified on admission, nutrition support initiated and continued for an adequate duration of time, probably beyond the period of admission. Similar poor outcomes have been reported in heart failure patients at nutritional risk, with patients experiencing unintentional weight loss being 2.5 times more likely to experience a cardiac event and have poorer survival [14].

5.6.4 Nutritional assessment

The identification of nutritional depletion in COPD and CHF is complex and requires comprehensive assessment. Due to the wasting nature of the disease, simple methods of nutrition screening may lack the sensitivity to identify patients at risk. Also, acute bouts of illness seriously compromise nutritional intake, which might precede any demonstrable changes in physical status. Unfortunately, current national and international guidelines for the management of these patients fail to formally recommend routine nutritional assessment and intervention [1,15].

Whilst a body mass index (BMI) of <20 kg/m² has been found to be an independent predictor of mortality and hospitalisation in COPD [16], it has limitations in both COPD and CHF that are characterised by wasting. Assessment of BMI alone will not detect clinically relevant losses of lean body mass. Most nutritional screening tools include BMI as a component but the exact cut-off to use in order to identify nutritional risk in COPD is unclear; various cut-offs include <20 kg/m² (MUST), <21 kg/m² [17] and <23 kg/m² (MNA®). A cross-sectional survey of 300 outpatients with COPD found 17% of outpatients to have a BMI <20 kg/m² but more than double (38%) were found to have fat-free mass depletion [18]. In a recent audit of COPD patients hospitalised for an acute exacerbation at an Australian tertiary hospital, simple nutritional screening alone failed to identify a significant number of patients, compared to a full nutritional assessment using the Subjective Global Assessment (SGA), which included a physical assessment of the patients' muscle stores by a dietitian [19]. Probably the only reliable way to promptly identify those at nutritional risk with COPD or CHF is to use nutritional assessment tools such as the SGA [20] or Patient Generated Subjective Global Assessment (PG-SGA) as they attempt to assess the losses of fat and muscle stores [21].

5.6.5 Nutrition management

Chronic obstructive pulmonary disease

Traditionally, weight loss was viewed as a symptom of COPD, considered an inevitable outcome due to the irreversible and progressive nature of the disease, and as such not amenable to intervention. In addition, it was even argued that nutrition support might be detrimental with increased substrate, particularly carbohydrate, placing additional demands on the respiratory system. However, recent systematic reviews and meta-analyses have demonstrated that undernutrition is treatable in COPD, and nutrition support significantly improves nutritional intake. This improvement leads to improved nutritional

status [22] and improvements in functional capacity and quality of life [23]. In addition, dietary quality may also play a role in the progression of the disease; consumption of a diet higher in antioxidants has been associated with a slower decline in respiratory function [24].

Energy requirements for COPD patients should be assessed individually, taking into consideration activity levels and disease state. It is unlikely that COPD patients require energy intakes beyond those of age-matched controls. However, due to the wasting associated with COPD, ensuring adequate protein is of clinical importance. Recent recommendations suggest that in the healthy elderly, the diet should provide at least 1.0–1.2 g protein/kg/body weight/day. In malnourished elderly or those with chronic illness, the diet should provide at least 1.2–1.5 g protein/kg/body weight per day [25]. The therapeutic effect of such intakes remains to be established but these are appropriate nutrition intervention targets based on the best available evidence.

Recent systematic reviews and meta-analyses exploring the effectiveness of nutrition support in the treatment of undernutrition in stable (non-exacerbating) COPD patients included 13 randomised controlled trials (RCTs) (439 stable COPD outpatients) [22]. Meta-analysis showed that nutrition support resulted in a significant increase in energy intake above baseline (+318 SD 157 kcal/day) and a significant increase in weight (+1.83 SE 0.26 kg; P<0.001) [22]. The significant improvements in respiratory (inspiratory and expiratory muscle strength) and non-respiratory (handgrip/quadriceps) muscle strength were accompanied with a significant increase in body weight of more than 2 kg (2.1–3.1 kg) [23]. Therefore, a therapeutic target for nutrition support in COPD should be an increase in weight of at least 2 kg.

Individualised dietary counselling

Only one study to date has investigated the effectiveness of tailored dietary counselling in malnourished COPD outpatients [26]. The intervention involved individualised dietary counselling by a dietitian and the provision of milk powder for 6 months. The intervention group gained approximately 2 kg in weight and this was associated with significant improvements in quality of life.

This study highlighted several key points of clinical relevance. First, simply providing patients with education material was ineffective as the control group went on to lose over 2 kg in weight over the 12-month study period. Second, the intervention group that received a 6-month supply of milk powder along with individualised dietary counselling by a dietitian maintained their 2 kg weight gain 6 months after the intervention. This suggests lasting behaviour change is associated with counselling strategies, and the resulting benefits persist beyond the period of intervention. This work shows the combination of milk powder with dietary counselling is effective, but it is not possible to know how much each element of this intervention contributed to the effects.

Oral nutritional supplements

The majority of the RCTs included in the recent systematic reviews and meta-analyses (11 trials, 374 outpatients) provided nutrition support by oral nutritional supplements (ONS), with most using ready-made liquid ONS. Three of the RCTs used ONS specifically formulated for use in COPD, two with the predominance of energy provided from carbohydrate (60% energy) [27,28] and one predominantly from fat (55% energy) [29]. Interestingly, the RCT that used the fat-rich ONS did not result in improvements in weight but the two studies using the carbohydrate-rich ONS did. However, the two studies using carbohydrate-rich ONS were done as part of an exercise programme and therefore direct comparisons with the fat-rich ONS study are not possible.

Previously, there was a belief that providing additional energy in the form of fat would be preferable in COPD as the metabolism of fat produces less carbon dioxide than carbohydrate, placing less demand on the respiratory system. Whilst this may be the case in patients who are ventilated or have respiratory failure, in ambulatory patients the rate of gastric emptying

is likely to be more important. The rationale for a carbohydrate-rich ONS is that it leaves the stomach faster and therefore is less likely to impair respiratory mechanics and to promote satiety. Currently there is no evidence to suggest that disease-specific ONS are preferable to standard ONS and avoidance of overfeeding is likely to be more important.

Recently, there has been an increased use of low-volume energy- and protein-dense ONS in clinical practice but to date no intervention studies have specifically used these in COPD and CHF. However, given the symptomatic and functional barriers encountered by these patients, low-volume, high-energy and -protein ONS do appear to lend themselves well to this patient group.

A recent study in the US retrospectively investigated the use of ONS in COPD patients and found ONS were associated with significant reductions in length of hospital stay, hospitalisation costs and early readmission [30]. Whilst changes in nutritional status were not reported, a plausible mechanism behind these improvements is the use of ONS leading to an attenuation of weight loss during the acute phase where requirements for certain nutrients are elevated at a time of worsening nutrition impact symptoms [31]. However, there is a need for prospective nutrition intervention studies demonstrating the clinical and cost-effectiveness of nutrition support with *a priori* hypotheses linked to primary outcomes such as quality of life, functional capacity, healthcare use and mortality. There is also an urgent need for studies in the patient group to explore the impact of cessation of supplementation and long-term effectiveness.

Enhancement of exercise programmes with ONS

In addition to the strong evidence for nutrition support in stable outpatients, there is also good evidence demonstrating the effectiveness of nutrition support in exercising patients with COPD. Two RCTs involving nourished patients found that nutrition support with ONS resulted in significant increases in body weight and performance [27,28]. These findings suggest a potential role for nutrition support beyond the treatment of undernutrition. However, exercise training in COPD patients could precipitate a negative energy balance, negatively impacting on the response to rehabilitation. This is of particular importance in undernourished patients where accrual of lean body mass is the target and an adequate intake of energy and protein is required. In this instance nutrition support may be needed throughout the rehabilitation programme.

More recently, research has shown that exercise programmes in a cohort of chronic respiratory failure patients, including COPD, resulted in significant improvements when combined with nutritional supplementation with ONS and oral testosterone. Although the mean BMI of the cohort was 21.5 SD 3.8 kg/m², they went on to gain 3 kg in body weight, of which half was lean body mass. Subsequently, there were significant improvements in functional capacity and improved survival [32].

Chronic heart failure

There is currently no evidence available demonstrating the effectiveness of nutrition support in treating undernutrition in CHF. However, as nutrition support has been effective in similar wasting diseases, it would appear to be a prudent recommendation in routine clinical practice. Routine nutritional screening and assessment should identify those at risk and subsequent initiation of nutrition support will help improve nutritional intake. If a similar causal pathway exists in CHF, this will lead to improvements in nutritional status and subsequent improvements in functional capacity and quality of life [4]. With an increasingly ageing population, growing levels of heart disease and sedentary lifestyles, the incidence of cardiac cachexia is predicted to rise [33]. It is therefore likely that nutrition support will have an increasingly important role to play in the management of cardiology patients. As such, there is an urgent need for more research into the nutritional management of CHF and whether nutrition can enhance exercise programmes in these patients.

5.6.6 Future directions and conclusions

Whilst there is good evidence for the nutritional management of stable (non-exacerbating) patients with COPD, it is unlikely we have seen the true effectiveness of nutrition support. There is a lack of published research exploring multimodal nutrition support strategies that are individualised. Often nutrition regimens are standardised across the intervention group without tailoring the intervention to overcome a particular nutritional deficit and achieve a therapeutic target. In addition, the evidence is scarce when looking for effectiveness during acute periods of illness with elevated inflammatory processes. Comparisons can be drawn with cancer in this clinical situation, since many of the nutritional and metabolic abnormalities are common to COPD and CHF. Thus, as for cancer cachexia, future work should focus on exploring multimodal interventions specifically aiming to treat the key issues of reduced food intake, abnormal metabolism and wasting. It is now important for future research to establish the best management of these patients in terms of nutrition, exercise and anti-inflammatory treatment [34].

In conclusion, nutrition support is effective at treating undernutrition in COPD, resulting in improvements in functional capacity and quality of life. It also appears to be associated with reductions in healthcare use and costs. However, the current evidence base is almost entirely based on ONS and is lacking for other methods of nutrition support. It appears that the true effectiveness of nutrition support in the management of chronic wasting diseases such as COPD and CHF is yet to be realised and further large, prospective, multimodal nutrition interventions of adequate duration are required.

References

1. Global Initiative for Chronic Obstructive Lung Disease (GOLD). Global strategy for diagnosis, management, and prevention of chronic obstructive pulmonary disease. *Am J Respir Crit Care Med* 2017; **195**: 557–582.

2. National Collaborating Centre for Chronic Conditions. Chronic obstructive pulmonary disease. National clinical guideline on management of chronic obstructive pulmonary disease in adults in primary and secondary care. *Thorax* 2004; **59**(Suppl 1): 1–232.

3. Schols AM. The 2014 ESPEN Arvid Wretlind Lecture: metabolism and nutrition: shifting paradigms in COPD management. *Clin Nutr* 2015; **34**(6): 1074–1079.

4. Anker SD, John M, Pedersen PU, et al. ESPEN guidelines on enteral nutrition: cardiology and pulmonology. *Clin Nutr* 2006; **25**(2): 311–318.

5. Stratton RJ, Green CJ, Elia M. Disease-Related Malnutrition: An Evidence-Based Approach to Treatment. Wallingford: CABI, 2003.

6. Vermeeren MA, Schols AM, Wouters EF. Effects of an acute exacerbation on nutritional and metabolic profile of patients with COPD. *Eur Respir J* 1997; **10**(10): 2264–2269.

7. Ambrosy AP, Fonarow GC, Butler J, et al. The global health and economic burden of hospitalizations for heart failure: lessons learned from hospitalized heart failure registries. *J Am Coll Cardiol* 2014; **63**(12): 1123–1133.

8. Katz A, Katz P. Disease of the heart in the works of Hippocrates. *BJM* 1962; **24**(3): 257–264.

9. Anker SD, Ponikowski P, Varney S, et al. Wasting as independent risk factor for mortality in chronic heart failure. *Lancet* 1997; **349**(9058): 1050–1053.

10. Wang Z, Ying Z, Bosy-Westphal A, et al. Specific metabolic rates of major organs and tissues across adulthood: evaluation by mechanistic model of resting energy expenditure. *Am J Clin Nutr* 2010; **92**(6): 1369–1377.

11. Tang NL, Chung ML, Elia M, et al. Total daily energy expenditure in wasted chronic obstructive pulmonary disease patients. *Eur J Clin Nutr* 2002; **56**(4): 282–287.

12. Toth MJ, Gottlieb SS, Goran MI, et al. Daily energy expenditure in free-living heart failure patients. *Am J Physiol* 1997; **272**(3 Pt 1): E469–475.

13. Hoong JM, Ferguson M, Hukins C, et al. Economic and operational burden associated with malnutrition in chronic obstructive pulmonary disease. *Clin Nutr* 2017; **36**(4): 1105–1109.

14. Song EK, Lee Y, Moser DK, et al. The link of unintentional weight loss to cardiac event-free survival in patients with heart failure. *J Cardiovasc Nurs* 2014; **29**(5): 439–447.

15. National Institute for Health and Care Excellence. Chronic Obstructive Pulmonary Disease in Over 16s: Diagnosis and Management (CG101). London: NICE, 2010. p. 62.

16. Chailleux E, Laaban JP, Veale D. Prognostic value of nutritional depletion in patients with COPD treated by long-term oxygen therapy: data from the ANTADIR observatory. *Chest* 2003; **123**(5): 1460–1466.

17. Celli BR, Cote CG, Marin JM, et al. The body-mass index, airflow obstruction, dyspnea, and exercise capacity index in chronic obstructive pulmonary disease. *N Engl J Med* 2004; **350**(10): 1005–1012.

18. Cano NJ, Roth H, Cynober L, et al., Nutritional depletion in patients on long-term oxygen therapy and/or home mechanical ventilation. *Eur Respir J* 2002; **20**(1): 30–37.

19. Stonestreet J, Masel PJ, Yang I, et al. Complexity of nutrition screening in patients admitted with an exacerbation of chronic obstructive pulmonary disease (COPD). *Respirology* 2015; **20**(2): 103.

20. Detsky AS, McLaughlin JR, Baker JP, et al. What is subjective global assessment of nutritional status? *J Parenter Enteral Nutr* 1987; **11**(1): 8–13.

21. Bauer JM, Egan E, Clavarino A. The scored patient-generated subjective global assessment is an effective nutrition assessment tool in subjects with chronic obstructive pulmonary disease. *e-SPEN* 2011; **6**(1): e27–e30.

22. Collins PF, Stratton RJ, Elia M. Nutritional support in chronic obstructive pulmonary disease: a systematic review and meta-analysis. *Am J Clin Nutr* 2012; **95**(6): 1385–1395.

23. Collins PF, Elia M, Stratton RJ. Nutritional support and functional capacity in chronic obstructive pulmonary disease: a systematic review and meta-analysis. *Respirology* 2013; **18**(4): 616–629.

24. Keranis E, Makris D, Rodopoulou P, et al. Impact of dietary shift to higher-antioxidant foods in COPD: a randomised trial. *Eur Respir J* 2010; **36**(4): 774–780.

25. Deutz NE, Bauer JM, Barazzoni R, et al. Protein intake and exercise for optimal muscle function with aging: recommendations from the ESPEN Expert Group. *Clin Nutr* 2014; **33**(6): 929–936.

26. Weekes CE, Emery PW, Elia M. Dietary counselling and food fortification in stable COPD: a randomised trial. *Thorax* 2009; **64**(4): 326–331.

27. Steiner MC, Barton R, Singh S, et al. Nutritional enhancement of exercise performance in chronic obstructive pulmonary disease: a randomised controlled trial. *Thorax* 2003; **58**(9): 745–751.

28. Schols AM, Soeters PB, Mostert R, et al. Physiologic effects of nutritional support and anabolic steroids in patients with chronic obstructive pulmonary disease. A placebo-controlled randomized trial. *Am J Respir Crit Care Med* 1995; **152**(4 Pt 1): 1268–1274.

29. DeLetter M. A Nutritional Intervention for Persons with Chronic Airflow Limitation. Kentucky: University of Kentucky, 1991.

30. Snider JT, Jena AB, Linthicum MT, et al. Effect of hospital use of oral nutritional supplementation on length of stay, hospital cost, and 30-day readmissions

among Medicare patients with COPD. *Chest* 2015; **147**(6): 1477–1484.

31. Saudny-Unterberger H, Martin JG, Gray-Donald K. Impact of nutritional support on functional status during an acute exacerbation of chronic obstructive pulmonary disease. *Am J Respir Crit Care Med* 1997; **156**(3 Pt 1): 794–799.

32. Pison CM, Cano NJ, Caron F, et al. Multimodal nutritional rehabilitation improves clinical outcomes of malnourished patients with chronic respiratory failure: a randomised controlled trial. *Thorax* 2011; **66**(11): 953–960.

33. Von Haehling S, Anker SD. Prevalence, incidence and clinical impact of cachexia: facts and numbers-update 2014. *J Cachexia Sarcopenia Muscle* 2014; **5**(4): 261–263.

34. Fearon KC. The 2011 ESPEN Arvid Wretlind lecture: cancer cachexia: the potential impact of translational research on patient-focused outcomes. *Clin Nutr* 2012; **31**(5): 577–582.

Chapter 5.7

Nutrition support in diabetes

Kevin Whelan[1] and Hilary McCoubrey[2]

[1]Department of Nutritional Sciences, King's College London, London, UK
[2]Birmingham Women's and Children's Hospital NHS Foundation Trust, Birmingham, UK

5.7.1 Introduction

People with diabetes, in particular type 2 diabetes, make up a disproportionately high percentage of hospital inpatients in many countries, including both the United States and the United Kingdom [1]. Currently, in the UK one in six hospitalised in-patients has diabetes [2]. This is unsurprising given that people with diabetes have an increased risk of disorders such as coronary artery disease, stroke, peripheral artery disease, chronic kidney disease, neuropathy and lower extremity infection, ulceration and amputation. Common causes of diabetes-related emergency admissions include diabetic ketoacidosis, hyperosmotic hyperglycaemic state and hypoglycaemia, but the UK National Diabetes Inpatient Audit (NaDIA) suggests that the majority of admissions in people with diabetes are not directly related to their diabetes but instead for other medical or surgical reasons [2].

Dietetic intervention is an essential component in the management of patient with diabetes requiring nutrition support. However, central to the management of nutrition support in diabetes is appropriate blood glucose management and the co-ordination of drug and insulin therapy, where necessary. The aims of inpatient dietetic care for patients with diabetes are to optimise glycaemic control, provide adequate nutrition to meet requirements, address individual needs and preferences, and provide a discharge plan for ongoing care [3,4]. This chapter explores the evidence for monitoring glycaemia, preventing and treating hyperglycaemia in hospitalised patients with diabetes and the challenges of treating or preventing undernutrition through nutrition support in this context.

5.7.2 Hyperglycaemia in hospitalised patients with diabetes

Hyperglycaemia is associated with an increased risk of adverse clinical outcomes in hospitalised patients with diabetes, including delayed healing of surgical wounds, foot ulcers and pressure sores [5]. Furthermore, patients with unstable blood glucose concentrations are likely to experience delayed discharge as it takes time to ensure safety at home in this potentially vulnerable population.

The mechanisms of hyperglycaemia in the hospitalised patient with diabetes are multifactorial. Infection and physical trauma including burns, surgery or stroke initiate a stress response that increase the production of proinflammatory cytokines and counterregulatory hormones, which in turn increase glucose production through gluconeogenesis and decrease cellular glucose uptake, resulting in hyperglycaemia [6]. The introduction of new medications, such as corticosteroids (which inhibit glucose uptake and thus significantly augment postprandial glycaemia), can also increase blood glucose concentrations in both diabetic and non-diabetic hospitalised patients [7]. This is often frustrating

Advanced Nutrition and Dietetics in Nutrition Support, First Edition. Edited by Mary Hickson and Sara Smith.
© 2018 John Wiley & Sons Ltd. Published 2018 by John Wiley & Sons Ltd.

for those with diabetes who previously had good glycaemic control and these patients are likely to need frequent monitoring and advice about dietary and medication changes.

Assessment and monitoring of glycaemia in diabetes

Optimising blood glucose concentrations can shorten recovery times in hospitalised patients [7]. In the UK, national initiatives such as 'Think Glucose' have highlighted the importance of improving the management of inpatients with diabetes, and offer a structured programme with resources to improve quality of care [8]. In patients in the intensive care unit, strict glycaemic control can be relatively easily achieved because more frequent blood glucose monitoring and insulin adjustment takes place.

There is controversy surrounding optimal blood glucose concentration targets for inpatients with diabetes. The key study from the University of Leuvan reported that blood glucose concentrations below 6.7 mmol/L (110 mg/dL) reduced hospital mortality by 34% in patients with diabetes [9]. However, a review of subsequent evidence suggests that general hospitalised patients do not benefit from very tight glycaemic control and that random blood glucose concentrations should be maintained only at <10 mmol/L (180 mg/dL) [7]. A Cochrane review of glycaemic control for prevention of surgical site infections recommended blood glucose concentrations <11 mmol/L (<200 mg/dL), concluding that there was insufficient evidence for strict glycaemic control compared with conventional management [10].

In terms of guidelines, the NaDIA defined acceptable glycaemic control as blood glucose concentrations 4–11 mmol/L [2]. However, the Joint British Diabetes Society (JBDS) guidelines state that evidence for target ranges is weak but expert opinion suggests targets of 6–12 mmol/L specifically during enteral nutrition in stroke patients with diabetes [11]. Therefore, although there is no consensus on exact targets from various research studies and guidelines, it is agreed that a strategy to avoid extremely high or low

blood glucose concentrations is important, and blood glucose targets should be individualised.

Medications for maintaining normoglycaemia

It is important to monitor renal function in hospitalised patients with diabetes as impaired glomerular filtration can reduce the clearance, and therefore increase circulation, of oral antihyperglycaemic agents and insulin. Liaison with the diabetes specialist team to monitor medication prescription is important under these circumstances. However, the American Association of Clinical Endocrinologists recommends that during acute illness, oral antihyperglycaemic agents should be switched to insulin, partly due to the slow onset of action and dissipation of oral medications and partly due to unsuitability in a number of acutely unwell groups [12].

Principles are very similar to those used in the DAFNE approach (Dose Adjustment for Normal Eating), which is widely utilised in Europe and Australia for those with type 1 diabetes. It recommends glucose monitoring before meals and at bedtime and suggests the calculation of a sensitivity or correction factor. This can be reached by the equation: 100/total daily dose of insulin and calculates the predicted mmol/L decrease in blood glucose concentration from administering one unit of insulin. Dietitians are well placed to support the multidisciplinary team (MDT) in providing correct information about insulin administration with appropriate carbohydrate intake, especially where the latter has been altered due to oral nutritional supplements (ONS), enteral or parenteral nutrition. In addition, advice regarding delaying insulin injections may be required in patients with reduced gastric emptying, such as those with gastroparesis.

Basal bolus insulin regimens

Basal bolus insulin regimens (rapid acting and background insulin) are superior to variable-rate intravenous insulin infusion (VRIII) for patients with oral intake, in terms of the numbers of patients reaching target blood glucose concentrations [13]. Basal bolus insulin regimens are also generally preferred to intravenous insulin for patients consuming food orally or via enteral nutrition, as they lessen the risk of hypoglycaemia. It has been recommended that basal bolus regimens based on 0.4–0.5 units of background insulin/kg/day combined with rapid-acting insulin with meals may provide improved glycaemic control compared with a VRIII approach [7].

Variable-rate intravenous insulin infusion

Variable-rate intravenous insulin infusion (formerly known as sliding scale insulin) is generally used perioperatively for patients receiving insulin and sometimes for those on oral antihyperglycaemic agents. VRIII requires regular blood glucose monitoring (usually 2–4 hourly) and adjusting the insulin dose given intravenously via a dedicated cannula, usually together with a glucose infusion [13]. Discontinuation of VRIII needs cautious management. As a patient's clinical condition improves, there may be decreased illness-related or surgery-related stress affecting glycaemia (thus reducing basal insulin requirements), at the same time as increased appetite will increase food intake (and thus the need for rapid-acting insulin).

5.7.3 Undernutrition in diabetes

Protein-energy undernutrition in hospitalised patients can be caused by increased nutrient requirements, increased losses or reduced intake, and can result in slower recovery, increased length of hospital stay and increased readmission, morbidity and mortality.

Obesity is a common precursor to type 2 diabetes (due to its impact on insulin resistance) and as a result, undernutrition can sometimes be overlooked. In fact, undernutrition has been shown to be prevalent in hospitalised patients with type 2 diabetes, especially in older adults. For example, one study in 146 consecutive patients with diabetes admitted to an older care hospital service administered detailed nutritional assessment [14]. Although mean BMI was in the overweight range (29.6 kg/m^2),

77.1% were at risk of 'possible undernutrition' following nutritional screening (≤11 on mini-nutritional assessment–short form), of whom 13.9% were diagnosed with undernutrition and 75.0% at risk of undernutrition following a full nutritional assessment [14]. Undernutrition is therefore highly prevalent in older hospitalised patients with diabetes and, paradoxically, may be associated with improved glycaemic control (HbA1c) [14].

In line with recommendations from clinical nutrition associations across the world, screening for undernutrition should be undertaken in all patients admitted to hospital, including those with obesity or diabetes, and where a risk of undernutrition is detected, a full and detailed nutritional assessment should be undertaken by a health professional with expertise in clinical nutrition, such as a dietitian, followed by appropriate nutrition intervention including oral, enteral and parenteral nutrition support as appropriate.

5.7.4 Oral nutrition support in diabetes

Hospital food service for diabetes

There is no consensus on the ideal meal plan for hospitalised patients with diabetes. Bantle et al. recommend consistent carbohydrate load across main meals and snacks but there is a lack of controlled trial evidence to demonstrate the clinical benefit of such an approach [15]. The American Association of Clinical Endocrinologists guidelines also recommend a consistent carbohydrate intake in hospitalised patients to optimise glucose control [12]. Such approaches require liaison with catering services and detailed information regarding the carbohydrate content of meals and snacks. Information regarding the type and quantity of carbohydrate in food should be available from hospital food services, and nutritional data regarding ONS, enteral formulas and parenteral nutrition are available from the manufacturers.

Complaints about meal choice and timings are common patient concerns. Amongst other areas, the NaDIA reported that only a marginal majority of patients considered the choice (54.4%) and timing of meals (63.4%) to be 'always' or 'almost always' suitable [2]. The Diabetes Inpatient Treatment Satisfaction study also investigated this area, and although its findings were similar, it did not gather qualitative information useful for shaping improvements in hospital food provision [16]. Food choices and flexibility for hospitalised patients are sometimes limited because food preparation may be off-site, with many hospitals purchasing off-site, ready-made meals.

Hospital meal provision usually aims to ensure adequate energy and macronutrient intake through a combination of main meal, dessert and sweet snacks (e.g. biscuits and cakes). Fats such as butter and cream are useful for energy fortification. These food choices do not necessarily match the advice given to people with diabetes in the outpatient setting. However, increased energy requirements relating to underlying illness, the prevalence of undernutrition and its associated complications, and potential taste preferences for sweet foods (e.g. in uraemic patients) mean that patients with diabetes should not be denied foods that would not traditionally be considered suitable while they are acutely unwell, as long as these do not induce hyperglycaemia. Working with the patient and the multidisciplinary team to re-educate on dietary recommendations in an inpatient setting is crucial to ensure food choices are not excessively restrictive and that medication changes are made when necessary to accommodate hospital food choices.

Oral nutrition supplements in diabetes

The majority of ONS contain carbohydrate in varying dose and form (e.g. disaccharides, polysaccharides). It is generally accepted that carbohydrates are absorbed more slowly when accompanied by fibre, protein and fat, due to delayed gastric emptying. Those ONS that are higher in protein or fibre, in theory, should affect blood glucose concentrations more gradually. However, there are no readily available data regarding the glycaemic index (GI) of all ONS.

Oral nutritional supplements with higher total carbohydrate content but low fibre, protein and fat, such as some juice-based ONS, are likely to have the greatest impact on blood glucose concentrations and should ideally be used in diabetes only as a last resort, or as suitable treatment for hypoglycaemia. If milk-based ONS are disliked, patients may consume higher carbohydrate ONS but in smaller doses.

Some ONS have been developed specifically for people with diabetes and such diabetes-specific ONS (DS-ONS) are available in some countries, although not globally. They vary in composition depending upon the manufacturer, but often contain lower doses of carbohydrate (which is replaced by fat) and by switching carbohydrates to those with lower glycaemic index. A systematic review, albeit published in 2005, at that time identified 16 controlled trials of DS-ONS with varying results and will be discussed below under Diabetes-specific enteral formulas [17].

Finally, in the absence of DS-ONS, various modular supplements (e.g. fat supplements, protein powders) are available in liquid and powder forms. These can be used as ONS or to fortify foods in order to reduce the carbohydrate intake associated with oral nutrition support. However, such modular supplements are not nutritionally complete in terms of micronutrients and the use of multivitamin and mineral tablets should be considered.

5.7.5 Enteral nutrition in diabetes

Monitoring and controlling glycaemia during enteral nutrition

Providing enteral nutrition to prevent or treat undernutrition in people with diabetes whilst maintaining glycaemic control can be challenging. It is important to calculate optimal enteral nutrition delivery regimes, including the volume and type of formula, the duration of feeding periods and rest periods and importantly to calculate the hourly dose of carbohydrate delivered by the formula.

Approaches to maintaining normoglycaemia include modifying the dose of carbohydrate (e.g. switching between formulas of varying carbohydrate content) or the rate of carbohydrate delivery (e.g. shortening or extending the duration of feeding). However, the evidence for success of these approaches is limited. Factors to be considered include the patient's individual nutritional requirements, suitability and tolerance of night-time enteral nutrition and the need for breaks in feeding for procedures or other events. The dietitian should work with the diabetes specialist team, particularly if hyperglycaemia occurs during feeding, and should advise the wider MDT on aspects of care such as prevention and treatment of hypoglycaemia and hyperglycaemia and the frequency of blood glucose monitoring.

The JBDS report is an important reference document outlining the roles and responsibilities of the MDT in ensuring that standards of care are being met at ward level during enteral nutrition [11]. In particular, great care should be taken in relation to monitoring blood glucose, use of medication and managing hypoglycaemia during enteral nutrition.

Blood glucose monitoring should take place at least every 4–6 hours while enteral nutrition is being delivered or hourly if feeding is unexpectedly stopped. However, recommendations for the timing and frequency of blood glucose monitoring vary depending on the delivery approach (continuous, intermittent, etc.) and

recommendations have been made specifically for patients with diabetes following stroke (Box 5.7.1) [11]. Dietetic reviews represent an ideal opportunity to monitor that these standards are being met.

Dehydration is an often overlooked cause of hyperglycaemia. Hydration status should therefore be routinely monitored and appropriate water flushes provided to maintain hydration during enteral nutrition.

Dietitians should be aware of appropriate medication regimes suited to different feeding rates and timings. Metformin powder is highlighted in the JBDS guidelines as being suitable for nasogastric administration, whereas other forms of oral medications in a crushed form are not recommended [11]. Different insulin regimens are detailed with a biphasic regimen of mixed insulin being used with continuous enteral nutrition, or basal bolus insulin regimes with short-acting insulin given at 6-hourly intervals. Where patients are receiving enteral nutrition as bolus feeds (e.g. in discrete 200 mL doses), the report suggests that rapid-acting insulin be administered as part of a basal bolus regime 20 minutes prior to the bolus of enteral nutrition (due to the rapid digestion and absorption of the nutrients in enteral formulas). Some guidance on insulin to carbohydrate ratios is provided depending on insulin sensitivity levels and usual total daily doses [11].

Box 5.7.1 Recommended frequency of bedside glucose monitoring in patients with diabetes who are receiving enteral nutrition following a stroke

- The frequency of bedside capillary blood glucose testing should be a clinical decision based on the stability of the patient, but as a general rule monitor blood glucose at least 4–6 hourly, both when feeding and during rest periods.
- There are specific recommendations depending upon whether enteral nutrition is continuous, intermittent or bolus.
  - If a patient is receiving continuous enteral nutrition and subcutaneous insulin, monitor blood glucose prior to initiating feeding and then 4–6 hourly.
  - If a patient is receiving intermittent enteral nutrition, monitor blood glucose prior to initiating feeding, 4–6 hourly during feeding, and 2 hourly post feeding.
  - If a patient is receiving bolus-only enteral nutrition, monitor blood glucose prior to the bolus of enteral nutrition, 2 hourly following the bolus and 4–6 hourly during prolonged intervals between feeding.
- If the patient is receiving variable-rate intravenous insulin infusion, monitor blood glucose hourly.
- Beware of the risk of hypoglycaemia during the 'fasting' period between feeding.
- Beware of hypoglycaemia as a cause of drowsiness in patients with stroke.

Source: Adapted from the Joint British Diabetes Societies for Inpatient Care [11].

The JBDS report highlights the risk of hypoglycaemia where insulin has been administered and enteral nutrition is then unexpectedly stopped (e.g. transfer to another unit, fasting for tests) [11]. Under these circumstances, the delivery of intravenous glucose is recommended to temporarily substitute enteral nutrition, but only where there is no alternative to stopping feeding. In patients with dysphagia, the treatment of hypoglycaemia involves administration of glucose-based liquids via the feeding tube or glucose gels and a water flush, to provide 15–20 g of rapidly absorbed carbohydrate followed by 15–20 g of carbohydrate from the enteral formula.

Diabetes-specific enteral formulas

Diabetes-specific enteral formulas (DS-EF) have been developed for use in enteral nutrition. Standard formulas are rich in complex carbohydrate (45–60%) with low lipid content (e.g. 30%). In contrast, many DS-EF reduce the carbohydrate content (e.g. 35–40% energy) and replace with fats (total fat 40–50% of energy), in particular monounsaturated fatty acids. Some DS-EF also modify the carbohydrate

source to focus on lower glycaemic index carbohydrates and some also include dietary fibre [18]. The decreased carbohydrate and increased fibre are thought to improve glycaemic control by delaying gastric emptying and decreasing the availability and rate of carbohydrate absorption.

Numerous studies of variable quality have investigated the effectiveness of DS-EF in comparison with standard enteral formulas. Many of these studies were included in a systematic review of both DS-ONS (16 trials) and DS-EF (6 trials) (Table 5.7.1) [17]. A meta-analysis synthesised results of both types of studies comparing DS-ONS/DS-EF in comparison with standard formulas. On average, DS-ONS/DS-EF reduced postformula blood glucose by 1.03 mmol/L, peak blood glucose by 1.59 mmol/L and glucose area under the curve by 7.96 mmol/L/min, that is, by 35% (see Table 5.7.1). Some studies demonstrated improved lipid profiles, although this was not consistently found in the meta-analysis [17].

However, the studies in this systematic review are difficult to synthesise due to variations in study design, the quantity and composition of the DS-ONS/DS-EF and the comparators used.

Table 5.7.1 Data from a meta-analysis of diabetes-specific formulas (DS-EF) versus standard formulas on glycaemic outcomes. Data represent the favourable effect of DS-EF over standard formulas, where they exist

Outcome	Number of RCTs	Total trial sizes (n)	Standardised mean difference (effect size)	Physiological difference, mean (95% CI)
Postprandial rise in blood glucose				
All studies	7	202	−0.52 (−0.81 to −0.24)	−1.03 mmol/L (−1.47 to −0.58)
Short-term studies only (<24 hours)	4	73	−0.71 (−1.14 to −0.27)	−1.18 mmol/L (−1.73 to −0.64)
Longer term studies only (5 d to 3 m)	3	129	−0.38 (−0.76 to −0.00)	−0.69 mmol/L (−1.49 to 0.10)
Peak blood glucose	2	22	−1.28 (−1.94 to −0.63)	−1.59 mmol/L (−2.32 to −0.86)
Glucose area under the curve	4	38	−1.19 (−1.69 to −0.7)	−7.98 mmol/L/min (−13.66 to −2.25)
Fasting blood glucose	2	68	−0.35 (−0.86 to 0.17)	Data not available

Source: Data taken from Elia et al. [17] with permission from the American Diabetes Association.
CI, confidence interval; RCT, randomised controlled trial.

In addition, the studies were all published prior to 2005, and numerous studies have been published since, and many were limited by their focus on short-term postformula response (rather than long-term glycaemic control).

Regarding longer term studies, a RCT of 105 patients with elevated HbA1c or fasting blood glucose at baseline compared a DS-EF to standard enteral formula for up to 84 days. Of the 55 patients who completed the study (analysed per protocol), there was a significantly greater reduction in total insulin requirements and fasting glucose in the DS-EF group compared with standard formula, although there was no difference in HbA1c [19].

A number of clinical guidelines have addressed the use of DS-EF in practice. ESPEN have reviewed the evidence and conclude that more evidence for clinical outcome benefits is needed to justify the additional economic cost of DS-EF [20]. The JBDS report also does not consider there to be sufficient evidence to recommend the use of DS-EF in the UK [11]. From a practical perspective, DS-EF may be of more importance outside the intensive care setting where less frequent blood glucose monitoring is carried out.

5.7.6 Parenteral nutrition in diabetes

Current guidelines do not make recommendations for management of patients with diabetes requiring parenteral nutrition (PN). Patients receiving exclusive PN have substantially higher insulin requirements to achieve the same blood glucose targets compared with those receiving enteral nutrition [21]. Nutrients enter the systemic circulation directly, thus bypassing the splanchnic circulation and the insulinotrophic effect of incretins. Thus, PN can commonly lead to hyperglycaemia, even in the absence of diabetes. Up to 75% of patients with type 2 diabetes who have not been previously treated with insulin may require insulin during PN.

Studies have shown that PN-associated hyperglycaemia is a risk factor for development of infection, cardiac and renal dysfunction and increased mortality in critically ill and non-critically ill patients [22]. For example, blood glucose concentrations of >10 mmol/L within 24 hours of initiation of PN have been associated with a greater possibility of mortality (odds ratio (OR) 2.80) [21]. It is hypothesised that immune function and inflammatory response may be the underlying mechanisms.

Guidelines from the American Association of Clinical Endocrinologists recommend 0.1 unit of insulin for every gram of carbohydrate administered, with daily increases of 80% of the previous day's correctional insulin. Intravenous insulin can be used to correct hyperglycaemia more rapidly [12]. Cyclical rather than continuous PN has been considered by some to allow insulin concentrations to drop, helping to prevent further insulin resistance. In addition, it may be possible to manipulate proportions of fat, protein and carbohydrate in PN infusions in order to reduce the impact on blood glucose concentrations.

5.7.7 Conclusion

The increasing population of people with diabetes, and its associated complications, mean that many patients requiring nutrition support will also have diabetes. Dietitians, doctors and nurses working in all areas need to have a good understanding of the guidelines for inpatients with diabetes and how these specifically apply to those receiving oral, enteral or parenteral nutrition support. Optimising blood glucose control during the delivery of appropriate nutrition support is beneficial in terms of wide range of clinical outcomes.

References

1. Jiang HJ, Stryer D, Friedman B, et al. Multiple hospitalisations for patients with diabetes. *Diabetes Care* 2003; **26**(5): 1421–1426.
2. NHS Digital 2017. National Diabetes Inpatient Audit. http://content.digital.nhs.uk/searchcatalogue?product id=24617 (accessed 4 September 2017).
3. American Diabetes Association. Standards of medical care in diabetes – 2011. *Diabetes Care* 2011; **34**(Suppl 1): S11–61.

4. Clement S, Braithwaite SS, Magee MF, et al. Management of diabetes and hyperglycaemia in hospitals. *Diabetes Care* 2004; **27**: 553–591.

5. Gosmanov AR, Umpierrez GE. Medical nutrition therapy in hospitalised patients with diabetes. *Curr Diab Rep* 2012; **12**(1): 93–100.

6. McDonnell ME, Umpierrez MD. Insulin therapy for the management of hyperglycaemia in hospitalised patients. *Endocrinol Metab Clin North Am* 2012; **41**(1): 175–201.

7. Sawin G, Shaughnessy AF. Glucose control in hospitalized patients. *Am Fam Physician* 2010; **81**(9): 1078–1080.

8. NHS Institution for Innovation and Improvement. Diabetes Inpatient Care: Think Glucose Programme. https://arms.evidence.nhs.uk/resources/qipp/1008647/attachment (accessed 4 September 2017).

9. Van den Berghe G, Wouters P, Weekers F, et al. Intensive insulin therapy in the critically ill patient. *N Engl J Med* 2001; **345**(19): 1359–1367.

10. Kao LS, Meeks D, Moyer VA, Lally KP. Perioperative glycaemic control regimens for preventing surgical site infections in adults. *Cochrane Database Sys Rev* 2009; **3**: CD006806.

11. Joint British Diabetes Societies (JBDS). Glycaemic management during the inpatient enteral feeding of stroke patients with diabetes. www.diabetes.org.uk/Documents/Position%20statements/JBDS-IP-Enteral-Feeding-Stroke.pdf (accessed 4 September 2017).

12. American Association of Clinical Endocrinologists and American Diabetes Association. Consensus statement on inpatient glycemic control. *Diabetes Care* 2009; **32**(6): 353–369.

13. Umpierrez GE, Palacio A, Smiley D. Sliding scale insulin use: myth or insanity? *Am J Med* 2007; **120**(7): 563–567.

14. Vischer UM, Perrenoud L, Genet C, Ardigo S, Registe-Rameau Y, Herrmann FR. The high prevalence of malnutrition in elderly diabetic patients: implications for anti-diabetic drug treatments. *Diabet Med* 2010; **27**(8): 918–924.

15. Bantle JP, Wylie-Rosett J, Albright AL, et al. Nutrition recommendations and interventions for diabetes: a position statement of the American Diabetes Association. *Diabetes Care* 2008; **31**(Suppl 1): S61–78.

16. Rutter CL, Jones C, Dhatariya KK, James J, Irvine L, Wilson EC, Singh H, Walden E, Holland R, Harvey I, Bradley C, Sampson MJ. Determining in-patient diabetes treatment satisfaction in the UK – the DIPSat study. *Diabet Med* 2013; **30**(6): 731–738.

17. Elia M, Ceriello A, Laube H, et al. Enteral nutrition support and use of diabetes-specific formulas for patients with diabetes: a systematic review and meta-analysis. *Diabetes Care* 2005; **28**: 2267–2279.

18. Via MA, Mechanick JI. Inpatient enteral and parenteral nutrition for patients with diabetes. *Curr Diab Rep* 2010; **11**: 99–105.

19. Pohl M, Mayr P, Mertl-Roetzer M, Lauster F, Haslbeck M, Hipper B, Steube D, Tietjen M, Eriksen J, Rahlfs VW. Glycemic control in patients with type 2 diabetes mellitus with a disease-specific enteral formula: stage II of a randomized, controlled multicenter trial. *J Parenter Enteral Nutr* 2009; **33**(1): 37–49.

20. Lochs H, Allison SP, Meier R, et al. Introductory to the ESPEN guidelines on enteral nutrition: terminology, definitions and general topics. *Clin Nutr* 2006; **25**: 180–186.

21. Pasquel FJ, Spiegelman R, McCauley M, et al. Hyperglycemia during total parenteral nutrition. An important marker of poor outcome and mortality in hospitalized patients. *Diabetes Care* 2010; **3**(4): 739–741.

22. McMahon M, Manji N, Driscoll D, Bistrian B. Parenteral nutrition in patients with diabetes mellitus: theoretical and practical considerations. *J Parenter Enteral Nutr* 1989; **13**(5): 461–464.

Chapter 5.8

Nutrition support in pancreatitis

Sinead N. Duggan[1] and Kevin Conlon[2]

[1]Trinity College Dublin, Dublin, Ireland
[2]Trinity College Dublin and St Vincent's University Hospital, Dublin, Ireland

5.8.1 Acute pancreatitis

Acute pancreatitis (AP) is an acute inflammatory process of the pancreas that frequently involves peripancreatic tissue and/or remote organ systems. The 2012 Atlanta Classification [1] defines AP as two of the following three features: abdominal pain consistent with AP, serum lipase/amylase above upper level of normal, characteristic features on imaging. In mild AP there is no organ failure or systemic complications. In moderately severe AP there is transient organ failure, or local systemic complications, without persistent organ failure [1]. Local complications include necrosis, acute fluid collections, pancreatic abscess and pseudocysts. In severe AP there is persistent single or multiple organ failure and a high mortality rate (36–50%) [1]. The two most common aetiological factors are gallstone disease and alcohol excess, together accounting for >80% of all cases. Other causes include metabolic abnormalities (e.g. hypertriacylglyceridaemia), duct obstruction (e.g. pancreas divisum), medications and trauma. Up to 20% of cases are classed as idiopathic. The incidence of AP is rising [2,3], most likely due to an increase in alcohol abuse.

Nutritional screening and assessment

As with other hospitalised patient groups, patients should undergo nutritional screening to identify those at nutritional risk and require a formal detailed nutrition assessment [4].

Nutritional requirements

Due to the systemic inflammatory response syndrome (SIRS), energy requirements will be increased in severe AP. Energy requirements of 15–25 kcal/g are recommended in early stages of complicated disease, and 25–35 kcal/kg in the recovery phase. Protein requirements are reported to be in the region of 1–1.5 g/kg/day [5,6].

Nutrition intervention in acute pancreatitis

The severity of disease informs nutrition intervention, but early prediction is difficult and often inaccurate. Commonly used scoring systems include the Glasgow-Imrie score (≥3 predictive of severe disease) and the Acute Physiological and Chronic Health Evaluation (APACHE) II score (≥8 predictive of severe disease). Single serum markers (C-reactive protein (CRP), amylase/lipase) may also guide management, with CRP reportedly being among the most useful (>150 mg/L predictive of severe disease) [7,8].

In patients with mild AP, oral diet is usually recommended within 3–7 days following a period of fasting. Nutrition support is not normally required, but a randomised controlled trial (RCT) which compared fasting and nasogastric (NG) enteral nutrition found that the latter may result in reduced abdominal pain and better food tolerance in mild-to-moderate AP [9]. Clinical judgement should be exercised where there is pre-existing undernutrition or prolonged fasting (>5 days).

In patients with severe AP, nutrition support is considered essential [10]. Parenteral nutrition (PN) was once recommended for 'pancreatic rest', but this concept is outdated and studies have demonstrated that enteral nutrition (EN) is safe and efficacious and is the preferred feeding mode [11]. Compared to PN, EN may maintain GI tract integrity, reduce intestinal permeability and downregulate the systemic immune response, thereby affecting clinical outcomes in severe AP.

Where feeding is indicated (in severe AP, complicated disease or prior to surgery), early EN is recommended, ideally as soon as fluid resuscitation is complete, or in <48 hours. EN via the NG route may be trialled if tolerated, and NG tubes are easily inserted by the bedside, conferring an obvious benefit over postpyloric tubes. Studies have suggested that NG feeding could be considered the first-line approach for patients with severe and critical AP [12–14]. If pain persists or augments with NG EN, consideration should be given to nasojejunal (NJ) EN, with placement of the tube tip 40–60 cm beyond the ligament of Treitz. Distal placement of the feeding tube results in less pancreatic stimulation [15]. Many studies on feeding in AP utilised the NJ route and therefore this route is known to be safe and effective [7]. NJ tubes may be inserted endoscopically or radiologically. Bedside insertion may also be employed by nurses and dietitians as well as doctors [16]. As most studies involved the use of peptide-based formulas, these are known to be safe [17]. However, standard formulas may be tolerated [18] but further research is required.

Pseudocysts and other complications are not contraindications to EN and the enteral route should be tried first. A meta-analysis of five RCTs has shown that PN may result in fewer gastrointestinal complications such as diarrhoea (odds ratio (OR) 0.20, 95% confidence interval (CI) 0.09–0.43) but greater episodes of hyperglycaemia (OR 2.59, 95% CI 1.13–5.94) [11]. Complications of EN include pain, nausea and diarrhoea, and may vary between patients. Where total EN fails, a combination of EN/PN may be required to prevent the effects of nutrient deprivation. Early research suggested that PN use should be avoided within 5 days of presentation (the peak inflammation period) [19] but more studies are needed, particularly with the availability of newer PN lipid mixes.

Contraindications to PN include triacylglycerol (TAG)-induced AP, or where TAG concentrations are >12 mmol/L. Further considerations for the nutritional management of AP are provided in Box 5.8.1.

Monitoring

Good glycaemic control is essential in AP (see Box 5.8.1), and blood glucose and TAG concentrations should be monitored during EN. The patient should be assessed frequently for symptoms of EN intolerance including pain, nausea and diarrhoea to pre-empt/prevent EN-related complications.

Box 5.8.1 Further considerations in the nutritional management of acute pancreatitis

- Glutamine should be given if patient is receiving PN (0.3–0.5 g/kg body weight of N(2) L-alanyl-L-glutamine dipeptide), as well as ensuring an adequate supply of micronutrients [17,19]
- Thiamine deficiency may occur, particularly in alcohol-induced AP or where there is risk of refeeding syndrome. IV supplementation is recommended [6]
- EN regimens should contain selenium [6]
- Probiotics are not recommended in AP [64]
- Good glycaemic control is essential; blood glucose concentration should be kept <10 mmol/L where possible [10]

5.8.2 Chronic pancreatitis

Chronic pancreatitis (CP) is classified by the Cambridge definition as a chronic inflammatory disease of the pancreas characterized by irreversible morphological changes and typically causing pain and/or permanent loss of function [20]. In CP, there is progressive loss of acinar and islet cells of the pancreas and the development of fibrous scar tissue. Loss of exocrine function results in maldigestion, malabsorption, nutrient deficiency and undernutrition. Loss of endocrine function results in eventual diabetes. Patients usually present with abdominal pain (epigastric, dull, constant) which may radiate towards the back. It may be difficult to distinguish between CP and pancreatic cancer.

Aetiology of chronic pancreatitis

The most common aetiology of CP is alcohol, thought to account for >80% of cases. The necrosis-fibrosis hypothesis describes CP as an initial acute process with ultimate progression to chronic permanent changes due to repeat attacks. In fact, the pathogenesis of CP is incompletely understood, and even in those who consume high levels of alcohol there may be an additional insult ('second hit') that precipitates the clinical onset of pancreatitis. Suggested factors are diet, pattern/volume/type of alcohol consumption, hyperlipidaemia, smoking and genetic predisposition. Abstinence from, or a marked reduction in, alcohol intake reduces the risk of developing CP in those with AP.

Epidemiological data for incidence and prevalence in CP are remarkably scarce, but in Europe the incidence is thought to be 6–7 per 100 000 population [21], and the data suggest increasing prevalence [22,23]. Approximately 20% of CP cases are classed as idiopathic (no identifiable causes) [24]. However, the number of idiopathic cases will diminish with the identification of putative genetic and environmental causes. Other common causes include pancreatic duct obstruction, pancreas divisum, cystic fibrosis, hypercalcaemia, auotimmuninty, gene mutations and hypertriglyceridaemia.

Tropical pancreatitis describes the type of CP observed in undernourished patients in tropical/subtropical countries. It tends to affect young adults (in the third and fourth decades) who seem to have an aggressive, progressive form of the disease with early diabetes [25]. Traditionally, it was thought to be related to the intake of the root vegetable cassava (*Manihot esculenta*) which contains cyanide-related compounds. However, it is now thought that the idiopathic CP seen in India and similar countries has a strong genetic predisposition [26]. Although not classed as an aetiology, smoking increases the risk of developing CP [27] and doubles the risk of pancreatic cancer [28].

Mechanisms of nutrient deficiency in chronic pancreatitis

Patients with CP are at a high risk of developing nutrient deficiency due to inadequate dietary intake, increased requirements and gastrointestinal malabsorption. Untreated steatorrhoea may result in deficiencies of fat-soluble vitamins A, D, E and K. Reports of the prevalence of biochemical deficiency vary considerably, from 14–40% for vitamin A to 10–75% for vitamin E and 11–86% for vitamin D [29–36]. Overt clinical manifestations have been described, mostly in case reports, and include photophobia, ocular pain, peripheral ulcerative keratitis and necrotising strand ulceration (vitamin A deficiency), brown bowel syndrome and neurological symptoms (vitamin E deficiency), and osteomalacia (vitamin D deficiency) [37–43]. Most cases were associated with an additional comorbidity such as diabetes, coeliac disease or gastrointestinal surgery. Clinical deficiency appears to take years to develop. Deficiencies of vitamin B12, folate, magnesium and zinc have also been reported [44–46]. Measurement of serum concentrations is recommended rather than the implementation of blanket supplementation [29]. Vitamin D deficiency (or insufficiency), smoking, poor diet and malabsorption, along with chronic inflammation render the CP patient at high risk of developing osteopenia or osteoporosis. A meta-analysis of 11 studies found that the pooled prevalence of osteoporosis was 23.4% and osteopenia 39.8% [47].

Exocrine dysfunction in chronic pancreatitis

The loss of acinar cells results in reduced production/secretion of pancreatic enzymes, causing maldigestion and malabsorption of macronutrients and micronutrients. Fat malabsorption may be problematic, driven by insufficient lipase secretion, destruction of lipase by acid (due to reduced bicarbonate excretion), precipitation of bile acids and impaired gastric empting. Lipase is especially vulnerable to destruction compared to other enzymes. While production of amylase and protease is also disrupted, there is also a degree of compensation due to the presence of intestinal brush border protease and oligosaccharides. Whilst studies from the 1970s [48] and 1980s [49] reported that there must be almost total destruction of the pancreas before exocrine impairment occurs, a review of the topic suggested that this is not the case, and that exocrine impairment occurs with even mild or moderate disease [50].

When diagnosing pancreatic exocrine insufficiency (PEI), clinical inspection of the stool is not reliable except in the case of gross fat malabsorption. Overt fat malabsorption is characterised by pale, formed, bulky stools that may float and are difficult to flush.

Tests that indirectly assess exocrine function are required as direct measurement is invasive and impractical [50]. A 72-hour faecal fat study requires the ingestion of a diet with a precisely measured quantity of fat for the 72-hour period, followed by laboratory analysis of stools collected for the duration [50]. This method is therefore painstaking, labour-intensive, expensive and impractical. Pancreatic elastase-1 (faecal elastase-1, FE-1) is a human-specific enzyme that does not degrade during intestinal transit and is enriched 5–6-fold in the faeces. Benefits of the FE-1 test include the fact that patients do not need to halt pancreatic enzyme replacement therapy (PERT), nor is there a need to ingest a special diet for testing. The test is inexpensive, widely available and simple, requiring a single sample of stool. A negative aspect of the FE-1 test is that it is not reliable in the diagnosis of mild insufficiency. Figure 5.8.1 details the FE-1 reference ranges and Box 5.8.2 provides suggestions on the management of PEI.

Endocrine insufficiency in chronic pancreatitis

Diabetes develops in late CP (about 30–50% of CP cases) due to the progressive loss of pancreatic islet cells, possibly due to micro-ischaemia and reduced secretion of certain hormones, including glucose-dependent insulinotrophic hormone and glucagon.

The type of diabetes that is associated with this patient group is termed pancreatogenic (or type 3c) diabetes and differs from types 1 and 2 [51]. Patients with type 3c diabetes are typically older than those with type 1, but younger than those with type 2. They are generally thinner than people with type 2 diabetes, and tend to suffer hypoglycaemic events more commonly although hyperglycaemia is usually less severe than that of type 1 diabetes. Patients with type 3c diabetes usually have lower glucagon concentration than either type 1 and 2 diabetes [52–54]. Despite the key differences, there are few guidelines relating to the management of type 3c diabetes, and awareness is low, even among health professionals [51,54].

In a patient with CP, fasting glucose and HbA1c should be measured as part of the overall nutritional assessment and any impairment warrants further evaluation (75 g oral glucose tolerance test) [53].

Dietary management is complicated by malabsorption, alcohol intake (for some) and erratic or poor dietary intake (often secondary to pain or other symptoms). The risk of hypoglycaemia is of particular concern [53,55]. This along with a significant risk of undernutrition means that those with severe CP complicated by diabetes require intensive dietetic input [53]. While profound hyperglycaemia in a catabolic patient with glycosuria and weight loss will probably require insulin therapy, lifestyle advice and other appropriate drug therapies should be optimised to reduce the requirement for insulin. Management of type 3c diabetes is likely to evolve as further research is published. Box 5.8.3 summarises the management priorities for the nutritional management of type 3c diabetes [53,55].

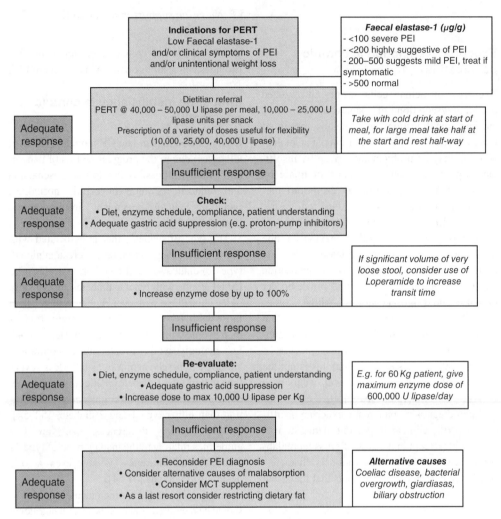

Figure 5.8.1 Algorithm for pancreatic enzyme replacement therapy in CP. Source: Adapted with permission from the Centre for Pancreatico-Biliary Diseases, Tallaght Hospital, Dublin, Ireland.

Box 5.8.2 Considerations for the management of pancreatic exocrine insufficiency in chronic pancreatitis

- PEI is often undertreated, and PERT underprescribed [66]
- Patients should be commenced on 40 000–50 000 U lipase with meals and 10 000–25 000 U lipase with snacks, increased in a step-wise manner according to symptoms to a maximum dose of 10 000 U lipase per kg body weight (see Figure 5.8.1)
- Patients should be taught to alter the PERT dose according to their own symptoms and requirements
- PERT should be taken at the beginning of a meal, and where more than 1 capsule is required, these may be spread throughout the meal
- Capsules are usually taken whole (not with a hot drink), but may be opened if required and mixed with an acidic, cold fruit purée and swallowed without chewing
- Acid suppression may be required
- Further medication may be required to manage symptoms, such as loperamide or codeine phosphate. Where patients are taking opiates for pain, laxatives may also be required
- PERT should be regularly reviewed in conjunction with a thorough nutritional assessment
- PERT may be administered with enteral formula if necessary [67]
- PERT should also be taken with fat-containing ONS

Box 5.8.3 Suggested principles of nutritional management of type 3c diabetes in chronic pancreatitis

Principles of management	Management strategies
Prevent: • Hypoglycaemia • Hyperglycaemia • Exacerbation of undernutrition • Malabsorption • Comorbidities associated with diabetes (e.g. retinopathy and renal disease)	• Regular meal pattern with regular starchy carbohydrates • Do not skip meals • Take small, frequent meals • Measure glucose concentration frequently, particularly after physical activity, if diet is poor, and if any hypoglycaemic symptoms • Avoid alcohol, smoking cessation • Ensure adequacy of enzyme therapy • Minimise high-sugar/high-glycaemic index food or fluids • Consider a diary to record diet, glucose concentration, enzymes, exercise, at least until acceptable glucose control is maintained • Routine dietitian assessment/monitoring

Source: Adapted from Duggan and Conlon [60].

5.8.3 Nutritional assessment in chronic pancreatitis

The nutritional management of CP has been described as 'a problem area' [56]. Therefore it is vital that a standardised framework is followed so that the complex issues may be adequately addressed. Figure 5.8.2 illustrates such a framework [57]. Patients should be assessed at baseline and regularly monitored. In severe CP (with concurrent exocrine and endocrine insufficiency), patients should maintain a food and symptoms diary so that the optimal regimen of PERT may be devised, along with adequate glycaemic control. Pancreatic exocrine and endocrine function is a cornerstone of nutrition assessment. Given the risk of osteoporosis in CP, at-risk patients should undergo a baseline bone density assessment (by dual-energy x-ray absorptiometry). At-risk groups include those with a prior low-trauma fracture, postmenopausal women, and men >50 years, as well as those with malabsorption [47,58].

5.8.4 Nutritional requirements

Limited data suggest that resting energy expenditure may be higher in (underweight) CP by 30–50%, so undernourished patients may require a high energy intake of 35 kcal/kg (146.5 kJ/kg) [59]. Regarding dietary composition, fat-free diets are neither recommended nor warranted [7,57,60]; rather, a moderate-fat diet (30% of energy) should be counselled, in conjunction with adequate PERT. However, there has been little research into the optimal diet for chronic pancreatitis, and the dietary guidelines are mostly expert opinion. Although recommended in European pancreatitis guidelines [6], there is no evidence that vegetable fat is better tolerated than animal fat [57]. A protein intake of 1–1.5 g/kg is usually well tolerated and adequate [6,61]. Generally, a higher carbohydrate diet is recommended (to ensure adequate energy intake where there is a reduction in fat intake), but this requires modification in the diabetic patient [6]. A very high fibre intake may bind pancreatic enzymes and therefore if PERT is suboptimal, dietary fibre intake may need to be reduced in those with high intakes [61,62].

5.8.5 Nutrition intervention in chronic pancreatitis

Whilst the majority of patients with CP will be maintained on normal diet with or without oral nutritional supplements, some will require specialised nutrition support [10]. Patients may also

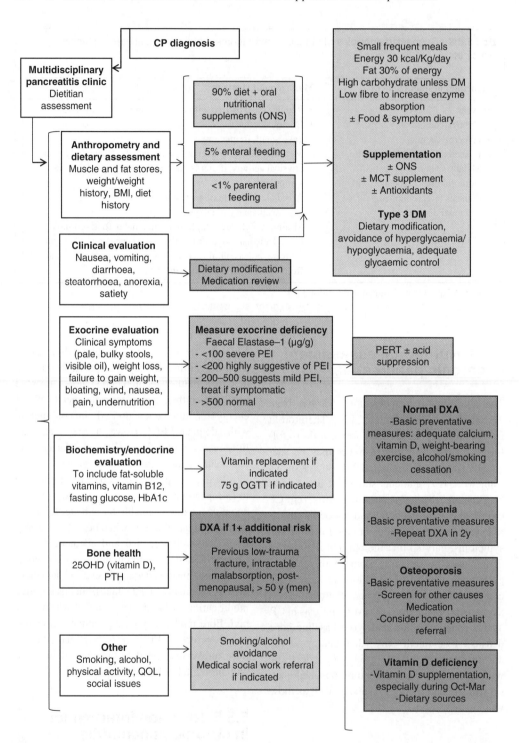

Figure 5.8.2 Algorithm for the nutritional management of chronic pancreatitis. Source: Adapted and modified from Duggan and Conlon [60] with permission from the Nature Publishing Group.

require vitamin or mineral supplementation, such as vitamin D, if deficiencies exist [29,30,57]. About 5% will need EN and indications include insufficient dietary intake, ongoing weight loss despite apparently adequate diet, where there are acute complications (including acute exacerbations of pancreatitis), and preoperatively in the undernourished patient [10]. Selected patients may benefit from long-term jejunal feeding. One study showed weight gain and a reduction in pain with minimal adverse events with this intervention. Fewer still will require PN (<1% of cases). Typical indications for PN are complex gastric fistulas, severe undernutrition preoperatively (where EN alone is insufficient/impossible), and gastric outlet obstruction (without jejunal access).

For those with PEI, small, frequent meals should be easier to tolerate and manage, as larger meals require large amounts of PERT and there may be inadequate mixing. ONS may be required for some patients, and whole-protein versions may be trialled first before progressing onto medium-chain triglyceride (MCT)-enriched or peptide-based versions [6]. MCT supplements may be a useful energy source in undernutrition, but should be increased slowly as they may be unpalatable and could cause cramping, nausea and diarrhoea [57].

Pain is a common complication of CP for which there are few medical options. Antioxidant supplements were initially promising, showing reduction in pain, quality of life and working days lost. Antioxidant supplements for CP are composed of selenium, β-carotene, L-methionine, vitamin C and vitamin E. A recent study showed that there was no reduction in pain or improvement in quality of life, despite an increase in serum antioxidant concentrations [63]. Nevertheless, several systematic reviews indicate a reduction in pain with antioxidant therapy. More research is required in this area, and large-scale studies are ongoing.

5.8.6 Monitoring

Figure 5.8.2 details the various factors to be considered in the monitoring of patients with chronic pancreatitis.

References

1. Banks PA, Bollen TL, Dervenis C, et al. Classification of acute pancreatitis – 2012: revision of the Atlanta classification and definitions by international consensus. *Gut* 2013; **62**(1): 102–111.
2. O'Farrell A, Allwright S, Toomey D, Bedford D, Conlon K. Hospital admission for acute pancreatitis in the Irish population, 1997 2004: could the increase be due to an increase in alcohol-related pancreatitis? *J Public Health* 2007; **29**(4): 398–404.
3. Goldacre MJ, Roberts SE. Hospital admission for acute pancreatitis in an English population, 1963–98: database study of incidence and mortality. *BMJ* 2004; **328**(7454): 1466–1469.
4. ASPEN Board of Directors, Clinical Guidelines Task Force. Guidelines for the use of parenteral and enteral nutrition in adult and pediatric patients. *J Parenter Enteral Nutr* 2002; **26**(1 Suppl): 1SA–138SA.
5. Meier R, Beglinger C, Layer P, et al. ESPEN guidelines on nutrition in acute pancreatitis. European Society of Parenteral and Enteral Nutrition. *Clin Nutr* 2002; **21**(2): 173–183.
6. Meier R, Ockenga J, Pertkiewicz M, et al. ESPEN guidelines on enteral nutrition: pancreas. *Clin Nutr* 2006; **25**(2): 275–284.
7. Todorovic V, Micklewright A. Pancreatic disease. In: A Pocket Guide to Clinical Nutrition, 4th edn. London: PENG, 2013.
8. Dambrauskas Z, Gulbinas A, Pundzius J, Barauskas G. Value of the different prognostic systems and biological markers for predicting severity and progression of acute pancreatitis. *Scand J Gastroenterol* 2010; **45**(7-8): 959–970.
9. Petrov MS, McIlroy K, Grayson L, Phillips AR, Windsor JA. Early nasogastric tube feeding versus nil per os in mild to moderate acute pancreatitis: a randomized controlled trial. *Clin Nutr* 2013; **32**(5): 697–703.
10. Meier R, Beglinger C, Layer P, et al. ESPEN guidelines on nutrition in acute pancreatitis. European Society of Parenteral and Enteral Nutrition. *Clin Nutr* 2002; **21**(2): 173–183.
11. Petrov MS, Whelan K. Comparison of complications attributable to enteral and parenteral nutrition in predicted severe acute pancreatitis: a systematic review and meta-analysis. *Br J Nutr* 2010; **103**(9): 1287–1295.
12. Eatock FC, Brombacher GD, Steven A, Imrie CW, McKay CJ, Carter R. Nasogastric feeding in severe acute pancreatitis may be practical and safe. *Int J Pancreatol* 2000; **28**(1): 23–29.
13. Eatock FC, Chong P, Menezes N, et al. A randomized study of early nasogastric versus nasojejunal feeding in severe acute pancreatitis. *Am J Gastroenterol* 2005; **100**(2): 432–439.
14. Petrov MS, Correia MI, Windsor JA. Nasogastric tube feeding in predicted severe acute pancreatitis. A

systematic review of the literature to determine safety and tolerance. *JOP* 2008; **9**(4): 440–448.

15. Kaushik N, Pietraszewski M, Holst JJ, O'Keefe SJ. Enteral feeding without pancreatic stimulation. *Pancreas* 2005; **31**(4): 353–359.

16. Duggan S, Egan SM, Smyth ND, Feehan SM, Breslin N, Conlon KC. Blind bedside insertion of small bowel feeding tubes. *Ir J Med Sci* 2009; **178**(4): 485–489.

17. Gianotti L, Meier R, Lobo DN, et al. ESPEN guidelines on parenteral nutrition: pancreas. *Clin Nutr* 2009; **28**(4): 428–435.

18. Petrov MS, Loveday BP, Pylypchuk RD, McIlroy K, Phillips AR, Windsor JA. Systematic review and meta-analysis of enteral nutrition formulations in acute pancreatitis. *Br J Surg* 2009; **96**(11): 1243–1252.

19. McClave SA, Chang WK, Dhaliwal R, Heyland DK. Nutrition support in acute pancreatitis: a systematic review of the literature. *J Parenter Enteral Nutr* 2006; **30**(2): 143–156.

20. Go VL, Dimagno EP, Gardner JD, Lebenthal E, Reber HA, Scheele GA. The Pancreas: Pathobiology and Disease, 2nd edn. New York: Raven, 1993.

21. Jupp J, Fine D, Johnson CD. The epidemiology and socioeconomic impact of chronic pancreatitis. *Best Pract Res Clin Gastroenterol* 2010; **24**(3): 219–231.

22. Hirota M, Shimosegawa T, Masamune A, et al. The seventh nationwide epidemiological survey for chronic pancreatitis in Japan: clinical significance of smoking habit in Japanese patients. *Pancreatology* 2014; **14**(6): 490–496.

23. Wang LW, Li ZS, Li SD, Jin ZD, Zou DW, Chen F. Prevalence and clinical features of chronic pancreatitis in China: a retrospective multicenter analysis over 10 years. *Pancreas* 2009; **38**(3): 248–254.

24. Whitcomb DC. Clinical practice. Acute pancreatitis. *N Engl J Med* 2006; **354**(20): 2142–2150.

25. Midha S, Khajuria R, Shastri S, Kabra M, Garg PK. Idiopathic chronic pancreatitis in India: phenotypic characterisation and strong genetic susceptibility due to SPINK1 and CFTR gene mutations. *Gut* 2010; **59**(6): 800–807.

26. Midha S, Singh N, Sachdev V, Tandon RK, Joshi YK, Garg PK. Cause and effect relationship of malnutrition with idiopathic chronic pancreatitis: prospective case-control study. *J Gastroenterol Hepatol* 2008; **23**(9): 1378–1383.

27. Imoto M, DiMagno EP. Cigarette smoking increases the risk of pancreatic calcification in late-onset but not early-onset idiopathic chronic pancreatitis. *Pancreas* 2000; **21**(2): 115–119.

28. Boyle P, Maisonneuve P, Bueno de Mesquita B, et al. Cigarette smoking and pancreas cancer: a case control study of the search programme of the IARC. *Int J Cancer* 1996; **67**(1): 63–71.

29. Duggan SN, Smyth ND, O'Sullivan M, Feehan S, Ridgway PF, Conlon KC. The prevalence of malnu-

trition and fat-soluble vitamin deficiencies in chronic pancreatitis. *Nutr Clin Pract* 2014; **29**(3): 348–354.

30. Sikkens EC, Cahen DL, Koch AD, et al. The prevalence of fat-soluble vitamin deficiencies and a decreased bone mass in patients with chronic pancreatitis. *Pancreatology* 2013; **13**(3): 238–242.

31. Nakamura T, Takebe K, Imamura K, et al. Fat-soluble vitamins in patients with chronic pancreatitis (pancreatic insufficiency). *Acta Gastroenterol Belg* 1996; **59**(1): 10–14.

32. Kalvaria I, Labadarios D, Shephard GS, Visser L, Marks IN. Biochemical vitamin E deficiency in chronic pancreatitis. *Int J Pancreatol* 1986; **1**(2): 119–128.

33. Moran CE, Sosa EG, Martinez SM, et al. Bone mineral density in patients with pancreatic insufficiency and steatorrhea. *Am J Gastroenterol* 1997; **92**(5): 867–871.

34. Joshi A, Reddy SV, Bhatia V, et al. High prevalence of low bone mineral density in patients with tropical calcific pancreatitis. *Pancreas* 2011; **40**(5): 762–767.

35. Marotta F, Labadarios D, Frazer L, Girdwood A, Marks IN. Fat-soluble vitamin concentration in chronic alcohol-induced pancreatitis. Relationship with steatorrhea. *Dig Dis Sci* 1994; **39**(5): 993–998.

36. Dujsikova H, Dite P, Tomandl J, Sevcikova A, Precechtelova M. Occurrence of metabolic osteopathy in patients with chronic pancreatitis. *Pancreatology* 2008; **8**(6): 583–586.

37. Benitez Cruz S, Gomez Candela C, Ruiz Martin M, Cos Blanco AI. Bilateral corneal ulceration as a result of caloric-protein malnutrition and vitamin A deficit in a patient with chronic alcoholism, chronic pancreatitis and cholecystostomy. *Nutr Hosp* 2005; **20**(4): 308–310.

38. Ruiz-Martin MM, Boto-de-los-Bueis A, Romero-Martin R. Severe bilateral ocular affection caused by vitamin A deficiency. *Arch Soc Esp Oftalmol* 2005; **80**(11): 663–666.

39. Reynaert H, Debeuckelaere S, de Waele B, Meysman M, Goossens A, Devis G. The brown bowel syndrome and gastrointestinal adenocarcinoma. Two complications of vitamin E deficiency in celiac sprue and chronic pancreatitis? *J Clin Gastroenterol* 1993; **16**(1): 48–51.

40. Yokota T, Tsuchiya K, Furukawa T, Tsukagoshi H, Miyakawa H, Hasumura Y. Vitamin E deficiency in acquired fat malabsorption. *J Neurol* 1990; **237**(2): 103–106.

41. Kurtulmus N, Yarman S, Tanakol R, Alagol F. Severe osteomalacia in a patient with idiopathic chronic pancreatitis. *Scott Med J* 2005; **50**(4): 172–173.

42. Kaur N, Gupta S, Minocha VR. Chronic calcific pancreatitis associated with osteomalacia and secondary hyperparathyroidism. *Indian J Gastroenterol* 1996; **15**(4): 147–148.

43. Shimazaki K, Kubota S, Chuman K. A case of chronic pancreatitis in whom osteomalacia due to malabsorption syndrome after a pancreaticoduodenectomy was recognized and treated. *IRYO Japn J Natl Med Serv* 1995; **49**(10): 837–841.

44. Glasbrenner B, Malfertheiner P, Buchler M, Kuhn K, Ditschuneit H. Vitamin B12 and folic acid deficiency in chronic pancreatitis: a relevant disorder? *Klin Wochenschr* 1991; **69**(4): 168–172.

45. Girish BN, Rajesh G, Vaidyanathan K, Balakrishnan V. Zinc status in chronic pancreatitis and its relationship with exocrine and endocrine insufficiency. *JOP* 2009; **10**(6):651–656.

46. Papazachariou IM, Martinez-Isla A, Efthimiou E, Williamson RC, Girgis SI. Magnesium deficiency in patients with chronic pancreatitis identified by an intravenous loading test. *Clin Chim Acta* 2000; **302**(1-2): 145–154.

47. Duggan SN, Smyth ND, Murphy A, Macnaughton D, O'Keefe SJ, Conlon KC. High prevalence of osteoporosis in patients with chronic pancreatitis: a systematic review and meta-analysis. *Clin Gastroenterol Hepatol* 2014; **12**(2): 219–228.

48. DiMagno EP, Go VL, Summerskill WH. Relations between pancreatic enzyme ouputs and malabsorption in severe pancreatic insufficiency. *N Engl J Med* 1973; **288**(16): 813–815.

49. Lankisch PG, Lembcke B, Wemken G, Creutzfeldt W. Functional reserve capacity of the exocrine pancreas. *Digestion* 1986; **35**(3): 175–181.

50. Duggan SN, Ni Chonchubhair HM, Lawal O, O'Connor DB, Conlon KC. Chronic pancreatitis: a diagnostic dilemma. *WJG* 2016; **22**(7): 2304–2313.

51. Ewald N, Kaufmann C, Raspe A, Kloer HU, Bretzel RG, Hardt PD. Prevalence of diabetes mellitus secondary to pancreatic diseases (type 3c). *Diabetes Metab Res Rev* 2012; **28**(4): 338–342.

52. Rickels MR, Bellin M, Toledo FG, et al. Detection, evaluation and treatment of diabetes mellitus in chronic pancreatitis: recommendations from PancreasFest 2012. *Pancreatology* 2013; **13**(4): 336–342.

53. Duggan SN, Ewald N, Kelleher L, Griffin O, Gibney J, Conlon KC. The nutritional management of type 3c (pancreatogenic) diabetes in chronic pancreatitis. *Eur J Clin Nutr* 2017; **71**(1): 3–8.

54. Ewald N, Bretzel RG. Diabetes mellitus secondary to pancreatic diseases (Type 3c) – are we neglecting an important disease? *Eur J Intern Med* 2013; **24**(3): 203–206.

55. Duggan SNC, Conlon K. A practical guide to the nutritional management of chronic pancreatitis. *Pract Gastroenterol* 2013; **118**: 24–32.

56. Lankisch PG. Chronic pancreatitis. *Curr Opin Gastroenterol* 2007; **23**(5): 502–507.

57. Duggan S, O'Sullivan M, Feehan S, Ridgway P, Conlon K. Nutrition treatment of deficiency and malnutrition in chronic pancreatitis: a review. *Nutr Clin Pract* 2010; **25**(4): 362–370.

58. Duggan SN, Conlon KC. Bone health guidelines for patients with chronic pancreatitis. *Gastroenterology* 2013; **145**(4): 911.

59. Hebuterne X, Hastier P, Peroux JL, Zeboudj N, Delmont JP, Rampal P. Resting energy expenditure in patients with alcoholic chronic pancreatitis. *Dig Dis Sci* 1996; **41**(3): 533–539.

60. Duggan SN, Conlon KC. A practical guide to the nutritional managment of chronic pancreatitis. *Pract Gastroenterol* 2013; Series **118**: 24–32.

61. Giger U, Stanga Z, DeLegge MH. Management of chronic pancreatitis. *Nutr Clin Pract* 2004; **19**(1): 37–49.

62. Petersen JM, Forsmark CE. Chronic pancreatitis and maldigestion. *Semin Gastrointest Dis* 2002; **13**(4): 191–199.

63. Siriwardena AK, Mason JM, Sheen AJ, Makin AJ, Shah NS. Antioxidant therapy does not reduce pain in patients with chronic pancreatitis: the ANTICIPATE study. *Gastroenterology* 2012; **143**(3): 655–663 e1.

64. Besselink MG, van Santvoort HC, Buskens E, et al. Probiotic prophylaxis in predicted severe acute pancreatitis: a randomised, double-blind, placebo-controlled trial. *Lancet* 2008; **371**(9613): 651–659.

65. Das SL, Singh PP, Phillips AR, Murphy R, Windsor JA, Petrov MS. Newly diagnosed diabetes mellitus after acute pancreatitis: a systematic review and meta-analysis. *Gut* 2014; **63**(5): 818–831.

66. Sikkens EC, Cahen DL, van Eijck C, Kuipers EJ, Bruno MJ. Patients with exocrine insufficiency due to chronic pancreatitis are undertreated: a Dutch national survey. *Pancreatology* 2012; **12**(1): 71–73.

67. Ferrie S, Graham C, Hoyle M. Pancreatic enzyme supplementation for patients receiving enteral feeds. *Nutr Clin Pract* 2011; **26**(3): 349–351.

Chapter 5.9

Nutrition support in inflammatory bowel disease

Miranda Lomer
Guy's and St Thomas' NHS Foundation Trust and King's College London, London, UK

5.9.1 Undernutrition in inflammatory bowel disease

The interaction between diet, nutrition and inflammatory bowel disease (IBD) is of great concern to patients and health professionals. Patients with IBD report food and nutrition problems as a result of their disease. Under_nutrition affects 20–85% of patients with IBD and weight loss is problematic in up to 83% of patients [1,2]. This wide variation may be due to differences in disease phenotype, disease activity and nutritional assessment methods used. Patients with ileal Crohn's disease appear to be most at risk. Undernutrition is often present at diagnosis and is an issue not only in active disease but also in remission. Increased body mass index (BMI), over 25 kg/m², is present in 10–30% of patients and may mask underlying protein-energy malnutrition and micronutrient deficiencies.

Causes and mechanisms

The causes of undernutrition in IBD are multifactorial and complex. Inadequate oral intake is the most commonly reported cause of undernutrition. It may be due to appetite suppression related to symptoms (e.g. nausea, vomiting, diarrhoea, abdominal pain), taste changes as a result of vitamin and/or mineral deficiencies, drug interactions and increased circulating proinflammatory mediators [3]. In addition, many patients self-restrict their diet to avoid symptoms.

Gastrointestinal losses are common and include diarrhoea, vomiting, bleeding and protein-losing enteropathy. Fluid, electrolytes and other nutrients (e.g. magnesium in chronic diarrhoea) may need to be replaced. Increased energy and nutrient intakes may be required due to systemic inflammation or extensive surgical resection. Chronic mucosal inflammation, extensive surgical resection, fistula formation or surgical bypass of healthy mucosa can result in blind intestinal loops and bacterial overgrowth, leading to malabsorption. If the terminal ileum is removed or inflamed, bile salts may not be reabsorbed which can lead to fat malabsorption and steatorrhoea.

Consequences

Inflammatory bowel disease has a major impact on people's lives, including disruption of daily activities, social interactions, intimacy, psychological function and physical health [4]. These social and psychological aspects are directly related to eating and drinking behaviour [2] and are associated with a high prevalence of reduced food-related quality of life [5].

Undernourished patients with IBD have high levels of anxiety and depression and their quality of life is decreased [4]. Over half of patients with Crohn's disease and 20–30% of patients with

Advanced Nutrition and Dietetics in Nutrition Support, First Edition. Edited by Mary Hickson and Sara Smith.

ulcerative colitis will have gastrointestinal surgery at some point. Impaired nutritional status preoperatively is associated with a greater risk of developing postsurgical complications and permanent stoma formation. It also increases health service costs, inpatient mortality rates and length of stay [6,7].

5.9.2 Assessment and diagnosis of undernutrition

Basic nutritional assessment measuring weight and BMI are insufficient to detect changes in nutritional status in IBD and there does not appear to be a consistent association between body composition and disease activity or disease phenotype [8]. In the absence of a gold standard IBD-specific nutritional assessment method, it is difficult to clarify what identifies an IBD patient to be at nutritional risk. Perhaps using one measure is inappropriate and multiple components including body composition, dietary intake, biochemical measurements, muscle function and energy expenditure are indicated, but how many is not known [9,10]. A recent systematic review of body composition in IBD recommends using a whole-body dual-energy x-ray absorptiometry (DEXA) scan at the time of bone densitometry to provide valuable body composition data alongside other anthropometric measurements, such as BMI, waist:hip circumference ratio and handgrip strength [8]. However, its potential for use in clinical practice is yet to be realised.

Micronutrient deficiencies are often reported in IBD and almost every vitamin, mineral and trace element has been reported as suboptimal [3,11]. However, measurements of circulating plasma concentrations in the presence of systemic inflammation are unlikely to provide any meaning due to the acute phase response. Thus, a reliable interpretation using plasma can only be measured when C-reactive protein (CRP) <20 mg/L for zinc, <10 mg/L for selenium, vitamin A and vitamin D, and <5 mg/L for vitamin B6 and vitamin C [12]. Alternative measurements, independent of inflammatory state (e.g. erythrocyte concentration), are needed to assess micronutrient status in IBD [9].

5.9.3 Dietary management

Anaemia

Anaemia of chronic disease and/or iron deficiency anaemia are common problems in IBD [13]. Gastrointestinal blood loss and increased disease severity are the major causes of anaemia, although low dietary iron intakes have been reported [14] and the quality and quantity of dietary iron are more predictive of iron status in IBD patients compared to healthy subjects [15]. Assessment of iron deficiency in IBD is difficult due to several contributing factors, such as inflammation and anaemia of chronic disease. Iron absorption is downregulated in patients with active IBD but in quiescent or mildly active IBD, iron absorption is normal but standard haematological parameters do not accurately predict iron requirements [16].

Oral iron supplementation often leads to gastrointestinal side effects (i.e. nausea, abdominal pain, diarrhoea). In iron deficiency without anaemia, large oral doses are best avoided but low doses, up to 60 mg elemental iron (e.g. one ferrous sulfate tablet per day) may be tolerable [3,13]. When iron deficiency coexists with anaemia in patients with clinically active IBD, intravenous iron, and possibly erythropoiesis-stimulating agents, are warranted [13].

Anaemia is also associated with folate or vitamin B12 deficiency. They may occur concurrently and be due to inadequate dietary intake. Folate supplementation is required in patients receiving methotrexate as it interferes with folate metabolism. Vitamin B12 deficiency is common in patients with terminal ileal Crohn's disease or surgical resection, but is rare in ulcerative colitis. Regular monitoring in patients at risk of deficiency and oral supplementation (folate) or intramuscular injection (vitamin B12) may be required [11].

Bone health

In IBD there is a 60–70% increased fracture risk compared to healthy subjects due to an increased incidence of osteoporosis. The cause of osteoporosis in IBD is multifactorial; contributing factors include systemic inflammation, inadequate vitamin D and calcium status, older age and corticosteroid use. Minimising the use of corticosteroids and ensuring an adequate intake of calcium and vitamin D, using supplementation when necessary, are vital in osteoporosis prevention. In particular, some patients may limit their dairy food intake due to concerns over lactose intolerance; dietary assessment and advice are important to ensure calcium intake can be maintained. Bone mineral density monitoring using DEXA is recommended in patients at high risk of osteoporosis but is often underutilised [17].

Crohn's disease

Almost half a century ago, interest developed in diet having a role in Crohn's disease and 'bowel rest' was considered important. Initially, nutrition was provided only as intravenous glucose, but patients developed protein-energy malnutrition. Parenteral nutrition (PN) was introduced but total GI tract rest led to atrophy and carried serious risks.

Exclusive enteral nutrition

In the 1970s, interest developed in using a chemically defined liquid 'elemental' diet, similar to those used in manned space programmes where they wanted minimal residue and nutrients provided in their simplest form. An elemental diet provides protein as free amino acids, carbohydrate as glucose or short-chain maltodextrins and fat as short-chain triglycerides and is complete with vitamins and minerals. It enables bowel rest, reducing faecal output, and has the advantage over PN in that it limits GI atrophy and is associated with fewer serious risks. However, the palatability of an elemental diet is limited. More recently, whole-protein (polymeric) and semi-elemental (peptide) formulas have been developed and in a Cochrane review of different types of enteral nutrition (EN), these more palatable formulas have been shown to be equally as efficacious as an elemental formula [18,19]. Altering the type of fat within EN has also been of great interest

due to the immune-modulatory effects of fats. It is postulated that altering the proportions and types of fats (e.g. ratio of long-chain to medium-chain triglycerides) within EN may have anti-inflammatory or proinflammatory effects [18,19]. However, the current limited evidence indicates that all types of EN formulas, independent of fat type and protein source, have similar efficacy [20].

Exclusive EN is a primary treatment for active Crohn's disease in paediatrics as it avoids the use of corticosteroids which can impair growth [21. However, in adults, exclusive EN is not as effective as corticosteroids [18,19]. In adherent adults, exclusive EN is more effective than placebo and as effective as corticosteroids [18,19]. Exclusive EN can be considered in adult patients where other primary treatments (e.g. immunosuppressive agents, biological therapy or corticosteroids) are not possible or where it is used as an adjunctive treatment, especially to address undernutrition and in presurgical optimisation [7,22–28].

The therapeutic mechanism for exclusive EN remains unclear, although evidence supports mucosal healing and downregulation of mucosal proinflammatory cytokines [29]. Nutrients are important to the gastrointestinal environment and diet has a profound effect on the gastrointestinal microbiota. There is growing interest in the effects that EN has on modulating the gastrointestinal microbiota, reducing inflammatory mediators and improving altered epithelial permeability [29].

Major barriers to successful exclusive EN are limited palatability, particularly with elemental diets, and high volumes required to meet nutritional requirements (usually 1500–2500 mL per day). Support and encouragement from all members of the IBD team are important to optimise the chances of successful treatment with EN [18]. Starter regimens are useful to improve initial tolerance of EN, gradually building up the target volume of EN over several days and reducing usual diet, unless normal food is contraindicated (e.g. in acute severe stricturing disease). Adherence is improved by using prescribable flavours and ensuring the EN is cold and taken from a closed beaker and a straw. Nasogastric tube feeding improves adherence in paediatrics and may also be appropriate for some adult patients.

Polymeric EN is generally more palatable and is advocated in preference to peptide or elemental EN [18,19]. However, patient taste and preference must be taken into consideration, especially when it comes to the volumes and duration of EN that are required. The optimal duration for exclusive EN is unknown; a clinical response (i.e. improvement in symptoms) can be achieved at 10 days but continuation for up to 8 weeks enables mucosal healing [18]. Exclusive EN is considered to be most effective in patients with ileal disease although good evidence to support this is lacking [19]. Quality of life can also be improved in patients receiving EN [19] and avoidance of hospital admission is possible where EN accounts for at least 900 kcal per day [30].

Partial enteral nutrition

A novel treatment using partial EN (up to 50% energy requirements) alongside an exclusion diet has recently been shown to induce disease remission in mild to moderately active Crohn's disease in children and young adults [31]. This case series showed that 33 out of 47 patients achieved clinical remission at 6 weeks. The exclusion diet was based on whole foods but reduced food components that have been associated with dysbiosis and impair innate immune mechanisms in cell line and animal models [31]. These preliminary data are interesting and a randomised controlled trial is under way.

Partial EN providing 35–50% of energy requirements from an elemental or polymeric diet for up to 12 months may achieve remission maintenance in 42–65% of cases although evidence is limited [32,33].

Since the introduction of biological agents (e.g. anti-TNF therapy) for the management of Crohn's disease, there have been several studies investigating the use of EN alongside a biological agent, with mixed results. A meta-analysis of four studies demonstrated that partial EN alongside infliximab was more effective at inducing and maintaining disease remission for at least a year than infliximab alone [34]. The studies predominantly used elemental EN but

two also used peptide and polymeric EN and were equally as efficacious. The energy intake from EN ranged from 600 to 1500 kcal per day. All of these studies were carried out in Japan where adherence to such dietary interventions is better than in other parts of the world so whether these data can be translated into clinical practice globally is unclear.

Reintroduction diets

Following a course of exclusive EN, gradual food reintroduction provides patients with a planned structure to introduce a nutritionally complete diet as quickly as possible and identifies potentially problematic foods. The Low Fat, Fibre Limited EXclusion (LOFFLEX) diet is a widely used food reintroduction plan and 56% of patients achieve remission maintenance at 2 years [18]. The diet involves a 2–4-week food reintroduction programme, initially introducing a wide variety of foods least likely to trigger symptoms while the volume of EN is tapered down and, if symptoms do not recur, discontinued. Following this, a systematic food reintroduction process occurs with one food being reintroduced back into the diet every few days.

Ulcerative colitis

There is little evidence to support a role for EN to treat ulcerative colitis beyond achieving and maintaining nutritional status [20]. One small study in severe pouchitis demonstrated that elemental diet did not induce disease remission despite improvement in gastrointestinal microbiota and symptoms [35].

5.9.4 Long-term impact

A summary of the nutritional problems and considerations is presented in Table 5.9.1. Inflammatory bowel disease is a chronic condition and thus the majority of patients with IBD have long-standing issues with diet and nutrition and how it affects their quality of life [1,2,4,18,36]. To ensure that the long-term nutritional and dietary needs are met, it is of

Table 5.9.1 Nutritional problems and considerations

Problem	Consideration
Undernutrition	Partial or exclusive EN can be used to optimise nutritional status, particularly in presurgical patients with Crohn's disease or ulcerative colitis [7,25]
Micronutrient monitoring	Systemic inflammation affects interpretation of plasma micronutrient concentration. Micronutrient status can be reliably interpreted when: CRP <20 mg/L for zinc CRP <10 mg/L for selenium, vitamin A, vitamin D CRP <5 mg/L for vitamin B6 and vitamin C [12]
Anaemia	Anaemia of chronic disease and/or iron deficiency anaemia are common in Crohn's disease and ulcerative colitis In iron deficiency only use oral iron supplementation doses up to 60 mg elemental iron (e.g. one ferrous sulfate tablet per day) [3,13] In iron deficiency anaemia and active IBD, use intravenous iron and, if appropriate, erythropoiesis-stimulating agents [13]
Bone health	Osteoporosis is common in Crohn's disease and ulcerative colitis Monitor vitamin D and calcium intake and status; supplementation may be appropriate
Active disease	Exclusive EN is used to induce disease remission in paediatric patients with Crohn's disease as primary therapy [21] In adults with Crohn's disease exclusive EN can be used as an adjunctive therapy or primary therapy where alternative treatments have failed or are contraindicated [7,25]
Remission maintenance	Partial EN up to 50% of energy requirements for up to 12 months in Crohn's disease may be appropriate but the evidence is limited [32,33]

CRP, C-reactive protein; EN, enteral nutrition; IBD inflammatory bowel disease.

paramount importance that patients are cared for by a specialist IBD team and have access to a dietitian who can provide expertise on all aspects of nutrition support and dietary management in IBD [37].

References

1. Lomer MC. Dietary and nutritional considerations for inflammatory bowel disease. *Proc Nutr Soc* 2011; **70**(3): 329–335.
2. Prince A, Whelan K, Moosa A, Lomer MC, Reidlinger DP. Nutritional problems in inflammatory bowel disease: the patient perspective. *J Crohns Colitis* 2011; **5**(5): 443–450.
3. Massironi S, Rossi RE, Cavalcoli FA, Della Valle S, Fraquelli M, Conte D. Nutritional deficiencies in inflammatory bowel disease: therapeutic approaches. *Clin Nutr* 2013; **32**(6): 904–910.
4. Ghosh S, Mitchell R. Impact of inflammatory bowel disease on quality of life: results of the European Federation of Crohn's and Ulcerative Colitis Associations (EFCCA) patient survey. *J Crohns Colitis* 2007; **1**(1): 10–20.
5. Hughes LD, King L, Morgan M, et al. Food-related quality of life in inflammatory bowel disease: development and validation of a questionnaire. *J Crohns Colitis* 2016; **10**(2): 194–201.
6. Mijac DD, Jankovic GL, Jorga J, Krstic MN. Nutritional status in patients with active inflammatory bowel disease: prevalence of malnutrition and methods for routine nutritional assessment. *Eur J Intern Med* 2010; **21**(4): 315–319.
7. Spinelli A, Allocca M, Jovani M, Danese S. Review article: optimal preparation for surgery in Crohn's disease. *Aliment Pharmacol Ther* 2014; **40**(9): 1009–1022.
8. Bryant RV, Trott MJ, Bartholomeusz FD, Andrews JM. Systematic review: body composition in adults with inflammatory bowel disease. *Aliment Pharmacol Ther* 2013; **38**(3): 213–225.
9. Gerasimidis K, Talwar D, Duncan A, et al. Impact of exclusive enteral nutrition on body composition and circulating micronutrients in plasma and erythrocytes of children with active Crohn's disease. *Inflamm Bowel Dis* 2012; **18**(9): 1672–1681.
10. Lomer MC, Gourgey R, Whelan K. Current practice in relation to nutritional assessment and dietary management of enteral nutrition in adults with Crohn's disease. *J Hum Nutr Diet* 2014; **27**(Suppl 2): 28–35.

11. Gerasimidis K. Inflammatory bowel disease: nutritional consequences. In: Lomer M, editor. Advanced Nutrition and Dietetics in Gastroenterology. Chichester: Wiley–Blackwell, 2014, pp. 180–190.

12. Duncan A, Talwar D, McMillan DC, Stefanowicz F, O'Reilly DS. Quantitative data on the magnitude of the systemic inflammatory response and its effect on micronutrient status based on plasma measurements. *Am J Clin Nutr* 2012; **95**(1): 64–71.

13. Dignass AU, Gasche C, Bettenworth D, et al. European consensus on the diagnosis and management of iron deficiency and anaemia in inflammatory bowel diseases. *J Crohns Colitis* 2015; **9**(3): 211–222.

14. Lomer MC, Kodjabashia K, Hutchinson C, Greenfield SM, Thompson RP, Powell JJ. Intake of dietary iron is low in patients with Crohn's disease: a case-control study. *Br J Nutr* 2004; **91**(1): 141–148.

15. Powell JJ, Cook WB, Chatfield M, Hutchinson C, Pereira D, Lomer MC. Iron status is inversely associated with dietary iron intakes in patients with inactive or mildly active inflammatory bowel disease. *Nutr Metab* 2013; **10**(1): 18.

16. Lomer MC, Cook WB, Jan-Mohamed HJ, et al. Iron requirements based upon iron absorption tests are poorly predicted by haematological indices in patients with inactive inflammatory bowel disease. *Br J Nutr* 2012; **107**(12): 1806–1811.

17. Etzel JP, Larson MF, Anawalt BD, Collins J, Dominitz JA. Assessment and management of low bone density in inflammatory bowel disease and performance of professional society guidelines. *Inflamm Bowel Dis* 2011; **17**(10): 2122–2129.

18. Lee J, Allen R, Ashley S, Becker S, et al. British Dietetic Association evidence-based guidelines for the dietary management of Crohn's disease in adults. *J Hum Nutr Diet* 2014; **27**(3): 207–218.

19. Zachos M, Tondeur M, Griffiths AM. Enteral nutritional therapy for induction of remission in Crohn's disease. *Cochrane Database Sys Rev* 2007; **1**: CD000542.

20. O'Sullivan M, Raftery T. Inflammatory bowel disease: dietary management. In: Lomer M, editor. Advanced Nutrition and Dietetics in Gastroenterology. Chichester: Wiley-Blackwell, 2014, pp. 191–201.

21. Day AS, Whitten KE, Sidler M, Lemberg DA. Systematic review: nutritional therapy in paediatric Crohn's disease. *Aliment Pharmacol Ther* 2008; **27**(4): 293–307.

22. Li G, Ren J, Wang G, et al. Preoperative exclusive enteral nutrition reduces the postoperative septic complications of fistulizing Crohn's disease. *Eur J Clin Nutr* 2014; **68**(4): 441–446.

23. Guo Z, Guo D, Gong J, et al. Preoperative nutritional therapy reduces the risk of anastomotic leakage in patients with Crohn's disease requiring resections. *Gastroenterol Res Pract* 2016; Article ID 5017856.

24. Li Y, Zuo L, Zhu W, et al. Role of exclusive enteral nutrition in the preoperative optimization of patients with Crohn's disease following immunosuppressive therapy. *Medicine* 2015; **94**(5): e478.

25. Dignass A, van Assche G, Lindsay JO, et al. The second European evidence-based consensus on the diagnosis and management of Crohn's disease: current management. *J Crohns Colitis* 2010; **4**(1): 28–62.

26. Forbes A, Escher J, Hebuterne X, et al. ESPEN guideline: clinical nutrition in inflammatory bowel disease. *Clin Nutr* 2017; **36**(2): 321–347.

27. Heerasing N, Thompson B, Hendy P, et al. Exclusive enteral nutrition provides an effective bridge to safer interval elective surgery for adults with Crohn's disease. *Aliment Pharmacol Ther* 2017; **45**(5): 660–669.

28. Patel KV, Darakhshan AA, Griffin N, Williams AB, Sanderson JD, Irving PM. Patient optimization for surgery relating to Crohn's disease. *Nat Rev Gastroenterol Hepatol* 2016; **13**(12): 707–719.

29. Day AS, Burgess L. Exclusive enteral nutrition and induction of remission of active Crohn's disease in children. *Expert Rev Clin Immunol* 2013; **9**(4): 375–383; quiz 384.

30. Watanabe O, Ando T, Ishiguro K, et al. Enteral nutrition decreases hospitalization rate in patients with Crohn's disease. *J Gastroenterol Hepatol* 2010; **25**(Suppl 1): S134–137.

31. Sigall-Boneh R, Pfeffer-Gik T, Segal I, Zangen T, Boaz M, Levine A. Partial enteral nutrition with a Crohn's disease exclusion diet is effective for induction of remission in children and young adults with Crohn's disease. *Inflamm Bowel Dis* 2014; **20**(8): 1353–1360.

32. Akobeng AK, Thomas AG. Enteral nutrition for maintenance of remission in Crohn's disease. *Cochrane Databse Sys Rev* 2007; **3**: CD005984.

33. Yamamoto T, Nakahigashi M, Umegae S, Matsumoto K. Enteral nutrition for the maintenance of remission in Crohn's disease: a systematic review. *Eur J Gastroenterol Hepatol* 2010; **22**(1): 1–8.

34. Nguyen DL, Palmer LB, Nguyen ET, McClave SA, Martindale RG, Bechtold ML. Specialized enteral nutrition therapy in Crohn's disease patients on maintenance infliximab therapy: a meta-analysis. *Therap Adv Gastroenterol* 2015; **8**(4): 168–175.

35. McLaughlin SD, Culkin A, Cole J, et al. Exclusive elemental diet impacts on the gastrointestinal microbiota and improves symptoms in patients with chronic pouchitis. *J Crohns Colitis* 2013; **7**(6): 460–466.

36. Hughes L, King L, Morgan M, et al. Food-related quality of life in inflammatory bowel disease: development and validation of a questionnaire. *J Crohn's Colitis* 2016; **10**: 194–201.

37. National Institute for Health and Care Excellence. Inflammatory Bowel Disease Quality Standard (QS81). London: NICE, 2015.

Chapter 5.10

Nutrition support in intestinal failure

Alison Culkin
St Mark's Hospital, Harrow, UK

5.10.1 Introduction

All patients with intestinal failure (IF) will need parenteral support (PS) but the route, type and duration of treatment will depend on the type of IF the patient experiences.

Definition and classification

Several definitions and classifications of IF have been reported in the literature over the last 40 years. Recently, the European Society of Parenteral and Enteral Nutrition (ESPEN) agreed a formal definition and classification and defined IF as 'the reduction of GI function below the minimum necessary for the absorption of macronutrients and/or water and electrolytes, such that intravenous supplementation is required to maintain health and/or growth' [1]. Patients who do not require parenteral nutrition (PN) are now considered to experience 'intestinal insufficiency'. The classification has been agreed utilizing functional, pathophysiological and clinical parameters.

The functional classification of IF is based on the onset, metabolic and expected outcomes and remains similar to previous reports (Box 5.10.1). The pathophysiological classification falls into five major conditions. The clinical classification is based on the volume and energy requirement of intravenous supplementation and contains 16 subtypes ranging from 0 kcal/kg/day and ≤1000 mL/day up to >20 kcal/kg/day and

>3000 mL/day [1]. Citrulline is a non-essential amino acid produced by the enterocytes of the small intestine, a marker of enterocyte mass, but has not been included by ESPEN. A study of 82 patients with <200 cm of small bowel 2 years post resection found plasma citrulline concentration significantly correlated with length of small bowel. Plasma concentrations of <20 μmol/L were prognostic of type 3 patients requiring long-term PN [2]. Type 1 and 2 are often referred to as acute intestinal failure. The prevalence is not known but estimates range from 10% to 15% of patients undergoing intestinal surgery in the UK [3]; worldwide data are unknown.

The Association of Surgeons of Great Britain and Ireland has published good principles on the management of patients with acute IF which include information on prevention and treatment. The detection and management of abdominal sepsis is a priority as this is the most common cause of death if not aggressively managed [3]. The introduction of enhanced recovery after surgery (ERAS) moderates the metabolic effects of surgery and prevents fluid and sodium overload and may minimise the development of type 1 IF in the future [4]. The worldwide incidence of type 3 IF remains unknown. Data collected as part of the British Artificial Nutrition Survey (BANS) estimate a prevalence of 10 per million which is likely to be an underestimate due to the voluntary nature of reporting [5]. Patients with type 3 are those requiring long-term parenteral support, usually at home.

Advanced Nutrition and Dietetics in Nutrition Support, First Edition. Edited by Mary Hickson and Sara Smith.
© 2018 John Wiley & Sons Ltd. Published 2018 by John Wiley & Sons Ltd.

Box 5.10.1 ESPEN recommendations: definition and classification of intestinal failure

Definition

Intestinal failure is defined as the reduction of GI function below the minimum necessary for the absorption of macronutrients and/or water and electrolytes, such that intravenous supplementation is required to maintain health and/or growth.

The reduction of GI absorptive function that doesn't require intravenous supplementation to maintain health and/or growth can be considered as 'intestinal insufficiency' (or 'intestinal deficiency' for those languages where 'insufficiency' and 'failure' have the same meaning).

Functional classification

On the basis of onset, metabolic and expected outcome criteria, intestinal failure is classified as:

- Type I – acute, short-term and usually self-limiting condition
- Type II – prolonged acute condition, often in metabolically unstable patients, requiring complex multidisciplinary care and intravenous supplementation over periods of weeks or months
- Type III – chronic condition, in metabolically stable patients, requiring intravenous supplementation over months or years. It may be reversible or irreversible.

Pathophysiological classification

Intestinal failure can be classified into five major pathophysiological conditions, which may originate from various gastrointestinal or systemic diseases:

- short bowel
- intestinal fistula
- intestinal dysmotility
- mechanical obstruction
- extensive small bowel mucosal disease.

Clinical classification of chronic intestinal failure

On the basis of the requirements for energy and the volume of the intravenous supplementation (IV), chronic intestinal failure is categorized into 16 subtypes.

IV energy supplementation[b] (kcal/kg body weight)	Volume of the IV supplementation[a] (mL)			
	≤1000 [1]	1001–2000 [2]	2001–3000 [3]	>3000 [4]
0 (A)	A1	A2	A3	A4
1–10 (B)	B1	B2	B3	B4
11–20 (C)	C1	C2	C3	C4
> 20 (D)	D1	D2	D3	D4

[a] Calculated as daily mean of the total volume infused per week=(volume per day of infusion×number of infusions per week)/7.
[b] Calculated as daily mean of the total energy infused per week=(energy per day of infusion×number of infusions per week)/7/kg.
Source: Reproduced with permission of the BMJ Publishing Group.

Consequences of short bowel intestinal failure

Patients with short bowel will have difficulties maintaining fluid and electrolyte balance, predominantly in the immediate postoperative period, with nutritional requirements increased as a result of malabsorption. The consequences of intestinal resection are dependent on the extent and site of resection plus the integrity and adaptation of the remaining bowel. Outcome post resection depends on the length of bowel remaining, with a residual small bowel length of

<200 cm considered short bowel which can lead to nutritional, fluid and electrolyte depletion if not adequately managed. It has been proposed that the following lengths of small bowel are required to avoid home parenteral nutrition, fluid and electrolytes [6]:

- >100 cm jejunum
- >75 cm jejunum
- >50 cm jejunum plus colon.

Prevalence of undernutrition

The prevalence of undernutrition in patients with type 1 and 2 IF is difficult to estimate as although it is usual for weight and/or body mass index (BMI) to be reported in clinical trials investigating PN, detailed information on body composition is rarely described.

A study of 56 patients with type 1 IF requiring PN for a mean length of 9 days demonstrated moderate or severe undernutrition in over half of patients using Subjective Global Assessment (SGA), Patient Generated SGA and the Nutrition Risk Screening 2002 questionnaire (NRS) [7]. A national IF unit in the UK reported that two-thirds of patients admitted had a BMI of <18.5 kg/m² [8]. Assessment of the nutritional status of 72 patients admitted to another UK IF unit demonstrated that 58% were undernourished or at risk of undernutrition on admission according to national guidelines [9]. Despite a mean BMI of 22.7 ± 5.5 kg/m², a wide range was observed (13.8–39 kg/m²) demonstrating the heterogeneity of patients experiencing IF [10]. Only a quarter of patients had a BMI <18.5 kg/m² in comparison to the study by Lal et al. [8], which may reflect improved care of patients receiving PN over the years. Mean percentage weight loss was 9.4% (range 0–35%) over the previous 3–6 months, mid-arm muscle circumference (MAMC) was <5th centile in 29% and handgrip dynamometry was below 85% of normal, indicating low lean body mass and poor functional capacity respectively [10]. Therefore, identification and treatment of undernutrition in this patient population are paramount as they are unable to rely on gastrointestinal function to meet nutritional requirements.

The negative impact of undernutrition on mortality in patients with fistulas is well known, with fistulas of the small bowel more likely to result in death compared to those arising from the colon [11].

Patients with type 3 IF on home parenteral nutrition (HPN) are often well nourished with a normal BMI after a period of repletion in hospital and years on HPN [12], in comparison with type 1 and 2 patients receiving PN in hospital. However, an observational study demonstrated that 34% of patients who had been on HPN a mean of 48 ± 36 months had a BMI <20 kg/m² with 30% having a MAMC <5th centile [13]. Nutritional status can deteriorate further during weaning from HPN and therefore close monitoring is an ongoing requirement [14].

Disease-specific causes of undernutrition

The causes of undernutrition in IF are multifactorial and include underlying inflammation (i.e. Crohn's disease, radiation enteritis); a lack of absorptive surface (short bowel, fistula); sepsis resulting in increased requirements; catheter-related bloodstream infection resulting in cessation of PN; nutrient losses from stomas/fistula/wounds [11,15]. All of these factors can result in significant underfeeding of patients if preventive measures are not taken, leading to poor outcomes including impaired wound healing, infections and reduced survival, especially in patients with an open abdomen.

Nutritional assessment and diagnosis of undernutrition

A thorough nutrition assessment is required at baseline as patients with IF can become dehydrated, electrolyte depleted and undernourished rapidly. This should be repeated regularly to assess the effectiveness of nutrition intervention.

Anthropometry

An accurate height and weight to calculate BMI and percentage weight loss over 3–6 months will help determine a baseline nutritional status. It is worth noting that if a patient is dehydrated or overhydrated then their weight may be several kilograms below or above their actual weight and this should be taken into account when assessing nutritional status and calculating requirements. Due to the significant fluid shifts experienced by patients, it is best practice to measure mid upper arm circumference and tricep skinfold thickness to calculate MAMC in order to monitor changes in body composition in response to nutrition support. Handgrip is also valuable in determining functional capacity. MAMC and handgrip should be repeated monthly in hospital in order to detect any deterioration in nutritional status so that amendments to nutrition support can be instigated [8]. It has also been demonstrated that ideal body weight is able to better predict resting energy expenditure compared to actual weight in malnourished patients with short bowel [16].

Biochemistry

It is important to identify and understand the underlying cause of any deranged biochemistry in relation to fluid balance. Electrolytes such as potassium, calcium and phosphate may be elevated due to dehydration whereas sodium and magnesium may be low due to excessive losses from the gastrointestinal tract. Urea and creatinine may be low in patients with reduced muscle mass and therefore dehydration can be difficult to identify [17]. A random urine sodium concentration of <20 mmol/L is a useful early warning sign that patients are becoming sodium depleted and dehydrated [18]. Patients with short bowel and a high-output stoma or fistula or profuse diarrhoea are at risk of micronutrient deficiencies and are likely to need parenteral replacement due to impaired absorption. A micronutrient screen including folate, iron, ferritin, selenium, zinc, copper, vitamins B12, A, D and E should be performed at baseline. It may be prudent to delay until CRP is <20 mg/L to avoid the influence of the acute phase response on serum concentrations [19].

No international guideline exists regarding the frequency of monitoring and replacement and therefore clinicians will need to establish protocols until robust evidence becomes available.

> **Box 5.10.2** Clinical assessment in intestinal failure
>
> - Physical assessment for dehydration and undernutrition
> - Symptoms including thirst, nausea, vomiting, pain, lethargy, dizziness, dry flaky skin
> - Fluid balance
> - Poor dentition can affect digestion and result in undigested food or blockage of stoma and fistula appliances
> - Signs and symptoms of micronutrient and/or essential fatty acid deficiency [20,21]
> - Mobility
> - Urinalysis to monitor for ketones, glucose, leucocytes and nitrates
> - Review of medications, including any over-the-counter or herbal preparations which may increase intestinal losses, e.g. medications containing sorbitol
> - Signs of sepsis

Essential fatty acid deficiency can occur in patients on lipid-free PN but can be prevented if 500 mL of lipid is infused once a week [20].

Clinical

The clinical assessment should, in view of the potential complications, incorporate the aspects outlined in Box 5.10.2 [19].

Dietary

A detailed diet history is required in order to establish the type and amounts of food consumed, eating patterns, food and fluid preferences, any modifications in diet or nutrition support previously tried including route, rate and formula and reason for failure to avoid the parenteral route. Dietary management of short bowel is complex and discussed in greater detail elsewhere [22].

Environment

The short bowel IF protocol is complex and a great deal of explanation, understanding and motivation is required to enable patients to maintain the protocol once discharged from hospital. Adherence to the protocol can result in reductions in parenteral dependence [23] and should be reinforced at every opportunity. Despite being a life-saving treatment for patients, Home parenteral nutrition (HPN) is known to adversely affect quality of life. A systematic review of 26 studies found that quality of life was similar to patients on dialysis, with fatigue, depression, anxiety and fear of complications common issues [24]. The development of a HPN-specific quality of life tool will enable future research in this area [25].

5.10.2 Nutrition interventions

Parenteral nutrition

Parenteral nutrition is a life-saving therapy for patients with IF. However, avoiding life-threatening complications is essential when providing PN. A UK report which aimed to audit the care process of 877 patients receiving PN in UK hospitals found good practice in only 19% (n = 171) [26]. Of the patients audited, 71% were experiencing IF including those with postoperative ileus, surgical complications, bowel obstruction, fistula and a leaking or perforated gastrointestinal tract. Inadequate consideration of enteral nutrition was found in 32.7%, with PN administered in patients considered not to be experiencing IF in 29%. There was an unreasonable delay in recognising the requirement for PN and starting PN in 16% and 6% of patients respectively. The study found that 39% of patients developed metabolic complications during PN administration, with hypophosphataemia and hypokalaemia the most common, and 49% avoidable with improved monitoring preferably from a dedicated nutrition support team. Furthermore, 15.5% were managed inappropriately after identification and the authors speculated that this was due to lack of knowledge or poor clinical care. These findings support the requirement for a thorough assessment by healthcare professionals who are familiar with PN and regular monitoring to minimise the risk of metabolic complications.

Hepatic complications

It is common for patients receiving short-term PN to develop abnormal liver function tests

---

Box 5.10.3 Patient-related factors

- Sepsis and inflammation
- Medication
- Underlying disease including liver and biliary disease
- Lack of enteral stimulation
- Bacterial overgrowth/translocation
- Bile acid secretion/composition

(LFTs). Abnormal LTFs have been reported in 25–100% of patients receiving PN [27]. PN is often prescribed for the sickest patients in hospitals and therefore abnormal LFTs are usually multifactorial in aetiology. A study by Baker and Nightingale (28) observed that 34% of patients already had pre-existing abnormal LFTs before the initiation of PN, with the presence of sepsis a major contributory factor. There are several factors which can contribute to the development of abnormal LFTs and they can be divided into two main aspects: patient related (Box 5.10.3) and parenteral nutrition related.

All of the factors in Box 5.10.3 need to be regularly reviewed and addressed in order to prevent and treat abnormal liver function. It is usual that once sepsis is identified and treated, abnormalities in liver function resolve.

The main PN-related causes are excessive glucose provision and excessive lipid provision. Previous reports have demonstrated that providing excess glucose and/or lipid can result in abnormal liver function [29]. Providing excessive glucose often results in steatosis whereby an excess of lipid can lead to cholestasis. Therefore, it is essential that an adequate assessment of energy requirements is completed to prevent overfeeding from either of these macronutrients.

The American Society of Parenteral and Enteral Nutrition (ASPEN) published a position paper in 2012 on the role of alternative lipid emulsions in PN due to concerns regarding the use of lipids high in potentially proinflammatory ω-6 fatty acids. They concluded that lipid emulsions containing significant amounts of anti-inflammatory and antioxidant ω-3 fatty acids will improve clinical outcomes [30]. A meta-analysis of lipid emulsions containing fish oil compared to standard emulsions demonstrated reduced length of stay and infections, and improvement in LFTs in postoperative surgical patients [31]. However, the number of patients with IF included in these trials is difficult to determine as although they included abdominal and gastrointestinal surgery, the diagnosis of IF and the requirement for PN are unknown.

Cyclical PN is also recommended to minimise abnormal LFTs, allow rehabilitation and enable monitoring if a patient requires HPN. Recommendations that cyclical PN is not stopped abruptly due to fear of hypoglycaemia are usually unfounded and a review including four studies comparing abrupt cessation verses gradually tapered PN in the short term was unable to demonstrate any adverse events [32]. More detail on complications can be found in Chapter 4.5.

Oral nutrition supplements and enteral nutrition

Oral intake, including clear liquids, can be initiated within hours after surgery in most patients undergoing colon resections [4]. The evidence is less clear after major gastrointestinal surgery where there is extensive resection of the small and large bowel, such as post resection due to mesenteric ischaemia or post fistula repair. The amount of initial oral intake should be adapted to the state of gastrointestinal function and to individual tolerance [33].

The general indications for nutrition support in surgery are for the prevention and treatment of undernutrition, that is, the correction of undernutrition before surgery and the maintenance of nutritional status after surgery, when periods of prolonged fasting and/or severe catabolism are expected. Morbidity, length of hospital stay and mortality are considered principal outcome parameters when evaluating the benefits of nutrition support [33]. After a small bowel resection, the GI tract undergoes adaptation, a process which is stimulated by the presence of nutrients in the gastrointestinal lumen. Therefore, the introduction of oral or enteral nutrition as soon as possible is of paramount importance [34]. The choice of formula is less clear due to a lack of randomised controlled trials (RCTs) (Table 5.10.1).

Table 5.10.1 Studies investigating the effect of oral nutrition supplements and enteral formula composition in short bowel intestinal failure

Reference	Number of patients and small bowel length	Method	Type	Results
McIntyre et al. 1986 [35]	7 stoma <150 cm	RCT Orally and NGT 2–3 days	Polymeric versus elemental	No difference in absorption
Rodrigues et al. 1989 [37]	4 stoma 1 JCA & 1 JRA 30–120 cm	RCT Oral 1 day	Fibre-containing versus fibre-free polymeric	Increased faecal wet weight and sodium with fibre formula
Cosnes et al. 1992 [36]	6 stoma 90–150 cm	RCT NGT 3 days	Polymeric alone Semi-elemental alone	Increased nitrogen absorption
Joly et al. 2009 [38]	11 JCA 4 stoma 25–130 cm	RCT NGT 3 days	Usual diet versus usual diet and polymeric	Increased energy, nitrogen and fat absorption with usual diet and polymeric

JCA, jejunocolic anastomosis; JRA, jejunorectal anastomosis; NGT, nasogastric tube; RCT, randomised controlled trial.

In the 1970s it was presumed that patients would be incapable of digesting a polymeric formula and that improved absorption would be demonstrated using elemental formula due to the lack of digestion required. However, in a comparative study, no significant differences in macronutrient absorption were observed between elemental and polymeric formulas [35]. A comparison between polymeric verses semi-elemental formulas demonstrated considerable variation regarding absorption of macronutrients between patients [36]. Nitrogen absorption was significantly improved on semi-elemental compared to polymeric although no other differences were observed. The contrasting results between the two studies are likely to be related to the composition of formulas [35,36]. Elemental has a higher osmolality and requires larger volumes to meet estimated energy requirements compared to polymeric and therefore, it is recommended that patients receive a polymeric formula. Fibre-containing ONS are not currently recommended as compared to fibre-free ONS, they resulted in higher faecal wet weight and sodium excretion [37].

One of the few trials of enteral nutrition in short bowel investigated the effect of continuous enteral feeding, randomising patients to usual diet or usual diet plus continuous enteral feeding using a polymeric formula [38]; this demonstrated an increase in energy, nitrogen and fat absorption whilst receiving continuous enteral feeding compared to those on diet alone with no detrimental increase in intestinal output. The continuous method of feeding may improve intestinal absorption to an extent that patients no longer require PN and should, therefore, be a treatment option for all patients with short bowel. In order to reach the optimum concentration of sodium in the jejunum (90 mml/L), additional sodium chloride is required to promote absorption in the small bowel and can be added to enteral nutrition. In practice, 10 mL of 30% sodium chloride containing 50 mmol of sodium is added to 1 L of formula.

Studies investigating the optimum ONS and enteral nutrition for patients with short bowel are few in number, underpowered and often include patients with differing anatomy which may adversely affect the results due to the presence or absence of the colon as a digestive organ. There is clearly a need for RCTs in this area of nutrition support although these would be difficult due to the relatively small numbers of patients affected.

Distal feeding or fistuloclysis

Distal feeding or fistuloclysis is the infusion of enteral nutrition into the distal small bowel via a loop stoma or enterocutaneous fistula respectively, which may allow cessation of PN. It can also be used to provide trophic feeding to the distal bowel preoperatively with the aim of improving gastrointestinal function postoperatively. Refeeding enteroclysis consists of collecting chyme from the proximal stoma and reinfusion down the distal stoma. A minimum of 75 cm of healthy small bowel distal to the fistula or stoma is required in order to fully establish the patient on enteral nutrition and withdraw PN [39]. Significant improvements in liver function tests have been demonstrated using this technique and during a 12-month follow-up, mortality was lower in the fistuloclysis group compared to the control group (2.9 versus 16.7%, P = 0.045) [40]. There are no RCTs comparing different formulas for this mode of feeding. Polymeric, semi-elemental and elemental formulas have all been described in the literature.

A proposed algorithm is shown in Figure 5.10.1 as the choice of formula depends on the intended outcome for the patient and whether or not chyme is reinfused as this will contain vital pancreatic enzymes and bile which may facilitate the digestion of a whole-protein formula.

Transition from parenteral to enteral nutrition

The decision to wean PN should be made by an experienced nutrition support professional, preferably a nutrition team. A thorough assessment of nutritional status, oral or enteral intake, fluid and electrolyte balance and gastrointestinal function is essential to aid this decision. It should be done in a step-wise process, balancing the

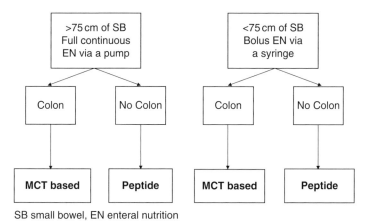

SB small bowel, EN enteral nutrition

Figure 5.10.1 Distal feeding algorithm.

need to ensure that requirements are met with the risk of malabsorption and undernutrition verses potential complications of ongoing PN [41].

There are two common approaches to weaning, a daily reduction in PN or omitting days of PN, but no clinical trials have compared these methods. Patients are usually keen to omit nights as the infusion often results in poor sleep and fatigue due to nocturia. During the early phase of weaning, it is prudent to avoid consecutive nights off to allow the patient to compensate orally. Whilst this can be done in hospital, it is frequently completed in the outpatient setting. Close attention should be paid to micronutrient status, especially B12, as many patients will have had their terminal ileum resected and regular intramuscular injections will be required to prevent pernicious anaemia. The American Gastroenterological Association has published guidelines on the provision of micronutrients in short bowel and states the importance of observing for clinical manifestation of deficiencies and regular monitoring of serum concentrations followed by suitable supplementation [42].

5.10.3 Intestinal transplantation

Patients with type 3 IF experiencing significant complications on HPN may be candidates for intestinal transplantation. Indications for intestinal transplantation vary worldwide due to differences in healthcare provision. In the USA,

the Center for Medicare and Medicaid Services has stated that transplantation is the standard of care for patients with type 3 IF with HPN, being viewed as a supportive treatment until a suitable donor can be found. In the UK and Europe, transplantation is only considered if HPN is failing due to complications such as lack of venous access, severe recurrent catheter sepsis, parenteral nutrition-related severe liver disease or poor quality of life. Survival rates are 76%, 56% and 43% at 1, 5 and 10 years respectively according to the most recent intestinal transplant registry report [43].

Strategies to reduce the indications for transplantation are of importance with interventions to improve liver function a priority as patients requiring a combined intestinal and liver transplant have a poorer outcome than those requiring intestine in isolation. Presently, the survival data comparing transplantation to HPN favour HPN, with early referral for those patients with deteriorating liver function and desmoid disease [44]. It is imperative that nutritional status is optimised before transplant as body weight can reduce by up to 25% in the first year post transplant, although this can be a challenge when liver function is deteriorating where the aim may be to avoid overfeeding [45].

There are no internationally agreed guidelines for postoperative management. Parenteral nutrition is used in the immediate postoperative stage to prevent deterioration in nutritional status and dehydration as several medications given to prevent rejection can be nephrotoxic. The early and progressive introduction of enteral nutrition using a polymeric formula is recommended in the USA once the stoma starts working, changing to a fibre-containing formula if a high output persists. Food is reintroduced 2 weeks post transplant with enteral nutrition weaned as oral intake increases to meet estimated requirements, with the ultimate aim of achieving nutritional autonomy. Long-term monitoring is important to prevent obesity and micronutrient deficiencies, especially vitamin B6 as deficiency has been demonstrated [46].

5.10.4 Future interventions

Teduglutide, an analogue of GLP-2, a peptide secreted from enteroendocrine L-cells in the distal small intestine, has been demonstrated to reduce parenteral dependence. In an international multicentre randomised placebo-controlled trial, patients with short bowel (n = 83) receiving a dose of 0.05 mg/kg/day demonstrated significant improvements in body weight and lean body mass as measured by DEXA scan, and reductions in parenteral volume, energy and frequency [47]. A short bowel syndrome quality of life questionnaire (SBS-QoL) developed in conjunction with the teduglutide trials demonstrated that reductions in parenteral support are associated with improvements in overall quality of life, including physical health, fatigue, diarrhoea/stoma output, gastrointestinal problems, sleep and social life [48].

Attempts to create intestinal tissue or an 'artificial gut' are still in their infancy and the complexities of creating an organ with all the functions of the human gastrointestinal tract (secretory, peristaltic, digestive, absorptive, hormonal and immunological) have meant that this technology remains at the experimental stage in animal models only [49]. The grafting of a tissue-engineered gastrointestinal tract would avoid complications faced after intestinal transplantation due to graft-versus-host rejection.

The ESPEN guidelines on chronic intestinal failure in adults highlight the significant lack of evidence supporting practice in this area. A total of 623 papers were identified with 16 meta-analyses and 58 RCTs. Of the 112 recommendations, the supporting evidence was high in 2%, moderate in 8%, low in 39% and very low in 51%, which reflects the difficulty of conducting quality research in a rare patient population [50].

References

1. Pironi L, Arends J, Baxter J, et al. ESPEN endorsed recommendations. Definition and classification of intestinal failure in adults. *Clin Nutr* 2015; **34**: 171–180.
2. Crenn P, Coudray-Lucas C, Thuillier F, Cynober L, Messing B. Postabsorptive plasma citrulline concentration is a marker of absorptive enterocyte mass and intestinal failure in humans. *Gastroenterology* 2000; **119**: 1496–1505.
3. Carlson G, Gardiner K, McKee R, MacFie J, Vaizey C. The Surgical Management of Patients with Acute Intestinal Failure. www.irspen.ie/wp-content/uploads/2014/10/ASGBA_The_surgical_management_of_patients_with_acute_intestinal_failure.pdf (accessed 4 September 2017).
4. Gustafsson UO, Scott MJ, Schwenke W, et al. Guidelines for perioperative care in elective colonic surgery: Enhanced Recovery After Surgery (ERAS) Society recommendations. *Clin Nutr* 2012; **31**: 783–800.
5. Smith T. Adult home parenteral nutrition (HPN). In: Smith T, editor. Annual BANS Report. Artificial Nutrition Support in the UK 2000–2010. Redditch: BAPEN, 2011, pp. 27–36.
6. Lennard-Jones JE. Review article: practical management of the short bowel. *Aliment Pharmacol Ther* 1994; **8**: 563–577.
7. Badia-Tahull MB, Cobo-Sacristán S, Leiva-Badosa E, et al. Use of subjective global assessment, patient-generated subjective global assessment and nutritional risk screening 2002 to evaluate the nutritional status of non-critically ill patients on parenteral nutrition. *Nutr Hosp* 2014; **29**: 411–419.
8. Lal S, Teubner A, Shaffer JL. Review article: intestinal failure. *Aliment Pharmacol Ther* 2006; **24**: 19–31
9. National Collaborating Centre for Acute Care. Nutrition Support in Adults. Oral Nutrition Support, Enteral Tube Feeding and Parenteral Nutrition. London: National Collaborating Centre for Acute Care.
10. Culkin A. The nutritional status and outcome of patients admitted to an intestinal failure unit. *Proc Nutr Soc* 2011; **70**(OCE5): E294.
11. Lloyd DA, Gabe SM, Windsor AC. Nutrition and management of enterocutaneous fistula. *Br J Surg* 2006; **93**: 1045–1055.

12. Van Gossum A, Vahedi K, Abdel-Malik, et al. ESPEN-HAN Working Group. Clinical, social and rehabilitation status of long-term home parenteral nutrition patients: results of a European multicentre survey. *Clin Nutr* 2001; **20**: 205–210.

13. Egger NG, Carlson GL, Shaffer JL. Nutritional status and assessment of patients on home parenteral nutrition: anthropometry, bioelectrical impedance or clinical judgement? *Nutrition* 1999; **15**: 1–6.

14. Chaer Borges V, Teixeira da Silva M de L, Gonçalves Dias MC, González MC, Linetzky Waitzberg D. Long-term nutritional assessment of patients with severe short bowel syndrome managed with home enteral nutrition and oral intake. *Nutr Hosp* 2011; **26**: 834–842.

15. Van Gossum A, Cabre E, Hébuterne X, et al. ESPEN guidelines on parenteral nutrition: gastroenterology. *Clin Nutr* 2009; **28**: 415–427.

16. Araújo EC, Suen VM, Marchini JS, Vannucchi H. Ideal weight better predicts resting energy expenditure than does actual weight in patients with short bowel syndrome. *Nutrition* 2007; **23**: 778–781.

17. Maroulis J, Kalfarentzos F. Complications of parenteral nutrition at the end of the century. *Clin Nutr* 2000; **19**: 295–304.

18. Duncan A, Talwar D, McMillan DC, Stefanowicz F, O'Reilly DS. Quantitative data on the magnitude of the systemic inflammatory response and its effect on micronutrient status based on plasma measurements. *Am J Clin Nutr* 2012; **95**: 64–71.

19. Nightingale J. Intestinal Failure. San Francisco: Greenwich Medical Media, 2001.

20. Jeppesen PB, Høy CE, Mortensen PB. Essential fatty acid deficiency in patients receiving home parenteral nutrition. *Am J Clin Nutr* 1998; **68**: 126–133.

21. Sriram K, Lonchyna VA. Micronutrient supplementation in adult nutrition therapy: practical considerations. *J Parenter Enteral Nutr* 2009; **33**: 548–562.

22. Culkin A. Intestinal failure and nutrition. In: Lomer M, editor. Advanced Nutrition and Dietetics in Gastroenterology. Chichester: Wiley-Blackwell, 2014, pp. 210–217.

23. Culkin A, Gabe SM, Madden AM. Improving clinical outcomes in patients with intestinal failure using individualised nutritional advice. *J Hum Nutr Diet* 2009; **22**: 290.

24. Huisman-de Waal G, Schoonhoven L, Jansen J, Wanten G, van Achterberg T. The impact of home parenteral nutrition on daily life – a review. *Clin Nutr* 2007; **26**: 275–288.

25. Baxter JP, Fayers PM, McKinlay AW. The clinical and psychometric validation of a questionnaire to assess the quality of life of adult patients treated with long-term parenteral nutrition. *J Parenter Enteral Nutr* 2010; **34**: 131–142.

26. Stewart JAD, Mason DG, Smith N, Protopapa K, Mason M. A Mixed Bag. An Enquiry into the Care of Hospital Patients Receiving Parenteral Nutrition. www.ncepod.org.uk/2010report1/downloads/PN_report.pdf (accessed 4 September 2017).

27. Quigley EM, Marsh MN, Shaffer JL, Markin RS. Hepatobiliary complications of total parenteral nutrition. *Gastroenterology* 1993; **104**: 286–301.

28. Baker M, Nightingale JMD. Abnormal liver function tests and parenteral nutrition. *Clin Nutr* 2004; **23**: 864.

29. Gabe SM, Culkin A. Abnormal liver function tests in the parenteral nutrition fed patient. *Frontline Gastroenterol* 2010; **1**: 98.

30. Vanek VW, Seidner DL, Allen P, Bistrian B, Collier S, Gura KM. A.S.P.E.N. Position paper: clinical role for alternative intravenous fat emulsions. *Nutr Clin Pract* 2012; **27**: 150–192.

31. Li NN, Zhou Y, Qin XP, et al. Does intravenous fish oil benefit patients post-surgery? A meta-analysis of randomised controlled trials. *Clin Nutr* 2014; **33**: 226–239.

32. Stout SM, Cober MP. Metabolic effects of cyclic parenteral nutrition infusion in adults and children. *Nutr Clin Pract* 2010; **25**: 277–281.

33. Lochs H, Dejong C, Hammarqvist F, Hebuterne X, Leon-Sanz M, Schutz T. ESPEN guidelines on enteral nutrition: gastroenterology. *Clin Nutr* 2006; **25**: 260–274.

34. Tappenden KA. Intestinal adaptation following resection. *J Parenter Enteral Nutr* 2014; **38**: S23–S31.

35. McIntyre PB, Fitchew M, Lennard-Jones JE. Patients with a high jejunostomy do not need a special diet. *Gastroenterology* 1986; **91**: 25–33.

36. Cosnes J, Evard D, Beaugerie L, Gendre JP, Le Quintrec Y. Improvement in protein absorption with a small-peptide-based diet in patients with high jejunostomy. *Nutrition* 1992; **8**: 406–411.

37. Rodrigues CA, Lennard-Jones JE, Thompson DG, Farthing MJ. The effects of octreotide, soy polysaccharide, codeine and loperamide on nutrient, fluid and electrolyte absorption in the short-bowel syndrome. *Aliment Pharmacol Ther* 1989; **3**: 159–169.

38. Joly F, Dray X, Corcos O, Barbot L, Kapel N, Messing B. Tube feeding improves intestinal absorption in short bowel syndrome patients. *Gastroenterology* 2009; **136**: 824–831.

39. Teubner A, Morrison K, Ravishankar HR, Anderson ID, Scott NA, Carlson GL. Fistuloclysis can successfully replace parenteral feeding in the nutritional support of patients with enterocutaneous fistula. *Br J Surg* 2004; **91**: 625e31.

40. Wu Y, Ren J, Wang G, et al. Fistuloclysis improves liver function and nutritional status in patients with high-output upper enteric fistula. *Gastroenterol Res Prac* 2014; **2014**: 1–10.

41. DiBaise JK, Matarese, LE, Messing B, Steiger E. Strategies for parenteral nutrition weaning in adult patients with short bowel syndrome. *J Clin Gastroenterol* 2006; **40**(Suppl 2): S94–98.

42. Buchman AL, Scolapio J, Fryer J. AGA technical review on short bowel syndrome and intestinal transplantation. *Gastroenterology* 2003; **124**: 1111–1134.

43. Grant D, Abu-Elmagd K, Mazariegos G, et al. Intestinal transplant registry report: global activity and trends. Intestinal Transplant Association. *Am J Transplant* 2015; **15**: 210–219.

44. Pironi L, Joly F, Forbes A, Colomb V, Lyszkowska M, Baxter J. Long-term follow-up of patients on home parenteral nutrition in Europe: implications for intestinal transplantation. *Gut* 2011; **60**: 17–25.

45. Middleton SJ, Pither C, Gao R, et al. Adult small intestinal and multivisceral transplantation: lessons through the "retrospecto-scope" at a single UK centre from 1991 to 2013. *Transplant Proc* 2014; **46**: 2114–2118.

46. Materese L. Nutritional interventions before and after adult intestinal transplantation: the Pittsburgh experience. *Pract Gastroenterol* 2010; Nov: 11–26.

47. Jeppesen PB, Gilroy R, Pertkiewicz M, Allard JP, Messing B, O'Keefe SJ. Randomised placebo-controlled trial of teduglutide in reducing parenteral nutrition and/or intravenous fluid requirements in patients with short bowel syndrome. *Gut* 2011; **60**: 902–914.

48. Jeppesen PB, Pertkiewicz M, Forbes A, et al. Quality of life in patients with short bowel syndrome treated with the new glucagon-like peptide-2 analogue teduglutide – analyses from a randomised, placebo-controlled study. *Clin Nutr* 2013; **32**: 713–721.

49. Nowocin AK, Southgate A, Shurey S, Sibbons P, Gabe SM, Ansari T. The development and implantation of a biologically derived allograft scaffold. *J Tissue Eng Regen Med* 2016; **10**: 140–148.

50. Pironi L, Arends J, Bozzetti F, et al. ESPEN guidelines on chronic intestinal failure in adults. *Clin Nutr* 2016; **35**: 247–307.

Chapter 5.11

Nutrition support in liver disease

Ronald L. Koretz
UCLA School of Medicine, Los Angeles, USA

5.11.1 Liver disease

Nutritional deficiencies in liver disease have been recognised for decades. This phenomenon is particularly obvious in those with decompensated cirrhosis; we have all encountered patients with large abdomens filled with litres of fluid (ascites) and marked reductions of peripheral musculature. In patients with cirrhosis, as the liver disease becomes more severe, so does the evidence of poor stores of both macro- and micronutrients [1]. It has been estimated that the prevalence of undernutrition in such patients ranges from 50% to 90% [1]. In addition, there are specific liver diseases that create certain nutrient deficiencies or have nutritional implications with regard to aetiology; these will be discussed in the material that follows.

5.11.2 Causes and consequences of undernutrition in liver disease

The proposed mechanisms that lead to these nutrient problems are discussed in detail in a review article from 2012 [1]. In summary, these mechanisms include hypermetabolism, malabsorption, altered macronutrient metabolism and poor intake. Undernutrition has been classically attributed to inadequate supplies of energy and protein. This is certainly the case when the underlying problem is famine or starvation. However, the situation becomes more complex when the manifestations of undernutrition are associated with a severe disease. Severe disease is accompanied by weight loss, decreased nutrient intake, hypermetabolism, hypoalbuminaemia, disordered immunological functioning and sarcopenia, but viewing all of this as being due to nutrient deprivation discounts the role of the underlying disease process. A new paradigm divides undernutrition according to its aetiology, into pure starvation (famine or short bowel), acute injury and chronic illness [2]. The latter two are cytokine dependent and the undernutrition is largely attributable to the underlying disease rather than to a lack of nutrients.

It has been well established that patients with cirrhosis and evidence of nutrient deficiency have poorer long-term clinical outcomes [1.3]. The excess morbidity, mortality and costs observed in these undernourished patients have been attributed to the poorer nutritional status [3]. However, it must be remembered that association cannot establish causation. The poorer prognosis and poorer nutritional status may both simply represent the presence of more advanced disease; if so, simply providing nutrients may not improve the prognosis [4].

5.11.3 Nutritional assessment of patients with liver disease

Assessment of undernutrition should employ the recently developed paradigm [5]. Serum albumin and prealbumin, negative nitrogen balance and increased resting energy are manifestations

Advanced Nutrition and Dietetics in Nutrition Support, First Edition. Edited by Mary Hickson and Sara Smith.
© 2018 John Wiley & Sons Ltd. Published 2018 by John Wiley & Sons Ltd.

of disease processes. Tests of nutritional status are limited to history of energy intake, weight loss, loss of muscle mass and/or subcutaneous fat, and fluid accumulation. Patients with end-stage liver disease (decompensated cirrhosis and/or hepatocellular carcinoma) present further challenges in this paradigm. The serum albumin concentration depends on the hepatocyte's capacity to manufacture this protein. Anthropometrics and body weight are complicated by ascites and peripheral oedema. Thus nutritional assessment is challenging in patients with end-stage liver disease.

On the other hand, why even assess such patients? At this stage of the liver disease, the prognosis is obviously poor without liver transplantation. If assessment is being done to identify candidates for nutrition support, what is the evidence that that intervention is helpful? We will discuss the randomised clinical trials (RCTs) comparing some form of artificial nutrition (oral nutritional supplements (ONS), enteral nutrition (EN) or parenteral nutrition (PN)) to no such therapy in the section that follows.

5.11.4 Nutrition support in liver disease

Oral diet

Late-evening feeding for patients with cirrhosis

It is believed that patients with cirrhosis more rapidly exhaust glucose stores (or have less available) and begin to burn fat for energy earlier than do normal individuals [6]. It has been speculated that late-evening feeding may allow them to 'normalise' energy consumption and reduce protein catabolism for gluconeogenesis. A number of RCTs summarised in Table 5.11.1 have addressed various aspects of 'late-evening feeding' [7–16] but none of the trials were at low risk of bias. The late-evening feedings appeared to improve a number of surrogate outcomes, although there was not a consistent effect on the same outcome when it was assessed in more than one RCT. On the other hand, there was no

convincing effect of this intervention with regard to improving mortality or morbidity. Thus, while there is much enthusiasm for providing late-evening feeding, the available data from RCTs cannot support such a recommendation.

Sodium restriction for ascites and oedema in decompensated cirrhosis

Since patients with ascites due to cirrhosis retain sodium, sodium-restricted diets are commonly prescribed [17]. In 1978 Reynolds et al. compared the use of an 'unrestricted' (albeit in a hospital setting) salt diet and less intense diuresis to a 250 mg/day sodium diet and more vigorous diuretic use [18]. The former patients were less likely to develop hyponatraemia and azotaemia as well as fewer episodes of hepatic encephalopathy. The downside to this regimen was patient dissatisfaction with the residual ascites and more diuretic use than might otherwise have been needed to reach whatever goal was intended. The actual amount of sodium consumed by the unrestricted patients was not reported and this management was not tested in outpatients.

A French trial employed the same diuretic regimen in patients consuming restricted (500 mg sodium/day) or unrestricted (not stated) sodium diets for 1 month [19]. No differences were seen in the incidences of total or partial ascites resolution. This French group then undertook a similar trial for 3 months [20]. Those consuming the higher sodium diet (not precisely stated, but probably 1–2 g/day during the 2-week period of hospitalisation) had a slower diuretic response and less improvement in their appetites in the first 14 days, but no significant differences were seen with regard to survival, duration of hospitalisation, cost, ascites resolution, appetite or nutritional status after 3 months. The investigators concluded in both trials that no benefit was observed with the unrestricted diet.

Finally an Italian group compared a 1 g to a 3 g sodium diet [21]. The ascites outcomes were similar and there were no differences in diuretic usage.

Table 5.11.1 Use of late-evening (nocturnal) feeding in cirrhosis

Comparison	Study	Nature of late-evening feeding	Control group feeding	Duration of trial	Surrogate outcomes assessed*	Clinical outcomes assessed*
Late-evening feeding *vs* no intervention	Swart 1989 [7]	4–6 meals daily	Breakfast, lunch, dinner	7 days	Nitrogen balance better	None described
	Yamanaka-Okumura 2010 [11]	Food at night	No food at night	12 months	1. No difference in weight, fat-free mass 2. No difference in prothrombin time, bilirubin, serum albumin, serum lipids, haemogram	1. Quality of life score improved in 1/8 domains at end of trial 2. No episodes of ascites in either group
	Morihara 2012 [12]	BCAA-enriched nutritional supplement at night	No supplement	12 weeks	1. Better serum albumin 2. No difference in serum bilirubin or prothrombin time	1. Better Child–Pugh score 2. No episodes of liver failure (encephalopathy, refractory ascites or Child–Pugh score ≥12) in either group 3. No apparent hepatocellular carcinoma recurrence in either group† (such patients were to be dropped out, but no dropouts in trial)
	Hou 2013 [15]	Lotus root starch supplement at night	No supplement	2 weeks	1. Higher resting energy expenditure 2. Higher respiratory quotient (suggesting more carbohydrate and less fat metabolism) 3. No differences in serum albumin, bilirubin, or MELD score	None described
Late-evening feeding *vs* daytime feeding	Fukushima 2003 [8]	BCAAs (4 g in morning, 8 g at night	BCAAs (4 g in morning, 4 g during day, and 4 g at night)	6 months	1. Serum albumin better 2. Serum bilirubin, prothrombin time, and serum ammonia not different	No episodes of ascites, encephalopathy, variceal bleeding, or need for hospitalisation in either group during trial
	Plank 2008 [10]	Nutritional supplement at night	Nutritional supplement during day	12 months	1. Improved fat-free mass and total body protein 2. No difference in plasma growth hormone, insulin-like growth factor-1 or its binding protein	No significant differences in mortality, liver transplantation or complications between the groups

(Continued)

Table 5.11.1 (Continued)

Comparison	Study	Nature of late-evening feeding	Control group feeding	Duration of trial	Surrogate outcomes assessed*	Clinical outcomes assessed*
	Nagata 2012 [13]	BCAAs (12 g during the day and 12 g at night	Mixed amino acids containing 5 g BCAAs (frequency of administration not provided)	6 months	Better serum albumin, total serum proteins, and body mass index	None described
	Tenda 2013 [14]	BCAA/L-ornithine L-aspartate combination in late evening	BCAA/L-ornithine L-aspartate combination during day	1 month	1. Better mid-arm muscle circumference, serum pre-albumin 2. Better critical flicker frequency test[§] 3. No difference in subjective global assessment	No comment in abstract regarding any episodes of frank encephalopathy
	Hidaka 2013 [16]	BCAAs (4 g after breakfast, 8 g before bedtime)	BCAAs (4 g after breakfast, lunch, and dinner)	3 months	No differences in serum albumin or bilirubin	1. Improvements in leg cramps in both groups, but no significant difference between groups 2. Quality of life scores improved in control group, but not in treatment group
Different late-evening feedings	Nakaya 2007 [9]	BCAA-enriched nutritional supplement at night	Food at night	3 months	Improved serum albumin	1. Quality of life improved in both groups with no significant differences between them 2. No differences in mortality or hepatic decompensation events

BCAA, branched-chain amino acid.

* Outcomes expressed in terms of effect on group labelled as 'nature of late-evening feeding' compared to control group.

[†] All patients recently treated for hepatocellular carcinoma.

[§] Surrogate marker for encephalopathy (all patients had subclinical hepatic encephalopathy).

None of these RCTs [18–21]was at low risk of bias. Also none of the patients had severe refractory ascites, so the data are not applicable to any patients with cirrhosis so severe that transplantation is going to be considered.

Sodium restriction in the patient with early decompensated cirrhosis has no well-established evidence base. Even if there was no advantage to more liberal sodium intake, there was no apparent disadvantage either. None of the trials was powered to show equivalency, or even non-inferiority. However, in the absence of well-designed and conducted RCTs to address this issue, it is unlikely that our current practice of sodium restriction is going to change.

Protein restriction in hepatic encephalopathy

Uncontrolled observations in the mid-20th century led to a practice of prescribing low-protein diets to patients with hepatic encephalopathy [22]. With the enthusiastic advent of nutrition support and a focus on 'undernutrition' in patients with end-stage liver disease, more recent concerns have arisen that protein deprivation was worsening the process. Unfortunately, only one RCT has been published [23]. In that trial, 30 cirrhotic patients admitted with acute episodes of encephalopathy and placed on enteral nutrition were randomised to a restricted protein formula (beginning with no protein and progressively advancing the protein content to 1.2 g/kg/day over the next 2 weeks) or a full protein (presumably 1.2 g/kg/day from the first day) formula. No differences were seen with regard to mortality, recovery from the encephalopathy, plasma ammonia, prothrombin time, bilirubin or serum albumin.

Based on this single RCT (which was not at low risk of bias and was small in size), recommendations have since appeared stressing the importance of maintaining protein intake, even in the face of encephalopathy [24]. From an evidence perspective, the question is still unresolved; the bias derived from old observational studies appears to have been replaced by the bias of individuals who are more focused on nutrition support.

Animal versus vegetable protein in hepatic encephalopathy

The use of vegetable rather than animal protein in cirrhotic patients with chronic encephalopathy is often recommended. Seven small cross-over trials (not all necessarily randomised) have addressed this issue and are summarised in Table 5.11.2 [25–31]. The earliest study showed dramatic differences in both the grade of encephalopathy and protein tolerance [25]. Unfortunately, the subsequent studies failed to validate these initial observations on both surrogate outcomes (EEG, psychometric tests, nitrogen balance, asterixis) and the grade of the encephalopathy.

The theoretical benefits from vegetable protein have been attributed to multiple factors. These include reduced amounts of methionine and mercaptan [25], increased amounts of BCAAs [26,27], better glucose metabolism [30] and increased amounts of fibre with consequent effects on stool pH and the colonic bacterial population [31].

While enthusiasm has been expressed for a policy of substituting vegetable protein for animal protein [32,33], the evidence does not seem to be as strong as the opinion.

Artificial nutrition

In 2012, we published a Cochrane systematic review that addressed the use of PN, EN or ONS in patients with liver disease [34]; 37 RCTs were included that compared one of these interventions to no nutritional therapy in patients with various liver diseases. Since then, three other RCTs [35–37] have been identified and are discussed here. Only one of these 40 trials [38] was at low risk of bias.

Oral nutrition supplements

Twenty RCTs assessed the use of ONS (namely, formulations containing at least a source of nitrogen and non-nitrogenous energy and consumed voluntarily by patients) [6,9]. Nine of these trials were conducted in cirrhotic patients [34]. In all but one of them [39], no effect was seen on mortality, hepatic morbidity, infections,

Table 5.11.2 Vegetable versus animal protein in cirrhosis and chronic encephalopathy

Study	Design	Number participants	Surrogate outcomes*	Clinical outcomes*	Comments
Greenberger 1977 [25]	Randomised cross-over	3 (one subject tested 3 times)	Improved EEG, arterial ammonia, fetor hepaticus, asterixis, psychometric test	Improved grade of hepatic encephalopathy	Confounded by use of lactulose and/or neomycin
Uribe 1982 [26]	Cross-over	10	Improved EEG, psychometric test. No difference – arterial ammonia	No difference – grade of hepatic encephalopathy	Sequence of protein challenges = 40 g animal, 40 g vegetable, 40 g animal, 80 g vegetable (not random)
Shaw 1983 [27]	Cross-over	5	No difference – nitrogen balance, plasma amino acids	No difference – manifestations of hepatic encephalopathy	Not stated that cross-over randomised, but different sequences in different subjects
De Bruijn 1983 [28]	Cross-over	8	Improved EEG, nitrogen balance. No difference – psychometric test	None reported	Not stated that cross-over randomised, but different sequences in different subjects
Keshavarzian 1984 [29]	Randomised cross-over	6	Improved EEG (only in 2/6 subjects)	Improved 'clinical performance' in 2/6 subjects	Only data from abstract available for analysis
Uribe 1985 [30]	Cross-over	8	No difference – asterixis, EEG, serum ammonia, psychometric test	No difference – grade of hepatic encephalopathy	Animal protein always given first. Only diabetic subjects evaluated and fasting blood sugar improved. The study was confounded by the fact that vegetable protein was supplemented with psyllium fibre and the animal protein was provided with neomycin
Bianchi 1993 [31]	Randomised cross-over	8	Improved nitrogen balance, serum ammonia, psychometric tests	? trend for better grade of hepatic encephalopathy (2 improved on vegetable protein and 1 got worse on animal protein)	No statistical analysis regarding changes in grades of hepatic encephalopathy

* Outcomes expressed as effect when vegetable protein provided compared to effect when animal protein provided.

serum bilirubin, duration of hospitalisation or quality of life scores. No cost data were available. In one trial, the use of a branched-chain amino acid (BCAA)-based preparation was more likely to lead to resolution of encephalopathy [39].

Four RCTs tested ONS in patients with hepatocellular carcinoma [34]; when the data were combined, the recipients of the intervention were less likely to develop ascites. No differences were seen with regard to intestinal bleeding, encephalopathy, infections or duration of hospitalisation; there were some equivocal benefits in some trials with regard to some aspects of quality of life scores. While no difference was seen in mortality when all the trials were combined, the single trial with low risk of bias reported that the recipients of the ONS had a significantly worse survival [38].

Two RCTs addressed ONS usage in patients undergoing liver transplantations [34]. One trial found no differences in mortality or postoperative complications and the other reported no differences in the appearance of encephalopathy. Four other RCTs assessed ONS in patients undergoing hepatic tumour resections [34]. No differences were observed in mortality or postoperative complication rates.

Finally, one RCT assessing the use of ONS and dietary counselling when hepatitis C treatment was begun found no differences in the response to antiviral therapy [37]. However, the treated patients reported better quality of life scores in this unblinded trial.

Enteral nutrition

Enteral nutrition had no effect on mortality, hepatic morbidity, infections or duration of hospitalisation in cirrhotic patients in four RCTs [34,36]; quality of life or cost data were not reported. EN had no effect on clinical outcomes in two trials of patients with alcoholic hepatitis [4]. Two small RCTs done in patients just before or after liver transplantation only reported data regarding encephalopathy, infections and duration of hospitalisation; no differences were seen [34]. One trial in patients with obstructive jaundice failed to demonstrate any differences in

mortality or individual postoperative complications, but there was a reduction in the total number of patients who had any such complication [40]. However, this observation was confounded by the fact that four sicker patients in the EN arm dropped out.

Parenteral nutrition

Four RCTs assessed PN in patients with alcoholic liver disease (alcoholic hepatitis and/or cirrhosis). PN had no effect on mortality, ascites, hepatic encephalopathy or infections [34]. No data were available regarding gastrointestinal bleeding, duration of hospitalisation or cost. PN did reduce serum bilirubin (a surrogate outcome) [34].

Parenteral nutrition was not shown to have any impact on mortality, cost, duration of hospitalisation or infections in three RCTs of patients undergoing liver transplantation [34,35]. The effect of PN on hepatic morbidity (ascites, intestinal bleeding or encephalopathy) was not reported.

Three RCTs evaluated patients undergoing various liver surgeries [34]. Only one of them described any benefit [41]; the PN recipients were less likely to develop ascites or postoperative complications. Overall, no differences were seen with regard to mortality, encephalopathy or gastrointestinal bleeding [34]. No data were available pertaining to quality of life, duration of hospitalisation or cost [34].

5.11.5 Specific aspects of nutritional management in liver disease

Branched-chain amino acids in hepatic encephalopathy

Patients with hepatic encephalopathy have low serum concentrations of BCAAs and a high ratio of aromatic amino acids to BCAAs. Since aromatic amino acids share transport mechanisms into the central nervous system, and since aromatic amino acids may be precursors of 'false neurotransmitters', the administration of BCAAs (enterally or parenterally) might ameliorate encephalopathy [42].

In the 2012 systematic review [34], BCAAs were not shown to have any beneficial effect on hepatic encephalopathy. However, only trials in which the BCAAs were part of a larger nutritional regimen were included; RCTs that tested pure BCAA supplements were excluded. A systematic review published in 2013 assessed eight RCTs of oral BCAAs (not necessarily provided as part of a nutritional supplement) [43]. When the data were combined, a beneficial effect on the clinical manifestations of hepatic encephalopathy was demonstrated; this effect was especially present in patients with overt (as opposed to subclinical or minimal) encephalopathy. The BCAAs did not have any effect on mortality, nitrogen balance or adverse events.

Thus, there is some evidence for the use of BCAAs in treating hepatic encephalopathy. However, this is a pharmacological intervention and not dependent on an entire programme of nutritional supplementation. BCAA preparations are relatively expensive and unpalatable when consumed orally, so BCAA therapy is a second-line treatment.

Non-alcoholic fatty liver disease

With the rise in the prevalence of obesity in the general population, hepatologists have become increasingly aware of non-alcoholic fatty liver disease (NAFLD). This entity is particularly associated with obesity, diabetes mellitus and hyperlipidaemia. In general, NAFLD is not considered to be a disorder that is associated with major hepatic complications. However, a minority of these patients develop non-alcoholic steatohepatitis (NASH); this lesion is very similar to alcoholic hepatitis histologically, but the patients deny significant alcohol consumption. NASH, unlike NAFLD, can progress to cirrhosis and subsequent decompensated disease. Thus, hepatologists are concerned with treatment opportunities. Unfortunately, from the perspective of evidence-based medicine, most of the RCTs that have been performed in this disorder have been relatively short term and surrogate outcomes (e.g. abnormal serum liver enzyme concentrations or liver histology) have been used to assess outcome. In this regard, vitamin E (800 IU per day) has

been shown to improve the histology in patients with NASH in a low risk of bias RCT [44].

An important consideration to make about NAFLD and NASH is that, unlike many of the other diseases that we have considered, this liver problem is not a primary hepatic one, but rather the consequence of other non-hepatic metabolic processes. In the absence of any convincing data that a liver-specific intervention will improve morbidity and/or mortality, the primary treatment should be directed at the underlying dysmetabolism (i.e. obesity, diabetes and/or hyperlipidaemia). The management of these conditions does have nutritional implications, but their discussion is beyond the scope of this chapter.

Bone disease associated with liver disease

Bone disease has been a recognised complication of cholestatic liver disease (primary biliary cirrhosis and primary sclerosing cholangitis in particular) for decades [45]. It has been attributed to multiple factors including malabsorption of fat-soluble vitamins and calcium, poor food intake and alterations in the hormone milieu. More recently, bone disease has been associated with liver disease in general [46]. The therapeutic nutritional approach has been to prescribe vitamin D and calcium [47]. However, there is only a limited evidence base that has addressed this recommendation. Four RCTs, only addressing surrogate outcomes, are summarised in Table 5.11.3 [48–51]. In two high risk of bias trials, calcium (for primary biliary cirrhosis) and 1,25 dihydroxyvitamin D (for cirrhosis) did have some benefit with regard to radiographic evidence of better bone health [48,49]. However, in two trials in inflammatory bowel disease patients [50,51], no benefit was seen from combined treatment (calcium and vitamin D). One of these trials [50] had much better methodology with regard to avoiding bias.

Given the lack of any indication that this intervention causes harm as well as its relatively low cost, it is likely that clinicians will continue to prescribe maintenance vitamin D and calcium for the foreseeable future.

Table 5.11.3 Calcium and/or vitamin D for liver disease-associated bone disease

Study	Liver disease	Intervention	Risk of bias	Duration of follow-up	Outcome assessment tool	Outcome
Epstein 1982 [48]	Primary biliary cirrhosis	Calcium supplementation* (all patients received vitamin D)	Not low	14 months	Cortical bone on x-ray	Both groups receiving calcium supplements did not demonstrate bone loss, which was seen in control group. Recipients of hydroxyapatite accumulated cortical bone
Shiomi 1999 [49]	Cirrhosis	1,25 dihydroxyvitamin D	Not low	>12 months (up to 3.5–4 years)	DXA	Bone mineral density better maintained in treated group
Bernstein 1996 [50]	Inflammatory bowel disease	Calcium/vitamin D supplement	Lower[†]	1 year	DXA	No differences between 2 groups with regard to bone mineral density
Benchimol 2007 [51]	Inflammatory bowel disease in children	Calcium/vitamin D in one treatment arm; calcium only in second treatment arm	Not low	1 year	DXA	No differences between 3 groups with regard to bone mineral density

DXA, dual-energy x-ray absorptiometry.

* Two different supplements used (hydroxyapatite and calcium gluconate).

[†] Major risks were 30% dropout rate during trial (all dropouts accounted for, but unable to do intention to treat analysis) and failure to do sample size calculation.

Copper restriction in Wilson's disease

Wilson's disease (hepatolenticular degeneration) is an infrequently encountered genetic disorder which typically presents with hepatic and neuropsychiatric signs and symptoms. It is characterised by excessive amounts of copper stored in the liver and the brain. The treatment is largely pharmacological and thus beyond the scope of this chapter. However, such patients are sometimes placed on copper-restricted diets. There is also some thought that zinc supplementation may be effective because it blocks copper absorption in the intestinal tract. However, there are no RCTs that have assessed either of these interventions [52].

Iron and haemochromatosis

Haemochromatosis is a more common genetic disorder that results in excessive iron accumulation. The iron accumulation can affect the liver (resulting in cirrhosis), heart (producing a cardiomyopathy), testes (with subsequent testicular atrophy and hypogonadism), pancreas (diabetes), skin (darkened colour), joints (arthritis) and thyroid gland (hypothyroidism). Since the actual effect of restricting iron intake is minimal, such a dietary intervention is not used [53]. The important nutritional issue to keep in mind is to avoid vitamin C supplementation, as this can cause iron mobilisation and, especially when other techniques are also being used to remove iron from the body (usually phlebotomy), problems with free radicals can be a threat [53]. Obviously, iron supplementation should be avoided.

Zinc

Zinc deficiency has been described in a number of liver diseases, especially alcoholic cirrhosis [54]. We have already considered its use in Wilson's disease. Zinc supplementation has been tested with RCTs in several other liver diseases, including hepatic encephalopathy, adjunctive therapy in the treatment of hepatitis C and in patients with various forms of cirrhosis.

Four RCTs, none with low risk of bias, addressed the use of zinc in patients with hepatic encephalopathy; they were combined in a systematic review [55]. Several different outcomes were reported, but each was usually unique to a single trial; meta-analysis could only be performed for two outcomes: recurrence of encephalopathy (no significant difference) and number connection test (better in the zinc recipients). One of the trials reported improvements in the grade of encephalopathy and quality of life scores in the zinc recipients over a 6-month period. However, a short-term randomised crossover trial not included in the systematic review [56] failed to see any improvement in the grade of encephalopathy after 2 weeks.

Six RCTs assessed the use of zinc in patients being treated for hepatitis C with interferon ± ribavirin [57–62]. While an improved rate of sustained virological response was seen in one of these trials [57], this phenomenon was not demonstrated in the other five [58–62]. No differences were seen with regard to any of the treatment-related toxicities.

Five RCTs assessed the use of zinc in patients with cirrhosis of various aetiologies [63–67]. Most of the outcomes were surrogate ones, blood tests in particular; serum albumin may [67] or may not [65] have improved. One trial found no impact on impotence or hypogonadism [66]. One trial found no difference in the incidence of hepatocellular carcinoma after 3 years [63]. One trial reported a modest reduction in the Child–Pugh score [67].

5.11.6 Lessons for practice

A number of recommendations for various nutritional interventions in patients with liver diseases have been made. Unfortunately, the evidence for most of them (sodium restriction for ascites, various interventions for hepatic encephalopathy (protein restriction, protein supplementation, vegetable protein, zinc), calcium and/or vitamin D for liver disease-associated bone problems, and zinc as an adjunctive intervention in the treatment of chronic hepatitis C or for cirrhosis) is limited and unconvincing.

Copper restriction is accepted for Wilson's disease but iron restriction is not used for haemochromatosis; neither practice is based on data from RCTs. Zinc for Wilson's disease and BCAAs for hepatic encephalopthy are both second-line treatments; in the former there is no evidence and in the latter the cost and intolerance for achieving a therapeutic response are high. Late-night feeding in patients with cirrhosis is difficult to justify in the face of the trials that have been performed. Non-alcoholic fatty liver disease entails treatment for the underlying metabolic disorders.

Perhaps most disappointing, evidence establishing benefit from any kind of nutrition support in patients with liver disease is virtually non-existent in spite of a large number of trials; this practice should not be undertaken until and unless future trials show a convincing effect on mortality or morbidity. If we are not going to employ nutrition support, there is no particular reason to be concerned about how to do nutritional assessment.

References

1. Cheung K, Lee SS, Raman M. Prevalence and mechanisms of malnutrition in patients with advanced liver disease, and nutrition management strategies. *Clin Gastroenterol Hepatol* 2012; **10** (2):117–125.

2. Jensen GL, Mirtallo J, Compher C, et al. Adult starvation and disease-related malnutrition: a proposal for etiology-based diagnosis in the clinical practice setting from the international consensus guideline committee. *J Parenter Enteral Nutr* 2010; **34**(2): 156–159.

3. Sam J, Nguyen GC. Protein-calorie malnutrition as a prognostic indicator of mortality among patients hospitalized with cirrhosis and portal hypertension. *Liver Int* 2009; **29**(9): 1396–1402.

4. Koretz RL. Death, morbidity, and economics are the only end points for trials. *Proc Nutr Soc* 2005; **64**(3): 277–284.

5. White JV, Guenter P, Jensen G, Malone A, Schofield M, Academy Malnutrition Work Group, A.S.P.E.N. Malnutrition Task Force, and A.S.P.E.N. Board of Directors. Consensus statement: Academy of Nutrition and Dietetics and American Society for Parenteral and Enteral Nutrition: characteristics recommended for the identification and documentation of adult malnutrition (undernutrition). *J Parenter Enteral Nutr* 2012; **36**(3): 275–283.

6. Chang WK, Chao YC, Tang HS, Lang HF, Hsu CT. Effects of extra-carbohydrate supplementation in the late evening on energy expenditure and substrate oxidation in patients with liver cirrhosis. *J Parenter Enteral Nutr* 1997; **21**(2): 96–99.

7. Swart GR, Zillikens MC, van Vuure JK, van den Berg JWO. Effect of a late evening meal on nitrogen balance in patients with cirrhosis of the liver. *BMJ* 1989; **299**(6709): 1202–1203.

8. Fukushima H, Miwa Y, Ida E, et al. Nocturnal branched-chain amino acid administration improves protein metabolism in patients with liver cirrhosis: comparison with daytime administration. *J Parenter Enteral Nutr* 2003; **27**(5): 315–322.

9. Nakaya Y, Okita K, Suzuki K, et al. BCAA-enriched snack improves nutritional state of cirrhosis. *Nutrition* 2007; **23**: 113–120.

10. Plank LD, Gane EJ, Peng S, et al. Nocturnal nutritional supplementation improves total body protein status of patients with liver cirrhosis: a randomized 12-month trial. *Hepatology* 2008; **48**: 557–566.

11. Yamanaka-Okumura H, Nakamura T, Miyake H, et al. Effect of long-term late-evening snack on health-related quality of life in cirrhotic patients. *Hepatol Res* 2010; **40**: 470–476.

12. Morihara D, Iwata K, Hanano T, et al. Late-evening snack with branched-chain amino acids improves liver function after radiofrequency ablation for hepatocellular carcinoma. *Hepatol Res* 2012; **42**: 658–667.

13. Nagata K, Iwakiri H, Oozono Y, et al. Nocturnal low-calorie BCAA supplementation may improve albumin metabolism in decompensated cirrhotic patients. *Hepatol Int* 2012; **6**: 299–300.

14. Tenda ED. Effect of BCAA and LOLA combination as late evening snacks on nutritional status and minimal hepatic encephalopathy in cirrhosis. *Hepatol Int* 2013; **7**(Suppl 1): S539.

15. Hou W, Li J, Lu J, et al. Effect of a carbohydrate-containing late-evening snack on energy metabolism and fasting substrate utilization in adults with acute-on-chronic liver failure due to hepatitis B. *Eur J Clin Nutr* 2013; **67**: 1251–1256.

16. Hidaka H, Nakazawa T, Kutsukake S, et al. The efficacy of nocturnal administration of branched-chain amino acid granules to improve quality of life in patients with cirrhosis. *J Gastroenterol* 2013; **48**: 269–276.

17. Gitlin N. The management of ascites in patients with cirrhosis of the liver. *S Afr Med J* 1970; **44**(26): 760–763.

18. Reynolds TB, Lieberman FL, Goodman AR. Advantages of treatment of ascites without sodium restriction and without complete removal of excess fluid. *Gut* 1978; **19**: 549–553.

19. Descos L, Gauthier A, Levy VG, et al. Comparison of six treatments of ascites in patients with liver cirrhosis. A clinical trial. *Hepatogastroenterology* 1983; **30**(1): 15–20.

20. Gauthier A, Levy VG, Quinton A, et al. Salt or no salt in the treatment of cirrhotic ascites: a randomized study. *Gut* 1986; **27**: 705–709.

21. Bernardi M, Laffi G, Salvagnini M, et al. Efficacy and safety of the stepped care medical treatment of ascites in liver cirrhosis: a randomized controlled clinical trial comparing two diets with different sodium content. *Liver* 1993; **13**: 156–162.

22. Madden AM. Changing perspectives in the nutritional management of disease. *Proc Nutr Soc* 2003; **62**: 765–772.

23. Cordoba J, Lopez-Hellin J, Planas M, et al. Normal protein diet for episodic hepatic encephalopathy: results of a randomized study. *J Hepatol* 2004; **41**: 38–43.

24. Merli M, Riggio O. Dietary and nutritional indications in hepatic encephalopathy. *Metab Brain Dis* 2009; **24**: 211–221.

25. Greenberger NJ, Carley J, Schenker S, Bettinger I, Stamnes C, Beyer P. Effect of vegetable and animal protein diets in chronic hepatic encephalopathy. *Dig Dis* 1977; **22**: 845–855.

26. Uribe M, Marquez MA, Garcia Ramos G, Ramos-Uribe MH, Vargas F, Villalobos A, Ramos C. Treatment of chronic portal-systemic encephalopathy with vegetable and animal protein diets. *Dig Dis Sci* 1982; **27**(12): 1109–1116.

27. Shaw S, Worner TM, Lieber CS. Comparison of animal and vegetable protein sources in the dietary management of hepatic encephalopathy. *Am J Clin Nutr* 1983; **38**: 59–63.

28. De Bruijn KM, Blendis LM, Zilm DH, Carlen PL, Anderson GH. Effect of dietary protein manipulations in subclinical portal-systemic encephalopathy. *Gut* 1983; **24**: 53–60.

29. Keshavarzian A, Meek J, Sutton C, Emery VM, Hughes EA, Hodgson HJ. Dietary protein supplementation from vegetable sources in the management of chronic portal systemic encephalopathy. *Am J Gastroenterol* 1984; **79**(12): 945–949.

30. Uribe M, Dibildox M, Malpica S, et al. Beneficial effect of vegetable protein diet supplemented with psyllium plantago in patients with hepatic encephalopathy and diabetes mellitus. *Gastroenterology* 1985; **88**: 901–907.

31. Bianchi GP, Marchesini G, Fabbri A, Rondelli A, Bugianesi E, Zoli M, Pisi E. Vegetable versus animal protein diet in cirrhotic patients with chronic encephalopathy. A randomized cross-over comparison. *J Intern Med* 1993; **233**: 385–392.

32. Conn HO. Animal versus vegetable protein diet in hepatic encephalopathy. *J Intern Med* 1993; **233**: 369–371.

33. Gumaste VV. Vegetable protein diet and hepatic encephalopathy. *Gastroenterology* 1993; **105**: 1578–1579.

34. Koretz RL, Avenell A, Lipman TO. Nutritional support for liver disease. *Cochrane Database Syst Rev* 2012; **5**: CD008344.

35. Zhu X, Wu Y, Qiu Y, Jiang C, Ding Y. Effects of ω-3 fish oil lipid emulsion combined with parenteral nutrition on patients undergoing liver transplantation. *J Parenter Enteral Nutr* 2013; **37**(1): 68–74.

36. Dupont B, Dao T, Joubert C, et al. Randomised clinical trial: enteral nutrition does not improve the long-term outcome of alcoholic cirrhotic patients with jaundice. *Aliment Pharmacol Ther* 2012; **35**: 1166–1174.

37. Huisman EJ, van Hoek B, van Soest H, van Nieuwkerk KM, Arends JE, Siersema PD, van Erpecum KJ. Preventive versus "on-demand" nutritional support during antiviral treatment for hepatitis C: a randomized controlled trial. *J Hepatol* 2012; **57**: 1069–1075.

38. Kobashi H, Morimoto Y, Ito T, et al. Effects of supplementation with a branched-chain amino acid-enriched preparation on event-free survival and quality of life in cirrhotic patients with hepatocellular carcinoma. A multicenter, randomized controlled trial (Abstract). *Gastroenterology* 2006; **130**: A497.

39. Hayashi S, Aoyagi Y, Fujiwara K, Oka H, Oda T. A randomized controlled trial of branched-chain amino acid (BCAA)-enriched elemental diet (ED-H) for hepatic encephalopathy (abstract). *J Gastroenterol Hepatol* 1991; **6**(2): 191.

40. Foschi D, Cavagna G, Callioni F, Morandi E, Rovati V. Hyperalimentation of jaundiced patients on percutaneous transhepatic biliary drainage. *Br J Surg* 1986; **73**(9): 716–719.

41. Fan ST, Lo CM, Lai EC, Chu KM, Liu CL, Wong J. Perioperative nutritional support in patients undergoing hepatectomy for hepatocellular carcinoma. *N Engl J Med*; **331**(23): 1547–1552.

42. Freund H, Dienstag J, Lehrich J, et al. Infusion of branched-chain enriched amino acid solution in patients with hepatic encephalopathy. *Ann Surg* 1982; **196** (2): 209–220.

43. Gluud LL, Dam G, Borre M, et al. Oral branched-chain amino acids have a beneficial effect on manifestations of hepatic encephalopathy in a systematic review with meta-analyses of randomized controlled trials. *J Nutr* 2013; **143**: 1263–1268.

44. Sanyal AJ, Chalasani N, Kowdley KV, et al. Pioglitazone, vitamin E, or placebo for non-alcoholic steatohepatitis. *N Engl J Med* 2010; **362**(18): 1675–1685.

45. Hay JE. Bone disease in cholestatic liver disease. *Gastroenterology* 1995; **108**(1): 276–283.

46. Carey E, Balan V. Metabolic bone disease in patients with liver disease. *Curr Gastroenterol Rep* 2003; **5**(1):71–77.

47. Collier JD, Ninkovic M, Compston JE. Guidelines on the management of osteoporosis associated with chronic liver disease. *Gut* 2002; **50**(Suppl 1): i1–i9.

48. Epstein O, Kato Y, Dick R, Sherlock S. Vitamin D, hydroxyapatite, and calcium gluconate in treatment of cortical bone thinning in postmenopausal women with primary biliary cirrhosis. *Am J Clin Nutr* 1982; **36**: 426–430.

49. Shiomi S, Masaki K, Hau D, et al. Calcitriol for bone disease in patients with cirrhosis of the liver. *J Gastroenterol Hepatol* 1999; **14**: 547–552.

50. Bernstein CN, Seeger LL, Anton PA, et al. A randomized, placebo-controlled trial of calcium supplementation for decreased bone density in corticosteroid-using patients with inflammatory bowel disease: a pilot study. *Aliment Pharmacol Ther* 1996; **10**: 777–786.

51. Benchimol EI, Ward LM, Gallagher JC, et al. Effect of calcium and vitamin D supplementation on bone mineral density in children with inflammatory bowel disease. *J Pediatr Gastroenterol Nutr* 2007; **45**: 538–545.

52. European Association for the Study of the Liver. EASL clinical practice guidelines: Wilson's disease. *J Hepatol* 2012; **56**: 671–685.

53. Bacon BR, Adams PC, Kowdley KV, Powell LW, Tavill AS. Diagnosis and management of hemochromatosis: 2011 practice guideline by the American Association for the Study of Liver Diseases. *Hepatology* 2011; **54**(1): 328–343.

54. Mohommad MK, Zhou Z, Cave M, Barve A, McClain CJ. Zinc and liver disease. *Nutr Clin Pract* 2012; **27**(1): 8–20.

55. Chavez-Tapia NC, Cesar-Arce A, Barrientos-Gutierrez T, Villegas-Lopez FA, Mendez-Sanchez N, Uribe M. A systematic review and meta-analysis of the use of oral zinc in the treatment of hepatic encephalopathy. *Nutr J* 2013; **12**: 74.

56. Riggio O, Ariosto F, Merli M, et al. Short-term oral zinc supplementation does not improve chronic hepatic encephalopathy. Results of a double-blind crossover trial. *Dig Dis Sci* 1991; **36**(9): 1204–1208.

57. Takagi H, Nagamine T, Abe T, et al. Zinc supplementation enhances the response to interferon therapy in patients with chronic hepatitis C. *J Viral Hep* 2001; **8**: 367–371.

58. Ko WS, Guo CH, Hsu GSW, Chiou YL, Yeh MS, Yaun SR. The effect of zinc supplementation on the treatment of chronic hepatitis C patients with interferon and ribavirin. *Clin Biochem* 2005; **38**: 614–620.

59. Suzuki H, Sato K, Takagi H, et al. Randomized controlled trial of consensus interferon with or without zinc for chronic hepatitis C patients with genotype 2. *World J Gastroenterol* 2006; **12**(6): 945–950.

60. Suzuki H, Takagi H, Sohara N, Kanda D, Kakizaki S, Sato K, Mori M. Triple therapy of interferon and ribavirin with zinc supplementation for patients with chronic hepatitis C: a randomized controlled clinical trial. *World J Gastroenterol* 2006; **12**(8): 1265–1269.

61. Murakami Y, Koyabu T, Kawashima A, et al. Zinc supplementation prevents the increase of transaminase in chronic hepatitis C patients during combination therapy with pegylated interferon α-2b and ribavirin. *J Nutr Sci Vitaminol* 2007; **53**: 213–218.

62. Kim KI, Kim SR, Sasase N, et al. Blood cell, liver function, and response changes by PEG-interferon-α-2b plus ribavirin with polaprezinc therapy in patients with chronic hepatitis C. *Hepatol Int* 2008; **2**: 111–115.

63. Matsuoka S, Matsumura H, Nakamura H, et al. Zinc supplementation improves the outcome of chronic hepatitis C and liver cirrhosis. *J Clin Biochem Nutr* 2009; **45**: 292–303.

64. Weismann K, Christensen E, Dreyer V. Zinc supplementation in alcoholic cirrhosis. A double-blind clinical trial. *Acta Med Scand* 1979; **205**: 361–366.

65. Hayashi M, Ikezawa K, Ono A, et al. Evaluation of the effects of combination therapy with branched-chain amino acid and zinc supplements on nitrogen metabolism in liver cirrhosis. *Hepatol Res* 2007; **37**: 615–619.

66. Goldiner WH, Hamilton BP, Hyman PD, Russell RM. Effect of the administration of zinc sulfate on hypogonadism and impotence in patients with chronic stable hepatic cirrhosis. *J Am Coll Nutr* 1983; **2**(2): 157–162.

67. Somi MH, Rezaeifar P, Rahimi AO, Moshrefi B. Effects of low dose zinc supplementation on biochemical markers in non-alcoholic cirrhosis: a randomized clinical trial. *Arch Iran Med* 2012; **15**(8): 472–476.

Chapter 5.12

Nutrition support in kidney disease

Katrina Campbell

Faculty of Health Sciences and Medicine, Bond University, Robina, Australia

5.12.1 Introduction

Kidney disease is characterised by derangements in the elimination of metabolic waste products and limitations in fluid, electrolyte and hormone homeostasis. Therefore, in the presence of kidney disease, nutritional and metabolic issues are common and play a major role in affecting clinical outcomes in this patient population [1].

This chapter will provide an overview of the latest evidence associated with the assessment and management of nutritional status in kidney disease. This will encompass acute kidney injury (AKI) and chronic kidney disease (CKD) not requiring dialysis (predialysis) and end-stage kidney disease (ESKD) requiring dialysis (peritoneal dialysis, haemodialysis).

5.12.2 Undernutrition in kidney disease

Acute kidney injury (AKI) is complex and heterogeneous in aetiology, often occurring alongside multiple organ syndrome, with significant mortality and morbidity, including undernutrition [2]. AKI represents an abrupt reduction in kidney function (i.e. within 48 hours) demonstrated by a >50% increase in creatinine and/or reduction in urine output [3]. Prevalence of undernutrition in AKI is estimated at ~40–50% and considered both a cause and consequence of the condition [4]. This highlights the critical need for effective nutritional management strategies in AKI.

Chronic kidney disease is defined as a progressive and irreversible reduction in kidney function [5] and it is not until kidney function falls below a glomerular filtration rate (GFR) of $30\,mL/min/1.73\,m^2$ that nutritional concerns begin to accumulate. At this stage, the focus of the medical treatment shifts to managing the metabolic disturbances and preparing the patient for renal replacement therapy. Ideally, this requires the provision of multidisciplinary care to prevent complications (such as anaemia, undernutrition and acidosis), treat comorbidities (including cardiovascular disease and diabetes) and manage symptoms (including nausea, hypertension and fluid balance).

Undernutrition, assessed using Subjective Global Assessment (SGA), is present in up to 50% of patients with chronic kidney disease predating dialysis commencement, increasing in prevalence with progressive deterioration of kidney function [6]. Studies show undernutrition rates of up to 52% close to the start of renal replacement therapy [7] and vary between 20% and 50% in patients on maintenance dialysis [6].

5.12.3 Aetiology of undernutrition in kidney disease

The development of anorexia, resulting in a reduction of dietary intake, together with increased requirements due to loss in dialysis, inflammation and metabolic changes with kidney disease work synergistically to compromise

Advanced Nutrition and Dietetics in Nutrition Support, First Edition. Edited by Mary Hickson and Sara Smith.
© 2018 John Wiley & Sons Ltd. Published 2018 by John Wiley & Sons Ltd.

nutrition status in kidney disease [8,9]. Appetite is typically driven by the endocrine system but in dialysis patients, factors related to the dialysis procedure, alterations in the gastrointestinal system as well as hedonic and social implications are also important to consider (Table 5.12.1).

In addition to the decrease in substrate availability from decreased dietary intake, nutritional status may be further compromised by other mechanisms of metabolic changes as a result of decreased renal function, including uraemic toxin accumulation, resulting in taste abnormalities, fatigue and anorexia [6]. Abnormal metabolic responses include a reduction in the activity of anabolic hormones, such as insulin and growth hormone, and an increase in cortisol

and glucagon which also contribute to a reduced capacity for protein synthesis [10].

5.12.4 Consequences of undernutrition in kidney disease

Undernutrition in kidney disease is associated with poor quality of life, infections, atherosclerosis, cardiovascular events, graft rejection and mortality [6].

The degree of impact undernutrition has been shown to have on clinical outcomes depends on the measure used to define nutritional status. Simple biomarkers, serum albumin, serum

Table 5.12.1 Summary of the potential mechanisms contributing to undernutrition in chronic kidney disease

Causes of undernutrition	Description
Diminished appetite	
Endocrine (appetite hormones and neuropeptide dysregulation)	Early satiety due to retention of cholecystokinin, leptin and peptide-YY and reduced function of ghrelin
Dialysis procedure	Inadequate dialysis; retention of uraemic by-products; peritoneal dialysis (early satiety due to fullness and effect of by-products of glucose degradation)
Alterations in gastrointestinal system	Smell and taste dysfunction
Risk of oral disease	Reduced salivary flow, salivary by-products and reduced buffering capacity (reduced pH)
Delayed transit time	Constipation, impaired gastric emptying and motility disorders ('dysbiosis'); diabetic gastroparesis
Inflammation	
Increased concentration of inflammatory cytokines and adipokines	Due to both reduced renal clearance and stimulation of increased production
Increased energy expenditure due to inflammation	Increased circulating proinflammatory cytokines; membrane bio-incompatibility, comorbid conditions, persistent infections
Dietary restrictions	With progressive deterioration of spontaneous reduction and/or unmonitored dietary restrictions
Metabolic acidosis	The accumulation of hydrogen directly stimulates protein catabolism and suppresses protein synthesis.
Reduced physical activity	Functional reductions and increase in sedentary lifestyle – reduced stimulus for muscle growth
Dialysis procedure	
Catabolic stimulus	Interaction between blood flow and dialysis membrane (inflammatory cascade); limited clearance of protein-bound uraemic toxins and GI ischaemia
Protein losses	Amino acid and protein losses during the dialysis session
Social	Food security, social isolation and depression

prealbumin or poor appetite, are strongly associated with the incidence of hospitalisations, but it is likely that these measures represent overall health, not nutritional status [11]. However, SGA ratings taken at commencement of dialysis have been shown to predict outcome of all-cause mortality, independent of albumin and body mass index (BMI) over a 10-year period [7], and have superior predictive ability of mortality over serum biomarkers, such as albumin [12].

5.12.5 Assessment of undernutrition in kidney disease

An overview of nutrition assessment parameters is provided in Table 5.12.2. Due to the high prevalence and significant consequences of undernutrition in kidney disease, a system of routine screening for undernutrition, followed by comprehensive assessment of

Table 5.12.2 Screening and assessment of undernutrition in kidney disease

Assessment	Tool/measure	Comments
Weight and weight change	Weight (kg); change over past 1, 3 and 6 months	Does not distinguish body compartments. Helps to assess fluid gains between dialysis Weight loss of >5% or more in 3 months clinically relevant
BMI	Weight/height^2	Does not distinguish body compartments. Evidence of reverse epidemiology, where high BMI results in reduced risk of poor clinical outcome over 3–4-year follow-up
Lean muscle mass (and/or fat mass)	Body composition instruments (e.g. bio-impedance, DEXA, total body potassium, total body nitrogen	High cost and/or challenging to undertake in the clinical setting. Research tools are expensive and not clinically applicable (e.g. total body potassium, total body nitrogen) or open to error due to indirect measure and body water fluctuations (bio-impedance, DEXA)
	Anthropometrics, i.e. skinfold thickness and mid-arm muscle circumference	Low cost and with training can optimise validity and reproducibility
Muscle function	Handgrip strength	Measure of muscle function, non-invasive. Unclear if longitudinal change. No current norms for renal population and cut-off values to indicate undernutrition
Serum proteins	Albumin, prealbumin	Affected by non-nutritional factors (i.e. inverse relationship with inflammation and hydration status; residual renal function and losses in dialysate)
Metabolic acidosis	Serum bicarbonate	Risk factor for poor appetite, hyperkalaemia, stimulation of protein breakdown and subsequent muscle wasting
Inflammation markers	C-reactive protein	Indicator of stress response, may decrease protein synthesis and raise energy expenditure
Clinical assessment tools	Subjective Global Assessment; Malnutrition Inflammation Score	Comprehensive and systematic assessment of summary of medical history and physical exam evaluating overall nutritional status
Dietary intake	Diet history	Requires training, but low cost and recommended to be undertaken routinely to inform assessment and intervention strategy
	Protein of nitrogen appearance (PNA)	Calculated by a standard equation to estimate the generation of urea nitrogen in blood (assumes clinically stable). Assumes nPNA = protein intake g/kg/day

BMI, body mass index; DEXA, dual-energy x-ray absorptiometry.

nutritional status, is essential across AKI and CKD populations.

Screening for undernutrition aims to identify potential nutrition risk early in the course of progression and may include weight change, appetite, biochemical parameters or ideally a combination [13]. Typically, nutrition assessment based on a combination of measures would follow nutrition screening, or be undertaken routinely in the dialysis setting, at least every 6 months.

Nutrition assessment tools

The SGA and the Malnutrition Inflammation Score (MIS) are the most comprehensive and validated nutrition assessment tools to evaluate undernutrition in kidney disease. These tools combine features of a medical history (weight change, gastrointestinal symptoms, dietary intake change, functional capacity and, in the case of MIS, biochemistry) as well as a physical examination (accounting for fat and muscle wasting). SGA differs from MIS because it does not require biochemistry, and is also based on a global rating rather than a summative score. Both tools have been shown to be prognostic indicators of all-cause mortality, although MIS and the scored SGA (7-point or patient-generated SGA) are likely to be more sensitive to detect small changes over time [14].

5.12.6 Nutritional management of undernutrition in kidney disease

Energy requirements

Adequate energy intake is imperative to the maintenance of nitrogen balance. Energy metabolism in CKD may be modified due to comorbidities such as insulin resistance, carnitine deficiency, hyperparathyroidism, metabolic acidosis, chronic inflammation and the dialysis procedure itself [15]. However, indirect calorimetry studies indicate that these abnormalities do not substantially affect resting energy expenditure, except in the case of critically ill patients [15]. Practice guidelines recommend an energy

intake for adults both dialysis and predialysis of 30–35 kcal/kg/day of ideal body weight [16,17] and considering age, gender and physical activity level. A level of 30–35 kcal/kg/day is recommended for individuals 60 years and over and for individuals with a sedentary lifestyle, or 35 kcal/kg for all other patients [16,18]. However, these guidelines are based on limited evidence, mainly observational studies.

In predialysis, it has been demonstrated that resting energy expenditure is not affected by change in renal function, but inflammation at levels typically seen in CKD may increase energy expenditure, and therefore requirements [19]. Regular monitoring of nutritional status should be conducted to determine the adequacy of an individual's energy intake.

Protein requirements

Table 5.12.3 provides a summary of protein intake recommendations from key international guidelines.

Protein requirements predialysis

Dietary protein restriction has been a time-honoured intervention for predialysis CKD. A significant number of studies have investigated the relationship between dietary protein restriction and progression of renal failure in diabetic and non-diabetic patients. Low protein diets result in modest reductions in the delay of kidney disease progression, have poor compliance and heighten risk of undernutrition. The recent NICE guidelines have recommended specifically against a low-protein diet, stating that protein intake less than 0.6–0.8 g/kg/day should be avoided in people with CKD [22] due to compliance issues and risk of undernutrition. Therefore, a controlled protein intake ~0.8 g/kg/day, aiming to reduce uraemic load without compromising nutritional status, may be most appropriate to aim for.

Protein requirements in dialysis

The process of dialysis is catabolic. One session can result in removal of amino acids (approximately 10–12 g/dialysis), peptides and glucose

Table 5.12.3 Protein intake recommendations across key guidelines and stages of chronic kidney disease

Organisation	Predialysis Stage 3–4	Haemodialysis Stage 5	Peritoneal dialysis Stage 5
National Kidney Foundation [16]	0.6–0.75 g/kg/day	>1.2 g/kg/day	1.2–1.3 g/kg/day
British Dietetic Association [20]	Not addressed	>1.1 g/kg/day	>1.2 g/kg/day
ESPEN [21]	0.6–0.8 g/kg/day	1.2–1.4 g/kg/day	1.2–1.5 g/kg/day
	Illness 1.0 g/kg	Illness >1.5 g/kg/day	
Ash et al. [18]	0.75–1.0 g/kg/day	1.2–1.4 g/kg/day	>1.2 g/kg/day
			1.5 g/kg peritonitis
NICE guidelines [22]	>0.75 g/kg/day (avoid <0.6–0.8 g/kg)	Not addressed	Not addressed

Table 5.12.4 General guidelines for fluid, potassium, phosphate and sodium recommendations on dialysis [35,37]

	Dialysis	Considerations
Fluid	Haemodialysis: 500 mL + UO Peritoneal dialysis: 800 mL + UO	Only if requiring fluid restriction
Potassium	1 mmol/kg IBW/day	Only if previously hyperkalaemic
Phosphate	800–1000 mg/d	Only if previously hyperphosphataemic
Sodium	<100 mmol/day	General advice for all patients with kidney disease. Especially to assist with fluid control

IBW, ideal body weight; UO, regular daily urine output.

(approximately 12–25 g/dialysis) which can all contribute to an imbalance between intake and requirements.

The most recent guidelines from the British Dietetic Association determined that (i) adults undergoing maintenance haemodialysis (HD) require a minimum protein intake of 1.1 g/kg per day, and (ii) adults undergoing maintenance peritoneal dialysis (PD) require a minimum protein intake of 1.0–1.2 g/kg per day, in conjunction with an adequate energy intake [20]. As with energy intake, there is consensus in recommending the use of ideal body weight (IBW) when calculating protein requirements.

Energy intake must also be sufficient, sparing available protein to support neutral or positive nitrogen balance. Regarding protein quality, K/DOQI guidelines originally stated that >50% of protein consumed should be of high biological value [16], which remains based on expert opinion [20].

Markers of protein intake include normalised protein nitrogen appearance (nPNA) or normalised protein catabolic rate (nPCR). These equations assume neutral nitrogen balance and are based on urea nitrogen appearance in the urine and/or dialysate. Based on evidence from a large cohort of haemodialysis patients in the United States, the nPNA should be at least 1.0 g/kg IBW/day, with best survival between 1.0 and 1.4 g/day [23].

Further considerations when managing undernutrition

The kidneys play a vital role in mineral metabolism, maintaining fluid balance and homeostasis between serum and tissue stores of essential minerals including phosphorus and potassium. Table 5.12.4 provides a summary of the guideline evidence for fluid, potassium and phosphorus intake.

On dialysis, excessive fluid gains are highly prevalent, and have significant implications for treatment and management. Psychological interventions, targeting fluid and sodium intake, have demonstrated benefit for reducing interdialytic weight gain (IDWG) [24].

Disturbance in potassium balance is a key challenge in kidney disease, due to disruption in aldosterone homeostasis. Muscular cells are highly sensitive to changes in intracellular concentrations of potassium, which may lead to potentially fatal cardiac arrhythmias. High serum potassium (hyperkalaemia) is associated with a two-fold increased risk of all-cause and cardiovascular mortality [25]. Therefore, in the event of hyperkalaemia (serum potassium >6 mmol/L) it is advised to restrict potassium to no more than 80 mmol/day or 1 mmol/kg IBW/day [18].

Excretion of phosphorus is progressively compromised with deterioration in kidney function, leading to hyperphosphataemia and hormonal disturbances. This results in an imbalance in calcium and phosphate minerals, augmented by derangements in parathyroid hormone, which can affect bone (low bone mineral density) and vasculature (calcium deposits and arterial stiffness) [26]. Despite a lack of intervention studies linking phosphorus manipulation to clinical outcomes, there is a practice imperative to optimise phosphate control by the use of phosphorus binders and control of phosphate intake to <1000 mg/day [16].

Micronutrient requirements

Dietary restrictions and dialysis losses can result in suboptimal balance of water-soluble vitamins in particular. However, a recent systematic review of the literature (1970 to 2014) examining vitamin supplementation needs in haemodialysis patients suggests a shift to a more individualised approach for individuals with suboptimal intake and/or established deficiency rather than routine supplementation [27].

However, guidelines suggest a multivitamin containing B vitamins and vitamin C (vitamin C not to exceed 500–1000 mg/day) [28] designed for adults with renal failure is recommended to meet requirements for these vitamins. In balance of recent findings, this is particularly pertinent to consider for individuals with suboptimal intake.

Considerations in acute kidney injury

Acute kidney injury is typically found as part of multiple organ failure and is thus managed as a critical care case. Energy intake is estimated to be up to 30 kcal/kg/day (non-protein) or 1.3 times basal energy expenditure [2,4]. Due to the heterogeneous nature of AKI presentation and critical care in general, the use of equations should be considered with caution, and ideally energy expenditure should be directly measured [4].

If receiving renal replacement therapy, recommendations for patients with AKI are 1.5 g/kg/day of protein with an additional 0.2 g/kg/day to compensate for loss of amino acids, especially with the use of continuous dialysis treatments [2,4].

Nutrition support in kidney disease

Deterioration in nutritional status often predates the onset of renal replacement therapy [7]. Individuals receiving nutritional management prior to dialysis clearly benefit in terms of quality of life [29] and nutritional status [8]. However, the effect of nutrition support on mortality and morbidity has not yet been investigated.

Nutrition support is a key strategy in the management of complications in kidney disease. Waste product accumulation and derangements in electrolyte, fluid and hormone homeostasis can all be limited through dietary modification, but ongoing monitoring is required throughout the stages of kidney disease and resultant treatments to ensure optimal management.

Dietary counselling

Nutrition interventions tailored to identify and manage patient-specific barriers, foster self-management and utilise behaviour change counselling strategies have been demonstrated to be effective in managing CKD [30] and are important considerations in the management of undernutrition.

Dietary counselling using a combination of face-to-face and phone intervention demonstrated a reduced rate of undernutrition despite a progressive deterioration in renal function in a randomised controlled trial [31]. This study determined that a structured nutrition intervention programme results in positive changes in dietary intake, albumin and quality of life, but it was underpowered to detect a difference in body composition [29,31]. More intense dietary intervention (monthly education and comprehensive materials) has also been evaluated and found to reduce protein intake on average to meet dietary recommendations (0.6–0.8 g/kg/day). However, there were no between-group differences with the control group, since that group also reduced protein intake, albeit insignificantly [32].

Group sessions delivered in addition to individualised counselling have also proved effective. Flesher et al. incorporated exercise sessions and building self-efficacy for dietary change by conducting a series of cooking skills workshops, provided in addition to individualised dietary care. These sessions improved dietary intake (reduction in protein and sodium intake to target), blood pressure and cholesterol [33]. Leon et al. investigated group intervention with dialysis patients tailored to identify and manage patient-specific barriers (such as poor nutritional knowledge, poor appetite, help with shopping or cooking, etc.) [34].

Evidence from the large multicentre trials in protein restriction, in particular the Modification of Diet in Renal Disease (MDRD) study, indicates that the most effective nutrition interventions involve frequent nutrition counselling, teaching patients self-management skills and frequent ongoing feedback and interventions with the nutrition team. A patient-centred, structured approach is supported by a systematic review of interventions that use regular feedback, routine follow-up and self-management strategies. This evidence shows that such strategies improved albumin, fluid balance and phosphate management [30].

Oral nutrition supplements

Oral nutrition supplements (ONS) can typically increase total energy and protein intake by 20–50% [1]. Renal disease-specific supplements are formulated as low-volume, high energy density (1.5–2.0 kcal/mL), with limited potassium, phosphate and sodium content. These are particularly necessary for patients who are fluid restricted, and with electrolyte derangements despite adequate dialysis. However, standard or generic formulations, particularly high-protein in dialysis or AKI, can be considered as first-line treatments, with renal disease-specific formulations introduced when the individual's requirements demand them. It is generally thought that this approach is more cost-effective, due to the lower cost of standard formulations and better adherence to them.

There is a paucity of evidence for the effectiveness of ONS on clinical endpoints. The only systematic review evaluating ONS in dialysis found that ONS increased serum albumin by 2.27 g/L (95% confidence interval (CI) 0.37–4.18 g/L) without compromising serum electrolyte concentrations [35]. This gradient of improvement in albumin observed in ONS studies (i.e. >2.0 g/L/day) is associated with improved survival [36]. Further details of these studies can be seen in Table 5.12.5.

The literature in this area is of limited quality. Trials to date are small, largely uncontrolled and report outcomes that are not solely related to nutritional status (i.e. albumin). Furthermore, many studies report per-protocol analyses, due to non-adherence to intention-to-treat protocols which limits evidence significantly. Evidence is mounting that interventions should be individualised, which provides a further challenge to researchers in this field reflecting the heterogeneous nature of nutrition support strategies for this patient group.

Although no controlled clinical trials have demonstrated long-term clinical improvements from ONS, recent large observational studies investigating hypoalbuminaemic haemodialysis patients show that those who received ONS had better outcomes compared with patients who did

Table 5.12.5 Randomised controlled trials and controlled clinical trials targeting undernutrition via oral nutrition support in chronic kidney disease

Reference	Study design	Design and duration	Intervention treatment	Results
Akpele 2004 [37]	n=41 HD **Supplement:** n=26 **Counselling:** n=14 Hypoalbuminaemia ≤3.5 g/dL	RCT; 14 months	**Supplement:** 1–2 cans of Nepro/day + normal diet **Counselling:** Normal diet + dietary counselling	Rate of change in serum alb> in non-supplement pts (dietary counselling alone) than supplement pts Albumin/month: ↑ counselling 0.06 vs ↓ supplement 0.04 g/L
Eustace et al. 2000 [38]	HD=29 PD=18 (n=47) Hypoalbuminaemia (≤38 g/L)	RCT; double-blind; 3 months	**Treatment:** Essential AA; 10.8 g/day **Control:** Placebo	Albumin ↑ 22 g/L (HD) P<0.02; NS (PD) Muscle strength: ↑ grip strength Compliance: 75% (1 mo); 70% (2 mo); 50% (3 mo)
Fouque et al. 2008 [39]	HD=86 nPNA <1 g/d	RCT; 3 months	**Supplement:** 2 × 125 mL Renilon 7.5®/day **Control:** Standard care	ITT: No significant differences 63% compliance. Per-protocol analysis: Intake: ↑energy and protein with supplements; regression in control; ↑ 2 of 8 QoL domains (General Health and Bodily Pain)
Gonzalez-Esinoza 2005 [40]	PD: n=28	RCT; 6 months	**Supplement:** Counselling + egg albumin supplement **Control:** Counselling only	Baseline to 6 mo ↑Supp: 1331 vs 1872 kcal; protein 1.0 vs 1.7 g/kg ↓Control: 1423 vs 1567 kcal; protein stable 1.0 g/kg Albumin: Suppl 26.4 to 30.5 g/L; Control 26.6 vs 28.0 g/L TSF and MAMC=NS Energy and protein intake Albumin muscle strength
Kalantar-Zadeh et al. 2005 [41]	HD; n=163 Reporting on hypoalbuminaemic groups only **Treatment:** n=21 (<3.8 g/dL) **Control:** n=20 (<3.8 g/dL)	CCT; 4-week pilot	**Supplement:** 1 × Nepro®; 1 × Oxepa @ 3 times/week **Control:** No supplements	Serum albumin ↑ 2.5 g/L Protein intake ↑ 0.1 g/kg Weight 1.7 kg (less weight loss) Oral supplements were associated with ↑albumin, no change control
Moretti et al. 2009 [42]	HD; PD (n=49) Hypoalbuminaemia	RCT; cross-over (1 yr); 6 month interventions	**Supplement:** Standard ONS **Control:** No supplement	nPCR: Supp ↑1.05 to 1.16 g/day; Control ↓1.11 to 0.98 Albumin: Supp: improvement by month 3, from 3.49 to 3.52 (P=0.035), not sustained to month 6

(Continued)

Table 5.12.5 (Continued)

Reference	Study design	Design and duration	Intervention treatment	Results
Sharma et al. 2002 [43]	n = 40 MHD non-diabetic pts BMI <20; Albumin <4.0 g/dL	RCT; 1 month	**G1:** Counselling **G2:** Home-made supplement **G3:** Clinical supplement	Dry weight G1 = ↑1.7 kg; G2 = ↑1.8 kg; G3 = NS Albumin G1 = NS; G2 = ↑6.0 g/L; G3 = ↑5.0 g/L Karnofsy G1 = NS, G2 = ↑0.4; G3 = ↑0.4 Intake (food-based): G1 = ↑236 kcal or 4 kcal/kg; G2 and 3 no change
Steiber 2003 [44]	n = 117 HD **High risk:** n = 26 **Low risk:** n = 91	CCT; 3 months	**High risk:** ONS daily **Low risk:** Usual care	Change in HD-PNI scores: ↓ 0.50 vs ↑ 0.21 Dietetic intervention with supplements ↓ pts HD-PNI and ↓ pts risk for hospitalisation
Stratton 2005 [35]	14 studies (2 RCTs, 5 CCTs, 6 historical control, 1 cohort) HD, PD, CKD	Systematic review	Oral supplements versus routine care	Albumin: ↑2.3 (0.4–4.2) g/L; OR 0.4 (0.1–0.8) Energy and protein intake ↑20–50% Weight ↑ ~3% in 3–4 months
Teixido-Planas 2005 [45]	PD: n = 65 SGA >5 out of 7	RCT; 6 months	**Protein 20 g/day, n = 35** **Control:** n = 30 (Proteinplus, n = 35) and group B (controls, n = 30), with evaluations at baseline and at 6 and 12 months	Treatment dropout Poor compliance n = 7 or side effects n = 8 NS results intention to treat

BMI, body mass index; CCT, clinical controlled trial; CKD, chronic kidney disease; HD, haemodialysis; ITT, intention to treat; MAMC, mid arm muscle circumference; MHD, maintenance haemodialysis; nPCR, normalised protein catabolic rate; nPNA, normalised protein nitrogen appearance; NS, not significant; ONS, oral nutritional supplement; OR, odds ratio; PD, peritoneal dialysis; PNI, Prognostic Nutrition Index; QoL, quality of life; RCT, randomised controlled trial; SGA, Subjective Global Assessment; TSF, triceps skinfold thickness.

not, including reduced hospitalisations [46] and improved survival [47]. Despite concerns with the methodology, including residual confounding and indication bias, these studies provide some promising data in the absence of intervention studies.

Benefits of intradialytic nutrition

An important distinction from general ONS provision is the provision of ONS during dialysis. A large case control study including 101 dialysis facilities and 2700 hypoalbuminaemic patients showed that provision of ONS during haemodialysis, upon diagnosis of hypoalbuminaemia with the aim of maintaining albumin within normal range, was associated with 20–30% reduced mortality compared to propensity-matched controls not receiving nutrition support during dialysis [48]. This type of intradialytic nutrition has been shown to counteract catabolism during haemodialysis, normalise metabolic derangement and increase serum albumin concentration. Concurrent amino acid supplementation throughout a haemodialysis session has also been demonstrated to prevent or reverse catabolism associated with the dialysis process [49]. This has given rise to a movement to support meal provision during dialysis as a key strategy for the prevention of undernutrition.

Intradialytic parenteral nutrition

Intradialytic parenteral nutrition (IDPN) provides nutrition support during the haemodialysis procedure directly via the venous access. IDPN is considered when oral supplements have been unsuccessful and oral intake is still considered inadequate (e.g. <20 kcal/kg/day) [50]. The largest and longest investigation of IDPN (2-year duration) was undertaken as the French Interdialytic Nutrition Evaluation Study (FINES). This study showed that there is no advantage of adding IDPN to ONS, compared with ONS alone, on serum albumin and body mass. However, regardless of the route of feeding, early response to reduced nutritional status resulted in reduced mortality and hospitalisation rates, in a *post hoc* analysis [50].

In peritoneal dialysis, the IDPN option consists of an amino acid-based dialysate solution (typically 1.1% amino acid). As with the FINES study, intraperitoneal nutrition has demonstrated benefits on nutritional parameters such as albumin, but not on survival [51]. Side effects include excess removal of potassium, hydrogen ions and phosphate, resulting in hypokalaemia, acidosis and hypophosphataemia respectively. This strategy therefore warrants close monitoring and is perhaps best suited to individuals who are metabolically stable but have insufficient oral intake.

When considering the option of IDPN, formulation and practicality are important. Formulations of IDPN include multi- or single macronutrients (dextrose, amino acids and/or lipids), and therefore may be individualised for the patient's needs [1]. The service also must be able to support IDPN in terms of resources and cost, for the equivalent delivery of approximately 10 kcal/kg/day. Although this has not been demonstrated to be more effective than ONS, it is considered to be a safe and convenient option for patients who cannot meet their needs orally.

Emerging interventions in kidney disease

There are a range of other interventions that warrant consideration in the prevention and care of undernutrition in kidney disease, including optimisation of dialysis, use of appetite stimulants and growth hormone. In addition, BCAA supplementation, exercise interventions and agents targeting inflammation and GI microbiota are increasing in interest. However, similar to the data on ONS and dietary counselling, the trials to date are short-term, proof-of-concept studies and typically measure albumin as the primary outcome. There is scope for longer term trials, including multimodal interventions, in this area.

5.12.7 Conclusions

Undernutrition is highly prevalent and associated with major implications in AKI, CKD and, in particular, at initiation of dialysis. Strategies to increase intake via both dietary counselling and

ONS have been shown to improve nutritional status and quality of life. Encouraging findings from observational studies demonstrate that intradialytic ONS provision has the potential to enhance survival and decrease both hospitalisations and inpatient expenditures. However, strategies to improve nutritional status need to be tested in the treatment and prevention of undernutrition long term (i.e. >6 months) to best investigate effect on clinical outcome and cost-effectiveness.

References

1. Ikizler TA, Cano NJ, Franch H, et al. Prevention and treatment of protein energy wasting in chronic kidney disease patients: a consensus statement by the International Society of Renal Nutrition and Metabolism. *Kidney Int* 2013; **84**(6): 1096–1107.
2. Fiaccadori E, Parenti E, Maggiore U. Nutritional support in acute kidney injury. *J Nephrol* 2008; **21**(5): 645–656.
3. Mehta RL, Kellum JA, Shah SV, et al. Acute Kidney Injury Network: report of an initiative to improve outcomes in acute kidney injury. *Crit Care* 2007; **11**(2): R31.
4. Fiaccadori E, Regolisti G, Maggiore U. Specialized nutritional support interventions in critically ill patients on renal replacement therapy. *Curr Opin Clin Nutr Metab Care* 2013; **16**(2): 217–224.
5. Levey AS, Coresh J, Balk E, et al. National Kidney Foundation practice guidelines for chronic kidney disease: evaluation, classification, and stratification. *Ann Intern Med* 2003; **139**(2): 137–147.
6. Carrero JJ, Stenvinkel P, Cuppari L, et al. Etiology of the protein-energy wasting syndrome in chronic kidney disease: a consensus statement from the International Society of Renal Nutrition and Metabolism (ISRNM). *J Ren Nutr* 2013; **23**(2): 77–90.
7. Chan M, Kelly J, Batterham M, Tapsell L. Malnutrition (subjective global assessment) scores and serum albumin levels, but not body mass index values, at initiation of dialysis are independent predictors of mortality: a 10-year clinical cohort study. *J Ren Nutr* 2012; **22**(6): 547–557.
8. Ikizler TA, Greene JH, Wingard RL, Parker RA, Hakim RM. Spontaneous dietary protein intake during progression of chronic renal failure. *J Am Soc Nephrol* 1995; **6**(5): 1386–1391.
9. Duenhas MR, Draibe SA, Avesani CM, Sesso R, Cuppari L. Influence of renal function on spontaneous dietary intake and on nutritional status of chronic renal insufficiency patients. *Eur J Clin Nutr* 2003; **57**(11): 1473–1478.
10. Pupim LB, Cuppari L, Ikizler TA. Nutrition and metabolism in kidney disease. *Semin Nephrol* 2006; **26**(2): 134–157.
11. Carrero JJ, Chen J, Kovesdy CP, Kalantar-Zadeh K. Critical appraisal of biomarkers of dietary intake and nutritional status in patients undergoing dialysis. *Semin Dial* 2014; **27**(6): 586–589.
12. De Mutsert R, Grootendorst DC, Boeschoten EW, et al. Subjective global assessment of nutritional status is strongly associated with mortality in chronic dialysis patients. *Am J Clin Nutr* 2009; **89**(3): 787–793.
13. Fouque D, Kalantar-Zadeh K, Kopple J, et al. A proposed nomenclature and diagnostic criteria for protein-energy wasting in acute and chronic kidney disease. *Kidney Int* 2007; **73**(4): 391–398.
14. Campbell KL, Ash S, Bauer J, Davies PSW. Critical review of nutrition assessment tools to measure malnutrition in chronic kidney disease. *Nutr Diet* 2007; **64**(1): 23–30.
15. Cuppari L, Ikizler TA. Energy balance in advanced chronic kidney disease and end-stage renal disease. *Semin Dial* 2010; **23**(4): 373–377.
16. National Kidney Foundation. Clinical practice guidelines for nutrition in chronic renal failure. K/DOQI, National Kidney Foundation. *Am J Kidney Dis* 2000; **35**(6 Suppl 2): S1–140.
17. Ash S, Campbell KL, Bogard J, Millichamp A. Nutrition prescription to achieve positive outcomes in chronic kidney disease: a systematic review. *Nutrients* 2014; **6**(1): 416–451.
18. Ash S, Campbell K, MacLaughlin H, et al. Evidence based practice guidelines for the nutritional management of chronic kidney disease. *Nutr Diet* 2006; **63**: S33–S45.
19. Avesani CM, Draibe SA, Kamimura MA, Colugnati FA, Cuppari L. Resting energy expenditure of chronic kidney disease patients: influence of renal function and subclinical inflammation. *Am J Kidney Dis* 2004; **44**(6): 1008–1016.
20. Naylor HL, Jackson H, Walker GH, et al. British Dietetic Association evidence-based guidelines for the protein requirements of adults undergoing maintenance haemodialysis or peritoneal dialysis. *J Hum Nutr Diet* 2013; **26**(4): 315–328.
21. Cano N, Fiaccadori E, Tesinsky P, et al. ESPEN guidelines on enteral nutrition: adult renal failure. *Clin Nutr* 2006; **25**(2): 295–310.
22. National Institute for Health and Care Excellence. Chronic Kidney Disease: Early Identification and Management of Chronic Kidney Disease in Adults In Primary and Secondary Care. London: National Institute for Health and Care Excellence, 2014.
23. Shinaberger CS, Kilpatrick RD, Regidor DL, et al. Longitudinal associations between dietary protein

intake and survival in hemodialysis patients. *Am J Kidney Dis* 2006; **48**(1): 37–49.

24. Bellomo G, Coccetta P, Pasticci F, Rossi D, Selvi A. The effect of psychological intervention on thirst and interdialytic weight gain in patients on chronic hemodialysis: a randomized controlled trial. *J Ren Nutr* 2015; **25**(5): 426–432.

25. Kovesdy CP, Regidor DL, Mehrotra R, et al. Serum and dialysate potassium concentrations and survival in hemodialysis patients. *Clin J Am Soc Nephrol* 2007; **2**(5): 999–1007.

26. London GM, Marty C, Marchais SJ, Guerin AP, Metivier F, de Vernejoul MC. Arterial calcifications and bone histomorphometry in end-stage renal disease. *J Am Soc Nephrol* 2004; **15**(7): 1943–1951.

27. Tucker BM, Safadi S, Friedman AN. Is routine multivitamin supplementation necessary in US chronic adult hemodialysis patients? A systematic review. *J Ren Nutr* 2015; **25**(3): 257–264.

28. Fouque D, Vennegoor M, ter Wee P, et al. EBPG guideline on nutrition. *Nephrol Dial Transplant* 2007; **22**(Suppl 2): ii45–87.

29. Campbell KL, Ash S, Bauer JD. The impact of nutrition intervention on quality of life in pre-dialysis chronic kidney disease patients. *Clin Nutr* 2008; **27**(4): 537–544.

30. Van der Veer SN, Jager KJ, Nache AM, et al. Translating knowledge on best practice into improving quality of RRT care: a systematic review of implementation strategies. *Kidney Int* 2011; **80**(10): 1021–1034.

31. Campbell KL, Ash S, Davies PS, Bauer JD. Randomized controlled trial of nutritional counseling on body composition and dietary intake in severe CKD. *Am J Kidney Dis* 2008; **51**(5): 748–758.

32. Paes-Barreto JG, Silva MI, Qureshi AR, et al. Can renal nutrition education improve adherence to a low-protein diet in patients with stages 3 to 5 chronic kidney disease? *J Ren Nutr* 2013; **23**(3): 164–171.

33. Flesher M, Woo P, Chiu A, Charlebois A, Warburton DE, Leslie B. Self-management and biomedical outcomes of a cooking, and exercise program for patients with chronic kidney disease. *J Ren Nutr* 2011; **21**(2): 188–195.

34. Leon JB, Albert JM, Gilchrist G, et al. Improving albumin levels among hemodialysis patients: a community-based randomized controlled trial. *Am J Kidney Dis* 2006; **48**(1): 28–36.

35. Stratton RJ, Bircher G, Fouque D, et al. Multinutrient oral supplements and tube feeding in maintenance dialysis: a systematic review and meta-analysis. *Am J Kidney Dis* 2005; **46**(3): 387–405.

36. Lacson E, Jr., Ikizler TA, Lazarus JM, Teng M, Hakim RM. Potential impact of nutritional intervention on end-stage renal disease hospitalization, death, and treatment costs. *J Ren Nutr* 2007; **17**(6): 363–371.

37. Akpele L, Bailey JL. Nutrition counseling impacts serum albumin levels. *J Ren Nutr* 2004; **14**(3): 143–148.

38. Eustace JA, Coresh J, Kutchey C, et al. Randomized double-blind trial of oral essential amino acids for dialysis-associated hypoalbuminemia. *Kidney Int* 2000; **57**(6): 2527–2538.

39. Fouque D, McKenzie J, de Mutsert R, et al. Use of a renal-specific oral supplement by haemodialysis patients with low protein intake does not increase the need for phosphate binders and may prevent a decline in nutritional status and quality of life. *Nephrol Dial Transplant* 2008; **23**(9): 2902–2910.

40. Gonzalez-Espinoza L, Gutierrez-Chavez J, del Campo FM, et al. Randomized, open label, controlled clinical trial of oral administration of an egg albumin-based protein supplement to patients on continuous ambulatory peritoneal dialysis. *Perit Dial Int* 2005; **25**(2): 173–180.

41. Kalantar-Zadeh K, Braglia A, Chow J, et al. An anti-inflammatory and antioxidant nutritional supplement for hypoalbuminemic hemodialysis patients: a pilot/feasibility study. *J Ren Nutr* 2005; **15**(3): 318–331.

42. Moretti HD, Johnson AM, Keeling-Hathaway TJ. Effects of protein supplementation in chronic hemodialysis and peritoneal dialysis patients. *J Ren Nutr* 2009; **19**(4): 298–303.

43. Sharma M, Rao M, Jacob S, Jacob CK. A controlled trial of intermittent enteral nutrient supplementation in maintenance hemodialysis patients. *J Ren Nutr* 2002; **12**(4): 229–237.

44. Steiber AL, Handu DJ, Cataline DR, Deighton TR, Weatherspoon LJ. The impact of nutrition intervention on a reliable morbidity and mortality indicator: the hemodialysis-prognostic nutrition index. *J Ren Nutr* 2003; **13**(3): 186–190.

45. Teixido-Planas J, Ortiz A, Coronel F, et al. Oral protein-energy supplements in peritoneal dialysis: a multicenter study. *Perit Dial Int* 2005; **25**(2): 163–172.

46. Cheu C, Pearson J, Dahlerus C, et al. Association between oral nutritional supplementation and clinical outcomes among patients with ESRD. *Clin J Am Soc Nephrol* 2013; **8**(1): 100–107.

47. Lacson E Jr, Wang W, Zebrowski B, Wingard R, Hakim RM. Outcomes associated with intradialytic oral nutritional supplements in patients undergoing maintenance hemodialysis: a quality improvement report. *Am J Kidney Dis* 2012; **60**(4): 591–600.

48. Weiner DE, Tighiouart H, Ladik V, Meyer KB, Zager PG, Johnson DS. Oral intradialytic nutritional supplement use and mortality in hemodialysis patients. *Am J Kidney Dis* 2014; **63**(2): 276–285.

49. Pupim LB, Majchrzak KM, Flakoll PJ, Ikizler TA. Intradialytic oral nutrition improves protein homeostasis in chronic hemodialysis patients with deranged nutritional status. *J Am Soc Nephrol* 2006; **17**(11): 3149–3157.

50. Cano NJM, Fouque D, Roth H, et al. Intradialytic parenteral nutrition does not improve survival in malnourished hemodialysis patients: a 2-year multicenter, prospective, randomized study. *J Am Soc Nephrol* 2007; **18**(9): 2583–2591.

51. Li FK, Chan LY, Woo JC, et al. A 3-year, prospective, randomized, controlled study on amino acid dialysate in patients on CAPD. *Am J Kidney Dis* 2003; **42**(1): 173–183.

Chapter 5.13

Nutrition support in critical care

Liesl Wandrag and Danielle Bear
Guy's and St Thomas' NHS Foundation Trust, London, UK

5.13.1 Overview of undernutrition in critical illness

There is limited robust evidence available for many nutritional practices in the intensive care unit (ICU) and consequently practice varies between units and countries. The lack of evidence is because there are huge difficulties in studying patients in the ICU environment. Patient populations are heterogeneous, and may include patients from medical (e.g. neurology, respiratory, renal, oncology), trauma (e.g. multiple trauma or isolated head injuries) or surgical (e.g. cardiac, hepatobiliary, gastrointestinal, orthopaedic, vascular) specialties. Recruitment and retention of patients in research studies is very difficult and consequently the sample size of studies is often small. Length of stay can also vary considerably and there are difficulties in generalising data from one patient group to another. Estimating nutritional requirements in the critically ill is notoriously difficult, which makes it hard to compare interventions and deliver an accurate nutrient intake. In addition, patients commonly do not meet their estimated nutritional requirements due to frequent feeding interruptions and the severity of their illness, which means that they may be underfed, adequately fed or overfed, which complicates understanding the clinical outcome.

Rates of undernutrition on the ICU are reported as being between 18% and 100% depending on the patient population studied and method used. For example, ICUs with a more medical population generally see higher rates of undernutrition compared to those with trauma patients due to the degree of comorbidities seen in the medical population. For this reason, standard nutrition screening tools are not recommended in critically ill patients and instead, nutrition risk scoring is used [1].

5.13.2 Mechanisms of undernutrition in critical illness

The metabolic response to stress, injury or critical illness is generally characterised by hypermetabolism, hypercatabolism, persistent muscle wasting and hyperglycaemia. This complex interaction involves numerous mediators, hormones and cytokines. The neuroendocrine response to stress or trauma is activated by the hypothalamic-pituitary-adrenal axis [2]. Adrenaline stimulates release of adrenocorticotrophic hormone and growth hormone from the anterior pituitary, vasopressin from the posterior pituitary and cortisol and aldosterone from the adrenal cortex [3]. Adrenaline furthermore stimulates glucagon release and mobilises liver substrates, where glycogen is converted into glucose. Triglycerides are oxidised into free fatty acids. Muscle glucagon is converted into pyruvate and lactate which is converted into glucose in the liver. The release of catecholamines and glucocorticoids after severe infection or

Advanced Nutrition and Dietetics in Nutrition Support, First Edition. Edited by Mary Hickson and Sara Smith.
© 2018 John Wiley & Sons Ltd. Published 2018 by John Wiley & Sons Ltd.

Table 5.13.1 Hormonal effects on protein metabolism

Hormone	Effect on protein metabolism
Insulin	↓ Protein catabolism, amino acid uptake
Insulin-like growth factors	Stimulate protein synthesis
Growth hormone	Stimulates protein synthesis
Testosterone	Stimulates protein synthesis
Glucagon	Stimulates amino acid catabolism
Glucocorticoids	Stimulate protein catabolism
Noradrenaline/adrenaline	Stimulatesamino acid catabolism
Thyroid hormones	Stimulate protein catabolism

injury results in proteolysis [4]. Table 5.13.1 shows the hormonal effect on protein metabolism. This hormonally driven metabolic response to critical illness leads to a rapid reduction in muscle mass, increased energy expenditure, hyperglycaemia and heightened inflammatory response.

5.13.3 Metabolic and nutritional consequences of critical illness

The burden of critical illness globally has been estimated as 13–20 million mechanically ventilated patients/year, 1–5.5 million acute lung injury patients/year and 15000–19000 sepsis patients/year [5]. In the UK approximately 110000 patients in England and Wales spend time in the ICU. Long-term sequelae after critical illness include physical disability (neuropathies, myopathies, joint stiffness, muscle wasting, pulmonary dysfunction and tracheostomy problems), neuropsychological problems (memory, hallucinations, delirium, disturbed sleep, depression and anxiety) as well as financial and physical burdens to families and carers.

Muscle wasting occurs at a staggering rate in the critically ill; patients lose 1–2% muscle mass per day [6]. Muscle weakness can lead to increased morbidity, duration of mechanical ventilation and ICU length of stay [7] and was confirmed to be the single greatest determinant of outcome [8]. Five-year follow-up showed that patients with acute respiratory distress syndrome were still markedly impaired in terms of physical function [9]. Delirium, low mood and low appetite [10] further characterise recovery from critical illness and have the potential to negatively affect nutritional status, physical function and quality of life.

The weakness associated with critical illness is referred to as ICU-acquired weakness. Several factors contribute to this weakness, including severity and duration of systemic inflammatory response syndrome, length of ICU stay, duration of mechanical ventilation, corticosteroid administration and use of neuromuscular blocking agents. Although the link is poorly understood, muscle wasting undoubtedly contributes. Rates of muscle wasting are higher in those patients with multiorgan failure compared with single organ failure [11] and this wasting occurs despite the provision of nutrition [6]. Studies indicate muscle protein breakdown to be the driving force with rates remaining high at the end of 7 days, whereas muscle protein synthesis appears to return to the level of a healthy fasted control [11].

Studies have explored the balance of whole-body protein synthesis and breakdown in different ICU patient groups and show that in trauma patients, synthesis and breakdown are both increased but breakdown exceeds synthesis, resulting in the overall negative balance [12]. Similarly, in patients with multiorgan failure, increased turnover is observed with increases in both synthesis and breakdown [13]. Conversely, in septic patients, tracer studies and muscle biopsies showed increased muscle protein breakdown with normal levels of muscle protein synthesis [14]. Tracer studies provide robust information on either whole-body or muscle protein turnover but can be time-consuming to perform. Muscle biopsies provide information on anabolic or catabolic pathways within the muscle but they are invasive to perform which is why such data are very limited in the ICU population. In addition, studies using whole-body protein turnover do not provide information specific to muscle mass itself.

5.13.4 Assessment and diagnosis of undernutrition in critical illness

Assessing the nutritional status of a critically ill patient is challenging because traditional screening tools and methods of assessment are not validated in the ICU setting. Nutritional assessment should include weight, height, body mass index (BMI), biochemistry, clinical history and nutritional intake history, but many of these variables are often not available, such as height, weight and dietary intake history.

Recently, the concept of 'nutrition risk' has been developed as a method to determine the patients who may benefit from aggressive nutrition support and those who may be harmed by its use [15]. This scoring system (NUTRIC score) includes variables for age, severity of illness, comorbidities and hospital length of stay prior to ICU admission. The NUTRIC score has been validated in a large group of patients and may be useful as the first step in nutritional assessment of the ICU patient as more appropriate variables have been included compared to traditional assessment tools. For the first time, the latest American Society of Parenteral and Enteral Nutrition and Society of Critical Care Medicine nutrition guidelines for ICU patients include a recommendation to undertake nutrition risk scoring in all patients and advocate its use in decision making regarding parenteral nutrition [1].

Traditional anthropometric measures such as weight, mid-arm circumference and skinfold thickness are inaccurate due to the enormous daily fluid shifts seen in these patients [16]. Obtaining an accurate height is limited by the supine positioning of the patient hence the use of surrogate measures, such as ulna length for predicting height and mid-arm circumference for predicting BMI, although their accuracy is in question. Additional methods may be available to assess lean body mass, such as muscle volume measurement via ultrasound or computed tomography [6,17] but these are limited to the research setting at present. As a result, anthropometric data are often estimated or obtained from previous medical notes, GP surgeries or the patient's relatives. Pre-ICU admission nutritional intake history may be difficult to obtain if relatives are not present and patients are unconscious.

Overall clinical assessment should include an assessment of the reason for admission, past medical and drug history and comorbidities along with the medical aspects of ICU management such as sedation, ventilation modes and assessment for drug–nutrient interactions. Biochemical parameters are available daily to assess inflammatory status, electrolyte status and renal function. Acute phase proteins are not a good marker of nutritional status in the critically ill and markers that are more sensitive, such as retinol-binding protein and serum transferrin, are not readily available in clinical settings, so serum albumin concentration should be interpreted with caution. Renal function and electrolyte status may only be helpful in monitoring the effects of nutrition support in more stable patients, since in the acute phase too many other variables may be affecting these factors.

5.13.5 Nutritional management and interventions in critical illness

Nutritional aims within the ICU should focus on commencing artificial nutrition support within 24–48 hours of ICU admission, choosing the most appropriate route (enteral (EN), parenteral (PN) or oral nutrition support), and on energy and protein prescription. Monitoring should include assessment of energy and protein delivered compared with requirements (including non-nutritional energy such as that from propofol, glucose and citrate) along with tolerance of enteral formula (gastric residual volumes, vomiting and diarrhoea), bowel and blood sugar management.

Currently, there are no known interventions, nutritional or otherwise, to prevent muscle wasting and the associated ICU-acquired weakness. Current treatment relies on reducing exposure to the known risk factors along with promoting early mobilisation and adequate nutrition. A systematic review on supplementation with amino acids or their metabolites on muscle wasting within critical illness found no evidence to support supplementation; however, leucine-enriched essential amino acid supplementation, β-hydroxy-β-methylbutyrate and creatine warrant further investigation [18].

There are many challenges to determining the optimum nutrition support for the ICU patient. The amount of energy and protein to provide along with timing and routes remain hotly debated topics. Underfeeding is associated with poorer outcomes, but it seems that there is no further mortality benefit above 80% of energy requirements [19]. However, undertargeting of nutrition prescription is not recommended due to the knowledge that ICU patients do not receive their full prescription, particularly over the first week of ICU stay.

Overfeeding may be associated with hypercapnia, hyperglycaemia, refeeding syndrome, hepatic steatosis and hypertriglyceridaemia and is as undesirable as underfeeding. Randomised controlled trials (RCTs) showing a benefit of nutrition support are limited but this is due in part to the heterogeneity of the population. It is also difficult to interpret clinical studies when nutrients and interventions are not studied in isolation. A summary of the available evidence is shown in Table 5.13.2.

Energy requirements

One of the current debates regarding energy provision in the critically ill is whether measured energy expenditure should be matched during the early catabolic stages of critical illness or whether patients should be underfed [20]. Feeding to measured energy expenditure has been associated with fewer infectious complications and lower mortality [21] but measurements are difficult to obtain in practice as indirect calorimeters are not compatible with modern ventilators and several limitations to the technique exist.

Indirect calorimetry

Indirect calorimetry, measuring O_2 consumption and CO_2 production to determine energy expenditure, is described as the 'gold standard' method in the critically ill [22]. The Deltatrac II metabolic monitor (Datex Ohmeda, Finland) has been validated [23] and widely used over the past few decades in mechanically ventilated patients, but it is now no longer manufactured. Comparisons between Deltatrac II and other indirect calorimeters have been made [24] but acceptable levels of agreement have not been demonstrated. This means that measuring energy expenditure is hampered by a lack of accurate equipment. The main problem is that indirect calorimetry equipment is generally not compatible with ventilators or dialysis machines and studies must exclude the sickest patients to ensure accuracy of the result (e.g. those with an FiO_2 above 60%).

Energy requirement prediction equations

Prediction equations are used as an alternative to indirect calorimetry in clinical practice. A multitude of equations are available, and many were designed specifically for use in the critically ill [22,25]. These equations are either simply weight based or regression equations which include physiological factors. Compher et al. assessed whether complex prediction equations, such as the Penn State equation, versus weight-only equations, such as 25 kcal/kg (American College of Chest Physicians (ACCP)), would affect mortality and time to discharge in 5672 critically ill patients from an international observational study [26]. No difference in mortality was observed, but time to discharge alive was shorter in patients fed according to weight-only equations. Data were limited due to the observational nature of the study and low actual energy intake achieved

Table 5.13.2 The most influential RCTs in critical care nutrition

	CALORIES (n = 2400) [44]	Early PN (n = 1372) [54]	SPN (n = 305) [55]	EPaNIC (n = 4640) [38]	EDEN (n = 1000) [39]	PermiT (n = 894) [40]
Patient population	Surgical 13%	Emergency surgery 45.85% Elective surgery 19.9%	45.5% surgical	~60% cardiac surgical	ALI	75% medical 3.45% surgical 21.5% non-operative trauma
Study design	Multicentre, 33 sites, Pragmatic RCT	Multicentre, 31 sites, RCT	Two-centre RCT	Single-centre RCT	Multicentre, 44 sites, RCT	Multicentre, 7 site, RCT
Age (mean)	63 years	68.5 years	60.5 years	64 years	52 years	50.6 years
BMI (mean)	28 kg/m²	28.2 kg/m²	25.9 kg/m²	>50% over 25 kg/m²	30.1 kg/m²	29.4 kg/m²
APACHE II	19.6	21	22.5	23	NR	21
Mortality	28% (ICU)	22.15% (60-day)	20% (ICU)	6.2% (ICU)	22.7% (60-day)	17.6%
LOS (ICU)*	7.7 days	9 days	13 days (mean)	3.5 days	NR	13 days
Provision of energy	21 kcal/kg PN 18.5 kcal/kg EN	Overall total not reported, but <1600 kcal/day	25 kcal/kg SPN 20 kcal/kg EN	Overall total NR, but >30 kcal/kg for early PN group and <20 kcal/kg for late PN group over the first week	1300 kcal/day full-feeding 400 kcal/day trophic feeding	835 kcal/day (46%) in permissive underfeeding group 1299 kcal/day (71%) in full-feeding group
Provision of protein	0.7 g/kg PN 0.6 g/kg EN	Total not reported, but 60 g/day	1.2 g/kg SPN 0.8 g/kg EN	<60 g/day in both groups	NR	57 g/day in permissive feeding group 59 g/day in full-feeding group
Outcomes	↑ Hypoglycaemia and vomiting in the EN group	↓ In mechanical ventilation ↑ SGA ↑ RAND-36 All favouring early PN	↓ Infections and days on antibiotics favouring the SPN group	↑ ICU and hospital survival ↓ Infections ↓ Days on mechanical ventilation ↓ Duration RRT ↓ Cholestasis All favouring late PN	↑ Vomiting, GRVs, use of prokinetics and antidiarrhoeals ↑ Average insulin administration All in full-feeding group	Less RRT requirement in the permissive underfeeding group (*post hoc* analysis)

* Median unless specified.

ALI, acute lung injury; BMI, body mass index; EN, enteral nutrition; GRV, gastric residual volume; ICU, intensive care unit; LOS, length of stay; NR, not reported; PN, parenteral nutrition; RCT, randomised controlled trial; RRT, renal replacement therapy; SGA, Subjective Global Assessment; SPN, supplemental parenteral nutrition.

(<70% of goal rate). Nevertheless, this study is a large dataset of patients which may promote the use of weight-only equations.

Indirect calorimetry versus prediction equations

Reid reported poor agreement between measured energy expenditure via indirect calorimetry and prediction equations (Harris–Benedict, Schofield and ACCP equations) in 27 critically ill patients during 192 days of measurement [27]. In Reid's study cohort, 35% of patients would have been inadequately fed (under- or overfed) if they had used one of the prediction equations. The study was limited by small sample size which did not allow subgroup analysis by range of BMI nor illness score of patients, but it was the first study of its kind comparing measured energy expenditure directly to prediction equations.

Frankenfield et al. systematically reviewed seven prediction equations (Harris–Benedict, Modified Harris–Benedict, Ireton-Jones 1992 and 1997, Penn State 1998 and 2003, and Swinamer) and the Fick method (determining whole-body oxygen consumption, or metabolic rate) for validation in critically ill patients [28]. Validation studies were limited either by small sample size or being studied in healthy individuals, thereby making it impossible to endorse one specific equation in this population. The authors then compared indirect calorimetry to eight prediction equations in 202 mechanically ventilated patients (Penn State equation, Faisy, Brandi, Swinamer, Ireton-Jones, Mifflin, ACCP and Harris–Benedict) and showed that accuracy rate was the highest (% of estimates ≤10% different from measured) for the modified Penn State equation (67%) [22]. This study was limited due to fairly small sample size. Because the sickest patients and those with burn injuries, penetrating trauma or spinal injuries were excluded, the results can only be applied to patients not represented in these aforementioned groups.

This means the calculation of energy requirements in ICU patients is severely hampered. Prediction equations are not as accurate as measuring energy expenditure, but equipment to measure energy expenditure may not be accessible in many institutions nor are there any indirect calorimeters currently on the market suitable for the ICU setting. Unfortunately, there is currently not one equation to recommend above another, although dietitians practising in critical care might use a combination of weight-based equations (25 kcal/kg) along with the modified Penn State equation.

Protein requirements

Currently there are no RCTs investigating optimum protein intake in critically ill patients, and research is urgently required, focusing on specific subgroups. Protein turnover is generally thought to be accelerated during critical illness, and patients are universally in negative nitrogen balance, but we do not know how much protein to provide to offset this effect. Nevertheless, early high protein provision is advocated [29], with current guidelines recommending a minimum intake of 1.2–1.5 g/kg/day protein [30,31]. A systematic and narrative review included 13 articles and suggested that 2–2.5 g protein/kg normal body weight may improve outcomes [32]. However, strong recommendations were not made due to the small number of studies available for inclusion and poor quality of available evidence.

Higher provision of protein and amino acids has been associated with lower mortality in ICU patients, whilst energy provision did not show this association [33]. These studies were limited by the observational design and small sample size; prospective RCTs would be required to assess dose of protein on outcomes such as mortality and length of stay. Meeting energy targets alone did not appear adequate in improving outcomes – meeting both energy and protein targets was necessary to achieve this.

Obesity requirements

Obese patients may experience more complications on the ICU than normal-weight patients. BMI does not appear to protect against muscle loss, with obese patients losing muscle depth in a similar manner to non-obese subjects [34]. Hypocaloric and high protein feeding in the obese is advocated, and in the absence of indirect calorimetry, either 50–70% of estimated energy needs or <14 kcal/kg actual weight with high protein feeding started at 1.2 g/kg actual weight or 2–2.5 g/kg ideal body weight [35]. The evidence base behind these recommendations is poor as all included studies were observational in design and the quality grading of each of these studies was low. Earlier guidance from the American Society of Parenteral and Enteral Nutrition and the Society of Critical Care Medicine [31] suggests that the nutritional goal should not exceed 60–70% of target energy requirements or 11–14 kcal/kg actual body weight should be used per day (or 22–25 kcal/kg ideal body weight per day). Protein recommendations are ≥2.0 g/kg ideal body weight per day for class I and II obesity (BMI 30–40) and ≥2.5 g/kg ideal bodyweight per day for class III obesity (BMI ≥40).

Measured energy expenditure is superior to prediction equations in the obese patient as prediction equation variability may be too large and lead to inaccurate estimates [36].

Early versus late feeding

Consensus statements recommend commencing EN within 24 hours of admission to the ICU to see the benefits of enhanced GI barrier function, and improved morbidity and mortality [20]. The difficulty with interpreting results of current studies is that 'early feeding' may have been initiated either within 24 hours or within 48 hours of ICU admission. One meta-analysis of patients fed within 24 hours included six RCTs with 234 patients. This review showed that early EN significantly reduced mortality (absolute risk reduction (ARR) 10%, P=0.02) and reduced pneumonia (ARR 27%, P=0.01) [37].

Energy and protein dose

Dosing studies are harder to perform in the heterogeneous critically ill population with the many confounding factors influencing ICU outcome. Although not consistent, observational data ultimately suggest a positive association between increased energy and protein intake and improved clinical outcome. However, these data are in contrast to large RCTs which have failed to show any outcome benefit with targeted energy intakes [38,39] and even when protein intakes were standardised across both groups [40]. However, each of these studies has limitations preventing generalisability to all ICU patients. Nonetheless, current recommendations support a degree of hypocaloric feeding (80% of energy target) in the first week of ICU stay with high protein intake, but the nutrition risk of the patient should be considered when determining the appropriateness of hypocaloric feeding at the bedside [1].

Parenteral nutrition versus enteral nutrition

There are four meta-analyses assessing outcomes between EN versus PN; two meta-analyses [41,42] showed no mortality difference between routes but EN patients had significantly fewer infections. In these studies patients were fed enterally within 48 hours. A later meta-analysis [43] showed that PN patients had significant reductions in mortality, and also significant fewer infections (in this updated review EN was started within 24 hours). In the latest meta-analysis which included the large CALORIES Trial [44], no mortality benefit was found between the two routes, but infections and ICU length of stay were significantly reduced in the EN group [45]. However, these results may be reflective of the macronutrient dose (e.g. underfeeding) rather than the route of feeding itself as target feeding is rarely reached in RCTs. Although the reviews had differing methodologies and inclusion criteria, the overall consensus remains that EN is still the first route of choice when the GI tract is functioning.

The recent multicentre UK-based CALORIES trial assessed early (within 36 hours of ICU admission) EN compared to early PN for 5 days [44]. Patients were randomised to either EN or PN despite having normal GI function. No difference was shown between groups for all-cause mortality at 30 days. Although this study had a strong design and adequate sample size, it is possible that 5 days of nutrition support is not enough to affect 30-day all-cause mortality. In addition, the dose of nutrition received in the PN group was lower than anticipated. This evidence supports the conclusion that, when considering mortality, EN is the most appropriate route, but PN can be considered in patients not tolerating EN without fear of increased infections if managed appropriately (e.g. overfeeding is avoided).

Supplemental parenteral nutrition

Supplemental PN is provided when EN energy or protein targets are not met during the early phases of critical illness and is given concurrently with EN. It may be initiated at any time and this ranges widely in studies from within 48 hours of ICU admission to day 8 of ICU admission. A systematic review [46] including four RCTs and two prospective observational studies reported that in one RCT (EPaNIC) [38], a higher percentage of patients were discharged alive from ICU at day 8 in the late supplemental PN group compared to early supplemental PN group, but no differences in overall ICU and in-hospital mortality were shown. None of the other RCTs demonstrated differences in ICU or in-hospital mortality rates. ICU length of stay was 1 day longer in the early PN group in one RCT. The heterogeneity in quality and design of the studies excluded any overall conclusion being drawn from this review.

Data suggest that there are no clinically relevant benefits from early PN compared with late PN when assessing morbidity or mortality endpoints [46]. The EPaNIC trial [38], a large RCT included in the systematic review, was limited by the fact that 60% of the cohort included cardiac surgery patients which may not be representative of most ICUs. Patients also received higher glucose loads than patients in the other RCTs included in the review.

Measuring gastric residual volume, gastrointestinal complications and impact on formula delivery

Patients on the ICU suffer frequent gastrointestinal (GI) complications which impact on formula delivery [47]. It is common practice to measure gastric residual volumes (GRVs) regularly, as a measure of poor gastric emptying, particularly

when enteral feeding is commenced. There is no consensus on the most appropriate GRV cut-off to define intolerance and indeed, whether they should be measured at all. Studies indicate no relationship between GRV cut-off and risk of ventilator-associated pneumonia, with cut-offs ranging between 150 mL and 500 mL every 4–6 hours. Given the poor clinical evidence surrounding GRV measurements, Reignier et al. investigated the impact of not measuring GRVs in critically ill patients and found no increased risk of developing ventilator-associated pneumonia [48]. The decision regarding measurement of GRVs needs to be balanced between minimising aspiration and ventilator-associated pneumonia risks with the ability to provide adequate feeding by improving formula delivery [20]. This decision should include the case mix of patients since surgical patients, a poorly represented group in the Reignier study, may be at higher risk of GI intolerances than medical patients.

Glucose control

Current recommendations are to maintain blood glucose concentration between 5 and 9 mmol/L. Tight glycaemic control (maintaining blood sugars between 4 and 6 mmol/L) was initially recommended for better outcomes in ICU patients, although evidence came predominantly from cardiac surgery patients. Subsequently, an international multicentre study in >6000 patients (NICE-Sugar Study) reported increased mortality rates in patients managed with tight glucose control and increased incidences of hypoglycaemia [49].

Immuno-nutrition

The concepts of 'immuno-nutrition' or 'pharmaco-nutrition' have been described as adding specific nutrients to EN or PN to enhance the immune system and improve clinical outcomes. Commonly studied nutrients include glutamine, arginine, ω-3 fatty acids and antioxidants. These are often studied in combination, making firm conclusions about individual nutrients difficult. There are three systematic reviews and meta-analyses which together show no evidence of benefit for glutamine, arginine (harm indicated in septic patients), nucleotides or ω-3 fatty acids and which highlight the many methodological problems with the included trials [2,50]. More recent evidence supports these conclusions; the MetaPlus study compared immune-enhancing high protein formula to normal high protein formula in 301 critically ill patients. No difference was seen in any outcome (new infections, ICU mortality, Sequential Organ Failure Assessment (SOFA) score, duration of ventilation and ICU and hospital length of stay) and the authors concluded that immune-enhancing feeds are not required [51].

There is also some evidence of harm. A large well-designed RCT (OMEGA Study) had to be stopped mid-trial because the patients receiving enteral ω-3 and antioxidants twice daily showed significantly higher ICU length of stay, ventilator dependency, mortality and diarrhoea [39]. Another RCT of intravenous and enteral glutamine and antioxidants in 1223 critically ill patients (REDOX Study) showed a higher 28-day mortality in the glutamine-supplemented group compared to those not receiving glutamine (32.4% vs 27.2%; adjusted odds ratio 1.28; 95% confidence interval 1.00–1.64; P=0.05) [52]. The Metaplus study showed higher 6-month mortality in the medical patient group [51]. This highlights the need for good evidence to support new nutritional strategies to prevent harm and ensure benefit.

The more recent SIGNET trial (not included in the systematic reviews mentioned above) investigated the effect of 7 days intravenous glutamine or selenium supplementation or both in 502 ICU patients. No effect was observed on new infections, mortality, ICU length of stay, antibiotic use or SOFA score but in a subgroup given selenium for >5 days, a significant reduction in new infections was shown. The authors commented that the selenium dose and timing may not have been optimal in their trial [53].

5.13.6 Summary

As many nutrition studies in the ICU are inconclusive or have conflicting results, it comes as no surprise that there are many areas of controversy amongst experts in the field, yet there are some areas of consensus. These include that overfeeding may be harmful, particularly in the acute phases of critical illness; early (within 24–48 hours of admission) EN is advocated, particularly once patients have received acute resuscitation; energy requirements are best determined by indirect calorimetry rather than predictive equations; and arginine supplementation is not recommended in septic patients. Controversy remains surrounding whether energy expenditure should be matched early during ICU stay or whether less energy should be provided in the acute stages; whether protein targets should meet estimated loss (1.2–1.5 g/day) or whether less protein should be provided in the acute stages; whether supplemental PN should be provided early in patients who do not meet EN targets or only after day 8 on ICU, and whether GRV monitoring up to 500 mL should be included in daily monitoring or abandoned in medical patients (not surgical patients).

Clearly, more high-quality studies are required to address many of the issues, particularly surrounding dose and timing of nutrition in these vulnerable patients.

References

1. McClave SA, Taylor BE, Martindale RG, Warren MM, Johnson DR, Braunschweig C, McCarthy MS, Davanos E, Rice TW, Cresci GA, Gervasio JM, Sacks GS, Roberts PR, Compher C. Guidelines for the provision and assessment of nutrition support therapy in the adult critically ill patient: Society of Critical Care Medicine (SCCM) and American Society for Parenteral and Enteral Nutrition (A.S.P.E.N.). *J Parenter Enteral Nutr* 2016; **40**(2): 159–211.
2. Marik PE, Zaloga GP. Immunonutrition in critically ill patients: a systematic review and analysis of the literature. *Intens Care Med* 2008; **34**(11): 1980–1990.
3. Desborough JP. The stress response to trauma and surgery. *Br J Anaesth* 2000; **85**(1): 109–117.
4. Hasselgren PO. Catabolic response to stress and injury: implications for regulation. *World J Surg* 2000; **24**(12): 1452–1459.
5. Adhikari NK, Fowler RA, Bhagwanjee S, Rubenfeld GD. Critical care and the global burden of critical illness in adults. *Lancet* 2010; **376**(9749): 1339–1346.
6. Reid CL, Campbell IT, Little RA. Muscle wasting and energy balance in critical illness. *Clin Nutr* 2004; **23**(2): 273–280.

7. Hough CL, Steinberg KP, Taylor TB, Rubenfeld GD, Hudson LD. Intensive care unit-acquired neuromyopathy and corticosteroids in survivors of persistent ARDS. *Intens Care Med* 2009; **35**(1): 63–68.

8. Cheung AM, Tansey CM, Tomlinson G, Diaz-Granados N, Matte A, Barr A, Mehta S, Mazer CD, Guest CB, Stewart TE, Al Saidi F, Cooper AB, Cook D, Slutsky AS, Herridge MS. Two-year outcomes, health care use, and costs of survivors of acute respiratory distress syndrome. *Am J Respir Crit Care Med* 2006; **174**(5): 538–544.

9. Herridge MS, Tansey CM, Matte A, Tomlinson G, az-Granados N, Cooper A, Guest CB, Mazer CD, Mehta S, Stewart TE, Kudlow P, Cook D, Slutsky AS, Cheung AM. Functional disability 5 years after acute respiratory distress syndrome. *N Engl J Med* 2011; **364**(14): 1293–1304.

10. Nematy M, O'Flynn JE, Wandrag L, Brynes AE, Brett SJ, Patterson M, Ghatei MA, Bloom SR, Frost GS. Changes in appetite related gut hormones in intensive care unit patients: a pilot cohort study. *Crit Care* 2006; **10**(1): R10.

11. Puthucheary ZA, Rawal J, McPhail M, Connolly B, Ratnayake G, Chan P, Hopkinson NS, Padhke R, Dew T, Sidhu PS, Velloso C, Seymour J, Agley CC, Selby A, Limb M, Edwards LM, Smith K, Rowlerson A, Rennie MJ, Moxham J, Harridge SD, Hart N, Montgomery HE. Acute skeletal muscle wasting in critical illness. *JAMA* 2013; **310**(15): 1591–1600.

12. Mansoor O, Breuille D, Bechereau F, Buffiere C, Pouyet C, Beaufrere B, Vuichoud J, Van't Of M, Obled C. Effect of an enteral diet supplemented with a specific blend of amino acid on plasma and muscle protein synthesis in ICU patients. *Clin Nutr* 2007; **26**(1): 30–40.

13. Liebau F, Sundstrom M, van Loon LJ, Wernerman J, Rooyackers O. Short term amino acid infusion improves protein balance in critically ill patients. *Crit Care* 2015; **19**(1): 106.

14. Klaude M, Mori M, Tjader I, Gustafsson T, Wernerman J, Rooyackers O. Protein metabolism and gene expression in skeletal muscle of critically ill patients with sepsis. *Clin Sci* 2012; **122**(3): 133–142.

15. Rahman A, Hasan RM, Agarwala R, Martin C, Day AG, Heyland DK. Identifying critically-ill patients who will benefit most from nutritional therapy: further validation of the "modified NUTRIC" nutritional risk assessment tool. *Clin Nutr* 2016; **35**(1): 158–162.

16. Sheean PM, Peterson SJ, Gurka DP, Braunschweig CA. Nutrition assessment: the reproducibility of subjective global assessment in patients requiring mechanical ventilation. *Eur J Clin Nutr* 2010; **64**(11): 1358–1364.

17. Casaer MP, Langouche L, Coudyzer W, Vanbeckevoort D, de Dobbelaer B, Guiza FG, Wouters PJ, Mesotten D, van den Berghe G. Impact of early parenteral nutrition on muscle and adipose tissue compartments during critical illness*. *Crit Care Med* 2013; **41**(10): 2298–2309.

18. Wandrag L, Brett SJ, Frost G, Hickson M. Impact of supplementation with amino acids or their metabolites on muscle wasting in patients with critical illness or other muscle wasting ilness: a systematic review. *J Hum Nutr Diet* 2015; **28**(4): 313–330.

19. Heyland DK, Cahill N, Day AG. Optimal amount of calories for critically ill patients: depends on how you slice the cake! *Crit Care Med* 2011; **39**(12): 2619–2626.

20. Preiser JC, van Zanten AR, Berger MM, Biolo G, Casaer MP, Doig GS, Griffiths RD, Heyland DK, Hiesmayr M, Iapichino G, Laviano A, Pichard C, Singer P, van den Berghe G, Wernerman J, Wischmeyer P, Vincent JL. Metabolic and nutritional support of critically ill patients: consensus and controversies. *Crit Care* 2015; **19**(1): 35.

21. Alberda C, Gramlich L, Jones N, Jeejeebhoy K, Day AG, Dhaliwal R, Heyland DK. The relationship between nutritional intake and clinical outcomes in critically ill patients: results of an international multi-center observational study. *Intens Care Med* 2009; **35**(10): 1728–1737.

22. Frankenfield DC, Coleman A, Alam S, Cooney RN. Analysis of estimation methods for resting metabolic rate in critically ill adults. *J Parenter Enteral Nutr* 2009; **33**(1): 27–36.

23. Takala J, Keinanen O, Vaisanen P, Kari A. Measurement of gas exchange in intensive care: laboratory and clinical validation of a new device. *Crit Care Med* 1989; **17**(10): 1041–1047.

24. Sundstrom M, Tjader I, Rooyackers O, Wernerman J. Indirect calorimetry in mechanically ventilated patients. A systematic comparison of three instruments. *Clin Nutr* 2013; **32**(1): 118–121.

25. Ireton-Jones C, Jones JD. Improved equations for predicting energy expenditure in patients: the Ireton-Jones Equations. *Nutr Clin Pract* 2002; **17**(1): 29–31.

26. Compher C, Nicolo M, Chittams J, Kang Y, Day AG, Heyland DK. Clinical outcomes in critically ill patients associated with the use of complex vs weight-only predictive energy equations. *J Parenter Enteral Nutr* 2015; **39**(7): 864–869.

27. Reid CL. Poor agreement between continuous measurements of energy expenditure and routinely used prediction equations in intensive care unit patients. *Clin Nutr* 2007; **26**(5): 649–657.

28. Frankenfield D, Hise M, Malone A, Russell M, Gradwell E, Compher C. Prediction of metabolic rate in critically ill adult patients: results of a systematic review of the evidence. *J Am Diet Assoc* 2007; **107**(9): 1552–1561.

29. Weijs PJM, Looijaard WGPM, Beishuizen A, Girbes ARJ, Oudemans-van Straaten HM. Early high protein

intake is associated with low mortality and energy overfeeding with high mortality in no-septic mechanically ventilated critically ill patients. *Crit Care* 2014; **18**(6): 701.

30. Kreymann KG, Berger MM, Deutz NE, Hiesmayr M, Jolliet P, Kazandjiev G, Nitenberg G, van den Berghe G, Wernerman J, Ebner C, Hartl W, Heymann C, Spies C. ESPEN guidelines on enteral nutrition: intensive care. *Clin Nutr* 2006; **25**(2): 210–223.

31. McClave SA, Martindale RG, Vanek VW, McCarthy M, Roberts P, Taylor B, Ochoa JB, Napolitano L, Cresci G. Guidelines for the provision and assessment of nutrition support therapy in the adult critically ill patient: Society of Critical Care Medicine (SCCM) and American Society for Parenteral and Enteral Nutrition (A.S.P.E.N.). *J Parenter Enteral Nutr* 2009; **33**(3): 277–316.

32. Hoffer LJ, Bistrian BR. Appropriate protein provision in critical illness: a systematic and narrative review. *Am J Clin Nutr* 2012; **96**(3): 591–600.

33. Allingstrup MJ, Esmailzadeh N, Wilkens KA, Espersen K, Hartvig JT, Wiis J, Perner A, Kondrup J. Provision of protein and energy in relation to measured requirements in intensive care patients. *Clin Nutr* 2012; **31**(4): 462–468.

34. Segaran E, Wandrag L, Stotz M, Terblance M, Hickson M. Does body mass index impact on muscle protein wasting and recovery following critical illness? A pilot feasibility study. *J Hum Nutr Diet* 2017; **30**: 227–235.

35. Choban P, Dickerson R, Malone A, Worthington P, Compher C. A.S.P.E.N. Clinical guidelines: nutrition support of hospitalized adult patients with obesity. *J Parenter Enteral Nutr* 2013; **37**(6): 714–744.

36. Anderegg BA, Worrall C, Barbour E, Simpson KN, DeLegge M. Comparison of resting energy expenditure prediction methods with measured resting energy expenditure in obese, hospitalized adults. *J Parenter Enteral Nutr* 2009; **33**(2): 168–175.

37. Doig GS, Heighes PT, Simpson F, Sweetman EA, Davies AR. Early enteral nutrition, provided within 24 h of injury or intensive care unit admission, significantly reduces mortality in critically ill patients: a meta-analysis of randomised controlled trials. *Intens Care Med* 2009; **35**(12): 2018–2027.

38. Casaer MP, Mesotten D, Hermans G, Wouters PJ, Schetz M, Meyfroidt G, van Cromphaut S, Ingels C, Meersseman P, Muller J, Vlasselaers D, Debaveye Y, Desmet L, Dubois J, van Assche A, Vanderheyden S, Wilmer A, van den Berghe G. Early versus late parenteral nutrition in critically ill adults. *N Engl J Med* 2011; **365**(6): 506–517.

39. Rice TW, Wheeler AP, Thompson BT, deBoisblanc BP, Steingrub J, Rock P. Enteral omega-3 fatty acid, gamma-linolenic acid, and antioxidant supplementation in acute lung injury. *JAMA* 2011; **306**(14): 1574–1581.

40. Arabi YM, Aldawood AS, Haddad SH, Al-Dorzi HM, Tamim HM, Jones G, Mehta S, McIntyre L, Solaiman O, Sakkijha MH, Sadat M, Afesh L. Permissive underfeeding or standard enteral feeding in critically ill adults. *N Engl J Med* 2015; **372**: 2398–2408.

41. Dhaliwal R, Jurewitsch B, Harrietha D, Heyland DK. Combination enteral and parenteral nutrition in critically ill patients: harmful or beneficial? A systematic review of the evidence. *Intens Care Med* 2004; **30**(8): 1666–1671.

42. Gramlich L, Kichian K, Pinilla J, Rodych NJ, Dhaliwal R, Heyland DK. Does enteral nutrition compared to parenteral nutrition result in better outcomes in critically ill adult patients? A systematic review of the literature. *Nutrition* 2004; **20**(10): 843–848.

43. Simpson F, Doig GS. Parenteral vs. enteral nutrition in the critically ill patient: a meta-analysis of trials using the intention to treat principle. *Intens Care Med* 2005; **31**(1): 12–23.

44. Harvey SE, Parrott F, Harrison DA, Bear DE, Segaran E, Beale R, Bellingan G, Leonard R, Mythen MG, Rowan KM. Trial of the route of early nutritional support in critically ill adults. *N Engl J Med* 2014; **371**(18): 1673–1684.

45. Elke G, van Zanten AR, Lemieux M, McCall M, Jeejeebhoy KN, Kott M, Jiang X, Day AG, Heyland DK. Enteral versus parenteral nutrition in critically ill patients: an updated systematic review and meta-analysis of randomized controlled trials. *Crit Care* 2016; **20**: 117.

46. Bost RB, Tjan DH, van Zanten AR. Timing of (supplemental) parenteral nutrition in critically ill patients: a systematic review. *Ann Intens Care* 2014; **4**: 31.

47. Martindale RG, McClave SA, Vanek VW, McCarthy M, Roberts P, Taylor B, Ochoa JB, Napolitano L, Cresci G. Guidelines for the provision and assessment of nutrition support therapy in the adult critically ill patient: Society of Critical Care Medicine and American Society for Parenteral and Enteral Nutrition: executive summary. *Crit Care Med* 2009; **37**(5): 1757–1761.

48. Reignier J, Mercier E, Le Gouge A, Boulain T, Desachy A, Bellec F, Clavel M, Frat JP, Plantefeve G, Quenot JP, Lascarrou JB. Effect of not monitoring residual gastric volume on risk of ventilator-associated pneumonia in adults receiving mechanical ventilation and early enteral feeding: a randomized controlled trial. *JAMA* 2013; **309**(3): 249–256.

49. Finfer S, Chittock DR, Su SY, Blair D, Foster D, Dhingra V, Bellomo R, Cook D, Dodek P, Henderson WR, Hebert PC, Heritier S, Heyland DK, McArthur C, McDonald E, Mitchell I, Myburgh JA, Norton R, Potter J, Robinson BG, Ronco JJ. Intensive versus conventional glucose control in critically ill patients. *N Engl J Med* 2009; **360**(13): 1283–1297.

50. Bollhalder L, Pfeil AM, Tomonaga Y, Schwenkglenks M. A systematic literature review and meta-analysis of randomized clinical trials of parenteral glutamine supplementation. *Clin Nutr* 2013; **32**(2): 213–223.

51. Van Zanten AR, Sztark F, Kaisers UX, Zielmann S, Felbinger TW, Sablotzki AR, de Waele JJ, Timsit JF, Honing ML, Keh D, Vincent JL, Zazzo JF, Fijn HB, Petit L, Preiser JC, van Horssen PJ, Hofman Z. High-protein enteral nutrition enriched with immune-modulating nutrients vs standard high-protein enteral nutrition and nosocomial infections in the ICU: a randomized clinical trial. *JAMA* 2014; **312**(5): 514–524.

52. Heyland D, Muscedere J, Wischmeyer PE, Cook D, Jones G, Albert M, Elke G, Berger MM, Day AG. A randomized trial of glutamine and antioxidants in critically ill patients. *N Engl J Med* 2013; **368**(16): 1489–1497.

53. Andrews PJ, Avenell A, Noble DW, Campbell MK, Croal BL, Simpson WG, Vale LD, Battison CG, Jenkinson DJ, Cook JA. Randomised trial of glutamine, selenium, or both, to supplement parenteral nutrition for critically ill patients. *BMJ* 2011; **342**: d1542.

54. Doig GS, Simpson F, Sweetman EA, Finfer SR, Cooper DJ, Heighes PT, Davies AR, O'Leary M, Solano T, Peake S. Early parenteral nutrition in critically ill patients with short-term relative con-traindications to early enteral nutrition: a randomized controlled trial. *JAMA* 2013; **309**(20): 2130–2138.

55. Heidegger CP, Berger MM, Graf S, Zingg W, Darmon P, Costanza MC, Thibault R, Pichard C. Optimisation of energy provision with supplemental parenteral nutrition in critically ill patients: a randomised controlled clinical trial. *Lancet* 2013; **381**(9864): 385–393.

Chapter 5.14

Nutrition support in burn injury

Rosemary Hayhoe, Katelynn Maniatis, Shahriar Shahrokhi and Marc Jeschke
Sunnybrook Health Sciences Centre, Toronto, Canada

5.14.1 Incidence and severity of burn

Worldwide, nearly 11 million people are burned severely enough to require medical attention annually. It is estimated that there are 265 000 deaths each year from flame burns alone [1].

The severity of thermal injury is dependent on the depth (i.e. superficial, partial thickness or full thickness) and percentage of total body surface area (TBSA) burned, with burns affecting ≥20% TBSA considered to be major [2]. Burn injury can be further complicated by presence of smoke inhalation [3]. Many burn patients undergo long hospital stays, including intensive care unit (ICU) admissions, and are left with lifelong physical and psychosocial challenges [1].

5.14.2 Pathophysiology and impact of undernutrition

The pathophysiology of burn injury is characterised by major endocrine, inflammatory, metabolic and immune alterations [2]. Increases in catecholamines, corticosteroids and inflammatory cytokines mediate the response, and concentrations can remain elevated for months after injury [4]. This hyperdynamic state is also characterised by increased heart rate, cardiac work and myocardial oxygen consumption [4]. The hypermetabolic and hypercatabolic responses are proportional to injury severity and include proteolysis, lipolysis and glycolysis, ultimately leading to reduced lean body mass (LBM), poor wound healing, immune dysfunction and multi-organ failure [2,4].

The principal goal of resuscitation is restoration and maintenance of tissue perfusion to prevent ischaemia and worsening injury [5]. Early excision of burn wounds and skin grafting is the primary mode of controlling the systemic response, but host response to injury can remain elevated despite adequate wound treatment [4,6]. Nutrition support can modulate the metabolic response and lead to improved outcomes [4,5].

Without intervention, burn patients would universally experience undernutrition. Cumulative energy deficits, especially in the first week of admission, are associated with many complications, including infection, sepsis, pressure sores and LBM loss, which further impair wound healing. Appropriate provision of nutrition and monitoring for adequacy of micro- and macronutrients are vital to burn recovery and help to prevent undernutrition, and subsequently reduce morbidity and mortality [5].

5.14.3 Nutrition assessment and monitoring

Nutrition assessment of the thermally injured patient requires a multifactorial approach and ongoing reassessment due to the dynamic nature

Advanced Nutrition and Dietetics in Nutrition Support, First Edition. Edited by Mary Hickson and Sara Smith.
© 2018 John Wiley & Sons Ltd. Published 2018 by John Wiley & Sons Ltd.

of the recovery process. Initial assessment should involve standard nutritional indicators, including anthropometrics, biochemical markers, clinical status and dietary history, with a focus on severity of burn injury and haemodynamic status [6,7]. A thorough nutrition assessment and ongoing monitoring are crucial to achieve the goal of mitigating the metabolic response, preserving LBM and preventing protein-energy undernutrition.

Numerous challenges limit accurate assessment of nutritional status in the acute phase. Pertinent anthropometric measurements include preinjury height and weight. Weight and weight changes are often skewed by fluid imbalance from resuscitation, oedema and fluid shifts [6].

Biochemical markers, such as visceral proteins, are not appropriate indicators of nutritional status in the acute phase due to the inflammatory response. Such markers better serve as prognostic indicators of disease status rather than undernutrition. Nitrogen balance (NB) as a marker of protein status is challenging as it is difficult to accurately quantify nitrogen losses via wounds [6].

Clinical factors, including burn size and severity, resultant metabolic response, timing of excision and grafting, use of occlusive wound dressing and haemodynamic stability, provide the foundation for initial nutrition assessment [6].

Due to the spontaneous nature of thermal injury, patients may present with varying dietary and environmental backgrounds. Baseline undernutrition significantly increases the risk of refeeding syndrome [6].

Despite the initial limitations of anthropometric and biochemical markers, these can be useful measures in ongoing monitoring and reassessment. For example, once fluid balance neutralises, weight trends over time may be indicative of adequacy of nutritional intake, but obtaining reliable weights in this population, as in any other acutely unwell population, is challenging. Clinical status (e.g. infections, ventilation status, wound healing), adequacy of intake and tolerance to nutrition support should also be considered in the ongoing reassessment of nutritional status and changing requirements [6,8]. To date, the assessment of muscle functional status, for example handgrip, has not been routinely undertaken in clinical practice.

5.14.4 Route and timing of nutrition support

Enteral nutrition (EN) is well established as the preferred route of nutrition support in patients with severe burns [5,8]. Early, aggressive EN prevents GI atrophy, decreases intestinal permeability and bacterial translocation, and can attenuate the inflammatory and hypermetabolic responses [4,9]. Gastric or small bowel EN should be initiated within 24 hours of injury, and even as early as 4–6 hours post injury [2,4,9–11]. Only when EN is not tolerated or contraindicated should PN be considered [2,11,12]. Complications of PN, including hyperglycaemia, increased proinflammatory response and infections related to both central lines and lack of GI stimulation, are of particular concern in the thermally injured patient [2,7,12].

Enteral nutrition strategies and protocols have become increasingly advanced to optimise nutrient delivery [4]. It is now common practice to continue EN infusion during perioperative and intraoperative periods, which has been demonstrated to decrease caloric deficit and infections [13].

Transitioning to oral intake

Meeting nutritional requirements via oral intake can be very challenging due to multiple factors inherent to postburn recovery, such as sedation, altered neurological status, intubation and high nutritional needs [7]. Given the fundamental role of nutrition in burn care, EN is typically discontinued only when a patient demonstrates the ability to meet requirements orally [8].

A small proportion of burn patients develop dysphagia; those with large burns, inhalation injury, and head and neck burns are at increased risk. Patients with dysphagia may require therapeutic texture-modified diets and the involvement of a speech-language pathologist. Most patients resume normal swallowing function by hospital discharge [14].

5.14.5 Energy and nutrient requirements

Energy

Energy requirements are significantly increased beyond normal basal resting energy expenditure (REE) due to the hypermetabolic and hypercatabolic response post burn. This increase is correlated with TBSA [2] and can approximate REE of 160% ± 30% [7]. Accurate assessment is crucial in avoiding undernutrition, meeting elevated energy needs and attenuating the hypermetabolic response, while simultaneously avoiding the risks associated with overfeeding [5]. The delicate balance of achieving optimal energy intake is further complicated by the dynamic nature of the hypermetabolic response, thus requiring ongoing reassessment throughout the recovery process [2].

According to the European Society for Parenteral and Enteral Nutrition (ESPEN), indirect calorimetry (IC) is the gold standard for determining energy requirements in thermally injured patients [2]. IC should be performed in the fed state, at rest, with a factor of 1.2–1.4 applied to account for activity, stress of wound care and other nursing tasks [12].

In the absence of IC, a number of burn-specific and non-burn-specific predictive equations are available to estimate REE [15]. The Toronto equation (Box 5.14.1), which considers anthropometrics, age, energy intake, temperature, TBSA and postburn days, is validated and recommended as an alternative to IC [2].

Macronutrients

Protein

The catabolic response post burn is characterised by proteolysis of up to 150 g/day of skeletal muscle [16], causing significant loss of LBM, which is associated with decreased wound healing and immune function. The catabolic state can last up to 2 years post burn, leading to significant negative NB in the setting of inadequate protein intake [7]. In order to attenuate the proteolytic response and minimise protein

---

Box 5.14.1 Toronto equation

$$REE = -4343 + (10.5 \times \% \, TBSA)$$
$$+ (0.23 \times caloric \, intake \, over \, 24 \, hours)$$
$$+ (0.84 \times Harris - Benedict \, REE)$$
$$+ (114 \times average \, temperature \, over \, 24 \, h)$$
$$- (4.5 \times postburn \, days)$$

---

catabolism and nitrogen loss post burn, protein requirements are estimated to be 1.5–2.5 g/kg/day [2,8,17].

Carbohydrate

Carbohydrates have a protein-sparing effect and should serve as the major energy source. Recent guidelines recommend providing 55–60% of energy from carbohydrates [2]. Similar to overall energy intake, carbohydrate delivery must be finely balanced. Excessive carbohydrate provision can lead to negative outcomes including hyperglycaemia, lipogenesis, polyuria, glucosuria and excessive carbon dioxide production, which is associated with difficulty weaning from ventilator support. In contrast, inadequate carbohydrate delivery can lead to increased rates of catabolism, infection and overall morbidity, as well as LBM loss and decreased wound healing [8]. A target glucose infusion rate of less than 5 mg/kg/min (7 g/kg/day) is recommended to achieve optimal carbohydrate balance [2,7,8,17]. ESPEN recommends close monitoring of blood glucose, particularly with PN administration, and continuous intravenous insulin infusion as appropriate to achieve targets between 4.5 and 8.0 mmol/L [2].

Fat

Dietary fat is required to prevent essential fatty acid (FA) deficiency and avoid excessive carbohydrate delivery, while still meeting increased energy requirements [8]. Due to alterations in fat metabolism post burn (e.g. increased breakdown of peripheral fat stores, β-oxidation of fat for use as energy) and risk of fat deposition in the liver, fat should be delivered at a minimum amount. Exogenous fat sources include enteral and parenteral nutrition (PN), and non-nutritional sources (e.g. propofol) [8]. Based on Grade C evidence, ESPEN guidelines recommend maintaining fat delivery at <35% of total energy intake [2]. Other literature suggests it may be beneficial to maintain fat delivery at <15% of total energy [7].

The type of fat provided should also be considered. It is recommended that essential FAs comprise 2–4% of total energy provided to thermally injured patients. ω-3 FAs have demonstrated immune-modulating effects and are associated with improved inflammatory response, reduced hyperglycaemia and overall improved outcomes. Conversely, ω-6 FAs may contribute to the proinflammatory response by converting into proinflammatory cytokines [8].

Micronutrients

Burn patients experience increased micronutrient requirements due to hypermetabolism, wound healing, oxidative stress and skin losses. The combination of inadequate micronutrient intake, heightened requirements and increased losses can contribute to poor wound healing, immune dysfunction and inflammation [8,18].

Antioxidants are required to stabilise reactive oxygen species produced during oxidative stress post burn [2,18]. Vitamins A, C and E function as antioxidants and play a role in decreasing oxidative stress and improving immunity. Vitamins A and C also contribute to wound healing [18]. Vitamin A is involved in epithelialisation, fibroplasia, angiogenesis and collagen synthesis but there is conflicting evidence with regard to improved outcomes with supplementation [18]. Vitamin C plays a role in collagen synthesis and cross-linking, and concentrations can decrease by up to 50% post burn [19]. In particular, a disproportionately high number of burn victims smoke or use alcohol in excess and therefore are already at risk of baseline vitamin C deficiency [18]. Vitamin C supplementation of 500 mg twice daily via the enteral route is suggested [2,18]. Vitamin E helps improve immune function, but specific dosing has not been recommended [18].

Thiamin and folate, both B vitamins, have been shown to be beneficial for burn patients. Thiamin contributes to decreased lactate and pyruvate concentrations. Folate contributes to protein and DNA synthesis and thus wound healing. Both can be adequately supplemented with a standard oral/enteral multivitamin [18].

Vitamin D deficiency may have immediate and long-term effects post burn. Initially, it can contribute to increased propensity for infection and poor glucose control [18]. In the long term, burn scar tissue has been shown to produce less vitamin D than healthy tissue [20], thus increasing susceptibility for vitamin D deficiency and associated risks. It is known that standard multivitamins contain inadequate amounts of vitamin D for repletion, but no specific dosing guidelines exist [18].

Supplementation of zinc, copper and selenium upon admission has been associated with reduced lipid peroxidation and infection, improved antioxidant defences and immunity, and shorter ICU stay. Larger burns require longer supplementation to accomplish these effects [2]. Their important roles in antioxidant function and wound healing, along with major losses of each from wound exudate, compound the significance of adequate supplementation. While trace element supplementation is recommended, exact dosing guidelines are not available [2,18].

Of note, IV antioxidant cocktails containing zinc, copper and selenium are increasingly popular in burn care. Berger proposed the use of an IV antioxidant cocktail (30 mg zinc, 4 mg copper, 500 μg selenium) for 2–3 weeks post burn after observing decreases in markers of oxidative stress, better graft take, reduced skin graft need and decreased rates of pneumonia [19].

5.14.6 Immuno-nutrition

Immuno-nutrition is of special interest in patients with thermal injury due to loss of skin barrier, hypermetabolic response-related suppression of normal host defences and subsequent immune suppression [21]. The use of immunonutrients in the general critically ill population has been called into question of late. Fish and borage oils for the management of acute respiratory distress syndrome and acute lung injury may be associated with increased mortality [22], and the use of glutamine for the management of oxidative stress has demonstrated increased mortality rates in the context of multiorgan failure [23]. Patients with thermal injury should be considered unique when determining the use of immune-modulating nutrients, given their hypermetabolic response and increased nutrient losses and requirements. Glutamine, ω-3 FAs, arginine, branched-chain amino acids (BCAAs) and dietary nucleotides remain of interest in burn care due to their role in immune function, wound healing, anti-inflammatory response and preservation of gastrointestinal tract integrity [21,24].

A recent Cochrane review investigated 16 randomised controlled trials involving at least one of glutamine, BCAAs, ω-3 FAs, combined immunonutrients or immunonutrient precursors and their use in burn care. Outcome measures included mortality, hospital length of stay (LOS) and rate of burn wound and non-wound infections. Only glutamine was found to have a significant effect on reducing mortality and LOS in burn patients. No effect was seen on rates of infection, wound related or otherwise [21]. Despite its contraindication in the general critically ill population, glutamine doses of 0.3–0.57 g/kg/day for 5–10 days or 30 g/day of glutamine precursor ornithine α-ketoglutarate should be considered in burn patients [2,7].

5.14.7 Non-nutritional management of hypermetabolism

Non-nutritional strategies can help mitigate the hypermetabolic, hypercatabolic response [2]. Early excision and grafting promotes wound closure and reduces fluid loss, inflammation,

Table 5.14.1 Summary of recommendations [2,7,8,18]

Topic	Recommendation
Route and timing	Unless contraindicated, EN should be initiated within 24 hours of injury
Energy	IC is the gold standard. In the absence of IC, the Toronto equation is recommended to predict REE
Macronutrients:	Both EN and PN:
• Protein	• 1.5–2.5 g/kg/day
• Carbohydrate	• 55–60% of total energy; glucose infusion rate <5 mg/kg/min (7 g/kg/day)
• Fat	• <35% of total energy from fat
Micronutrients:	EN/oral (unless specified otherwise):
• Vitamin A	• No consensus; consider 10 000–15 000 IU/day for major burns
• Vitamin C	• 500 mg twice daily
• Vitamin D	• No consensus; consider 600–1000 IU/day
• Vitamin E	• No consensus; consider 800–3000 IU/day for major burns
• Thiamin	• No consensus; consider 5–10 mg/day
• Folate	• No consensus; consider 1–2 mg/day
• Zinc	• No consensus; consider 25–50 mg/day
• Copper	• No consensus; consider up to 4 mg/day
• Selenium	• No consensus; consider 400–1000 µg/day
• Antioxidant cocktail (i.e. zinc, copper, selenium)	• IV cocktail containing 30 mg zinc, 4 mg copper, 500 µg selenium for 2–3 weeks post burn
Immune-modulating nutrients	• Arginine, BCAAs, ω-3 FAs or dietary nucleotides not recommended
	• No consensus on glutamine administration. Consider glutamine doses of 0.3–0.57 g/kg/day or 30 g/day ornithine α-ketoglutarate

BCAA, branched-chain amino acid; EN, enteral nutrition; FA, fatty acid; IC, indirect calorimetry; IU, international unit; IV, intravenous; PN, parenteral nutrition; REE, resting energy expenditure.

risk of infection and REE [25,26]. Whilst there is a lack of consensus and practices vary globally, oxandrolone, an anabolic androgenic steroid, has been shown to moderate postburn hypermetabolism and promote protein synthesis, LBM maintenance, wound healing and decreased hospital LOS and mortality [27–29]. In addition, non-specific β-blockade using propranolol has been shown to impede catecholamine surges, improve wound healing and decrease heart rate, cardiac index, cytokine release and thermogenesis post burn. Additional strategies to attenuate the hypermetabolic response include thermoregulation of ambient temperature, pain control and early rehabilitation [2,26].

5.14.8 Summary

Nutrition support is a cornerstone of modern burn care. Early initiation of EN and ongoing, accurate nutritional assessment are crucial to meet increased requirements, attenuate the hypermetabolic response, and prevent LBM loss and undernutrition. Non-nutritional therapies to reduce the hypermetabolic response should also be employed when appropriate. Micronutrient deficiencies are common and supplementation should be considered (Table 5.14.1). Nutritional status should be closely monitored throughout the recovery process to meet the continuously changing requirements of the thermally injured patient.

References

1. World Health Organization. Burns. Fact Sheet No. 365. www.who.int/mediacentre/factsheets/fs365/en/ (accessed 5 September 2017).
2. Rousseau AF, Losser MR, Ichai C, Berger MM. ESPEN endorsed recommendations: nutritional therapy in major burns. *Clin Nutr* 2013; **32**: 497–502.
3. Barrow RE, Spies M, Barrow LN, Herndon DN. Influence of demographics and inhalation injury on burn mortality in children. *Burns* 2004; **30**(1): 72–77.
4. Mandell SP, Gibran NS. Early enteral nutrition for burn injury. *Adv Wound Care* 2014; **3**(1): 64–70.
5. Gibran NS, Wiechman S, Meyer W, et al. American Burn Association consensus statements. *J Burn Care Res* 2013; **34**(4): 361–385.
6. Prelack K, Dylewski M, Sheridan RL. Practical guidelines for nutritional management of burn injury and recovery. *Burns* 2007; **33**: 14–24.
7. Rodriguez NA, Jeschke MG, Williams FN, Kamolz LP, Herndon DN. Nutrition in burns: Galveston contributions. *J Parenter Enteral Nutr* 2011; **35**(6): 704–714.
8. Hall KL, Shahrokhi S, Jeschke MG. Enteral nutrition support in burn care: a review of current recommendations as instituted in the Ross Tilley Burn Centre. *Nutrients* 2012; **4**: 1554–1565.
9. Kovacic-Vicic V, Radman M, Kovacic V. Early initiation of enteral nutrition improves outcomes in burn disease. *Asia Pac J Clin Nutr* 2013; **22**(4): 543–547.
10. Mosier MJ, Pham TN, Klein MB, et al. Early enteral nutrition in burns: compliance with guidelines and associated outcomes in a multicenter study. *J Burn Care Res* 2011; **32**(1): 104–109.
11. McClave SA, Martindale RG, Vanek VW, et al. Guidelines for the provision and assessment of nutrition support therapy in the adult critically ill patient: Society of Critical Care Medicine (SCCM) and American Society for Parenteral and Enteral Nutrition (A.S.P.E.N.). *J Parenter Enteral Nutr* 2009; **33**(3): 277–316.
12. Ahrenholz DH, Cope N, Dimick AR, et al. Practice guidelines for burn care. Chicago: American Burn Association, 2001.
13. Jenkins ME, Gottschlich MM, Warden GD. Enteral feeding during operative procedures in thermal injuries. *J Burn Care Rehabil* 1994; **15**(2): 199–205.
14. Rumbach AF, Ward EC, Cornwell PL, Bassett LV, Muller MJ. Clinical progression and outcome of dysphagia following thermal burn injury: a prospective cohort study. *J Burn Care Res* 2012; **33**(3): 336–346.
15. Machado NM, Gragnani A, Ferrieria LM. Burns, metabolism and nutritional requirements. *Nutr Hosp* 2011; **26**(4); 692–700.
16. Saffle JR, Graves C. Nutritional support of the burned patient. In: Herndon DN, editor. Total Burn Care, 3rd edn. London: Saunders Elsevier, 2007, pp. 398–419.
17. Williams FN, Branski LK, Jeschke MG, Herndon DN. What, how, and how much should patients with burns be fed? *Surg Clin North Am* 2011; **91**: 609–629.
18. Nordlund MJ, Pham TN, Gibran NS. Micronutrients after burn injury: a review. *J Burn Care Res* 2014; **35**: 121–133.
19. Berger MM. Antioxidant micronutrients in major trauma and burns: evidence and practice. *Nutr Clin Pract* 2006; **21**: 438–449.
20. Klein GL, Chen TC, Holick MF, et al. Synthesis of vitamin D in skin after burns. *Lancet* 2004; **363**: 291–292.
21. Tan HB, Danilla S, Murray A, et al. Immunonutrition as an adjuvant therapy for burns (review). *Cochrane Database Syst Rev* 2014; **12**: CD007174.

22. Rice TW, Wheeler AP, Thompson BT, et al. Enteral omega-3 fatty acid, γ-linolenic acid, and antioxidant supplementation in acute lung injury. *JAMA* 2011; **306**(14): 1574–1581.

23. Heyland D, Muscedere J, Wischmeyer PE, et al. A randomized trial of glutamine and antioxidants in critically ill patients. *N Engl J Med* 2013; **368**(16): 1489–1497.

24. Kurmis R, Parker A, Greenwood J. The use of immunonutrition in burn injury care: where are we? *J Burn Care Res* 2010; **31**: 677–691.

25. Orgill DP. Excision and skin grafting of thermal burns. *N Engl Med* 2009; **360**(3): 893–901.

26. Williams FN, Jeschke MG, Chinkes DL, Suman OE, Branski LK, Herndon DN. Modulation of the hypermetabolic response to trauma: temperature, nutrition and drugs. *J Am Coll Surg* 2009; **208**(4): 489–502.

27. Latenser BA. Critical care of the burn patient: the first 48 hours. *Crit Care Med* 2009; **37**(10): 2819–2826.

28. Wolf SE, Edelman L, Kemalyan N, et al. Effects of oxandrolone on outcome measures in the severely burned: a multicenter prospective randomized double blind trial. *J Burn Care Res* 2006; **27**(2): 131–139.

29. Jeschke MG, Finnerty CC, Suman OE, Kulp G, Mlcak RP, Herndon DN. The effect of oxandrolone on the endocrinologic, inflammatory, and hypermetabolic responses during the acute phase postburn. *Ann Surg* 2007; **246**(3): 351–362.

Chapter 5.15

Nutrition support in orthopaedics

Jack J. Bell
Prince Charles Hospital, Brisbane, Australia

5.15.1 Introduction

Orthopaedic patients requiring nutrition intervention range from outpatients requiring weight loss prior to elective orthopaedic surgery through to those with acute hip fracture. The latter condition is noted as the most common cause of injury-related death internationally and costs the UK approximately £2 billion per annum [1]. This chapter focuses on the nutritional management of undernutrition.

5.15.2 Undernutrition in orthopaedic inpatient populations

Prevalence and incidence

Undernutrition prevalence in orthopaedic populations is wide-ranging due to the heterogeneity across orthopaedic populations, the lack of gold standards for nutrition screening and diagnosis, and other methodological issues [2–5]. Approximately 25% of elective orthopaedic populations are likely to be undernourished on admission to hospital, increasing up to half of those with traumatic or hip fractures [5,6]. Undernutrition is a significant concern requiring further investigation, particularly in those with acute hip fracture [6,7].

Pathogenesis of undernutrition

The pathogenesis of undernutrition in orthopaedic inpatients can be attributed to unintentional lean body mass loss in the context of inadequate protein or energy intake or absorption, the acute or chronic inflammatory effects of stress or disease or a combination of these [7]. Identification of these underlying causes can help overcome the challenge of differentiating between undernutrition, sarcopenia and frailty in older orthopaedic patients [8].

Barriers to adequate nutrition intakes have been reported under the themes of medical (physiological, physical and medical), psychosocial, environmental and population perceptions [7]. Poor dietary intakes are most commonly identified in hip fracture patients who are predominantly older, female, with multiple comorbidities, and prone to postoperative complications, polypharmacy, functional and cognitive impairment, depressive symptoms, dysphagia, poor dentition and undernutrition [2,9,10].

Consequences of undernutrition

Undernutrition has been identified as an independent predictor of mortality after adjusting for relevant covariates in hospitalised orthopaedic patients (odds ratio 2.4; 95% confidence interval (CI) 1.3–4.7) [11]. A recent prognostic study investigated the impact of comorbidities on hospitalisation costs in 32 440 hip fracture patients [12]. This study concluded that the comorbidity with the largest associated hospitalisation cost was weight loss or undernutrition. Findings also demonstrated that weight loss or undernutrition was the comorbidity most likely to prolong

Advanced Nutrition and Dietetics in Nutrition Support, First Edition. Edited by Mary Hickson and Sara Smith.
© 2018 John Wiley & Sons Ltd. Published 2018 by John Wiley & Sons Ltd.

hospital stay (2.5 days, 95% CI 2.2–2.8 days). Other studies demonstrate associations between undernutrition and delayed mobility or functional status, quality of life, pressure injuries, recurrent falls-related injuries, postoperative infections or delayed wound healing, other postoperative complications, hospital readmissions and unfavourable discharge destination [3,5,8,13–19].

5.15.3 Nutrition screening in orthopaedic settings

Nutrition screening tools demonstrate a wide range of reported risk rates across orthopaedic studies, and may particularly lack sensitivity in predicting undernutrition in hip fracture inpatients [4,20]. In a recent study of a 142 older acute hip fracture patients, the Mini Nutritional Assessment Short-Form (MNA-SF) demonstrated the highest sensitivity (89%), but lowest specificity (49%) when compared with a broad variety of other screening tools (including the Malnutrition Universal Screening Tool), anthropometric measures or other markers [4]. The poor performance of all the nutrition screening tools, combined with high undernutrition rates, routinely observed inadequate intakes, and the patient and healthcare cost implications of undiagnosed undernutrition have resulted in recommendations that nutrition screening should be replaced with routine nutrition assessment in hip fracture [4,21]. In lower risk orthopaedic populations or where resource limitations preclude routine assessment, clinicians need to consider the target population, context and treatment aims and outcomes when considering which screening tool is most appropriate to apply [4].

5.15.4 Nutrition assessment and nutritional diagnosis

Systematic routine assessment, for example using an ABCDE format, should be undertaken (Box 5.15.1) [22,23]. In the absence of a gold standard, clinicians should combine clinical judgement with relevant and available nutrition

assessment parameters to ensure correct nutritional diagnoses to guide the provision of appropriate nutrition intervention in orthopaedic inpatients [22].

Anthropometry

Body mass index (BMI) is the most commonly reported anthropometric measure utilised for the diagnosis of undernutrition in orthopaedic populations [4,20]. A low BMI is associated with increased risk of falls with fracture, post-fracture reduced mobility, functional status and quality of life, and increased postoperative complications, residential care placement and mortality [24–27].

However, relying on BMI or other anthropometric factors (see Table 5.15.1) as a stand-alone diagnostic measure of undernutrition is not ideal [5]. A key limitation of BMI is its failure to identify those who are overweight but at risk of undernutrition, which may represent a growing population of concern in orthopaedic inpatients [26,28]. The potential impact of fluid shifts and kyphosis, prostheses, casts and bulky dressings, changes in fat distribution, suitability of described norms or reference ranges, the need to utilise surrogate measures, and the skills and training of those undertaking measurements on anthropometric measures should also be considered. Despite these limitations, routine anthropometric measurements should be integrated into care pathways and systematic, multidisciplinary processes, in addition to ensuring adequate access to specialised equipment where required, for example weigh beds.

Biochemical assessment

Serum albumin, transferrin or other 'nutritional proteins' and immunological markers should also not be considered as stand-alone nutrition assessment parameters in orthopaedic inpatients. Reductions in these parameters are commonly observed following severe trauma, sepsis or inflammation, or major surgery, and consequently predict postoperative orthopaedic outcomes but not necessarily nutrition status [5,20].

Box 5.15.1 Commonly applied nutrition assessment parameters in orthopaedic practice [32]

Anthropometry
- Weight (reported/ measured)
- Height or surrogate height measure
- Usual weight
- Weight change
- BMI
- Calf circumference
- Mid-arm circumference
- Mid-arm muscle area, corrected mid-arm muscle area*
- Skinfolds**
- BIA‡**
- Dual-energy x-ray absorptiometry**

Biochemistry and functional measures
- Electrolytes
- Vitamins†
- LFTs
- Osmolarity
- Glucose concentration
- Albumin/transthyretin/ insulin-like growth factor-1, retinol binding protein, transferrin, haemoglobin/total protein*
- Nitrogen balance**
- Grip strength
- Delayed cutaneous hypersensitivity*
- Total lymphocyte count*

ClinicalDiet
- Reason for referral
- Current medical/surgical issues
- Medical/surgical history
- Gastrointestinal symptoms and bowel output
- Intake barriers

Medications
- Antidepressants
- Antiemetics/prokinetics
- Aperients
- Electrolytes
- Insulin/oral hypoglycaemic agents
- Lipids
- Narcotics
- Vitamin/mineral supplements

Diet
- Current diet
- Usual diet
- Assistance required
- Texture modification or other dietary therapy/restriction/ intolerance/allergy
- Estimated usual intake (macro/ micronutrient excess or deficiency evaluation)
- Estimated current intake (macro/ micronutrient excess or deficiency evaluation)

Psychosocial
- Usual place of residency
- Food access/preparation
- Employment/income
- Social support network
- Cultural/religious preferences
- Cognitive state
- Knowledge/literacy

Estimated requirements
- Energy§
- Protein§
- Fluid
- Other (specify)

Global assessments/index scores results
- MNA/MNA-SF score
- Subjective Global Assessment
- ICD9/10-AM undernutrition diagnostic criteria
- ASPEN adult malnutrition consensus statement characteristics

* Single markers of nutritional status including 'dietary proteins', anthropometric and functional measures should be interpreted cautiously in acute inpatient settings and are not considered reliable as stand-alone measures of nutritional status.
† Vitamin D, B12 and folate deficiencies are commonly observed in older, multimorbid orthopaedic populations. Other deficiencies should be considered dependent on client history.
§ Estimates of energy requirements vary considerably across individuals and orthopaedic inpatient types. Higher estimates (e.g. 125–145 kJ/kg/day and 1.2–1.5 g/kg/day protein should be considered for hip fracture or multitrauma inpatients as a starting point).
‡ Bioelectrical impedence results should be interpreted cautiously in patients with substantial fluid or electrolyte shifts.
** Less commonly applied in routine practice.
ASPEN, American Society for Parenteral and Enteral Nutrition; BIA, bioelectric impedance analysis; BMI, body mass index; ICD, International Classification of Diseases; LFT, liver function test; MNA-SF, Mini Nutritional Assessment Short-Form.

Clinical and functional assessment

Functional measures such as handgrip strength have also been applied in orthopaedic inpatient populations as measures of nutritional status. Whilst hip fracture studies have reported associations between handgrip strength and weight loss, pressure injuries and mortality, these do not routinely demonstrate statistical significance following adjustment for confounders [29,30]. The predisposition of hip fracture patients to osteoarticular disease, delirium, dementia or cognitive impairment may limit the applicability of handgrip strength in routine practice [10].

Clinical assessment of elective orthopaedic inpatients will routinely consider factors detailed in Table 5.15.1. Cognitive impairment in non-elective orthopaedic populations is common [7,10]. Consequently, patient-reported data can be lacking, inaccurate, skewed or misrepresented. Appropriate alternative information sources, including relatives and carers, should be utilised in such circumstances [7]. A comprehensive 'geriatric' assessment should be considered as part of routine care for these patients [1,21,31].

Dietary assessment

Routine dietary assessment methods should consider both macronutrient and micronutrient evaluation (see Table 5.15.1). Again, triangulation of data from multiple sources is recommended for complex, older inpatients, particularly in acute hip fracture cohorts where delirium, dementia or cognitive impairment prevalence approximates 60% of all admitted patients [10].

Environmental assessment

In addition to identifying physiological, physical, medical, psychosocial and environmental barriers and facilitators to nutrition care (see Table 5.15.1), high priority should be given to exploring and addressing the perceptions of orthopaedic patients and those who care for them [7]. In addition, as part of discharge planning, consideration should be given to social and financial circumstances.

Global approaches to undernutrition diagnosis

A small number of studies report the concurrent or predictive validity of index scores and global assessments such as the MNA-SF, Subject Global Assessment, ICD10-AM criteria or the Academy of Nutrition and Dietetics' undernutrition diagnostic criteria in elective orthopaedic or hip fracture inpatient populations [3,5,7]. The ICD10-AM undernutrition diagnostic criteria recently demonstrated the highest predictive and concurrent validity in diagnosing undernutrition in hip fracture inpatients when compared with the MNA-SF and a number of other measures [7].

5.15.5 Estimating requirements for orthopaedic conditions

Given conflicting evidence and a lack of consensus guidelines, a starting point of 125–145 kJ/kg/day (30–35 kcal/kg/day) and 1.2–1.5 g/kg/day protein is suggested for hip fracture, multitrauma patients or others with suspected increased energy requirements or existing undernutrition [33]. Others, for example those with head injuries, may exceed these estimates [20]. Elective orthopaedic patients, particularly those receiving minimally invasive surgery with an absence of other processes or disease states, may only require 25–30 kcal/kg/day and normal protein requirements [33,34]. Attention should also be given to adjusting initial estimates in response to monitoring and evaluation parameters.

5.15.6 Approaches to the management of undernutrition in orthopaedic patients

Common goals of nutrition interventions

Nutrition interventions for undernutrition in orthopaedics can be broadly themed around food and nutrient delivery, education and counselling,

Table 5.15.1 Key monitoring and outcome measures in orthopaedic inpatients [32]

Measure	
Intake	Individual: Macronutrient and micronutrient intake adequacy considering: • Food and beverage intake • Oral nutritional supplement intake • Enteral and parenteral tube feeding intake Health service/population based: • Food wastage audits • Meal/tray audit data • Supplement and tube feeding usage • Patient satisfaction surveys
Physiological/medical	Individual: • Anthropometric changes • Biochemical/medical tests/medication changes • Bowels/gastrointestinal symptoms • Losses (vomiting, malabsorption, drug–nutrient interactions, drains/ exudate) • Metabolic changes • Changes in physical examination or global nutrition score/status Health service/population based: • 'Nutrition day' audit data • Wound infections or dehiscence audit data • Pressure injury audit data • Postoperative infections or complications • Acute and subacute length of stay • Postoperative functional status (eg. activities of daily living) • Grip strength/mobility measures/mobility aides • Need for support/assistance post discharge • Discharge destination • Unplanned readmission rates • Refracture rates • Inpatient and postdischarge mortality
Psychosocial, cultural, behavioural, environmental	Individual: • Nutrition-related knowledge • Nutrition behaviours, perceptions, beliefs and attitudes • Adherence to recommendations • Quality of life measures Health service/population based: • Benchmarking and adherence to key policies, standards, guidelines, and/or legislation • Staff surveys/focus group results • Compliments and complaints register • Quality-adjusted life-years • Proportion of healthcare budget allocated to nutrition care • Occasions of service/activity metrics • Healthcare costs/cost-effectiveness analysis • Nutrition governance infrastructure • Research and knowledge base outputs

and co-ordination of care to facilitate an adequate protein and energy intake [22]. Limitations in study design and inconsistency of outcomes to date have precluded the routine recommendation of nutrition intervention strategies in hip fracture management guidelines [1,2,21,31,32].

Food and oral nutrition supplements

Nutrition intervention studies in orthopaedic settings predominantly target provision of oral nutrition supplements, with a limited number of studies investigating food fortification or modifications to food provision methods [32]. Many intervention studies have demonstrated a significant increase in energy or protein intake; however, the impact of these increases in intake remains slanted towards non-significant versus positive patient and healthcare outcomes [2,32]. Whether oral nutrition supplements should be selective or prescribed remains unclear, although there may be benefit in considering and prescribing 'supplements as medicine' rather than as a selective food choice in hip fracture inpatients [7,35].

A recent Cochrane review concluded that there was low-quality evidence to support the use of oral supplements started before or soon after surgery to prevent complications after hip fracture in older people; however, their use has no clear influence on mortality [2]. Only randomised and quasi-randomised controlled trials of nutrition interventions in hip fracture patients were included (41 studies and 3881 patients). The review acknowledged poor study designs and the impact of confounding variables as key determinants and as a consequence recommended that further adequately sized randomised studies with better study designs should be carried out. The review also suggested that the role of dietetic assistants, peripheral venous feeding or nasogastric feeding in very undernourished patients required further evaluation.

Enteral nutrition

In the recent Cochrane review, hip fracture studies involving enteral nutrition were among those demonstrating the highest increase in protein or energy intakes, but no clear effect of nasogastric feeding on outcomes was evident [2]. Enteral nutrition in the absence of a supportive orthopaedic team environment has demonstrated difficulties with administration and adherence, and appears poorly tolerated [2,7]. There is some suggestion that enteral nutrition may be associated with increased mortality and this area remains a priority for ongoing research [2,36].

Parenteral nutrition

Multinutrient parenteral nutrition with oral nutritional supplementation has demonstrated a reduction in complications but not in mortality in the orthopaedic setting [37]. However, evidence more broadly supports limiting parenteral nutrition to those with an inability to feed via the gastrointestinal tract [34].

Nutrition education or counselling

Nutrition education and counselling of patients or those who care for them may improve intakes and outcomes in orthopaedic inpatients [7,9,30,35]. Increased problem recognition and consciousness raising may also liberalise unwarranted dietary restrictions in older inpatients, resulting in improved patient and healthcare outcomes [7]. Demanding clinical environments and poor multidisciplinary team engagement are recognised as barrier to interventions in this patient group; education strategies may be helpful to focus staff towards the delivery of nutrition care [7].

Nutrition assistants

Orthopaedic studies including nutrition assistants to facilitate nutrition care have demonstrated a positive impact on patient satisfaction, energy intake, anthropometric measures, nutrition status, discharge destination and mortality [30,35]. The role of nutrition assistant staff in orthopaedic settings is recommended as an area for ongoing research [2].

Limiting unnecessary preoperative and postoperative dietary restrictions

Extended or overnight fasts or the use of highly restrictive postoperative diets such as clear fluids, free fluids or surgical light diets are historical practices applied for the management of aspiration, nausea, vomiting, ileus or intestinal pseudo-obstruction [34,38]. Short fasting times with the early commencement of oral fluids and diet in combination with multidisciplinary interventions may be more appropriate [34,35].

Multimodal, multidisciplinary care and enhanced recovery after surgery (ERAS) programmes

Adopting a multidisciplinary, multimodal approach to nutrition care has demonstrated improved patient and healthcare outcomes when compared with individualized care [9,34,35].

Enhanced recovery programmes in elective orthopaedic populations include preoperative patient education, multimodal pain control, minimally invasive or computer-assisted surgery and/or advanced perioperative multidisciplinary techniques. These have demonstrated improved patient and healthcare outcomes both with and without inclusion of preoperative carbohydrate drinks, and currently provide limited evidence base for recommendations to routinely include carbohydrate drinks within ERAS programmes in orthopaedic inpatients [39].

Whilst preoperative administration of carbohydrates appears safe, high-quality studies are still required to substantiate dosing, timing and the overall utility of perioperative carbohydrate loading in improving patient and healthcare outcomes in both elective and traumatic orthopaedic patients [40].

Micronutrient requirements

The potential for micronutrient deficiency states should not be overlooked, particularly in older, multiple comorbidity type patients or those with gastrointestinal disorders, recurrent infections or surgeries, chronically inadequate intakes, high-dose diuretics or moderate-to-severe undernutrition.

Managing medical comorbidities

Dysphagia, pain, constipation, medications/polypharmacy, delirium and other medical comorbidities and complications are highly prevalent in older orthopaedic inpatients and are associated with poor oral intake and undernutrition [7,10,27]. Overly restrictive diets should be avoided and instead individualised systematic strategies should be provided to actively manage associated medical comorbidities in nutritionally vulnerable orthopaedic inpatients [7,9].

5.15.7 Monitoring and evaluation in orthopaedic patients

Lack of diagnostic gold standards, population-specific reference ranges and evidence-based guidelines for nutrition care of orthopaedic inpatients has contributed to the heterogeneity in nutritional monitoring and outcome measures to date [32]. Table 5.15.1 provides a list of commonly reported monitoring and outcomes measures for consideration by clinicians, researchers and health service managers to evaluate and improve the delivery of nutrition care [22]. A careful approach to interpretation is advised; measurements may be inaccurate, unreliable, skewed or require considerable clinical skill or resources when applied within the scope of routine clinical practice.

References

1. National Institute for Health and Clinical Excellence. The Management of Hip Fracture in Adults. NICE Clinical Guideline No. 124. London: NICE, 2011.
2. Avenell A, Handoll HH. Nutritional supplementation for hip fracture aftercare in older people. *Cochrane Database Syst Rev* 2016; **11**: CD001880.
3. Ozkalkanli MY, Ozkalkanli DT, Katircioglu K, Savaci S. Comparison of tools for nutrition assessment and screening for predicting the development of complications in orthopedic surgery. *Nutr Clin Pract* 2009; **24**(2): 274–280.

4. Bell JJ, Bauer JD, Capra S, Pulle RC. Quick and easy is not without cost: implications of poorly performing nutrition screening tools in hip fracture. *J Am Geriatr Soc* 2014; **62**(2): 237–243.

5. Bell JJ, Bauer JD, Capra S, Pulle RC. Concurrent and predictive evaluation of malnutrition diagnostic measures in hip fracture inpatients: a diagnostic accuracy study. *Eur J Clin Nutr* 2014; **68**(3): 358–362.

6. Dwyer AJ, John B, Mam MK, Antony P, Abraham R, Joshi M. Relation of nutritional status to healing of compound fractures of long bones of the lower limbs. *Orthopedics* 2007; **30**(9): 709–712.

7. Bell JJ, Bauer J, Capra S, Pulle CR. Barriers to nutritional intake in patients with acute hip fracture: time to treat malnutrition as a disease and food as a medicine? *Can J Physiol Pharmacol* 2013; **91**(6): 489–495.

8. Lloyd BD, Williamson DA, Singh NA, et al. Recurrent and injurious falls in the year following hip fracture: a prospective study of incidence and risk factors from the sarcopenia and hip fracture study. *J Gerontol A Biol Sci Med Sci* 2009; **64**(5): 599–609.

9. Hoekstra JC, Goosen JHM, de Wolf GS, Verheyen CCPM. Effectiveness of multidisciplinary nutritional care on nutritional intake, nutritional status and quality of life in patients with hip fractures: a controlled prospective cohort study. *Clin Nutr* 2011; **30**(4): 455–461.

10. Sivakumar BS, McDermott LM, Bell JJ, Pulle CR, Jayamaha S, Ottley MC. Dedicated hip fracture service: implementing a novel model of care. *Aust NZ J Surg* 2013; **83**(7-8): 559–563.

11. Bell JJ, Pulle RC, Crouch AM, Kuys SS, Ferrier RL, Whitehouse SL. Impact of malnutrition on 12-month mortality following acute hip fracture. *Aust NZ J Surg* 2016; **86**(3): 157–161.

12. Nikkel LE, Fox EJ, Black KP, Davis C, Andersen L, Hollenbeak CS. Impact of comorbidities on hospitalization costs following hip fracture. *J Bone Joint Surg Am* 2012; **94**(1): 9–17.

13. Ponzer S, Tidermark J, Brismar K, Soderqvist A, Cederholm T. Nutritional status, insulin-like growth factor-1 and quality of life in elderly women with hip fractures. *Clin Nutr* 1999; **18**(4): 241–246.

14. Koren-Hakim T, Weiss A, Hershkovitz A, Otzrateni I, Grosman B, Frishman S, Salai M, Beloosesky Y. The relationship between nutritional status of hip fracture operated elderly patients and their functioning, comorbidity and outcome. *Clin Nutr* 2012; **31**(6): 917–921.

15. Miyanishi K, Jingushi S, Torisu T. Mortality after hip fracture in Japan: the role of nutritional status. *J Orthop Surg* 2010; **18**(3): 265–270.

16. Bastow MD, Rawlings J, Allison SP. Undernutrition, hypothermia, and injury in elderly women with fractured femur: an injury response to altered metabolism? *Lancet* 1983; **1**(8317): 143–146.

17. Gumieiro DN, Rafacho BPM, Gonçalves AF, et al. Mini Nutritional Assessment predicts gait status and mortality 6 months after hip fracture. *Br J Nutr* 2013; **109**(9): 1657–1661.

18. Foster MR, Heppenstall RB, Friedenberg ZB, Hozack WJ. A prospective assessment of nutritional status and complications in patients with fractures of the hip. *J Orthop Trauma* 1990; **4**(1): 49–57.

19. Baumgarten M, Margolis DJ, Orwig DL, et al. Pressure ulcers in elderly patients with hip fracture across the continuum of care. *J Am Geriatr Soc* 2009; **57**(5): 863–870.

20. Cross MB, Yi PH, Thomas CF, Garcia J, Della Valle CJ. Evaluation of malnutrition in orthopaedic surgery. *J Am Acad Orthop Surg* 2014; **22**(3): 193–199.

21. Australian and New Zealand Hip Fracture Registry (ANZHFR) Steering Group. Australian and New Zealand Guideline for Hip Fracture Care. 2014. https://acem.org.au/getattachment/91169f29-890e-47c8-a4db-03e1ae0b716e/Australian-New-Zealand-Hip-Fracture-Registry-(ANZH.aspx (accessed 6 September 2017).

22. Writing Group of the Nutrition Care Process/Standardized Language Committee. Nutrition care process and model part I: the 2008 update. *J Am Diet Assoc* 2008; **108**(7): 1113–1137.

23. White JV, Guenter P, Jensen G, Malone A, Schofield M. Consensus statement: Academy of Nutrition and Dietetics and American Society for Parenteral and Enteral Nutrition: characteristics recommended for the identification and documentation of adult malnutrition (undernutrition). *J Parenter Enteral Nutr* 2012; **36**(3): 275–283.

24. Batsis JA, Naessens JM, Keegan MT, Wagie AE, Huddleston PM, Huddleston JM. Impact of body mass on hospital resource use in total hip arthroplasty. *Public Health Nutr* 2009; **12**(8): 1122–1132.

25. Bruce D, Laurance I, Ng L, Goldswain P. Undernourished patients with hip fracture: poor outcome is not due to excess infections. *Australas J Ageing* 1999; **18**(3): 119–123.

26. Di Monaco M, Vallero F, di Monaco R, Mautino F, Cavanna A. Body mass index and functional recovery after hip fracture: a survey study of 510 women. *Aging Clin Exp Res* 2006; **18**(1): 57–62.

27. Juliebo V, Bjoro K, Krogseth M, Skovlund E, Ranhoff AH, Wyller TB. Risk factors for preoperative and postoperative delirium in elderly patients with hip fracture. *J Am Geriatr Soc* 2009; **57**(8): 1354–1361.

28. Murphy MC, Brooks CN, New SA, Lumbers ML. The use of the Mini-Nutritional Assessment (MNA) tool in elderly orthopaedic patients. *Eur J Clin Nutr* 2000; **54**(7): 555–562.

29. Gumieiro DN, Rafacho BPM, Gradella LM, Azevedo PS, Gaspardo D, Zornoff LAM, Pereira GJC, Paiva SAR, Minicucci MF. Handgrip strength predicts pressure ulcers in patients with hip fractures. *Nutrition* 2012; **28**(9): 874–878.

30. Duncan DG, Beck SJ, Hood K, Johansen A. Using dietetic assistants to improve the outcome of hip fracture: a randomised controlled trial of nutritional support in an acute trauma ward. *Age Ageing* 2006; **35**(2): 148–153.

31. Scottish Intercollegiate Guidelines Network. Management of Hip Fracture in Older People. A National Clinical Guideline. 2009. www.sign.ac.uk/assets/sign111.pdf (accessed 6 September 2017).

32. Bell JJ. Identifying and Overcoming Barriers to Nutrition Care in Acute Hip Fracture Inpatients. PhD thesis, University of Queensland, Brisbane, 2014.

33. Dietitians/Nutritionists from the Nutrition Education Materials Online Team. Estimating Energy, Protein and Fluid Requirements for Adult Clinical Conditions. www.health.qld.gov.au/nutrition/resources/est_rqts.pdf (accessed 6 September 2017).

34. Deren ME, Huleatt J, Winkler MF, Rubin LE, Salzler MJ, Behrens SB. Assessment and treatment of malnutrition in orthopaedic surgery. *JBJS Rev* 2014; **2**(9): e1.

35. Bell JJ, Bauer JD, Capra S, Pulle RC. Multidisciplinary, multi-modal nutritional care in acute hip fracture inpatients – results of a pragmatic intervention. *Clin Nutr* 2014; **33**(6): 1101–1107.

36. Hartgrink HH, Wille J, Konig P, Hermans J, Breslau PJ. Pressure sores and tube feeding in patients with a fracture of the hip: a randomized clinical trial. *Clin Nutr* 1998; **17**(6): 287– 292.

37. Eneroth M, Olsson UB, Thorngren KG. Nutritional supplementation decreases hip fracture-related complications. *Clin Orthop* 2006; **451**: 212–217.

38. Traviss KA, Barr SI. Rethinking postoperative diets for short-stay orthopedic surgery patients. *J Am Diet Assoc* 1997; **97**(9): 971–974.

39. Ibrahim MS, Twaij H, Giebaly DE, Nizam I, Haddad FS. Enhanced recovery in total hip replacement: a clinical review. *Bone Joint J* 2013; **95-B**(12): 1587–1594.

40. Li L, Wang Z, Ying X, Tian J, Sun T, Yi K, Zhang P, Jing Z, Yang K. Preoperative carbohydrate loading for elective surgery: a systematic review and meta-analysis. *Surg Today* 2012; **42**(7): 613–624.

Chapter 5.16

Nutrition support in HIV infection

Alastair Duncan

Guy's and St Thomas' NHS Foundation Trust and King's College London, London, UK

5.16.1 Background and prevalence of undernutrition in HIV

Following the identification of the human immunodeficiency virus (HIV) in 1983, the link between profound immunodeficiency and HIV was made, and the term 'acquired immune deficiency syndrome' (AIDS) coined to describe it. AIDS presents with wasting – protein energy undernutrition – and in Africa those with AIDS were referred to as having 'slim disease'. For many people an enduring image of a person ill with HIV is someone experiencing severe undernutrition. More than 30 million people died from the consequences of AIDS in the 1980s and 1990s. Fear of HIV and AIDS was widespread, and stigma for those living with HIV was, and sadly continues to be, a pervasive consequence. The development of highly active antiretroviral therapy (HAART) in the late 1990s, and its widespread use in recent years, has led to HIV becoming, for most, a chronic, manageable condition [1].

An asymptomatic phase of variable length follows transmission of HIV, sometimes months, and often years in duration, where viral replication is largely controlled, with immune function remaining relatively normal. Eventually, the HIV viral load increases along with a decline in immune function, signalled by reducing CD4 cell numbers. Opportunistic infections take hold once the CD4 count falls below 200 cells/mm^2 [1].

People unaware of being HIV positive may remain asymptomatic for some time, presenting late in the course of infection profoundly immunosuppressed. Even with modern effective antiretroviral therapy, late presenters experience higher rates of morbidity and mortality, therefore early diagnosis of HIV is essential.

Highly active antiretroviral therapy consists of several antiretrovirals used in combination, targeting viral replication at different sites in the pathway. Treatment regimens continually evolve; current information and guidelines can be found online through resources listed in Section 5.16.7 of this chapter. Therapeutic drug concentrations must be maintained to both prevent development of viral resistance, which may prevent future use of several medications, and avoid toxicities. Adherence to sometimes complicated regimens is therefore vital, and can prove challenging, especially when medications must be taken with or without food, and within certain time windows [1].

The HIV epidemic is stabilising worldwide, with new infection rates predicted to decline as adults and children living with HIV respond successfully to HAART. Taken as a whole, the cohort of people living with HIV is an ageing population, as survival improves [1]. The most recent epidemiology data can be accessed through resources listed in Section 5.16.7.

Individuals immunocompromised through HIV infection experience a range of AIDS-defining infections and conditions, often

Advanced Nutrition and Dietetics in Nutrition Support, First Edition. Edited by Mary Hickson and Sara Smith.
© 2018 John Wiley & Sons Ltd. Published 2018 by John Wiley & Sons Ltd.

Table 5.16.1 Common AIDS-defining conditions and their nutritional consequences

AIDS-defining condition	Nutritional consequences
Burkitt's lymphoma	Cachexia, development or exacerbation of undernutrition during treatment
Candida in the oesophagus	Painful or difficult swallowing leading to reduced nutritional intake
Cytomegalovirus (CMV) retinitis	Failing sight or blindness can limit usual activities including shopping and cooking
Cryptococcal meningitis	Headaches, nausea and vomiting can lead to reduced nutritional intake
Cryptosporidial or microsporidial diarrhoea > 1 month duration	Dehydration, electrolyte imbalance, malabsorption and undernutrition
HIV-associated dementia	Cognitive decline can limit usual activities including shopping and cooking
Kaposi's sarcoma	Internal tumours can lead to gastrointestinal obstruction
Mycobacterium avium complex (MAI)	Gastrointestinal infection can lead to diarrhoea and malabsorption
Pneumocystis pneumonia (PCP)	Increased energy expenditure and loss of appetite can lead to undernutrition
Progressive multifocal leucoencephalopathy (PML)	Cognitive decline can limit activities of daily living such as shopping and cooking
Salmonella septicaemia	Acute illness, electrolyte imbalance, reduced nutritional intake and undernutrition
Toxoplasmosis	Acute illness, reduced nutritional intake and undernutrition
Wasting: involuntary weight loss >10%	Can present in isolation with no other symptoms, or together with other opportunistic infections

treatable but debilitating, with mortality increasing in likelihood as both the duration of HIV infection and the degree of immunosuppression increase [1]. Table 5.16.1 describes the most commonly presenting AIDS-defining illnesses and conditions, and consequences for undernutrition associated with these.

The stigma associated with HIV infection should not be underestimated, and can lead to negative attitudes, prejudice, discrimination and psychological damage. It usually stems from incorrect beliefs regarding behaviours that can lead to HIV transmission, onward transmission of the virus itself, and disease progression. People living with HIV can self-isolate as a result, and rates of poor mental health are high; there is potential for undernutrition to be exacerbated as a result [1].

Both HIV infection and antiretroviral therapy may lead to long-term side effects, including redistribution of subcutaneous fat (lipodystrophy), dyslipidaemia, insulin resistance, osteoporosis, cognitive decline and renal disease [1]. It is postulated that these long-term consequences are a result of chronic inflammation, metabolic toxicities associated with historic and current use of certain antiretrovirals, an increasing prevalence of obesity in HIV, and the ageing of the cohort taken as a whole.

Historically, severe undernutrition was prevalent in HIV; a review of 27 papers describes lower than expected levels of lean body mass (LBM) in HIV patients [2]. Prior to the widespread use of HAART in the late 1990s, rates of undernutrition were high, for example 37.9% in France [3] and 38.1% of infants in Tanzania [4]. More recently, rates of undernutrition have declined, and indeed in well-resourced countries, most people living with HIV are overweight or obese [5]. Selected reports of nutritional status in HIV published between 2012 and 2015 are summarised in Table 5.16.2.

Undernutrition remains most prevalent in those with immunosuppression. People presenting late in the natural history of HIV infection, those not prescribed HAART, and those with a persistently low CD4 count are most at risk [6–8]. In well-resourced countries [5] and in those prescribed HAART in less well-resourced countries [8], the prevalence of undernutrition

Table 5.16.2 Prevalence of undernutrition in HIV

Reference	Cohort	Period data collected	Rates of undernutrition	Comments
Tate et al. [6]	681 outpatients, USA	2008	8%	Rate declined to 4% after 24 months of HAART
Andrade et al. [7]	Hospitalised patients, Brazil	2009–2010	43%	33% were diagnosed with HIV on admission, and 16% died
Wrottesley et al. [8]	149 female outpatients, South Africa	2011–2012	1% (CD4 ≥ 350) 11% (CD4 ≤ 200)	Undernutrition significantly higher in those with the greatest immunosuppression
Duncan et al. [5]	338 outpatients, London, UK. 94% are prescribed HAART	2014–2015	3%	Significantly associated with white ethnicity and detectable HIV viral load

has declined to 3% or less. The World Health Organization is supporting less well-resourced countries to achieve a target of 90% of people living with HIV treated with HAART by 2020. Working towards this goal will further limit undernutrition in HIV [1].

5.16.2 Causes of undernutrition in HIV

An unfortunate constellation of factors leads to undernutrition in HIV. Historically, this has been described as a vicious cycle since these factors can exacerbate one another.

HIV

The retrovirus HIV can itself cause undernutrition through direct damage to the gastrointestinal tract, resulting in malabsorption of nutrients, impaired cognition and dementia, and pain from its direct effects on body systems, for example in HIV arthropathy [2].

Opportunistic and HIV-related infection and disease

Brain infections are relatively common in untreated HIV infection and much rarer in those treated with HAART. They can lead to impaired cognitive and neurological function. This in turn can negatively affect appetite and

satiety, and can reduce the ability to shop and cook. Oral and gastrointestinal opportunistic infections and HIV-related disease, including oral hairy leucoplakia and oesophageal candida, can lead to changes in perception of taste, pain, loss of appetite, diarrhoea and malabsorption of nutrients. Cryptosporidial and microsporidial diarrhoea can lead to widespread damage to the lining of the gastrointestinal tract, reducing absorptive surface area. Kaposi's sarcoma can occasionally be found in the gastrointestinal tract and can lead to obstruction. A warning sign for this rare condition is the presence of Kaposi's sarcoma lesions in the oral cavity [2].

Metabolic change

Hypogonadism (low testosterone concentration) has been reported in up to 50% of those with untreated HIV infection, with a prevalence of 20–30% in those treated with HAART. It can lead to an inability to gain lean body mass, or even result in wasting, and is associated with multiple comorbidities and frailty [9,10]. Futile cycling of triglycerides has been described, where impaired clearance of lipoproteins in both the fed and fasting state is observed – an inefficient use of energy at a metabolic level [9]. This futile cycling is observed in untreated HIV infection, and also in those with lipodystrophy; the aetiology is unclear and requires further research.

Increased resting energy expenditure

Studies using indirect calorimetry have observed that following HIV infection, resting energy expenditure (REE) increases by at least 10% [9]. Even in those treated with HAART and achieving suppression of HIV replication, REE remains raised, particularly in those experiencing lipodystrophy or those with a higher HIV viral load. It has been argued that this increase in REE is offset by reduced physical activity when unwell, and can be balanced by usual energy intake levels. However, following recovery from a period of ill health, raised total energy expenditure may increase, energy intake may not meet increased needs, and undernutrition can result. Hypermetabolism and raised REE have been reported in those with opportunistic infections, higher HIV viral loads, and in those with lipodystophy [9]. Further research is now needed given the use of newly developed antiretrovirals, their initiation at higher CD4 counts, and the potential for lower levels of cytokine disturbance.

Social and psychological consequences of HIV

A diagnosis of HIV can lead to enforced or self-isolation, stigma and poor mental health. Some may find themselves unable to work or perform usual activities. These factors can lead to a reduced opportunity to shop for food and a loss of interest in cooking or eating, resulting in the development of undernutrition [2,7,11].

5.16.3 Consequences of undernutrition in HIV

Mortality and morbidity

In people living with HIV, the consequences of undernutrition include increased morbidity and mortality. In 1989, a seminal paper by Donald Kotler [12] was published correlating loss of LBM with time from death. In this pre-HAART era, it was observed that most people with AIDS were experiencing undernutrition – specifically wasting of muscle mass – in the weeks and months before death. Kotler and his team made serial measurements of both total body mass and LBM, using the labelled potassium method. At the point of death, LBM had declined to approaching 50% of its predicted normal value for the individual, whereas decline in total body mass was less significantly associated. They concluded that preservation of LBM would prevent death from AIDS. Weight loss remains an independent predictor of mortality in the era of HAART [13].

Undernutrition in HIV is associated with progression from HIV to AIDS, development of comorbidities and opportunistic infections, frailty and reduced survival, and these are all independent of CD4 count and HIV viral load [9]. In infants and children impaired growth and development can also result.

Long-term health

Most people treated with HAART are expected to achieve near-normal longevity [1]. However, there appears to be an increased prevalence and early onset of diseases associated with the ageing process, including cardiovascular disease, osteoporosis, chronic kidney disease, type 2 diabetes, cancer and cognitive decline. A risk factor for the development of osteoporosis in HIV is previous and current undernutrition [14] whereas weight gain following initiation of HAART is associated with later development of cardiovascular disease and type 2 diabetes [5]. Further research is needed to clarify the most appropriate methods for reversing undernutrition in HIV given the risk to long-term health of weight gain.

5.16.4 Nutritional assessment and diagnosis of undernutrition in HIV

Nutritional assessment should be individualised according to stage of presentation of HIV. Suspicion or confirmation of a range of conditions may present during nutritional assessment, including malabsorption, hypermetabolism, hypogonadism, lipodystrophy, poor adherence

Table 5.16.3 Anthropometry in HIV

Routine measurements: perform regularly, at every assessment	Additional measurements for those at risk of undernutrition	Additional measurements for those on antiretrovirals: perform annually to monitor for lipodystrophy
• Height • Weight • Waist circumference • Hips circumference	• Mid-arm circumference • Triceps skin fold *Consider bioelectrical impedance analysis (BIA)*	• Mid-arm circumference • Triceps skinfold • Biceps skinfold • Subscapular skinfold • Suprailiac skinfold • Chest circumference • Mid-thigh circumference • Mid-thigh skinfold

to antiretroviral therapy and metabolic side effects; these should be discussed with the multidisciplinary healthcare team at the first opportunity [2].

A medical history should be taken from the patient, with particular note made of any recent development of illness. With patients experiencing undernutrition, there should be a high suspicion for infection, and therefore the history should include a whole-body assessment of symptoms, including questioning regarding pain, gastrointestinal involvement and difficulty in breathing, history of changes in anthropometry and physical assessment.

Anthropometry

Given the importance of maintaining LBM irrespective of HIV stage, regular monitoring for the development or progression of lipodystrophy, and the increasing prevalence of obesity in HIV patients, routine anthropometry should include measurements as outlined in Table 5.16.3 [2].

Biochemistry

There are specific biochemistry tests to consider in people living with HIV, which should be assessed in addition to the biochemical information collected in people without HIV [2]. These include CD4 count and HIV viral load, which allow an assessment of disease progression and immune function. In infants and children, CD4 percentage is a more useful measure. In addition,

serum testosterone concentration should be monitored in those experiencing wasting, general undernutrition or difficulty in gaining body mass.

People on long-term HAART are at risk of cardiovascular disease and type 2 diabetes; fasting lipids and glucose should be performed annually. HbA1c may be underestimated in those on HAART, particularly where protease inhibitors are used [15].

Clinical assessment and diagnosis of undernutrition

Assessment should include asking about general symptoms such as gastrointestinal issues, appetite and fatigue. Symptoms such as low libido, fatigue and inability to gain LBM can all indicate hypogonadism. Night sweats can indicate hypermetabolism, as well as being a sign of infection. A physical examination should include assessment for vitamin or mineral deficiencies, signs of wasting and dehydration. Taking note of changes in physical appearance can aid monitoring of lipodystrophy. The patient should be asked to self-assess for body shape changes, including facial wasting, but this should be carried out sensitively as others may have already commented on this to the patient. It is possible that lipodystrophy may be mistaken for undernutrition, but in lipodystrophy there is a preservation of LBM, with loss of subcutaneous fat the principal presentation. Bioelectrical impedance analysis (BIA) can help diagnose loss of LBM in HIV patients [2].

Finally, the development of type 2 diabetes should be considered as a potential contributing factor to weight loss in people living with HIV; diabetes is up to four times more common compared to the general population [5]. There are currently no specific assessment tools designed for use with patients who have HIV but there are tools under development.

Dietary intake

Dietary intake should be assessed in the usual way, but diet histories should be extended to elicit a wider range of information to support care in HIV patients. Adherence to HAART regimens can be challenging; antiretrovirals may need to be taken with very specific timing, some have to be taken with food, whilst others must be without food. Nutritional supplements and complementary and alternative medicines are commonly used by HIV patients; care should be taken to ask about these [2]. Finally, there is potential for negative interactions between antiretrovirals and a range of supplements and complementary and alternative medicines, including garlic capsules, ascorbic acid in doses ≥1000 mg, St John's wort, African potato, and *Sutherlandia*; further details can be found using resources in Section 5.16.7.

Nutritional requirements

Calculation of nutritional requirements in HIV should take account of the potential for raised REE, hypermetabolism, malabsorption, opportunistic infections and comorbidities, and changes in physical activity. Specific predictive equations correlated with indirect calorimetry have not been produced for people living with HIV, and so usual methods for calculation of energy requirements should be used. However, during recovery following opportunistic infections, nutritional requirements in both children and adults may be increased by 20%, and up to 50% in cases of severe multiple opportunistic infections [16,17].

Protein requirements in HIV are thought to be no different to the general population, but in those experiencing opportunistic infections and immunosuppression, stable isotope studies have demonstrated positive nitrogen balance when intake of protein is increased to between 1.2 and 1.8 g/kg body weight/day [17]. Current practice recommendations are to follow protein requirements for the general population unless the patient is unwell with opportunistic infections [2], when increased protein intake may be required.

Economic, ethical and social considerations

Most people living with HIV experience happy normal lives, but there remains a potential for negative economic, ethical and social considerations. Current clinical practice recommendations [2] suggest that care should be taken to widen any clinical nutritional assessment to account for unemployment or financial hardship, poor mental health, fear, stigma, isolation or loneliness, all of which could lead to reduced or poor-quality nutritional intake [11].

5.16.5 Clinical and nutritional management of undernutrition in HIV

Clinical management of undernutrition

Guidelines for treatment of common HIV-related infections can be found through resources listed in Section 5.16.7. Clinicians should take account of the social and psychological effects of a recent HIV diagnosis; multidisciplinary care is key [2].

If hypogonadism is suspected and confirmed by blood test, testosterone replacement therapy needs to be considered. Suboptimal testosterone concentration can limit the effectiveness of nutrition support in the treatment of undernutrition [18]. Testosterone replacement ameliorates hypogonadism, and can be delivered by injection, but more commonly through application of dermal patches. However, it has been suggested that the use of testosterone replacement in frail HIV patients may be counterproductive, where lower testosterone concentration might be an adaptive response to reduce energy expenditure during illness [10]. Further research is needed.

Appetite stimulants such as cannabinols and megestrol acetate have historically been used for chronic symptom control, but they are no longer routinely used in clinical practice. Side effects from megestrol acetate in particular have outweighed benefit, for example the development of permanent dysglycaemia, and any weight gained is largely fat mass [18].

During the 1990s, anabolic steroids were researched as a potential therapy for loss of or inability to gain LBM in HIV patients. Studies demonstrated limited efficacy, with small gains in LBM when anabolic agents were used in combination with nutrition support and progressive resistance exercise (PRE), and also in combination with testosterone replacement. However, a Cochrane review [17] suggests these gains in LBM were only marginally more than with PRE alone, and not sustained once the anabolic agents were stopped.

Nutritional management of undernutrition

Food safety

Patients with a CD4 count less than 200 are deemed to be at higher risk for food- and waterborne infection, and should be counselled regarding food safety [19]. Evidence for this risk predates the modern HAART era, but current practice guidelines continue to recommend the same advice given in pregnancy [2]. Specific education resources can be found through links in Section 5.16.7.

Oral nutrition support

The first-line therapy for undernutrition is nutritional counselling to improve usual food intake to achieve an adequate energy and protein intake [20,21]. When patients cannot meet their requirements through food alone, oral nutrition supplements (ONS) can be provided and have been shown to increase energy intake by 20% in people with HIV [18]. ONS can meet the pharmacokinetic requirements for those antiretrovirals requiring food to aid absorption and

metabolism, for example rilpiverine, eviplera, atazanavir and darunavir. ONS should be taken at the same time as these particular antiretrovirals, and equally should be avoided when medication has to be taken on an empty stomach, for example didanosine. Additionally, liquid formulations of certain antiretrovirals taken by infants or those unable to tolerate tablets may be relatively unpalatable, and oral nutritional supplements with a stronger taste can help with administration [2].

Enteral nutrition

Studies of enteral nutrition administered by tube feeding in people unwell with HIV have demonstrated increased nutritional intake and weight gain, but this was principally fat mass. Nocturnal tube feeding to supplement oral intake has been described as the most common type of enteral feeding for undernutrition in HIV [18], although given the lack of controlled intervention trials of enteral nutrition in HIV patients, this practice is based on expert opinion only. Formula containing peptides and/or medium chain triglycerides and soluble fibre has been shown to be beneficial in malabsorptive states [18].

When planning enteral feeding, antiretroviral pharmacokinetics should be considered [2]; medications to be taken on an empty stomach should be administered during a break in feeding, whereas those requiring food for absorption should be taken during feed delivery. Antiretroviral pharmacokinetics can be checked using resources listed in Section 5.16.7 – please note that liquid formulations of certain antiretrovirals may have different pharmacokinetics from tablets. For example, Kaletra tablets can be taken with or without food, whereas Kaletra liquid must be coadministered with food to prevent suboptimal absorption.

Parenteral nutrition

The use of supplementary and total parenteral nutrition (PN) has been investigated in people living with HIV, and there do not appear to be specific contraindications [18]. Weight gained with parenteral nutrition in HIV is predominantly fat mass [15]. A Cochrane review of home

PN as a treatment for undernutrition in HIV concluded that it did not improve mortality or prevent readmission to hospital [22].

Refeeding syndrome

As with all people experiencing undernutrition, the possibility of refeeding syndrome should be considered as a consequence of nutrition support. In regions where the staple diet is rich in carbohydrate compared to protein and fat, there may be a higher risk of refeeding syndrome in people living with HIV, in common with all undernourished patients [21].

5.16.6 Future research needs

Further research is needed investigating macronutrient intake *in vivo* in HIV-positive people receiving HAART, particularly the ratio of saturated to unsaturated fats and fibre intake. This research should investigate those with undernutrition as well as those with obesity, since published research has a focus on lipodystrophy alone. There is a need to develop HIV-specific predictive equations for energy requirements using indirect calorimetry, taking into account the diversity of the population, with a wide range of resting energy expenditures observed. Finally, given the increasing prevalence of obesity in people living with HIV, the focus of nutrition-related research should switch from undernutrition, which is becoming less common and less of a clinical priority, to the management of obesity and its consequences [5,6].

5.16.7 Resources

- Pandemic statistics, policy and guidelines: www.unaids.org
- Pharmacokinetics of HAART, including food–drug interactions: www.hiv-druginteractions.org
- UK Dietitians in HIV Care: www.dhiva.org.uk
- News and information resources: www.aidsmap.com
- UK Clinical Guidelines: www.bhiva.org
- European Clinical Guidelines: www.eacsociety.org

References

1. Maartens G, Celum C, Lewin SR. HIV infection: epidemiology, pathogenesis, treatment, and prevention. *Lancet* 2014; **384**: 258–271.
2. Fields-Gardner C, Campa A, American Dietetic Association. Position of the American Dietetic Association: nutrition intervention and human immunodeficiency virus infection. *J Am Diet Assoc* 2010; **110**: 1105–1119.
3. Niyongabo T, Bouchaud O, Henzel D, et al. Nutritional status of HIV-seropositive subjects in an AIDS clinic in Paris. *Eur J Clin Nutr* 1997; **51**(9): 637–640.
4. Kawo G, Karlsson K, Lyamuya E, et al. Prevalence of HIV type 1 infection, associated clinical features and mortality among hospitalized children in Dar es Salaam, Tanzania. *Scand J Infect Dis* 2000; **32**(4): 357–363.
5. Duncan A, Goff L, Peters B. The association of HAART-related weight gain with type 2 diabetes and impaired glucose tolerance in a UK HIV cohort – a longitudinal study. *HIV Med* 2015; **16**(S2): 34.
6. Tate T, Willig A, Willig J, et al. HIV infection and obesity: where did all the wasting go? *Antivir Ther* 2012; **17**(7): 1281–1289.
7. Andrade C, Jesus R, Andrade T, et al. Prevalence and characteristics associated with malnutrition at hospitalization among patients with acquired immunodeficiency syndrome in Brazil. *PLoS One* 2012; **7**(11): e48717.
8. Wrottesley S, Micklesfield L, Hamill M, et al. Dietary intake and body composition in HIV-positive and -negative South African women. *Public Health Nutr* 2014; **17**(7): 1603–1611.
9. Chang E, Sekhar R, Patel S, Balasubramanyam A. Dysregulated energy expenditure in HIV-infected patients: a mechanistic review. *Clin Infect Dis* 2007; **44**: 1509–1517.
10. Rochira V, Diazzi C, Santi D, et al. Low testosterone is associated with poor health status in men with human immunodeficiency virus infection: a retrospective study. *Andrology* 2015; **3**: 298–308.
11. Erlich A, Jones H, Nicholls D, Duncan A, Smith K. Exploring need: a cross-sectional study of people accessing nutritional support from The Food Chain. *HIV Med* 2012; **13**(S1): 27.
12. Kotler D, Tierney A, Want J, Pearson R. Magnitude of body-cell-mass depletion and the timing of death from wasting in AIDS. *Am J Clin Nutr* 1989; **50**(3): 444–447.
13. Tang A, Forrester J, Spiegelman D, Knox T, Tchetgen E, Gorbach S. Weight loss and survival in HIV-positive patients in the era of highly active antiretroviral therapy. *J Acquir Immune Defic Syndr* 2002; **31**(2): 230–236.

14. Peters B, Perry M, Wierzbicki A, et al. A cross-sectional randomised study of fracture risk in people with HIV in the PROBONO 1 study. *PloS One* 2013; **8**(10): e78040.

15. Slama L, Palella F, Abraham A, et al. Inaccuracy of haemoglobin A1c among HIV-infected men: effects of CD4 cell count, antiretroviral therapies and haematological parameters. *J Antimicrob Chemother* 2014; **69**: 3360–3367.

16. Hsu J, Pencharz P, Macallan D, Tomkins A. Macronutrients and HIV/AIDS: A Review of Current Evidence. Consultation on Nutrition and HIV/AIDS in Africa: Evidence, Lessons and Recommendations for Action. Geneva: WHO, 2005.

17. Johns K, Beddall M, Corrin R. Anabolic steroids for the treatment of weight loss in HIV-infected individuals. *Cochrane Database Syst Rev* 2005; **4**: CD005483.

18. Ockenga J, Grimble R, Jonkers-Schuitema C, Macallan D, Melchior J-C, Sauerwein H, Schwenk A. ESPEN guidelines on enteral nutrition: wasting in HIV and other chronic infectious diseases. *Clin Nutr* 2006; **25**: 319–329.

19. Houtzager L. Food and water safety. In: Pribram V, editor. HIV Nutrition. Hoboken: Wiley-Blackwell, 2011, pp. 360–382.

20. Grinspoon S, Mulligan K. Weight loss and wasting in patients infected with human immunodeficiency virus. *Clin Infect Dis* 2003; **36**(S2): 69–78.

21. Koethe J, Chi B, Megazzini K, Heimburger D, Stringer J. Macronutrient supplementation for malnourished HIV-infected adults: a review of the evidence in resource-adequate and resource-constrained settings. *Clin Infect Dis* 2009; **49**: 787–798.

22. Young T, Busgeeth K. Home-based care for reducing morbidity and mortality in people infected with HIV/AIDS. *Cochrane Database Syst Rev* 2010; **1**: CD005417.

Chapter 5.17

Nutrition support in oncology

Clare Shaw
Royal Marsden NHS Foundation Trust, London, UK

5.17.1 Introduction

Cancer is the unregulated growth of cells that ultimately leads to significant morbidity and mortality in the person affected. 14.1 million adults were diagnosed with cancer and there were 8.2 million deaths from cancer in the world in 2012 [1]. One in three people will be affected by cancer and it contributes to the death of one in four people.

Cancer can be divided into over 200 different types of disease which are classified depending on the type of tissue from which they originate. The five main types are as follows [1].

- **Carcinoma** – cancer that begins in the skin or in tissues that line or cover internal organs. There are a number of subtypes, including adenocarcinoma, basal cell carcinoma, squamous cell carcinoma and transitional cell carcinoma
- **Sarcoma** – cancer that begins in the connective or supportive tissues such as bone, cartilage, fat, muscle or blood vessels
- **Leukaemia** – cancer that starts in blood-forming tissue such as the bone marrow and causes large numbers of abnormal blood cells to be produced and go into the blood
- **Lymphoma and myeloma** – cancers that begin in the cells of the immune system
- **Brain and spinal cord cancers** – these are known as central nervous system cancers

Survival rates for cancer have improved significantly and now 50% of those with a diagnosis of cancer can expect to survive longer than 10 years [10].

Nutritional status before, during and after treatment may influence tolerance to treatment and ultimately the amount of treatment provided for the person with cancer. Studies have consistently demonstrated that poorer outcomes, such as reduced survival, occur in those who are malnourished at the start of treatment and continue to be malnourished during treatment [2,3].

5.17.2 Background to undernutrition in cancer

Cancer is often associated with significant changes in body composition and nutritional status. These changes can include loss of body weight and muscle wasting leading to reduced physical functioning, low performance status, reduced tolerance to anticancer therapy and reduced survival.

Undernutrition is common amongst patients with cancer, 14–70% being undernourished or at risk [4,5]. Prevalence of undernutrition varies depending on the type of cancer, stage of disease and whether the study was undertaken in the inpatient or outpatient setting (Table 5.17.1). Prevalence rates in the literature also vary depending on the screening or assessment tool used. For example, screening tools that assess nutrition impact symptoms, as well as weight loss, may detect more patients at risk of

Advanced Nutrition and Dietetics in Nutrition Support, First Edition. Edited by Mary Hickson and Sara Smith.

Table 5.17.1   Prevalence of undernutrition in different diagnostic groups from studies of nutrition screening or nutritional assessment in cancer [4,45]

Diagnosis	Well nourished (%)	Moderately malnourished or at risk (%)	Severely malnourished (%)
Upper digestive tract	15	63	22
Haemato-oncology	17	72	10
Gynae-oncology	27	58	16
Lower digestive tract	28–59	25–62	10–17
Head and neck	30	46	25
Lung and pleura	34	56	9
Soft tissue and bone	46	36	18
Breast	49	42	8
Central nervous system	50	50	0
Urological	51	39	10
Skin	55	36	9
Endocrine	83	17	0
All tumours	29–38	50	13–21

undernutrition since such symptoms are common in people undergoing treatment. Simple undernutrition may occur due to an inadequate dietary intake, but in cancer additional metabolic changes may be present which further exacerbate the situation.

Cancer cachexia is a multifactorial syndrome which includes a continuum of changes in body composition and clinical condition. An international consensus described three clinically relevant stages as precachexia, cachexia and refractory cachexia [6] (Figure 5.17.1). The definition is based on changes in body weight, low body mass index (BMI), reduced food intake, systemic inflammation and sarcopenia.

The development of precachexia and cachexia is complex and is influenced by a number of factors including the type and stage of cancer, systemic inflammation, alterations in food intake and response to cancer treatment. The term refractory cachexia is used when the cancer is not responding to anticancer treatment, nutrition support is unable to halt or reverse the changes in body composition and performance status continues to deteriorate. This is generally associated with a poor prognosis.

Factors that contribute to the development of cancer cachexia

Factors that contribute to cancer cachexia can be divided into three broad categories that are described in detail in the following sections: reduced food intake, changes in body composition and metabolism, and changes to function. These factors are likely to be present together and influence each other.

Reduced food intake

Food intake is controlled by an interaction of neural, metabolic and humoral factors which are received and processed by the hypothalamus in the brain [7]. These include short-, medium- and long-term signals which influence desire to both commence and stop eating. Short-term signals include the sight and smell of food and a rise in the concentration of ghrelin, an appetite-stimulating peptide secreted by the stomach in response to fasting. Gastric distension during eating and circulating hormones including cholecystokinin secreted by the duodenum,

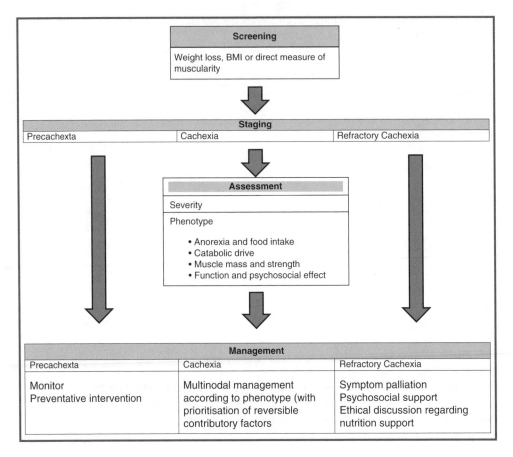

Figure 5.17.1 Management algorithm for cancer cachexia [6]

polypeptide YY secreted by the colon, in addition to circulating products of digestion all signal satiety and contribute to cessation of eating.

There has been much deliberation as to whether the anorexia observed in cancer is a result of changes in the peripheral signals responsible for appetite or whether it is due to an inappropriate response to these signals by the hypothalamus [7]. Proinflammatory cytokines, including interleukin (IL)-1 IL-6 and tumour necrosis factor α (TNF-α), may contribute to increased activity in the pro-opiomelanocortin (POMC) area of the hypothalamus. It is thought that this activation of the POMC neurons leads to a suppression of food intake.

From a clinical perspective, loss of appetite is a common symptom of cancer and is often associated with spontaneous reduction in food intake. Other symptoms may occur in cancer prior to diagnosis which may have an effect on food intake. These may be specifically related to the site of the tumour or they may occur due to the systemic effect of the tumour. They include dysphagia, taste changes, early satiety, altered bowel habits and nausea (Table 5.17.2).

Changes in metabolism

A key component of cachexia is a potential increase in catabolism caused by tumour metabolism, systemic inflammation (often measured as an increase in C-reactive protein) or other tumour-mediated effects [6]. Additional metabolic changes that may be present include insulin

Table 5.17.2 Symptoms affecting food intake in cancer [11,46]

Symptom	Prevalence*	Comments
Anorexia	26–38%	Can occur prior to diagnosis and as a result of treatment Inflammatory cytokines may play a role in its development Contributory factors include psychological factors associated with diagnosis of cancer
Early satiety	27%	Feeling full quickly can occur in many diagnostic groups. Particularly common in cases of gastric outflow obstruction, ascites and bulky pelvic tumours
Nausea	18–35%	Can occur as a result of medication, chemotherapy and radiotherapy May occur if GI tract obstructed
Vomiting	8–11%	Can occur as a result of chemotherapy or radiotherapy. Also occurs in cases of intestinal obstruction
Pain	23–27%	Pain may occur in any site although pain related to the GI tract is likely to have a more significant effect on food intake
Dysphagia	7–9%	Higher in some diagnostic groups such as oesophageal and head and neck cancer
Sore mouth/ mucositis	75% (high-dose chemotherapy) 40–50% (less intense regimens)	Clinical signs include erythema and ulceration which can result in difficulty speaking, swallowing, reduced oral intake of food and fluids Occurs during radiotherapy to oral cavity
Taste changes	26–75%	Associated with high levels of distress Particularly associated with chemotherapy and radiotherapy to head and neck Variety of taste changes experienced, including reduced sensitivity to all tastes, metallic taste, bitter taste, specific food aversions such as tea, coffee, meat
Dry mouth (xerostomia)	17–38%	May be related to toxicity from radiotherapy to head and neck Also related to use of some medications, e.g. hyosine
Constipation	14–27%	May be exacerbated by inadequate dietary intake, use of opioids or compression of the lower GI tract
Diarrhoea	11–30%	May occur during chemotherapy or radiotherapy to the abdomen or pelvis

* Prevalence refers to the presence of symptom. Impact on dietary intake not recorded.

resistance, changes in protein, fat and carbohydrate metabolism, and changes in overall energy expenditure.

As with anorexia, the proinflammatory cytokines IL-1, IL-6 and TNF-α are thought to be important mediators of the metabolic changes that occur in cancer cachexia. Changes in protein metabolism, including increased catabolism that is not offset by an increase in anabolism, may lead to a loss of muscle mass and muscle function. This has important implications for the person since a loss of muscle mass is associated with increased toxicity of chemotherapy and overall reduced survival [8].

Changes in both carbohydrate and lipid metabolism have been observed in cancer cells. Preferential anaerobic metabolism of glucose may occur with an enhanced glycolytic pathway occurring, despite adequate oxygen being available. This preference for cancer cells to metabolise glucose anaerobically, with subsequent processing of the lactate produced back to glucose, occurs via the Cori cycle. This presents a possible mechanism for increased energy expenditure via the energy-dependent Cori cycle.

Loss of fat stores is frequently observed in cancer patients, which may not be explained by reduced food intake alone. Metabolic changes and circulating cytokines may stimulate activity of the hormone-sensitive lipase resulting in the lipolysis and loss of subcutaneous fat on the trunk, legs and arms [7].

The changes in metabolism and body composition described may not be apparent in pre-cachexia and cachexia. The extent to which they develop will depend on the progression of the cancer, the response to cancer treatment, and individual factors, such as dietary intake, exercise and use of medication to manage symptoms.

Some studies have failed to show an increase in energy expenditure in those with cancer when measured at rest. Accurate measurement of metabolic rate in this patient group is difficult and is also influenced by changes in lean body tissue and overall physical activity. For example, a decrease in resting metabolic rate may be compensated for by a decrease in physical activity, resulting in a stable total energy expenditure [9].

Changes to physical and psychosocial function

Physical and psychosocial functioning can be profoundly affected by cancer and the associated changes that occur. Measurement of performance status using internationally recognised tools, such as the Karnofsky score, is essential as part of the holistic patient assessment to ascertain patient need and may influence the choice of cancer treatment.

Quality of life tools such as the European Organisation for Research and Treatment of Cancer (EORTC) Quality of Life Questionnaire (QLQ)-C30 may be used to capture data on quality of life in both a clinical and research environment. The psychosocial needs of the patient must be assessed at diagnosis and regularly during cancer treatment, allowing appropriate intervention when necessary.

5.17.3 Causes and mechanisms of undernutrition during cancer treatment

Cancer treatment is planned following extensive assessment of the patient's performance status, the histology, staging of local tumour, local spread or distant, metastatic spread and other baseline investigations. Early-stage disease is usually treated with radical or curative intent with the aim of producing long-term remission. More advanced disease, characterised by local or distant spread, may necessitate palliative treatment whereby the aim is to control the disease, manage symptoms and improve survival, although it may not be possible to produce long-term remission.

All decisions about the planned course of treatment should be made with a multidisciplinary team and should be based on the results of clinical trials which demonstrate the most effective methods of treatment. Often a treatment plan will include different treatment modalities given simultaneously or sequentially. All treatments have the potential to affect nutritional status and symptoms that affect food intake.

Surgery

The use of surgery underpins the management of a significant number of cancers. Surgery may be used with curative intent; that is, to remove the cancer and immediate surrounding healthy tissue margin to ensure complete removal of the tumour. Data suggest that 49% of all cancers are cured by surgery [10]. In addition, surgery may be used to reconstruct tissues or organs where cancer has been removed, to reduce tumour bulk or for symptom relief, such as formation of a stoma to relieve bowel obstruction. Minor surgical procedures may also be required, for example insertion of a central venous access device, such as a Port-a-cath, for administration of fluids, nutrition or chemotherapy.

Surgery can influence dietary intake and nutritional status through limited oral intake, transient GI failure and increased requirements due to the catabolic response to trauma.

Chemotherapy

Cytotoxic drugs are used as single agents or in combination, with the aim of reducing the rate of cell growth and division more effectively than in normal, non-cancerous tissues [10]. If effective, they reduce tumour growth, resulting in the tumour becoming stable or shrinking. Some tumours may be resistant to chemotherapy, with growth progressing through the administration of planned courses of treatment, or resistance may be acquired after an initial response to treatment. The dose of chemotherapy that can be administered is limited by the effect on normal tissue. Side effects such as the immunosuppressive effect on bone marrow, stomatitis and diarrhoea as a result of effect on the gastrointestinal (GI) tract require periods of time between administrations of chemotherapy cycles to enable normal tissue to recover.

Chemotherapy can profoundly influence nutritional status due to its effect on appetite, nausea, taste changes, stomatitis, diarrhoea and increased episodes of neutropenic sepsis. Studies that have assessed the prevalence of nutrition impact symptoms during and after treatment have demonstrated that these can occur in up to 79% of patients during treatment and may still be present in 49% of patients a year after starting treatment [11].

Targeted therapy

Newer treatments are being trialled which aim to slow the growth of cancer cells or cause cell death through different mechanisms. Some are dependent on targeting very specific cellular receptors such as EGFR, HER2 or Kit and therefore are only effective in tumour types that have such receptors. Examples include monoclonal antibodies and tyrosine kinase inhibitors. Often these drugs are much better tolerated than chemotherapy and do not exhibit the same toxicities. As a result, they are less likely to influence dietary intake and nutritional status compared

with other chemotherapeutic regimens [10]. There are a few exceptions where novel therapies have been implicated in the cause of specific disorders of absorption, such as bile acid malabsorption in the case of lenolidamide [12].

Radiotherapy

Radiotherapy is a common treatment modality used on its own or in combination with chemotherapy. The most commonly used form is external beam radiotherapy where ionising radiation is produced outside the body with beams being directed towards the tumour. More recent techniques include conformal, stereotactic and intensity-modulated radiotherapy which allow the radiotherapy to be contoured more closely to the tumour, thereby reducing the dose received by normal adjacent tissues and organs. Generally, treatment is given over a number of weeks to achieve a maximum dose.

Side effects commonly include generalised symptoms, such as fatigue and anorexia, with additional symptoms arising dependent on the site of the treatment. For example, radiotherapy to the oesophagus is likely to cause dysphagia and pain on swallowing, whereas in the pelvic area it is likely to cause diarrhoea.

Endocrine therapy

Hormonal manipulation is used as a treatment in some hormone-dependent cancers, such as breast and prostate cancer. Hormones such as oestrogen, progesterone and androgens may stimulate tumour growth. Endocrine therapy uses drugs that block cellular hormone receptors, block the enzymes responsible for the conversion of androgens to active hormones, or block luteinizing hormone-releasing hormone. The latter is produced by the hypothalamus and acts on the pituitary to stimulate the release of hormones from the ovary or testis.

The nutritional effects of endocrine therapy are that it can influence appetite and body composition, favouring weight gain and fat deposition, especially abdominal fat. It also facilitates loss of bone density with a subsequent increased risk of osteoporosis and osteopenia [13].

5.17.4 Consequences of undernutrition in cancer

Undernutrition in cancer has been associated with worse clinical outcomes for patients undergoing different treatment modalities. It has been linked to increased mortality, morbidity, increased length of hospital stay and higher healthcare-related costs [14]. Early surgical studies identified that all patients, not just those with cancer, had a worse outcome if they were undernourished.

Weight loss at diagnosis may reduce tolerance to treatment [2,3,15]. For example, GI cancer patients required more breaks in treatment and dose reduction, resulting in the administered chemotherapy being less when compared to those who had not lost weight. Patients who continued to lose weight also had a poorer outcome with increased mortality compared to those who did not lose further weight [3]. Similarly, lung cancer patients who had lost weight failed to complete more than three courses of chemotherapy more frequently and experienced a greater incidence of anaemia. Weight loss was an independent predictor of shorter overall survival [15].

5.17.5 Assessment and diagnosis of undernutrition in cancer

Many studies have used generic nutrition screening tools such as the Malnutrition Universal Screening Tool which use measurements such as BMI, weight loss and changes in food intake [16]. Other studies have used tools that are oncology specific and include symptoms that are known to affect food intake in oncology patients. Nutrition screening tools aimed at oncology patients tend to show greater sensitivity and specificity in detecting the risk of undernutrition [4]. A full nutritional assessment using the Patient-Generated Subjective Global Assessment (PG-SGA) has been shown to be a useful tool in oncology as it is linked with patient outcome and therefore provides more detailed and holistic nutritional assessment. The PG-SGA includes an extensive assessment of weight history, dietary intake, the presence of nutrition impact symptoms and an assessment of the patient's functional capacity. A physical examination provides information on muscle and adipose tissue changes and enables the dietitian or clinician to categorise the patient as normally nourished, mildly malnourished or at risk of malnutrition or severely malnourished. A disadvantage of this tool is that it takes time and a skilled assessor to use it appropriately.

The use of nutrition screening tools at diagnosis and regularly during cancer treatment allows those who are undernourished or at risk of undernutrition to be identified and a suitable nutrition care plan to be decided as part of the multidisciplinary assessment and treatment plan. Nutrition screening should be undertaken regularly, for example weekly during inpatient hospital stay and at every outpatient consultation, enabling changes in nutritional risk to be identified [17].

5.17.6 Interventions for nutrition support in cancer

The provision of nutrition support in cancer patients should be considered in the context of undernutrition prior to diagnosis and anticipated problems that may arise as a result of planned cancer treatment. The presence of nutrition impact symptoms (see Table 5.17.2) can have a profound effect on dietary intake and can cause distress to the patient and be associated with a poorer quality of life [11,12,18–20]. As weight loss can influence tolerance to cancer treatment, there is much interest in whether nutrition support, either as dietary counselling oral nutritional supplementation (ONS) or enteral (EN) or parenteral nutrition (PN), can influence nutritional status and ultimately patient outcome, including morbidity and mortality. A number of studies have highlighted that although undernutrition is common in cancer, a significant number of patients do not receive advice on appropriate food intake or other methods of nutrition support [16].

Oral intake and oral nutrition support

Specific dietary approaches may be required for particular diagnoses, particularly those where the presence of a tumour may impact on the ingestion or digestion of food. Dysphagia is common at diagnosis in upper GI and head and neck cancer. Such patients require individualised advice about texture modification, food fortification and the use of high-energy fluids or ONS to enable them to achieve their nutritional requirements. Specific dietary counselling is also helpful in managing symptoms, enabling patients to maintain an adequate dietary intake despite eating difficulties [19]. The insertion of GI stents to maintain patency of the GI tract, for example in cases of oesophageal or pyloric stenosis, requires a nutritional assessment and appropriate advice to ensure patients are confident and able to maintain a good dietary intake.

In patients who are neutropenic and at high risk of infection due to high-dose chemotherapy, there may be restrictions imposed on certain foods to reduce the risk of food-borne organisms. The research evidence that this is essential is weak, due in part to the ethical issues involved in planning a suitable study. Nevertheless, the use of these restrictions is common practice, with 68% of registered dietitians working in this specialist area endorsing such dietary changes [20].

Haematological malignancy is the most common condition for which neutropenic diets are used and often restrictions are imposed when neutrophils are below $0.5–2.0 \times 10^9$/L. Patients are advised to avoid unpasteurised dairy products, raw or lightly cooked meat, fish or shellfish, blue vein or soft ripened cheese, raw or lightly cooked eggs and paté, which are all believed to be more likely to carry pathogenic food-borne organisms. Additional restrictions in hospital may be placed on unpeeled and dried fruit, uncooked nuts and spices, food from large packets such as cereal and bottled still water due to the risk of contamination from fungal spores, cross-contamination from food handling and the potential presence of Gram-negative bacteria such as *Stenotrophomonas maltophilia* in bottled water. Dietary restrictions of this type derive from an assessment of risk and exposure to food-borne pathogens, so the advice may change over time or with the introduction of new methods of food handling and preparation.

The use of dietary counselling by registered dietitians during radiotherapy treatment for colorectal cancer has been demonstrated to improve dietary intake when compared to protein supplementation or *ad libitum* dietary intake [21]. Protein supplementation in this patient group also showed some benefit in terms of nutritional status and quality of life although this was lower than in the dietary counselling group. Dietary counselling given to 37 patients was the only intervention to sustain a significant impact on patient outcomes compared to protein supplements or usual care. A follow-up study, with a median follow-up of 6.5 years, compared survival and late radiotherapy toxicity in the three groups of patients [22]. Patients who had received the period of individualised dietary counselling from a registered dietitian during radiotherapy had improved survival, quality of life and decreased radiotherapy toxicity compared to the two other groups. Worse radiotherapy toxicity, quality of life and mortality were associated with deterioration in nutritional status and intake [22].

Whilst this provides evidence for the use of dietary counselling by a dietitian in this patient group, not all studies support the effect of dietary interventions on these outcomes. A systematic review of studies that used dietary counselling in malnourished cancer patients demonstrated that dietary intake and nutritional status can be improved with appropriate and timely interventions but collectively these studies did not influence survival [23].

In the study undertaken by Um et al., 87 patients receiving radiotherapy to the head and neck, thorax or abdomen were randomised to receive intensive dietary counselling from a registered dietitian within 4 days of commencing radiotherapy, aiming to achieve energy and protein requirements, or to a control group. It was not clear whether any patients in the control group received dietary counselling if deemed essential nor whether the study was powered to detect a difference in nutritional status between the two groups. Energy and protein intake did not differ significantly between the two groups during the course of radiotherapy. At the end of period of radiotherapy, a greater proportion of the intervention group were classified as being normally nourished compared to the control group but this was not significant [24].

Studies undertaken during chemotherapy have also failed to demonstrate any significant benefit from dietary intervention. A four-arm study examining the use of dietary counselling and/or ONS for a 6-week period failed to demonstrate any impact of these interventions on quality of life or survival in GI and lung cancer patients at 1 year. A limitation of this study was compliance with the dietary counselling and ONS, with a significant number of patients being unable to comply with the amount of ONS prescribed by the end of the 6-week study period. Poor completion rates of dietary diaries also meant that there was uncertainty around implementation of dietary counselling and how effective this was in changing dietary intake [25].

A systematic review of oral nutrition interventions in malnourished patients with cancer identified 13 studies of varying quality in a number of diagnostic groups. Overall, oral nutrition interventions were effective at increasing nutritional intake and improving some aspects of quality of life in those who were undernourished or at risk of undernutrition, but did not appear to improve mortality [25].

Enteral nutrition

The indications for EN in cancer are the same as for those in non-malignant conditions; the person is unable to meet their nutritional requirements via oral intake of diet and fluids and the GI tract is functioning. Neither the European or American recommendations on the use of nutrition support in cancer support the routine use of EN [26,27]. All patients should undergo appropriate assessment with support planned as part of their overall cancer treatment, if required.

In some circumstances, when it can be anticipated that a patient's oral intake will be compromised, for example during radiotherapy to the head and neck, an enteral feeding tube is placed before treatment. This is in anticipation of the side effects from radiotherapy which will affect dietary intake. In such circumstances, the patient should receive information about the benefits and risks of tube placement to allow them to participate in the final decision [17].

The use of ONS or enteral formulas containing nutrients such as arginine and glutamine, usually referred to as immunonutrition, has generated interest in the area of surgical oncology. Immunonutrition can be taken as a flavoured drink orally or as an enteral formula. Various formulations of immunonutrition have been studied, with the most common components including arginine, glutamine, n-3 fatty acids and ribonucleic acid (RNA) in various combinations and doses [28].

The diagnostic groups selected for studies have been primarily in upper GI cancer patients, including oesophageal, gastric and pancreatic cancer, with some including colorectal cancer.

Increasingly, immunonutrition is used as part of an enhanced recovery after surgery (ERAS) programme where a number of interventions are used with the aim of improving patient outcome in terms of morbidity and length of stay. It is not clear from early studies whether immunonutrition was being used as part of an ERAS programme or was being used in isolation. Overall studies indicate a beneficial effect of immunonutrition on both infectious and total postoperative complications in upper abdominal surgery, for example, gastric, oesophageal and pancreatic surgery, when used preoperatively in normally nourished patients, and pre- and post-operatively in malnourished patients [29]. Its use is recommended by ESPEN for upper GI cancer and by the ERAS Society for pancreatic surgery. However, in other areas (e.g. gastrectomy), the ERAS Society has highlighted that whilst immunonutrition may be of benefit, studies are lacking to support a recommendation for its use in this patient group [30].

Parenteral nutrition

The indications for use of PN in patients with cancer are the same as for those without malignant disease. Its use should be reserved for those with intestinal failure as a result of disease or treatment. EN should always be considered as first line for nutrition support [17]. There is no therapeutic benefit for the use of PN in patients with cancer; that is, it is unable to treat any underlying metabolic changes that occur. Its use is therefore solely as a means of support for those who are unable to tolerate enteral nutrition or for whom there is no access to the GI tract.

Parenteral nutrition may be used in a number of circumstances. Intestinal obstruction can occur in a number of diagnoses, with intrinsic or extrinsic compression of the GI tract at many possible sites from oesophagus to rectum. It may be possible to access the GI tract for enteral feeding, for example, with a gastrostomy or jejunostomy, by stenting the GI tract or by alleviation of the obstruction with a temporary or permanent stoma. PN may be required prior to obtaining access to the GI tract or prior to surgery. Other examples of its use may be in circumstances of intractable diarrhoea, ileus or intractable vomiting [31].

Management of cancer cachexia

The metabolic changes that occur in cancer cachexia put a different perspective on its management when compared to simple undernutrition. Cachexia is characterised by hypercatabolism caused by tumour metabolism directly, by systemic inflammation or by other tumour-mediated effects. Intermediary metabolites, such as IL-6 and TNF-α, have been implicated as the drivers for the metabolic changes. As yet, there is no evidence-based treatment for cancer cachexia although Fearon recommends that early intervention when the patient has precachexia or cachexia is preferable to trying to manage refractory cachexia [32]. It has been recommended that the management of cachexia should be via a multiprofessional approach that addresses all aspects of cachexia, including food impact symptoms, reduced food intake, reduced performance, anaemia and sarcopenia [32]. Treatment of the inflammation that occurs would be helpful in managing the condition but there are no widely approved drugs currently available. Steroids, such as dexamethasone, have been shown to improve appetite although subsequent weight gain may be body fat rather than lean body tissue.

There has been much interest in the potential of n-3 fatty acids to reduce the inflammatory response in cachexia. Randomised studies of energy and protein supplements with and without fish oils, fish oil supplementation alone or use of fish oil supplementation with an appetite stimulant have failed to demonstrate a benefit in terms of body composition [33]. More recently, studies have supported their role in maintenance of weight and muscle mass in lung cancer patients undergoing chemotherapy [34].

Vitamin and mineral status

Assessment of vitamin and mineral requirements and status during cancer and its treatment is difficult. Metabolic changes, including low albumin, may alter vitamin and mineral concentrations and it is not clear whether a correction of such levels may improve patient outcome. There has been much interest in the potential value of vitamins, particularly antioxidants, as potential anticancer agents and also to reduce oxidative damage from chemotherapy and radiotherapy. Whilst some studies have demonstrated that antioxidant supplements can reduce toxicity of radiotherapy, there is also evidence that their use can reduce the effectiveness of radiotherapy. This results in an increased risk of overall recurrence and mortality, as demonstrated in head and neck cancer patients [35]. Studies of vitamin supplementation during chemotherapy, including vitamin E, selenium and vitamin C, have provided mixed results. Whilst some have shown reduced toxicity, others have shown no effect [36]. The long-term effects of antioxidant supplementation during chemotherapy on recurrence and survival have not been studied.

Some diagnostic groups require particular attention to vitamin and mineral status. Examples include those with intestinal failure and pelvic radiation disease which may impact on a range of vitamins and minerals, particularly fat-soluble vitamins and vitamin B12 [37]. Other situations, for example post gastrectomy, require specific supplementation with vitamin B12 due to loss of intrinsic factor.

5.17.7 Undernutrition and living with and beyond cancer

Changes in nutritional status may persist long after treatment has finished. This is particularly apparent in patients with upper GI, head and neck, and haemato-oncology cancers, particularly those who have undergone a bone marrow transplant. In addition, some patients who have undergone pelvic radiotherapy will experience long-term nutritional consequences [38]. Exacerbation of poor nutritional status or difficulty in reversing weight loss may arise due to persistent symptoms affecting taste, appetite, ability to chew and swallow, or as a result of changes in absorptive capacity of the GI tract. This may be particularly apparent in patients who have undergone bone marrow transplantation and developed graft-versus-host disease of the GI tract, in those who have undergone pelvic radiotherapy (pelvic radiation disease) and/or intestinal resection. GI symptoms can have a major impact on the patient's quality of life. Referral to a specialist multiprofessional service, including a gastroenterologist and dietitian with the appropriate medical and dietary investigations and treatment, can improve GI symptoms in this patient group [39].

Some patients may require medium- or long-term nutrition support in terms of using ONS and EN. It should not be assumed that nutritional status returns to normal following treatment for cancer. Symptoms such as small bowel obstruction, diarrhoea or fistulas may occur many years after treatment, particularly following pelvic radiotherapy [40]. Such patients require medical and dietary management which involves the use of appropriate methods of nutrition support, including home PN in a small proportion of people [40].

5.17.8 Palliative care

As disease progresses, there may be a continued deterioration in nutritional status in some patients, ultimately with progression to refractory cachexia [6]. In such circumstances, the provision of nutrition support has a reduced capacity to influence body composition. It may be able to stabilise the deterioration in nutritional status but ultimately will be unable to prevent this occurring when malignant disease is advanced and progressing. The psychological effect of being able to eat and drink should not be underestimated and this has a profound influence on quality of life. It is important to address weight changes, nutrition impact symptoms, weight loss and the interventions that are useful to help patients, their families and carers to cope with the impact of these changes. By addressing them in a timely fashion, there is an opportunity to help maintain physical strength, limit the deterioration in nutritional parameters and improve quality of life [41].

The use of EN or PN may be appropriate in some patients who are unable to meet their requirements due to dysphagia or intestinal failure, for example, due to bowel obstruction. All cases should be assessed on an individual basis with a multiprofessional team, with the patient at the centre of the decision-making process. In the UK, EN and PN are classified as a treatment and if commenced should have a clear aim, have an assessment of the potential benefits and risks and should be reviewed on a regular basis to ensure that the aims of treatment are being met [42]. If this support is considered not to be of benefit then it should be stopped. Such a decision can be difficult for the patient and carers due to the emotional component attached to the provision of food, including when being given via an artificial method.

European guidance supports the use of PN in palliative care if patients have intestinal failure, EN is not possible or is insufficient, the expected survival is longer than 2–3 months, there is an expectation that PN can stabilise or improve performance status and quality of life, and the patient is involved in the decision regarding this method of support [43,44].

5.17.9 Summary

A significant proportion of cancer patients are undernourished or at risk of undernutrition at diagnosis or during treatment. The undernutrition is compounded further by metabolic changes that occur in cancer. The presence of nutrition impact symptoms, many of which arise because of cancer treatment, can have a profound effect on nutritional status, performance status and quality of life. The provision of appropriate and timely nutrition support is essential to enable patients to withstand cancer treatment. Whilst the effect of nutrition support on morbidity and mortality in surgical patients is well established, the effect of nutrition support on patient outcomes whilst undergoing chemotherapy and radiotherapy is less clear. Evidence is emerging, however, that suitable nutrition support can improve nutritional parameters and quality of life and possibly influence long-term outcomes such as morbidity and survival.

References

1. Cancer Research UK. Types of Cancer. www.cancer researchuk.org/about-cancer/what-is-cancer/how-cancer-starts/types-of-cancer (accessed 6 September 2017).
2. Langius JA, Bakker S, Rietveld DH, et al. Critical weight loss is a major prognostic indicator for disease-specific survival in patients with head and neck cancer receiving radiotherapy. *Br J Cancer* 2013; **109**(5): 1093–1099.
3. Andreyev H, Norman A, Oates J, Cunningham D. Why do patients with weight loss have a worse outcome when undergoing chemotherapy for gastrointestinal malignancies? *Eur J Cancer* 1998; **34**(4): 503–509.
4. Shaw C, Fleuret C, Pickard JM, Mohammed K, Black G, Wedlake L. Comparison of a novel, simple nutrition screening tool for adult oncology inpatients and the Malnutrition Screening Tool (MST) against the Patient-Generated Subjective Global Assessment (PG-SGA). *Support Care Cancer* 2014; **23**(1): 47–54.
5. Bozzetti F, Group SW. Screening the nutritional status in oncology: a preliminary report on 1,000 outpatients. *Support Care Cancer*; **17**(3): 279–284.
6. Fearon K, Strasser F, Anker SD, et al. Definition and classification of cancer cachexia: an international consensus. *Lancet Oncol*; **12**(5): 489–495.
7. Allessandro L, Preziosa I, Fanellie FR. Cancer and nutritional status. In: Shaw C, editor. Nutrition and Cancer. Oxford: Wiley Blackwell, 2011, pp. 13–24.
8. Prado CM, Baracos VE, McCargar LJ, et al. Sarcopenia as a determinant of chemotherapy toxicity and time to tumor progression in metastatic breast cancer patients receiving capecitabine treatment. *Clin Cancer Res*; **15**(8): 2920–2926.
9. Weekes C. Nutritional requirements of patients with cancer. In: Shaw C, editor. Nutrition and Cancer. Oxford: Wiley-Blackwell, 2011.
10. Popat S. Treatment of cancer. In: Shaw C, editor. Nutrition and Cancer. Oxford: Wiley-Blackwell, 2011, pp. 27–44.
11. Tong H, Isenring E, Yates P. The prevalence of nutrition impact symptoms and their relationship to quality of life and clinical outcomes in medical oncology patients. *Support Care Cancer* 2009; **17**(1): 83–90.
12. Pawlyn C, Khan MS, Muls A, Sriskandarajah P. Lenalidomide-induced diarrhea in patients with myeloma is caused by bile acid malabsorption that responds to treatment. *Blood* 2014; **124**(15): 2467.
13. Khan NF, Mant D, Carpenter L, Forman D, Rose PW. Long-term health outcomes in a British cohort of breast, colorectal and prostate cancer survivors: a database study. *Br J Cancer* 2011; **105**(Suppl 1): S29–37.
14. Arends J, Bodoky G, Bozzetti F, et al. ESPEN guidelines on enteral nutrition: non-surgical oncology. *Clin Nutr* 2006; **25**(2): 245–259.
15. Ross PJ, Ashley S, Norton A, et al. Do patients with weight loss have a worse outcome when undergoing chemotherapy for lung cancers? *Br J Cancer* 2004; **90**(10): 1905–1911.
16. Hebuterne X, Lemarie E, Michallet M, de Montreuil CB, Schneider SM, Goldwasser F. Prevalence of malnutrition and current use of nutrition support in patients with cancer. *J Parenter Enteral Nutr* 2014; **38**(2): 196–204.
17. National Collaborating Centre for Acute Care. Nutrition Support in Adults. Oral Nutrition Support, Enteral Tube Feeding and Parenteral Nutrition. London: National Collaborating Centre for Acute Care, 2006.
18. Khalid U, Spiro A, Baldwin C, et al. Symptoms and weight loss in patients with gastrointestinal and lung cancer at presentation. *Support Care Cancer* 2007; **15**(1): 39–46.
19. Shaw C. The Royal Marsden Cancer Cookbook. London: Kyle Books, 2015.
20. Carr SE, Halliday V. Investigating the use of the neutropenic diet: a survey of UK dietitians. *J Hum Nutr Diet* 2015; **28**(5): 510–515.

21. Ravasco P, Monteiro-Grillo I, Vidal PM, Camilo ME. Dietary counseling improves patient outcomes: a prospective, randomized, controlled trial in colorectal cancer patients undergoing radiotherapy. *J Clin Oncol* 2005; **23**(7): 1431–1438.

22. Ravasco P, Monteiro-Grillo I, Camilo M. Individualized nutrition intervention is of major benefit to colorectal cancer patients: long-term follow-up of a randomized controlled trial of nutritional therapy. *Am J Clin Nutr* 2012; **96**(6): 1346–1353.

23. Baldwin C, Spiro A, Ahern R, Emery PW. Oral nutritional interventions in malnourished patients with cancer: a systematic review and meta-analysis. *J Natl Cancer Inst* 2012; **104**(5): 371–385.

24. Um MH, Choi MY, Lee SM, Lee IJ, Lee CG, Park YK. Intensive nutritional counseling improves PG-SGA scores and nutritional symptoms during and after radiotherapy in Korean cancer patients. *Support Care Cancer* 2014; **22**(11): 2997–3005.

25. Baldwin C, Spiro A, McGough C, et al. Simple nutritional intervention in patients with advanced cancers of the gastrointestinal tract, non-small cell lung cancers or mesothelioma and weight loss receiving chemotherapy: a randomised controlled trial. *J Hum Nutr Diet* 2011; **24**(5): 431–440.

26. Loser C, Aschl G, Hebuterne X, et al. ESPEN guidelines on artificial enteral nutrition – percutaneous endoscopic gastrostomy (PEG). *Clin Nutr* 2005; **24**(5): 848–861.

27. Huhmann MB, August DA. Review of American Society for Parenteral and Enteral Nutrition (A.S.P.E.N.) clinical guidelines for nutrition support in cancer patients: nutrition screening and assessment. *Nutr Clin Pract* 2008; **23**(2): 182–188.

28. Cerantola Y, Hubner M, Grass F, Demartines N, Schafer M. Immunonutrition in gastrointestinal surgery. *Br J Surg* 2011; **98**: 37–48.

29. Burden S, Todd C, Hill J, Lal S. Pre-operative nutrition support in patients undergoing gastrointestinal surgery. *Cochrane Database Syst Rev* 2012; **11**: CD008879.

30. Mortensen K, Nilsson M, Slim K, et al. Consensus guidelines for enhanced recovery after gastrectomy: Enhanced Recovery After Surgery (ERAS(R)) Society recommendations. *Br J Surg* 2014; **101**(10): 1209–1229.

31. Bozzetti F, Arends J, Lundholm K, et al. ESPEN guidelines on parenteral nutrition: non-surgical oncology. *Clin Nutr* 2009; **28**(4):445–454.

32. Fearon KCH. Cancer cachexia: developing multimodal therapy for a multidimensional problem. *Eur J Cancer* 2008; **44**(8): 1124–1132.

33. Dewey A, Baughan C, Dean T, Higgins B, Johnson I. Eicosapentaenoic acid (EPA, an omega-3 fatty acid from fish oils) for the treatment of cancer cachexia. *Cochrane Database Syst Rev* 2007; **1**: CD004597.

34. Murphy RA, Mourtzakis M, Chu QS, Baracos VE, Reiman T, Mazurak VC. Nutritional intervention with fish oil provides a benefit over standard of care for weight and skeletal muscle mass in patients with nonsmall cell lung cancer receiving chemotherapy. *Cancer* 2011; **117**(8): 1775–1782.

35. Bairati I, Meyer F, Jobin E, et al. Antioxidant vitamins supplementation and mortality: a randomized trial in head and neck cancer patients. *Int J Cancer* 2006; **119**(9): 2221–2224.

36. Harvie M. Nutritional supplements and cancer: potential benefits and proven harms. *Am Soc Clin Oncol Educ Book* 2014: e478–486.

37. Andreyev J. Gastrointestinal symptoms after pelvic radiotherapy : a new understanding to improve management of symptomatic patients. *Lancet* 2007; **8**: 1007–1017.

38. Andreyev HJN, Wotherspoon A, Denham JW, Hauer-Jensen M. "Pelvic radiation disease": new understanding and new solutions for a new disease in the era of cancer survivorship. *Scand J Gastroenterol* 2011; **46**(4): 389–397.

39. Andreyev HJ, Benton BE, Lalji A, et al. Algorithm-based management of patients with gastrointestinal symptoms in patients after pelvic radiation treatment (ORBIT): a randomised controlled trial. *Lancet* 2013; **382**(9910): 2084–2092.

40. Andreyev HJN. Gastrointestinal problems after pelvic radiotherapy: the past, the present and the future. *J Clin Oncol* 2007; **19**(10): 790–799.

41. Shaw C, Eldridge L. Nutritional considerations for the palliative care patient. *Int J Palliat Nurs* 2015; **21**(1): 7–8, 10, 12–15.

42. British Medical Association. Withholding and Withdrawing Life-prolonging Medical Treatment: Guidance for Decision Making, 3rd edn. Hoboken: Blackwell Publishing, 2007.

43. Staun M, Pironi L, Bozzetti F, et al. ESPEN guidelines on parenteral nutrition: home parenteral nutrition (HPN) in adult patients. *Clin Nutr* 2009; **28**(4): 467–479.

44. Braga M, Ljungqvist O, Soeters P, Fearon K, Weimann A, Bozzetti F. ESPEN guidelines on parenteral nutrition: surgery. *Clin Nutr* 2009; **28**(4): 378–386.

45. Cunha SFC, Tanaka LS, Salomao RG, Macedo DM, Santos TD, Peria FM. Nutritional screening in a university hospital: comparison between oncologic and non-oncologic patients. *Food Nutr Sci* 2015; **6**: 75–82.

46. Shaw C, Power J. Nutritional support for the cancer patient. In: Shaw C, editor. Nutrition and Cancer. Oxford: Wiley-Blackwell, 2011, pp. 130–154.

Chapter 5.18

Nutrition support in palliative care

Denise Baird Schwartz

Providence Saint Joseph Medical Center, Burbank, USA

5.18.1 Introduction

The World Health Organization (WHO) defines palliative care as 'an approach that improves the quality of life of patients and their families facing the problems associated with life-threatening illness, through the prevention and relief of suffering by means of early identification and impeccable assessment and treatment of pain and other problems, physical, psychosocial and spiritual' [1]. Box 5.18.1 provides an expanded list of palliative care functions.

Palliative care-trained specialists involved in the earlier stages of diseases can improve the quality of life and medical decision making throughout an individual's illness [2]. Decision making should involve shared decision making, with the clinician educating the patient and family on realistic options [3]and making medical decisions based on the informed patient's quality-of-life goals.

Essentially, the goal of palliative care is the achievement of the best quality of life for patients and their families throughout an illness, with a focus on patient-centred care, which shifts the focus away from disease and back to the patient and family members. Healthcare should be respectful and responsive to the individual's preferences and needs and all clinical decisions should be guided by the patient's values [4]. Whilst respect for the individual's dignity and autonomy is the goal, palliative care in different countries can vary dependent on law, healthcare processes, local policy, culture, religion and financial limitations.

The WHO estimates that each year around 20 million people need palliative end-of-life care and around 20 million more individuals require palliative care in the years before death [5]. Using the National Hospice and Palliative Care Organisation (NHPCO) data and the number of known palliative care teams by country, the estimated numbers of patients who die while receiving palliative care services is approximately 3 million, 14% of those needing palliative care at the end of life worldwide [5].

Palliative care is for all age groups and as the proportion of older adults increases globally, the need for palliative care is growing further. Unfortunately, palliative care is only reliably available in Western Europe, North America, Australia and New Zealand [6]. In 2011, 136 of the world's 234 countries (58%) had at least one palliative care service, an increase of 21 (9%) from 2006, with the most significant gains having been made in Africa. Advanced integration of palliative care has been achieved in only 20 countries (8.5%) [7].

Both supportive care and palliative care are often provided by the patient's family and other caregivers, and not exclusively by healthcare professionals. Use of supportive care can have implications in various care settings throughout the world [8]. Supportive care can include pallia-

Advanced Nutrition and Dietetics in Nutrition Support, First Edition. Edited by Mary Hickson and Sara Smith.
© 2018 John Wiley & Sons Ltd. Published 2018 by John Wiley & Sons Ltd.

Box 5.18.1 Palliative care functions [1]

- Provides relief from pain and other distressing symptoms.
- Affirms life and regards dying as a normal process.
- Intends neither to hasten nor postpone death.
- Integrates the psychological and spiritual aspects of patient care.
- Offers a support system to help patients live as actively as possible until death.
- Offers a support system to help the family cope during the patient's illness and in their own bereavement.
- Uses a team approach to address the needs of patients and their families, including bereavement counselling, if indicated.
- Will enhance quality of life, and may also positively influence the course of illness.
- Is applicable early, in conjunction with other therapies that are intended to prolong life, such as chemotherapy or radiation therapy, and includes the need to better understand and manage distressing clinical complications.

Box 5.18.2 Definition of types of care

- Supportive care – involves all services that may be required for a person, including nutrition therapies, from diagnosis of an individual's disease process, and the patient's journey to end of life [8]
- Palliative care – improves the quality of life of patients and their families facing life-threatening illness, with prevention and relief of suffering with early identification, assessment and treatment of pain, physical, psychosocial and spiritual concerns [1]
- End-of-life care – can mean any period between the presumed last year of a person's life with chronic and progressive disease, to the last hours or days of life [9]

---

tive care, and palliative care includes end-of-life care. Supportive care should be given equal priority with other aspects of care and be integrated with the diagnosis, treatment, prevention and management of the adverse side effects of treatment, relief of symptoms and the complications, and ease the emotional burden for the patient and caregivers leading up to end of life [8,9]. Box 5.18.2 provides a brief explanation of the different types of care.

Future optimum use of nutrition support in palliative care may require a culture change, from the clinician, patient and family perspective [10]. Modern medicine and healthcare have become increasingly technology driven in some countries, compared to others where individuals lack basic healthcare needs, including palliative care. Nutrition support is a medical therapy, yet patients and their family members may attribute this artificial means of substrate delivery through tubes with the same characteristics as food. Values attributed to food may include love, caring and essentially a sense of normalcy with family gatherings. Early use of palliative care in a person's illness optimises the patient-centred focus to the care and incorporates available evidence-based medicine in the shared decision-making process.

Understanding of an individual's religious perspective on palliative care and nutrition interventions is important to provide optimum communication with patients and family members. Healthcare clinicians should recognise religious diversity in order to tailor the information required to facilitate understanding and the ability of the decision maker to achieve care based on the patient's wishes. However, the clinician should be aware that the perspective attributed to one religion is not meant to be inclusive for everyone in that religious or cultural group [11]. Numerous recommendations, guidelines and reports have been published on nutrition support addressing ethical issues and palliative care principles [12–20]. An understanding of palliative care, incorporating the benefits for the patient, family and clinicians and integrating an interdisciplinary approach is beneficial [21]. A formal process with physician engagement and administration support is needed to establish a healthcare institution communication practice for a consistent healthcare team approach to obtain advance directives, if available, and early discussion with the patient and family on healthcare wishes [16,22].

5.18.2 Undernutrition in palliative care

Undernutrition is a common complication for patients at the end-of-life stage of many disease processes. Nutrition support (enteral or parenteral nutrition) can reduce morbidity and mortality, for example, during the medical treatment period for cancer patients, and improve quality of life [23], but the disease entity that results in undernutrition is unlikely to abate. However, initiation of nutrition support is controversial, when other medical treatments are discontinued due to the clinical status of the patient. Introduction of nutrition support in all cases of undernutrition, especially if the individual's life expectancy is shorter than 2 months, is not recommended. Addressing the risk versus benefit ratio is beneficial in the decision-making process for initiation of nutrition support. Unfortunately, weight loss and appetite deficit are often indicated as reasons for nutrition support initiation, even if the individual is able to consume an oral diet. In the end-of-life stage, nutrition support initiation may be more as a result of subjective considerations dealing with beliefs, cultural or religious traditions [23].

5.18.3 Nutrition support in palliative care

A Cochrane systematic review examining the effectiveness of medically assisted nutrition for patients receiving palliative care on their quality of life and length of life identified no randomised controlled trials (RCTs) or prospective controlled trials that met the inclusion criteria [19]. The few included studies did not have

well-defined palliative care populations and as a consequence lacked sufficient consideration of nutrition therapy goals, which would be different for an individual in the last few days or weeks of life versus a longer period. However, performing an RCT in this area may be difficult. Withholding of nutrition support, despite lack of data for improved outcomes at the presumed end-of-life period, may be emotionally directed rather than by scientific evidence-based medicine. Additionally, an RCT would require the physician to provide an early prognosis for the patient's disease process. Future studies, if feasible, should focus on well-defined patient populations and stratify participants according to their functional status/activities of daily living [19].

Nutrition support in end-of-life care

For the purpose of this section, end-of-life care will be interpreted as being in the last months to weeks of life. Having a *good death* is one of the most important goals of palliative care. The concept of a good death may differ among and within different cultures. Therefore, starting discussions early about healthcare treatment options, including nutrition support, between clinicians, patient and family members is important. Components of a good death used for a study in Japan consisted of 57 attributes generated by qualitative and quantitative information [24]. None of these components specifically addressed receiving nutrients orally or through tubes at the end of life. Bridging the person's components of a good death compared to decision options that may be required during this phase of someone's life will require engagement, empowerment and education of individuals, family members and healthcare clinicians. Dietitians have a unique role in the process of understanding the person's view on nutrition and explaining alternative feeding routes. Nutrition in palliative care can have implications for oral diet, enteral nutrition and parenteral nutrition (Table 5.18.1). Patients and family members may feel more comfortable addressing their concerns about nutrition with the dietitian compared to the physician.

Table 5.18.1 Nutrition interventions in palliative care

Problems to address	Nutrition intervention action steps
Appetite alterations	
Food and eating perception	1. Liberalise unnecessary diet restrictions that limit food intake. 2. Offer small frequent meals with nutrient-dense favourite foods and fluids. 3. Alter food texture, cohesiveness, viscosity, temperature and density. 4. Encourage sense of food control, be respectful of food choices and rekindle eating pleasure. 5. Decrease the feeling of *pressure to eat* and more acceptance of whatever was able to be eaten. 6. Change posture to achieve the most efficient position while eating. 7. Adjust dentures or address other dental concerns. 8. Assess medication side effects affecting food intake. 9. Achieve environmental comfort while eating to optimise oral intake.
Functional deficits	

Swallowing impairment	1. Modify food texture (mechanical soft, chopped foods, extra gravy to purée) and fluid consistency (nectar, honey to pudding).
	  a. Eat small bites, avoid talking and distractions while eating.
	  b. Sit upright and eat when most alert.
	2. Assess and communicate potential benefits versus risk/burdens of short-term (nasogastric tube) and long-term (gastrostomy or jejuostomy tube) feeding, if aspiration with any oral intake.
	  a. Include evidence-based medicine in decision process.
	  b. Provide interprofessional approach to person-centred care.
	  c. Differentiate concepts of food from nutrient solutions delivered via tubes (medical therapy) for individuals and family members.
	  d. Comprise person's wishes for quality-of-life goals in shared decision making.
	3. Optimise foods for pleasure and not cause distress, if tube feeding declined.
	  a. Focus on sense of comfort with food and fluid consumption by person, rather than total daily protein and kcal intake.
	  b. Recognise that the manner of how food is served by family and caregivers may connote a sense of caring and respect more than the actual food and fluid intake.
	  c. Redirect emphasis on joyful eating, rather than food functionality for living.

Gastrointestinal obstruction	1. Determine if partial or complete gastrointestinal obstruction.
	2. Assess and communicate potential benefits versus risk/burdens of short-term (peripheral parenteral nutrition) and long-term (central parenteral nutrition) feeding.
	  a. Include evidence-based medicine in decision process.
	  b. Provide interprofessional approach to person-centred care.
	  c. Differentiate concepts of food from artificial nutrition via tubes (medical therapy) for individual and family.
	  d. Determine person's wishes for quality-of-life goals in shared decision making process.

5.18.4 Palliative care and nutrition support decision making

Shared decision making and health literacy

As part of shared decision making, patients should be educated on their own essential role. Individuals should be given effective tools incorporating evidence-based medicine to help them understand options and consequences of decisions. Patients should also receive emotional support to express their values and preferences and ask questions without censure from clinicians. Shared decision making is the pinnacle of patient-centred care and incorporates health literacy [25]. Health literacy acknowledges that there can be significant issues for patients in understanding what healthcare providers say to them. It involves the capacity for the person to obtain, process and understand basic health information, and services needed to make appropriate decisions [26].

Informed consent

Informed consent is a widely accepted legal, ethical and regulatory requirement for most healthcare interventions. Laws and regulations, in different countries, dictate the current informed consent requirement [27]. Generally, the focus is on respect for a person's autonomy and their right to define their own goals and make choices designed to achieve those goals. These rights apply to health-related interventions, including life-sustaining interventions, such as placement of long-term enteral feeding devices and access lines for parenteral nutrition. Although informed consent is widely accepted in the UK, Europe, United States and many other countries, understanding of and emphasis on an individual right to self-determination vary according to culture [27]. Cultural differences are evident in the practice of informed consent, involving what is told to whom and who makes decisions. Additionally, cultural differences can influence the understanding of the informed

consent as respect for individual autonomy [27]. The World Medical Association Declaration of Lisbon on the Rights of the Patient emphasises that patients everywhere have a right to information and to self-determination [28].

5.18.5 Food and hydration at the end of life

Management of dysphagia in patients choosing to continue oral nutrition

Managing dysphagia requires an interprofessional approach, to evaluate and recommend other strategies, comprising a modified diet to reduce the potential of aspiration [29]. A thorough discussion should take place with the patient, family, significant others, caregivers, and/or surrogate decision makers to cover the most up-to-date evidence-based information regarding the possibility of aspiration with or without oral feedings and the potential benefit versus burden/risks. Emphasis should be placed on the functional status of the individual and quality-of-life goals [18].

Comfort feeding

Patients suffering from advanced dementia with swallowing difficulties frequently do not receive the care that is consistent with their desires or best interest [30]. A suggested approach is comfort feeding only (CFO) [30]. CFO through careful hand feeding, by a nurse or trained caregiver, offers an alternative to nutrition via a tube and eliminates the apparent care or no care contrast imposed by current orders to forego artificial nutrition and hydration. The CFO approach highlights the goals of careful hand feeding. These goals aim to draw the focus back to the patient by providing a care plan that emphasises the patient's comfort and wishes for care. CFO avoids the misleading contradiction of care *versus* no care. It can facilitate continued attempts at careful hand feeding as long as the patient is not in distress, avoid unwanted feeding tube discussions with families and highlights that the comfort of the patient during feeding is of primary importance [30].

5.18.6 Decision-making tools and options for nutrition interventions

Decision-making process involving surrogate decision makers

Surrogate decision makers are individuals selected by the patient to make healthcare choices for them, when the patient may not be able to speak for themselves. Ideally, the patient and the surrogate decision maker have discussed the healthcare options based on the patient's wishes and the information would be documented in an advance directive [31]. If a patient has an advance directive, the goal is that the healthcare providers determine the intent of the wishes documented, including nutrition support. In a study of Western European countries, advance directives were considered as an instrument that supports a broad concept of patient autonomy [32]. Some of the countries enacted national legislation on end-of-life decisions. All countries emphasised the importance of the patient's right to self-determination. Variation may have occurred due to the interpretation of the physician in charge, with some countries having a physician-centred versus patient-centred approach [32].

Individuals who designate a decision maker and discuss their wishes prior to becoming non-competent are more likely to receive medical therapies based on their wishes. A qualitative study of 35 surrogates, with a recent decision-making experience for an inpatient aged 65 or older, found that, in addition to the patient's wishes and best interests, surrogates also consider other factors such as their own wishes, interests, emotional needs, religious beliefs and past experiences with healthcare [31]. Whilst the study involved a small number of participants, it provides some insight into additional items that should be considered when a surrogate is required to make decisions on an patient's behalf [31].

Decision making in advanced dementia

Individuals with advanced dementia generally lose interest in food and fluids, are unable to focus on meals, and may refuse to eat. Numerous studies have found no evidence that enteral nutrition provides benefit for individuals with advanced dementia in terms of survival time, mortality risk, quality of life, nutrition parameters, physical function or improvement or reduced incidence of pressure ulcers [14,16,33]. Current scientific evidence suggests that the potential benefits of enteral nutrition do not outweigh the possible burden/risks of treatment in persons with advanced dementia [14,34–36]. Advanced dementia should be seen by the healthcare team as a terminal illness, that cannot be cured or adequately treated and that is reasonably expected to result in the death of the patient within a short period of time. This perspective should be communicated to the patient's family, significant others, caregivers and/or surrogate decision makers [18]. The recommended approach for patients with advanced dementia or near end-of-life conditions considering long-term enteral feeding access device placement is provided in Table 5.18.2.

5.18.7 Early communication and application to nutrition practice

Early communication of preferences for life-sustaining healthcare options, including nutrition support, is not always a standard process. There is a stark difference between what individuals focus on at the end of life compared to the medical therapy choices that they may face. This difference and inadequate early communication between individuals, their family members and the healthcare professionals may result in ethical dilemmas involving nutrition support.

Initiatives have been developed to start these conversations about healthcare wishes, along with other tools and resources [37–47]. Furthermore, the Institute for Healthcare

Table 5.18.2 Recommended approach for patients with advanced dementia or near end-of-life conditions considering long-term enteral nutrition access devices

Category	Recommended approach for patient care
Scientific evidence	Decision to withhold/withdraw long-term enteral nutrition in end-stage illness is supported by current scientific evidence
Communicate terminal illness perspective	Advanced dementia should be seen by healthcare team as a terminal illness and this perspective should be clearly communicated to patient's family, significant others, caregivers and/or surrogate decision makers
Discussion components	Discuss the most up-to-date evidence-based findings regarding short-term and long-term potential benefits and risk/burdens
Feeding alternatives	Assisted oral feeding and other innovative oral interventions should be thoroughly explored and discussed with patient, family, significant others, caregivers and/or surrogate decision makers
Respect for autonomy	Essential aspect of care involves cultural, religious, social and emotional sensitivity to the patient's value system. A time-limited trial of nasogastric enteral nutrition may be considered. Emphasis should be placed on functional status and quality of life
Patient-centred approach	Final informed decision should be reached via a patient-centred approach, including family, significant others, caregivers and/or surrogate decision makers
Process development	Clinicians in hospitals and long-term care facilities should develop an interdisciplinary, collaborative, proactive, integrated and systematic process to engage in decision making with the patient, family, significant others, caregivers and/or surrogate decision makers. Process should promote advance directives that could optimise healthcare based on patient's wishes and best interest

Source: Reproduced from Schwartz et al. [18] with permission from Sage Publications.

Improvement (IHI) has developed an initiative to target providers and institutions so that when patients want to talk about wishes for end-of-life care, healthcare providers are ready to have that conversation. The initiative is based on the following core principles.

- Engage with our patients and families to understand what matters most to them at the end of life.
- Respect patients' wishes for care at the end of life by partnering to develop shared goals of care.
- Connect in a manner that is culturally and individually respectful of each patient.
- Steward this information as reliably as we do allergy information.
- Exemplify this work in our own lives so that we understand the benefits and challenges [48].

Whilst countries may have alternative approaches to discussing end-of-life support and decisions, the adoption of a 'conversation readiness' strategy, independent of the cultural, religious and social behaviours, is important to provide the most adequate care with respect for the patient's autonomy [49]. Dietitians involved in recommending and prescribing nutrition support should provide care based on a patient's wishes and as part of the healthcare team should be appropriately educated to integrate clinical ethics within the nutrition care process [50].

References

1. World Health Organization. WHO Definition of Palliative Care. www.who.int/cancer/palliative/definition/en/ (accessed 7 September 2017).
2. Quill TE, Abernethy AP. Generalist plus specialist palliative care – creating a more sustainable model. *N Engl J Med* 2013; **368**: 1173–1175.
3. Barry MJ, Edgman-Levitan S. Shared decision making – the pinnacle of patient-centered care. *N Engl J Med* 2012; **366**: 780–781.

4. Barrocas A, Geppert C, Durfee SM, et al., A.S.P.E.N. Board of Directors. A.S.P.E.N. ethics position paper. *Nutr Clin Pract* 2010; **25**(6): 672–679.

5. World Health Organization. Global Atlas of Palliative Care at the End of Life www.who.int/nmh/Global_Atlas_of_Palliative_Care.pdf (accessed 7 September 2017).

6. Connor SR. International palliative care initiatives. In: Ferrell BR, Coyle N, Paice JA, editors. Oxford Textbook of Palliative Nursing, 4th edn. New York: Oxford University Press, 2015, pp. 1056–1057.

7. Lynch T, Connor S, Clark D. Mapping levels of palliative care development: a global update. *J Pain Symptom Manage* 2013; **45**(6): 1094–1106.

8. National Institute for Health and Care Excellence. Improving Supportive and Palliative Care for Adults with Cancer. Cancer Service Guideline No. 4. www.nice.org.uk/guidance/csg4 (accessed 7 September 2017).

9. Gillespie L, Raferty AM. Nutrition in palliative and end-of-life care. *Br J Commun Nurs* 2014; Suppl: S15–20.

10. Schwartz DB, Olfson K, Babak B, Barrocas A, Wesley JR. Incorporating palliative care concepts into nutrition practice: across the age spectrum. *Nutr Clinc Pract* 2016; **31**: 305–315.

11. Schwartz DB. Ethical considerations in the critically ill patient. In: Cresci G, editor. Nutritional Therapy for the Critically Ill Patient: A Guide to Practice, 2nd edn. Boca Raton: Taylor & Francis, 2015, pp. 635–652.

12. Körner U, Bondolfi A, Bühler E, et al. Introduction part to the ESPEN guidelines on enteral nutrition: ethical and legal aspects of enteral nutrition. *Clin Nutr* 2006; **25**(2): 196–202.

13. Volkert D, Berner YN, Berry E, et al. ESPEN guidelines on enteral nutrition: geriatrics. *Clin Nutr* 2006; **25**(2): 330–360.

14. Sampson EL, Candy B, Jones L. Enteral tube feeding for older people with advanced dementia. *Cochrane Database Syst Rev* 2009; **2**: CD007209.

15. Barrocas A, Geppert C, Durfee SM, et al., A.S.P.E.N. Board of Directors. A.S.P.E.N. ethics position paper. *Nutr Clin Pract* 2010; **25**(6): 672–679.

16. Schwartz DB, Posthauer ME, O'Sullivan Maillet. J. Ethical and legal issues of feeding and hydration. www.eatright.org/positions (accessed 7 September 2017).

17. O'Sullivan Maillet J, Schwartz DB, Posthauer ME. Position of the Academy of Nutrition and Dietetics: ethical and legal issues of feeding and hydration. *J Acad Nutr Diet* 2013; **113**; 828–833.

18. Schwartz DB, Barrocas A, Wesley JR, Kliger G, Pontes-Arruda A, Arenas Márquez H, James RL, Monturo C, Lysen LK, DiTucci. A.S.P.E.N. Special report: gastrostomy tube placement in patients with advanced dementia or near end of life. *Nutr Clin Pract* 2014; **29**: 829–840.

19. Good P, Richard R, Syrmis W, Jenkins-Marsh S, Stephens J. Medically assisted nutrition for adult palliative care patients. *Cochrane Databyse Syst Rev* 2014; **4**: CD006274.

20. Schwartz DB. Ethics in action column: applying dietetics practitioner's code of ethics to ethical decisions for withholding/withdrawing medically assisted nutrition and hydration. *J Acad Nutr Diet* 2015; **115**: 440–443.

21. Barrocas A, Schwartz DB. Ethical considerations in nutrition support in critical care. In: Van Way C, Seres D, editors. Nutrition Support for the Critically Ill. Marlton: Springer, 2015, pp. 195–227.

22. Geppert CMA, Barrocas A, Schwartz DB. Ethics and law. In: Mueller C, McClave SA, Schwartz DB, Kovacevich D, Miller SJ, editors. The A.S.P.E.N. Adult Nutrition Support Core Curriculum, 2nd edn. Springfield: American Society for Parenteral and Enteral Nutrition, 2012, pp. 656–676.

23. Pazart L, Cretin E, Grodard G, et al. and the ALIM-K Study Investigational Group. Parenteral nutrition at the palliative phase of advanced cancer: the ALIM-K study protocol for a randomized controlled trial. *Trials* 2014; **15**: 370.

24. Miyashita M, Kawakami S, Kato D, et al. The importance of good death components among cancer patients, the general population, oncologists, and oncology nurses in Japan: patients prefer "fighting against cancer". *Support Cancer Care* 2015; **23**: 103–110.

25. Barry MJ, Edgman-Levitan S. Shared decision making – the pinnacle of patient-centered care. *N Engl J Med* 2012; **366**: 780–781.

26. Carbone ET, Zoellner JM. Nutrition and health literacy: a systematic review to inform nutrition research and practice. *J Acad Nutr Diet* 2012; **112**: 254–265.

27. Grady C. Enduring and emerging challenges of informed consent. *N Engl J Med* 2015; **372**: 855–862.

28. World Medical Association. WMA Declaration of Lisbon on the Rights of the Patient. http://dl.med.or.jp/dl-med/wma/lisbon2005e.pdf (accessed 7 Septemer 2017).

29. Schwartz DB, DiTucci A, Goldman B, Gramigna GD, Cummings B. Achieving patient-centered care in a case of a patient with advanced dementia. *Nutr Clinc Pract* 2014; **29**; 556–558.

30. Palecek JE, Teno JM, Casarett JD, Hanson KC, Rhodes RL, Mitchell SL. Comfort feeding only: a proposal to bring clarity to decision-making regarding difficulty with eating for persons with advanced dementia. *J Am Geriatr Soc* 2010; **58**(3): 580584.

31. Fritch J, Petronio S, Helft PR, Torke A. Making decisions for hospitalized older adults; ethical factors considered by family surrogates. *J Clin Ethics* 2013; **24**(2): 125–134.

32. Veshi D, Neitzke G. Advance directives in some western European countries: a legal and ethical comparison between Spain, France, England, and Germany. *Eur J Health Law* 2015; **22**: 321–345.

33. Casarett D, Kapo J, Caplan A. Appropriate use of artificial nutrition and hydration-fundamental principles and recommendations. *N Engl J Med* 2005; **353**(24): 2607–2612.

34. Hanson LC. Tube feeding versus assisted oral feeding for persons with dementia: using evidence to support decision-making. *Ann Longterm Care* 2013; **21**(1): 36–39.

35. Teno JM, Gozalo PL, Mitchell SL, et al. Does feeding tube insertion and its timing improve survival? *J Am Geriatr Soc* 2012; **60**(10): 1918–1921.

36. Givens JL, Selby K, Goldfield KS, Mitchell SL. Hospital transfers of nursing home residents with advanced dementia. *J Am Geriatr Soc* 2012; **60**(5): 905–909.

37. Aging With Dignity. *Five Wishes*. www.agingwith dignity.org/five-wishes.php (accessed 7 September 2017).

38. The Conversation Project. www.theconversation project.org (accessed 7 September 2017).

39. House of Commons Health Committee End of Life Care, Fifth Report of Session 2014–15. www. publications.parliament.uk/pa/cm201415/cmselect/ cmhealth/805/805.pdf (accessed 7 September 2017).

40. Institute of Healthcare Improvement. Conversation Ready Health Care Community. www.ihi.org/ Engage/Initiatives/ConversationProject/Pages/ ConversationReady.aspx (accessed 7 September 2017).

41. Institute of Medicine. Dying in America: Improving Quality and Honoring Individual Preferences Near the End of Life. www.nationalacademies.org/hmd/ Reports/2014/Dying-In-America-Improving-Quality-and-Honoring-Individual-Preferences-Near-the-End-of-Life.aspx (accessed 7 September 2017).

42. International Association for Hospice and Palliative Care. www.hospicecare.com (accessed 7 September 2017).

43. International Observatory on End of Life Care. www.lancaster.ac.uk/shm/research/ioelc/ (accessed 7 September 2017).

44. National Healthcare Decisions Day – April 16 annually. www.nhdd.org (accessed 7 September 2017).

45. Physician Orders for Life-Sustaining Treatment (POLST). www.polst.org (accessed 7 September 2017).

46. Speak Up campaign. www.advancecareplanning.ca (accessed 7 September 2017).

47. World Medical Association Declaration of Lisbon on the Rights of the Patient. www.wma.net/en/30publications/ 10policies/l4/ (accessed 7 September 2017).

48. Institute for Healthcare Improvement. Collaboratives Conversation Ready Health Care Community. www. ihi.org/Engage/collaboratives/Conversation ReadyCommunity/Pages/default.aspx (accessed 7 September 2017).

49. Schwartz DB, Pontes-Arruda A. Ethics column integrating the "conversation ready" initiative into nutrition practice. *Nutr Clin Pract* 2014; **29**; 406–408.

50. Schwartz DB, Armanios N, Cheryl M, Frankel EH, Wesley JR, Patel M, Goldman B, Kliger G, Schwartz E. Clinical ethics and nutrition support practice: implications for practice change and curriculum development. *J Acad Nutr Diet* 2016; **116**: 1738–1746.

Index

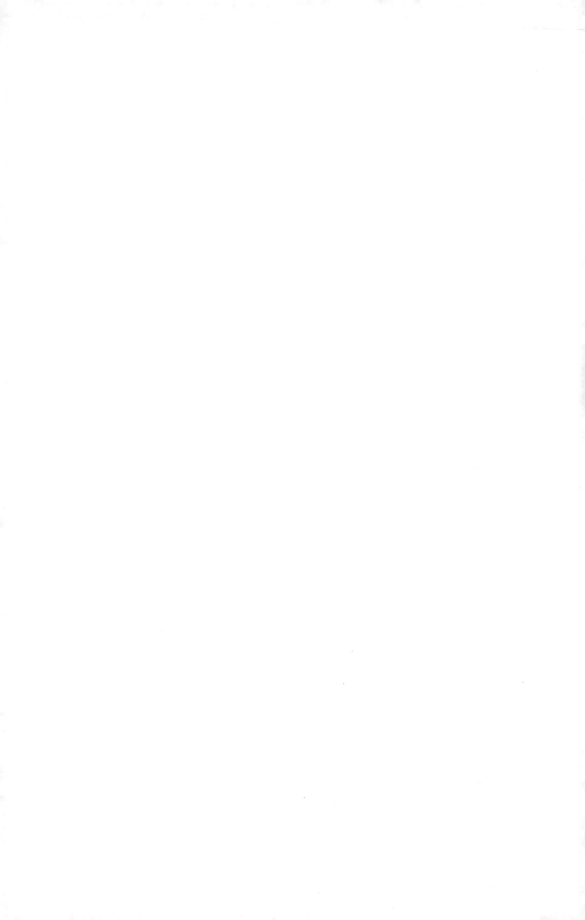